FOUNDATIONS OF PEDIATRIC PRACTICE

for the Occupational Therapy Assistant

FOUNDATIONS OF PEDIATRIC PRACTICE

for the Occupational Therapy Assistant

Edited by

Amy Wagenfeld, PhD, OTR/L
Lasell College
Newton, MA

Jennifer Kaldenberg, MSA, OTR/L
New England College of Optometry
New England Eye Institute
Boston, MA

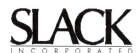

An innovative information, education, and management company
6900 Grove Road • Thorofare, NJ 08086

Published by: SLACK Incorporated
                  6900 Grove Road
                  Thorofare, NJ 08086 USA
                  Telephone: 856-848-1000
                  Fax: 856-853-5991
                  www.slackbooks.com

Contact SLACK Incorporated for more information about other books in this field or about the availability of our books from distributors outside the United States.

Foundations of pediatric practice for the occupational therapy assistant / [edited by] Amy Wagenfeld, Jennifer Kaldenberg.
    p. ; cm.
  Includes bibliographical references and index.
  ISBN 1-55642-629-1 (alk. paper)
  1. Occupational therapy for children--Outlines, syllabi, etc. 2. Occupational therapy assistants--Outlines, syllabi, etc.
  [DNLM: 1. Occupational Therapy--Child. WS 368 F771 2005] I. Wagenfeld, Amy. II. Kaldenberg, Jennifer.

RJ53.O25F68 2005
615.8'515'083--dc22
                              2004029296

For permission to reprint material in another publication, contact SLACK Incorporated. Authorization to photocopy items for internal, personal, or academic use is granted by SLACK Incorporated provided that the appropriate fee is paid directly to Copyright Clearance Center. Prior to photocopying items, please contact the Copyright Clearance Center at 222 Rosewood Drive, Danvers, MA 01923 USA; phone: 978-750-8400; website: www.copyright.com; email: info@copyright.com

Printed in the United States of America.

For further information on CCC, check CCC Online at the following address: http://www.copyright.com.

Last digit is print number: 10 9 8 7 6 5 4

A Note About the Cover

Everywhere and everyday, across the world, children engage in occupations. While the nature and meaning of these occupations or purposeful activities may differ according to culture, gender, and age, children engage in occupations to learn new skills, to practice skills that are emerging, to perfect what has been learned, and to prepare them for future roles.

The four photographs on the cover of this text represent four boys ages 17, 10, 6, and 4, all engaged in different age-appropriate occupations of childhood. David is walking his dog Glacier, an Instrumental Activity of Daily Living; Tyler is practicing his piano, a Leisure Activity; Tristan is riding his bicycle, a Play Activity; and Nolan is building with blocks, another Play Activity.

What makes these photographs special is that they are of our sons, and it is to them that we dedicate this book.

Contents

Major Infant Reflexes chart (back cover)
Normal Developmental Milestones chart (pullout)

Foundations of Pediatric Practice for the Occupational Therapy Assistant, Instructor's Manual, is also available from SLACK Incorporated. Don't miss this important companion to *Foundations of Pediatric Practice for the Occupational Therapy Assistant*. To obtain the *Instructor's Manual*, please visit www.efacultylounge.com.

Acknowledgments

It is truly amazing to believe that what began as one of those middle of the night inspirations at the 2001 AOTA National Conference in Philadelphia, came to fruition. As we sit down in front of the computer composing these acknowledgments, it is not without some tears of joy, accomplishment, and yes, a bit of relief to realize that we finished what we started out to achieve.

First and foremost to our contributors; what can we say, but THANK YOU! We feel that we assembled a team of accomplished, talented, committed, and enthusiastic authors who made this book what it is. For those of you writing for the first time, to those of you who are "more seasoned," hats off to you. Because of your insights and commitment to the occupational therapy profession, our job of blending your words into a seamless product was a joy. Thank you so much for being part of this exciting process.

Without the invaluable help, assistance, caring, and compassion afforded to us by the staff at SLACK Incorporated, this project would never have reached completion. We would like to acknowledge John Bond, Vice President, Book Publishing; Amy McShane, Editorial Director; Lauren Biddle Plummer, Executive Editor; Debra Toulson, Editor; and James Pennewill, Marketing Coordinator for their important parts in seeing this project from proposal to publication. For John, Amy, Lauren, Debra, and Jim, your wisdom, humor, encouragement, and unwavering commitment to this important project kept us afloat throughout this process. For that we are most grateful.

Thank you to those of you who read, reread, and offered helpful comments and insights into preparing the initial proposal and the end product for this text. Extra eyes always help to hone in on developing the best product possible.

We would also like to acknowledge and thank other people who provided us with assistance at various stages of the preparation process. We appreciated your interest in this project and would like our readers to know who you are, in alphabetical order, with specialties listed parenthetically.

Darragh Callahan (Child Development)
Gary Chu (Optometry)
Anne Corn (Optometry)
Richard Dodds (Instructional Technology)
Louis Frank (Optometry)
Karen Jacobs (Occupational Therapy)
Richard Jamara (Optometry)
Leslie Jones (Permissions Editor American Occupational Therapy Association, Inc.)
Lauren Knott (Optometry)
Teresa May-Benson (Occupational Therapy)
Jaclyn Pfeil (Physical Therapy)
Jacqueline Schaffer (Medical Illustrator)
Jeanne Wagenfeld (Psychology)
Morton O. Wagenfeld (Medical Sociology and Public Health)
Mary Warren (Occupational Therapy)

PERSONAL ACKNOWLEDGMENTS

Amy would like to thank Kate Blumberg and Lauren Fox, both masters in their respective professions. Deepest thanks to my parents, Morton Wagenfeld and Jeanne Wagenfeld, as well as my siblings, Eric Wagenfeld, David Wagenfeld, and Ellen-Wagenfeld-Heintz, for being there for me. Most of all, to my husband Jeffrey Hsi, our beloved son David, and our adored Glacier, you represent the best part of my life, and I thank you for always.

Jennifer would like to thank all those who supported us. Deepest thanks to my parents John & Paula Brodie, to my in-laws Russell Kaldenberg and Judyth Reed and Bill and Danielle Torrance, as well as my siblings Heather Perry and John Brodie. Thank you for your love and support. Most of all to my husband Casey, and our sons, Tyler, Tristan, and Nolan, thank you for your love and support; you truly are my inspiration.

We welcome feedback from you and invite you to contact either of us via SLACK Incorporated.

About the Authors

Amy Wagenfeld received a BS in occupational therapy, an MA in human development, and a PhD in education. Amy has 20 years of clinical experience, with a majority of those years spent in various pediatric contexts, including school systems, outpatient pediatric rehabilitation clinics, and private practice. Amy is on the faculty at Lasell College in Newton, MA. In addition to her teaching and mentoring duties, Amy is the Clinical Director of Children's Therapy Connections, which provides consultative services and workshops to parents, administrators, teachers, and childcare providers.

Amy's research interests include the influence of music on the development of early attachment connections between babies and primary caregivers as well as the human-animal connection. Amy has presented her work on occupational therapy, human development, and attachment at local, state, and national conferences. Amy is also involved with several state and local nonprofit advocacy and community service organizations and is in the process of writing several other books on topics related to occupational therapy, attachment, and animal-assisted therapy.

In addition to her professional responsibilities, Amy is a passionate organic gardener. Amy, her husband Jeff, their wonderful and amazing 17-year-old son David, and incredibly spoiled dog Glacier live in suburban Boston, where they all enjoy traveling, long walks, trips to the beach, and tennis.

Jennifer Kaldenberg is Director of Occupational Therapy Services at New England College of Optometry and the New England Eye Institute. She received her BS in occupational therapy from the University of New Hampshire and an MSA in Administration with a concentration in Health Care Administration from Central Michigan University. Jennifer has over 10 years of clinical experience, with a majority of those years spent in neurological and visual rehabilitation. Jennifer previously was an assistant professor at Lasell College in Newton, MA and currently lectures at the New England College of Optometry.

Jennifer's research interests include the impact of vision on functional independence, visual perception, and neurological visual impairment. She has spoken extensively on the role of occupational therapy in vision rehabilitation to occupational therapy practitioners, optometrists, and the general public.

In addition to her professional pursuits, Jennifer and her husband Casey are the proud parents of three wonderful boys who all enjoy participating in sporting activities and traveling together. In her free time, Jennifer enjoys painting, drawing, and cooking.

About the Contributors

Olga Baloueff, ScD, OTR/L, PT, BCP is an Associate Professor of Occupational Therapy at Tufts University in the Boston School of Occupational Therapy. Her clinical expertise and teaching include early intervention services for families and young children with developmental deviations.

Sue Berger, MS, OTR/L is Clinical Assistant Professor at Boston University Sargent College. She does clinical work with older adults in the community with low vision and has a strong interest in occupational therapy's role in hospice care.

Donna Buckland Gallen, MS, OTR/L works as an occupational therapist for a local school district in St. Louis County, Missouri. Her professional interests include pediatric practice and hand grasps.

Darragh Callahan, EdD spent many years teaching elementary school on a Native American Pueblo. She later moved to Europe, where she worked with the U.S. Army as a Child Development Services Coordinator in Germany and Italy. After a long career with the U.S. Government, Darragh returned to her native Massachusetts where she is currently a part-time faculty member in the Schools of Education at Boston University and Walden University.

Linda Cammaroto, OTR/L is a school-based therapist in Northern New Jersey. With over 30 years in the field, she is currently working for both the Hackettstown and Fredon School Districts.

Molly Campbell, MS, OTR/L, ATP coordinates the Assistive Device Center at Perkins School for the Blind in Watertown, MA. She also teaches Assistive Technology at Tufts University and provides consultation services to day programs for adults with developmental disabilities. She is the co-author of *Creative Constructions: Technologies That Make Adaptive Design Accessible, Affordable, Inclusive and Fun.*

Rachel B. Diamant, MS, OTR/L, BCP has worked with children and their families for over 20 years in clinical practice. Currently, she is an associate professor at the Arizona School of Health Sciences, a division of A.T. Still University.

Lisa A. Dixon, PhD, JD is an attorney in Cambridge, Massachusetts.

Sandra J. Edwards, MA, OTR, FAOTA is a Professor of Occupational Therapy at Western Michigan University. She is certified in administration of the Sensory Integration and Praxis Test (SIPT) and NDT with children. Her professional interests include children's hand function and grasps and interdisciplinary research with engineers using haptic robot devices to develop evaluation and intervention for children's hand skills.

Tara J. Glennon, EdD, OTR/L, BCP, FAOTA is an Associate Professor of Occupational Therapy at Quinnipiac University and owner of the Center for Pediatric Therapy in Connecticut. Her commitment to professional and community education is reflected in her lectureship, authorship of numerous pediatric works, and the creation of the web resource OTforKids.

Cynthia Haynes, MEd, MBA, OTR/L is an Assistant Professor and Fieldwork Coordinator in the Occupational Therapy Program at Philadelphia University. Cyndi has worked extensively with children in early intervention and school system service delivery models and currently consults with a suburban school district outside of Philadelphia. She has presented at conferences on best practice for children and innovative methods of OT student instruction.

Priscilla Hayden-Sloane, MHA, OTR/L, LEND Fellow provides evaluation, consultation, and support services to the Norwood Public Schools, Norwood, MA as a member of the Early Childhood Assessment Team. Priscilla developed a 10 hour hands-on learning module for teachers and early childhood providers addressing sensory processing and behavioral self-regulation in a classroom environment entitled *Sensory Integration and Learning Readiness.*

Joylynn Holladay, MS, OTR/L is a pediatric therapist at Children's Memorial Hospital in Chicago, IL.

Jan Hollenbeck, MS, OTR/L has been a practicing occupational therapist for 20 years. She is currently the Coordinator of Occupational Therapy, Physical Therapy, Vision Services, and Assistive Technology for the Medford Public School District in Massachusetts.

DeLana Honaker, PhD, OTR, BCP worked as staff and Lead Occupational Therapist for the Lubbock Independent School District in Texas for 10 years. She currently consults with several school districts and is an invited presenter for workshops nationwide on school-based practice. She teaches as adjunct faculty for Texas Woman's University in their online advanced MA program and is an Associate Professor at Elizabethtown College in Elizabethtown, PA. DeLana is Sensory Integration & Praxis Test (SIPT) certified. Her other publications include: *Ready, Set, Write!* video/manual program and the book, *Writing Goals and Objectives in School-based Practice* (www.theschooltherapistsbag.com).

Nicole Jacobs, OTR/L, CHT, a Hand Therapist at New England Medical Center in Boston, MA, has authored several papers/publications including topics on splinting, arthritis and the management of mallet finger. Recently, she co-authored a chapter on Neoprene splinting and an abstract on the rehabilitation protocol following cruciate repair of Zone II flexor tendon injuries. Nicole is also a member of the American Society of Hand Therapists, and is currently involved with the Education Committee and is Co-editor of the *ASHT Times*.

David L. Lee, MS, OTR/L is a Doctor of Science (D.S.) student in Occupational Health–Ergonomics and Injury Prevention, at the Harvard School of Public Health and is an occupational therapist at Spaulding Rehabilitation Hospital in Boston, MA. He also consults in office ergonomics and assistive technology.

Jean Lyons Martens, MS, OTR/L is NDT trained in pediatrics and certified to administer the SIPT. She is currently in private practice and teaches in the OT program at Worcester State College in Worcester, MA.

Teresa A. May-Benson, MS, OTR/L is Clinical Specialty Director at Occupational Therapy Associates–Watertown, P.C., Research Director of the Spiral Foundation at OTA–Watertown and a well-known lecturer on sensory integration theory and intervention. She has authored two book chapters on praxis. Ms. May-Benson has a special interest in and extensive experience with autism, particularly with older students and adults. She is a doctoral candidate and Maternal and Child Health Fellow at Boston University in Boston, MA.

Jenna McCoy-Powlen, MS, OTR/L is an occupational therapist at a pediatric therapy clinic in Southern California. Her professional interests include early intervention and sensory integration.

Christina Monaco, COTA/L is an occupational therapy assistant at New England Pediatric Care, a nursing home for children and young adults with severe needs, in Billerica, MA.

Cindee Quake-Rapp, PhD, OTR is Professor and Chair, Department of Occupational Therapy, Western Michigan University. A specialist in occupational therapy for children, she has published widely and presented internationally on such topics as children's handwriting, executive functioning of children with ADHD, and child assessment.

Michael Roberts, MS, OTR/L is currently splitting his time between home care in the Boston area, following developments in oncology rehabilitation, and teaching at Tufts University.

Catherine Verrier Piersol, MS, OTR/L is Assistant Professor and Program Director in the Occupational Therapy Program at Philadelphia University. Ms. Piersol co-edited and authored a manual for home care occupational therapy practitioners and maintains a private practice in home health care. She is active in both state and national occupational therapy association activities.

Sidney Michael Trantham, PhD is employed full time at Lasell College in Newton, MA as an assistant professor in the department of social science and part-time as a psychotherapist at Fenway Community Health in Boston, MA. His professional interests include neuropsychology, child abuse, and psychotherapy.

Christy Halpin Wright, OTR/L, CHT is Senior Hand Therapist at New England Medical Center in Boston, MA and is assistant editor of the *ASHT Times*. Christy has authored papers/publications on the management of flexor tendon repairs, tendon transfers, and splinting. Recently she co-authored a chapter on Neoprene splinting and an abstract on flexor tendons. Christy has presented at several New England Hand Society annual meetings and organized and presented workshops on various hand therapy and splinting topics, teaches splinting techniques at several New England colleges, and developed a rehabilitation protocol following cruciate repair of Zone II flexor tendon injuries.

Foreword

Pediatrics is "the medical science relating to the care of children and treatment of their disease" (Venes, 2001, p. 1598). In the United States, over 22% of occupational therapy practitioners work in school systems and this number increases if non-school based pediatric settings are included. Without a doubt, pediatrics is an important area of practice in occupational therapy. Therefore, the question arises, how does one best prepare our students to work in this area? *Foundations of Pediatric Practice for the Occupational Therapy Assistant* provides an exceptional resource for occupational therapy assistants in their journey to develop a clinical foundation in pediatrics as well as being able to reinforce their learning with practical application activities.

Foundations of Pediatric Practice for the Occupational Therapy Assistant was skillfully conceived and edited by Amy Wagenfeld and Jennifer Kaldenberg, two exceptional occupational therapists with over 30 years of combined experience in occupational therapy. More specifically, Amy has 15 years of experience in pediatrics and Jennifer, with 10 years of experience in vision and neurological rehabilitation. Above and beyond their experience, they make a dynamic team, with the determination and enthusiasm to do a superlative job with such an undertaking as editing a textbook on such a vast subject as pediatrics. Amy and Jennifer have joined forces with other experts, too. Well-known authorities in the areas of occupational therapy, child development, and psychology wrote the 24 comprehensive chapters contained in the textbook.

I know readers will enjoy and treasure *Foundations of Pediatric Practice for the Occupational Therapy Assistant* and keep it within arm's reach!

Karen Jacobs, EdD, OTR/L, CPE, FAOTA
Clinical Professor
Boston University
Sargent College of Health and Rehabilitation Sciences

Reference

Venes, D. (Ed.) (2001). *Taber's Cyclopedic Medical Dictionary* (19th ed.). Philadelphia: F.A. Davis Company.

Chapter 1

INTRODUCTION

Amy Wagenfeld, PhD, OTR/L
Jennifer Kaldenberg, MSA, OTR/L, CLVT

"The quality of life is determined by its activities" (Aristotle).

A Beginning

This is an exciting time to be embarking on a career as an occupational therapy assistant (OTA). Today, through continued commitment to engage those we work with in "occupation" or purposeful activity, occupational therapy practitioners actively function in traditional and nontraditional roles in nearly every sector of society. Our unique skills enable us to enrich the lives of many people in equally as many creative ways. How we enrich the lives of others is part of an exciting developmental process.

When we step back and recognize the common denominator in advancements in technology, medicine, and even the occupational therapy profession, it is arguably *development*. As we move society forward, be it through committed individual practice, exciting technological advancements, or medical breakthroughs, we are doing so based on a developmental foundation. It is a developmental foundation of pediatric practice that we are presenting to you, for without a good beginning, the middle and the end are more difficult to achieve.

When we set out to write this book, it was with the intention of providing OTA students and certified occupational therapy assistants (COTAs) with a developmental foundation from which to work with children and their families and caregivers. By assembling an amazing cadre of experienced and skilled professionals from disciplines such as occupational therapy, child development, psychology, and law, we think we have succeeded in presenting you with a book that

will serve you well in the classroom and out in the field. We hope you enjoy reading and using *Foundations of Pediatric Practice for the Occupational Therapy Assistant* as an ongoing reference just as much as we enjoyed editing it.

The Format

Every chapter in the book provides pediatric clinical foundations and practical application activities for the OTA student, as well as the entry level and experienced COTA. One of the unique organizational features of this text is that it begins with foundational concepts and skills and then moves to specific treatment and practice areas. The following is a brief description of the chapters and their content.

CHAPTER 2

Foundations of Occupational Therapy provides a brief history and foundation of occupational therapy, which includes discussion of the uniqueness of the field of occupational therapy as applicable to pediatric practice, role delineation, AOTA *Practice Framework*, standards of practice, and best practice in relationship to pediatric occupational therapy.

CHAPTER 3

A Brief Overview of Occupational Therapy Theories, Models, and Frames of Reference provides an introduction to occupational therapy frames of reference commonly used in pediatric practice. Each is discussed in terms of historical context, theoretical foundations, and clinical applications for the pediatric OTA.

CHAPTER 4

Collaborative Models of Treatment provides an introduction to the conceptualization and relevance of various treatment models commonly seen in pediatric practice. This chapter also examines the environments and team member compositions in which the various collaborative treatment models are commonly employed, and the importance of communication and collaborative team building in pediatric occupational therapy practice.

CHAPTER 5

Legal Mandates for Pediatric Practice provides an introduction to laws impacting the practice of occupational therapy, including PL 94-142/ IDEA, and the ADA. A brief overview of the *Occupational Therapy Code of Ethics*, a discussion of role delineation and supervisory requirements for OTAs in various service environments, and a discussion of patient (child) rights as pertaining to occupational therapy are also discussed.

CHAPTER 6

Documentation provides a discussion of the purpose of documentation, including note writing, goals, and objectives in clinical practice. Various documentation procedures, including SOAP notes, narrative note, and goal writing within specific treatment areas, are explored. An overview of the role of the OTA in evaluation, re-evaluation, discharge, and program (home and clinic) development is also included.

CHAPTER 7

An Overview of Early Development provides an introduction to theories of development and an overview of the nature and theoretical foundations of development, specifically the fundamentals and implications of gross, fine, cognitive, and social emotional development. An introductory discussion of motor milestones and their application to normal development from birth through adolescence is also presented.

CHAPTER 8

An Overview of Developmental Assessments provides a historical overview of developmental assessments, discussion of the purpose of developmental assessments, an introduction to various developmental assessments, and an examination of various professionals trained to administer and interpret developmental assessments.

CHAPTER 9

Interacting With Families provides a discussion of the importance of early caregiver-child relationships as an integral part of the developmental spectrum. Concepts of attachment and relationship building as they apply to family structure are also discussed. The chapter examines the family from both historical and contemporary perspectives and explores methods and strategies to encourage development of effective therapeutic relationships between OTAs and the families with whom they interact.

CHAPTER 10

Diagnoses Commonly Associated With Childhood provides an overview of diagnoses commonly associated with childhood, and a discussion of the functional implications and/or limitations secondary to the specific diagnoses. The role of the OTA in working with children diagnosed with various disabilities, diseases, and syndromes is also explored.

CHAPTER 11

Positioning in Pediatrics: Making the Right Choices provides an examination of normal reflex development and its implications for development. A discussion of the development and range of postural control and dysfunction and its importance in motor development, and discussion of the nature of atypical development and its implications for postural control are also provided. Alternative seating options such as wheelchairs, bolsters, and innovative seating systems as well as an overview of treatment strategies and the role of the OTA in working with children and their families to enhance postural skills and develop alternative seating programs are explored in this chapter.

CHAPTER 12

An Introduction to Sensory Integration provides a discussion of the history and theory of Sensory Integration; an introduction to sensory motor development, praxis, and sensory processing challenges; an examination of the nature of disorders of Sensory Integration; and an overview of the nature of Sensory Integration assessment and treatment.

CHAPTER 13

Oral Motor Skills and Feeding provides an overview of the oral motor structures and their application to feeding and language development; an overview of the development of normal oral motor function progressing from the early suck swallow reflex to a mature chewing pattern; an overview of oral motor and feeding assessments; and a discussion of oral motor feeding treatment teams, implementation protocols, and the role of the OTA in the facilitation of oral motor and feeding skills with children.

CHAPTER 14

Childhood Occupations provides an examination of the nature of occupations specific to childhood, an overview of the historical context of play, and a discussion of the foundations of play and its implications for development throughout childhood. The chapter also explores the unique perspective that occupational therapy brings to the facilitation of play skills and the OTAs role in enhancing play skills in children who are developing atypically.

CHAPTER 15

Self-Care provides an overview of ADL and IADL tasks associated with childhood, an exploration of family influences on the development and progression of ADL/IADL skills, an examination of compensations and adaptations of self-care skills for the child with developmental challenges, and a discussion of the role of the OTA in the facilitation of the self-care skills associated with childhood.

CHAPTER 16

Visual Perceptual Dysfunction and Low Vision Rehabilitation provides an introduction to the visual system, an overview of common visual problems of childhood, discussion of pertinent terms for the OTA to use in study and practice, a discussion of treatment strategies for enhancing visual and visual perceptual skills in children, and an examination of developmentally appropriate goals and objectives of vision intervention.

CHAPTER 17

Hand Development provides an introduction to integrated development of hand skills encompassing motoric, cognitive, social, and sensory domains; a discussion of the typical developmental progression of hand skills; an examination of prehension skills (grasp and release, in-hand manipulation skills); and strategies for the OTA to enhance the hand skills of children.

CHAPTER 18

Handwriting provides an introduction of the developmental progression of prewriting and writing skills; an examination of treatment strategies for enhancing underlying writing skills such as positioning, grasp alteration, and use of alternative writing paper; discussion of goals and expectations of handwriting based therapy as pertaining to specific age groups (i.e., 3 to 5, 5 to 12, 12+ years); and discussion of age-appropriate prewriting and writing activities for the OTA to implement.

CHAPTER 19

Early Intervention provides an introduction to early intervention, historical, and legal background information; IDEA Part C; discussion of the population identified and served through early intervention services; examination of the serv-

ice models associated with early intervention; discussion of the context in which early intervention services are disseminated; discussion of the composition of the team members serving the early intervention population; discussion of the IFSP; and a discussion of the role of the OTA and the OT in early intervention.

CHAPTER 20

Preschool and School-Based Therapy presents an introduction to preschool and school-based practice; historical and legal background information; discussion of the population identified and served (and challenges associated with) through school-based services (K-12); examination of the service models associated with school-based practice; discussion of the context in which school-based services are disseminated; and a discussion of the IEP and the 504 Accommodation Plan. A discussion of the roles of the OTA and the OT in school-based therapy; an overview of standard measures used by OTs in school-based services; discussion of prevocational and transitional planning issues pertinent to occupational therapy practitioners; and discussion of goal development, documentation procedures, and treatment strategies associated with school based-practice are also presented.

CHAPTER 21

Pediatric Hospital Based, Outpatient Clinic, Home Health, Hospice, and Private Clinical Practice Treatment provides an introduction to hospital and outpatient clinic based, home health, hospice, and private clinical practice, and a discussion of the population identified and served through these contexts. This chapter also examines the service models and systems associated with hospital, outpatient clinic practice, home health, hospice, and private clinical practice contexts and discusses the composition of the team members serving the child receiving services in these practice areas. The role of the OTA with evaluation and treatment are also discussed.

CHAPTER 22

Pediatric Psychosocial Therapy provides an introduction to psychosocial based practice, historical, and legal background information. A discussion of the population identified and served through psychosocial clinical services, examination of the service models associated with psychosocial clinical practice and the context through which psychosocial services are disseminated are explored. An overview of the role of the OTA and the OT in psychosocial therapy, standard measures used by Occupational Therapists in psychosocial practice, and a discussion of goal development, documentation procedures, and treatment strategies associated with psychosocial practice are also presented.

CHAPTER 23

Adaptive Equipment and Assistive Technology provides an introduction to adaptive equipment, assistive technology and occupational therapy and a discussion and rationale for the use of adaptive equipment and assistive technologies in pediatric occupational therapy treatment. An exploration of the planning and implementation of adaptive equipment or assistive technology in the therapy milieu, as well as in the other environments that a child occupies is presented. Examination of the role of the OTA in the entire process of fabrication and/or ordering of equipment is included. Discussion of the role of the OTA in educating the child, family, and other significant adults regarding the indications and contraindications of specifically prescribed adapted equipment and assistive technology; exploration of the reimbursement procedures for obtaining specific equipment or assistive technology devices; and a discussion of goal development, documentation procedures, and treatment strategies associated with monitoring of the efficacy of adapted equipment or assistive technology is also explored in this chapter.

CHAPTER 24

Orthotics provides an introduction to orthotics in occupational therapy, a discussion and rationale for the use of orthotics in pediatric occupational therapy treatment, and an exploration of the planning and implementation of orthotics in the therapy milieu, as well as in other environments that a child occupies. Examination of the role of the OTA in the entire process of fabrication and/or ordering of orthotics is included. A discussion of the role of the OTA in educating the child, family, and other significant adults regarding the indications and contraindications of specifically prescribed orthotics, goal development, documentation procedures, and treatment strategies associated with monitoring orthotics, and reimbursement procedures is also presented.

Developmental Milestones Chart

Towards the end of the book you will find an extensive Developmental Milestones chart that you can remove and use both when you are a student as well as out in the field. To make it withstand the rigors of much use, we suggest that you laminate it.

Chapter 2

FOUNDATIONS OF OCCUPATIONAL THERAPY

Catherine Verrier Piersol, MS, OTR/L
Cynthia Haynes, MEd, MBA, OTR/L

Chapter Objectives

- Describe the therapeutic nature of *occupation* as it relates to occupational therapy.
- Describe the development and history of the occupational therapy assistant.
- Discuss the unique contributions of occupational therapy in pediatric practice settings.
- Delineate the role of the occupational therapist and occupational therapy assistant.
- Define the relationship between the occupational therapist and occupational therapy assistant and the associated supervisory requirements.
- Explain the terminology used in occupational therapy practice, including the *Occupational Therapy Practice Framework: Domain and Process*.
- Describe best practice in pediatric occupational therapy.
- Apply the concepts of occupation, role delineation, best practice, and professional terminology through case analysis.

Introduction

The foundation of occupational therapy practice is grounded in the therapeutic nature of "occupation" or purposeful activity. The history of occupational therapy reflects a profession that has undergone expansion and refinement. However, the practice of engaging clients in purposeful and meaningful activities in order to promote their ability to participate in daily life remains the central focus of occupational therapy. *The Philosophical Base of Occupational Therapy* (AOTA, 1979) states, "Occupational therapy is based on the belief that purposeful activity (occupation), including its interpersonal and environmental components, may be used to prevent and mediate dysfunction, and to elicit maximum adaptation" (p. 785).

In all practice settings, using occupations to facilitate a person's occupational performance, or function, is the cornerstone of occupational therapy. Occupational performance is the "result of the dynamic relationship between person, environment and occupation" (CAOT, 1997, p. 45). The interplay between these human and nonhuman aspects of occupational performance is summarized below.

> A person constantly engages in occupations in interactions with an environment. The environment provides the context within which occupations are accomplished. Occupational performance represents the actual execution or carrying-out of occupation and is the experience of a person engaged in occupation within an environment (CAOT, 1997, p. 45).

As a profession, occupational therapy is built on a unique knowledge base that enables practitioners to provide a variety of services to the pediatric population. This knowledge base embodies the *Occupational Therapy Practice Framework* (AOTA, 2002), which guides the Occupational Therapy Assistant (OTA) in the clinical reasoning and problem solving processes necessary to address the unique needs of each child and his/her family/caregiver. The occupations most frequently facilitated though pediatric practice are related to developmentally appropriate *play*. Both the

Occupational Therapist (OT) and the OTA are responsible for facilitating these play related occupations of childhood. In day-to-day practice, the relationship between the OT and OTA must be one of mutual respect and collaboration. When providing pediatric occupational therapy services, the OT and OTA work as a team, as both strive to achieve successful outcomes for the child. In the area of pediatric practice, the OTA is expected to implement what is known as a *best practice* approach to therapy in order to facilitate the child(ren's) intervention plan and to use clinical reasoning to make appropriate decisions during ongoing treatment. This chapter examines these foundational issues of pediatric occupational therapy and its application to the OTA.

The Emergence of the Role of the Occupational Therapy Assistant

In the 1950s, the role of the OTA emerged, and in 1958, educational guidelines and supervisory requirements providing a structure for the practice roles of the OTA were established (Carr, 2001). Beginning in the early 1960s, the role and practice scope of the OTA began to expand to include contributing articles for the *American Journal of Occupational Therapy* and election of officials to the AOTA executive board (Carr, 2001). Please refer to Figure 2-1 for a complete chronology of OTA professional developmental milestones.

Today, the OTA plays a vital role in the provision of occupational therapy services in a variety of practice settings. This role is guided by federal practice standards, state licensure mandates, and supervisory requirements. Federal and state guidelines and facility based supervisory requirements provide a structure for the practice of occupational therapy. For instance and as stated in the AOTA *Guide for Supervision of Occupational Therapy Personnel in the Delivery of Occupational Therapy Services*, OTs are responsible for the directing service delivery (AOTA, 1999). Specifically,

> *The level of supervision required for an OTA is determined by the supervising OT and is based on an assessment of the OTA's skills, the demands of the job, the needs of the service recipients, and the service setting requirements. The ultimate criteria used in selecting the level of supervision is related to the ability of the OTA to safely and effectively provide those interventions that are delegated by the OT. When new aspects of practice are delegated to the assistant, service competency must be established between the supervising OT and the OTA.* (AOTA, 1999b, p.3)

The Uniqueness of the Field of Occupational Therapy in Pediatric Practice

The foundation of occupational therapy embraces the ideal that individuals achieve *role fulfillment* through occupational performance (Pedretti & Early, 2001). Pediatric-based occupational therapy practice reflects the concept that children achieve role fulfillment through occupational performance, maturation and development, and within the confines of social, cultural, and personal factors. Collectively, these factors must be considered in order to maintain a best practice approach when working with children and their families/caregivers. The demands and expectations of the child's context or environment, the child's and caregiver's hopes and dreams, as well as barriers that impact role fulfillment also feature prominently in developing a treatment plan. The treatment plan should incorporate the child's strengths and needs as well as the challenges of current and future environments in order to encourage occupational competence.

Childhood occupations are a visible set of responses and/or actions to an environment, which includes many settings, situations, and activities. Occupation also encompasses activities that are culturally valued, interesting, or desired by the child, or those that the child is expected to perform (Humphry, 2002). Play is a primary occupation of childhood (Law, Missiuna, Pollack, & Stewart, 2001). Play is the medium through which children expand their knowledge base, become socialized, practice roles, reflect their culture, and expand *cognition* (Parham & Primeau, 1997). Play includes exploration and interaction. Play is fun! Regardless of the setting in which therapy is provided, OTAs may develop effective play interventions that facilitate turn-taking, chaining newly acquired movement sequences, or that require problem-solving. These skills facilitate the occupational performance of a child. Play may be used to help a child become goal-directed, and motivated to challenge him/herself in occupational and role performances (please refer to Chapter 14: Childhood Occupations). Respecting the child and his/her unique spirit, strengths, and needs through thoughtful development of individual treatment plans cannot be stressed enough. This theme will be reflected throughout this text.

The ultimate developmental goal for any child is to participate within their natural environment (Case-Smith, 2001). This is particularly true for children with special needs. Active participation in one's natural environment implies fulfillment of various occupational roles that are appropriate and feasible for a child irrespective of his/her unique needs and developmental status. As a child grows

1949	AOTA Board of Management discussed a proposal to the AMA for a one-year training program for "assistants" by Guy Morrow, OTR, of Ohio.	1975	Award of Excellence created for COTA.
		1975	COTAs became eligible to receive the Eleanor Clarke Slagle Lectureship Award and the Award of Merit.
1956	AOTA Board of Management approved a task force to investigate OT aides and supportive personnel.	1976	First COTA elected member-at-large of the Executive Board.
1956	AOTA Board of Management changed name of Committee on Recognition of Non-professional Personnel to Committee on Recognition of OT Aides to avoid use of term "non-professional" in all correspondence. In October of the same year, the name was changed to Committee on Recognition of Occupational Therapy Assistants.	1977	First national certification examination administered to OTAs.
		1978	ROH award established.
		1979	Policy adopted that the acronym "COTA" can be used only by assistants currently certified by AOTA.
		1980	Funding for two year (later refunded) COTA advocacy position for AOTA office.
1957	AOTA Board of Management accepted the committee's plan and agreed to implement plan in October, 1958.	1981	COTA Task Force established.
1958	First Essentials and Guidelines of an Approved Educational Program for Occupational Therapy Assistants adopted.	1981	Eight COTAs are faculty members of professional OT curricula.
1958	Plan implemented.	1981	Entry-level OTR and COTA role delineations adopted.
1958	Grandfather clause established.	1982	Career mobility plan terminated.
1959	First OT assistant education program approved at Westborough State Hospital in Massachusetts.	1982	"COTA Share Column" introduced in OT newspaper.
1960	336 COTAs certified through grandfather clause.	1983	Representative Assembly agreed a COTA member-at-large elected to the assembly would have voice and vote.
1961	First general practice program approved at Montgomery County, Maryland.	1985	First COTA representative and alternate to serve in the Representative Assembly elected.
1962	First COTA directory published.	1987	AOTA Bylaws Revision allowed no distinction between COTA and OTR in running for or holding office, including president of the Association.
1963	Board of Management established COTA membership category.		
1965	First paper authored by a COTA published in the *American Journal of Occupational Therapy*.	1989	Twenty-one full-time and 20 part-time COTAs employed in OTA education programs.
1966	All future educational programs must prepare OTA students as generalists, including both psychosocial and general practice input.	1989	Six full-time and 20 part-time COTAs employed in professional OT curricula.
		1989	Nine COTAs are members of state regulatory boards.
1967	First COTA meeting held at AOTA Annual Conference.	1990	New guidelines for supervision of COTAs adopted by the Representative Assembly.
1968	Eight COTAs served on various AOTA committees.		
1969	Tenth anniversary of COTAs noted in Schwagmeyer paper.	1991	Treatment in Groups: A COTA Workshop was sponsored by the AOTA as the association's first continuing education program specifically for COTAs.
1970	Effort to change name of COTA to "associate" or "technician" failed in Delegate Assembly.		
1971	Military OT technicians eligible for certification as COTAs.	1991	First AOTA COTA/OTR Partnership Award received by Ilenna Brown and Cynthia Epstein.
1972	Fifth Annual COTA Workshop held in Baltimore on subject of COTA/OTR relationship.	1991	AOTA's Executive Board invites COTA participation.
1972	First book review written by COTA published in the *American Journal of Occupational Therapy*.	1992	17,000 COTAs certified by AOTCB.
		1998	AOTA establishes Advanced Practitioner (AP) credential and awards first 26 APs.
1973	Career mobility plan endorsed by Executive Board.		
1974	First COTAs take certification examination as part of career mobility plan to become OTRs.	1998	Theresa Letois is elected first COTA as state president for Indiana. Terry Olivas De La O became the first voting COTA representative member on AOTA's Executive Board.
1974	COTAs get *American Journal of Occupational Therapy* as a membership benefit.		

Figure 2-1. Chronology of COTA developmental milestones. Reprinted from Ryan, S. E. & Sladyk, K. (2001). *Ryan's occupational therapy assistant: Principles, practice issues, and techniques.* 3rd ed. Thorofare, NJ: SLACK Incorporated.

and develops, the interrelationship between the child and his/her roles in various environments changes. For instance, throughout childhood, occupational roles change in complexity and may include:

- An infant who can now tolerate position changes and interact with his/her siblings as they play with him/her on the floor.
- A preschooler who learns to take off his/her coat and hang it in her cubby in a timely manner so he/she may play with friends in the kitchen play center.
- A primary school age boy who can successfully stand in line and walk with the class to the library, keeping his hands to himself and off other children, or bulletin boards in the hallway.
- A young adolescent who adheres to the timelines for class changes and gets from gym to the next class period along with his/her peers.

Inherent with children is the ongoing process of adaptation to environmental demands and assimilation of opportunities as they grow and develop from *infancy* to adulthood. Childhood is a unique time of exploration, joy, inquisitiveness, energy and endless possibilities. As *occupational therapy practitioners*, we have the unique opportunity to interface with the child and his/her spirit (Case-Smith, 2001).

Best Practice in Pediatric Occupational Therapy

Occupational therapy practitioners and/or occupational therapy intervention may have a profound impact on the competencies a child takes forward in life. As OT practitioners strive to facilitate a child's many occupations, consider the concept of best practice as a means to most effectively work with a child. Best practice in pediatrics describes an OT practitioner's decisions and actions as it relates to childhood occupations. It is based on sound clinical judgment that reflects and puts into practice, current and innovative ideas (Dunn, 2000). When working with children, occupational therapy best practice reflects an understanding of a child's interactions within his/her environment. Based on a systems model, a child's environment may include:

1. The immediate physical environment: A neighborhood where the child lives, and the places the child frequents such as friend's and relative's homes, stores, school, daycare or outpatient clinics.
2. The *social* and *cultural context*: The unique practices of the child's family/caregiver as influenced by religious or spiritual practices, ethnic heritage, and socioeconomic status.

3. Beliefs and values of the child's family/caregivers. Beliefs and values that influence decisions, including access to services, levels of participation and roles within the family, acceptance of a child with a special needs and the support network available to the family/caregivers (Dunn, 2000).

In response to the *Individuals With Disabilities Education Act (IDEA)* (1999), best practice guidelines were developed for providing occupational therapy services to children with special needs (Maruyama, Chandler, Frolek Clark, West Dick, Lawlor, & Lewis Jackson, 1999). These guidelines specifically focus on children receiving services in *Early Intervention* and educational settings. Although best practice guidelines do not address every practice setting associated with provision of OT services to children, they can be used to guide the OT practitioner with the clinical reasoning and professional problem solving processes necessary for working with all children.

In addition to federal and state guidelines, service provision also depends on the type and location of the facility. Service provision involves the evaluation process, determining the length and type of intervention sessions, and actual therapeutic intervention. The creative efforts of the OTA will determine, in part, how restrictive, limiting, or facilitating the setting is. Best practice guidelines help the OTA working with children and their families/caregivers in a variety of settings to provide the most effective, professional, and meaningful service provision possible. Regardless of the setting, best practice guidelines also encourage occupational therapy services be provided within a *family-centered care philosophy*.

Family-centered care, as applied to occupational therapy intervention, includes meaningful involvement of families/caregivers in the planning and implementation of occupational therapy services (Salisbury & Dunst, 1977). Family-centered care insures that the OT practitioner will acknowledge, respect, and embody the family/caregiver's priorities, and their hopes and dreams for the child. Ideally and regardless of the treatment environment, a family-centered care model should guide most occupational therapy interventions with children. While each OT practitioner's interpretation of family-centered care principles may differ slightly, and despite individual differences and interpretations, the guiding principles of family-centered care are as follows:

- Parents know their children the best and want the best for their children.
- Each family is different and unique.
- Optimal child function occurs within a supportive family and community context.
- Families and professionals are equal in the partnership.

- Families define the priorities for intervention.
- Interventions must be based on the family's values, culture, and visions for their child.
- Evaluation and interventions must be unique to the specific needs of the family and the child (Dunn, 2000).

In terms of a family-centered care philosophy, OTAs must:

- Enable the child to successfully participate in inclusive settings.
- Provide services in natural *contexts* or in *least restrictive environments*.
- Participate in communications that promote family/caregiver participation and understanding.
- Include consultation with and education to families/caregivers and others involved with the child to support generalization across environments and promote optimal *growth and development* as part of the intervention process.
- Engage in *person first language* to demonstrate respect and acknowledgment of the child as a person first regardless of other manifestations or characteristics relevant to occupational therapy (Dunn, 2000; Case-Smith, 2001).

Current research indicates that a family-centered philosophy results in greater family satisfaction with services and perceived changes in their child (Law, et. al., 2001). Family-centered care occurs when the family takes an active role during treatment planning and intervention. A recent survey of OT practitioners working with parents of preschool children with developmental disabilities revealed that OT practitioners using a family-centered care philosophy felt their therapeutic intervention to be effective (Hinojosa, Sproat, Mankhetwit, & Anderson, 2002). Occupational therapy practitioners also suggested that participation in family-centered care had the greatest impact on successful outcomes of a child with disabilities (Hinojosa, Sproat, Mankhetwit, & Anderson, 2002). Additionally, development of parent-therapist relationships directed towards supporting parents perceived needs of their child led to more positive therapeutic outcomes (Hinojosa et al, 2002). Better perceived therapy outcomes, better follow through on home activities, and indication of being able to overtly enjoy their child were all reported outcomes of participation in a family-centered care model (Mayer, White, Ward, & Barney, 2002).

Intervention evolves from the collaborative efforts of family members and professionals involved with the family and child (Law, Missiuna, Pollack, & Stewart, 2001; Dunst, Trivette, & Deal, 1988). Application of a family-centered care model is evident through the careful and sensitive planning and implementation of best practice oriented intervention services. To maintain a positive therapeutic relationship with a child and the family/caregiver, the OTA must maintain a standard of best practice by constantly monitoring changes and modifying treatment approaches to meet a child's ever-changing needs (Case-Smith, 2001).

The Role of the OTA in Pediatric Practice

According to AOTA guidelines (Maruyama et al, 1999), OT practitioners should consider the following when working with children:

1. To provide an essential, individualized, and culturally relevant service to children whose development and occupational performance have been influenced by disease, disability, or vulnerability.
2. To offer services derived via partnerships with the child, family/caregivers, and other service providers from various disciplines.
3. As a member of a team, the OT practitioner is responsible for:
   - Addressing the priorities of the family and child that will support learning and ongoing skill acquisition within identified occupational roles.
   - Facilitating the person–environment fit unique to each child and their family/caregiver.
   - Preparing the child and family/caregiver for new environments and the challenges they will present.
   - Fostering team collaboration via open communication with team members that facilitate understanding of, respect for and integration of input from other team members (Maruyama et al, 1999. p. 4).

The AOTA (Maruyama et al, 1999) has established guidelines explaining the roles and responsibilities of both the OT and the OTA. These guidelines apply to the provision of OT services for the pediatric population in a unique way. The guidelines are discussed below.

SUPERVISION

According to AOTA guidelines (AOTA, 1999), the OTA works under the supervision of the OT, who is ultimately responsible for the overall delivery of services to a child. As an OTA gains experience, the level of supervision provided by the OT changes. AOTA (2002) defines supervision as a cooperative process that will maintain or elevate the level of the OTAs competency in the provision of occupational therapy services to a child. There are four levels of supervision suggested by the AOTA. They are:

1. Close supervision: includes direct, daily contact between the OTA and OT.

2. Routine supervision: includes direct contact between the OT and OTA at approximately biweekly intervals. Additional contact may occur through telephone consultation and emails.

3. General supervision: includes at least once monthly direct contact with interim contacts on an as-needed basis.

4. Minimum supervision: occurs solely on an as indicated basis and may include direct and indirect contact (AOTA, 2002; Rainville, Cermack & Murray, 1996).

The level of supervision provided by the OT is also determined by state regulations, the facility, and payer or funding sources.

SERVICE COMPETENCY

In order for an OTA to provide a specific service for a child, he/she must first demonstrate *service competency*. Service competency pertains to the OTAs ability to demonstrate clinical reasoning, and administer specific evaluations or treatment techniques commensurate with standardization guidelines, facility or accreditation requirements, and OT supervisor discretion. Service competency provides a means for determining the reliability of the OTAs skills. Achieving service competency suggests that equivalent or same procedures will produce equivalent or same results when comparing the service provision of an OTA with the OT. The OTAs competencies must be monitored, reassessed, and documented on a regular basis (AOTA, 1999b). Demonstration of service competency may be achieved for a specific skill area through ongoing training by an OT or by attending continuing education courses.

COLLABORATION

Collaboration is a key element in the successful partnership between the OT and OTA for delivery of occupational therapy services (Commission on Practice, 2002). Ongoing communication is an important aspect of the collaboration process. In order to develop a successful collaboration, it is the responsibility of the OT to maintain regular and frequent communication with the OTA regarding client status. Intervention planning and implementation are two means through which the OT and the OTA may collaborate. To achieve this level of collaboration, the OTA must demonstrate competency in specific interventions, and must be monitored on a regular basis by the OT through observation of intervention sessions, written documentation, and ongoing dialogue and communication. Ongoing monitoring, communication and collaboration between the OT and the OTA also provides a foundation from which the OT determines the extent of the OTA's competency with regards to thoughtful, sound, clinical practice. For example, in a school-based setting where the OT and OTA share responsi-

bilities for caseloads, the OTA may implement and carry out a feeding program with a child. The OT designs the program in collaboration with the OTA and the child's team, which is then carried out by the OTA. When minor program changes, such as a utensil modification, positioning adaptations, or slight increases in food texture are called for, if competency has been already established in these intervention areas, the OTA implements these changes and reports back to the supervising OT on the efficacy of the program.

EVALUATION AND INTERVENTION

A child's current and emerging performance skills are dependent upon the child's context or environment. Context, including cultural, physical, social, personal, spiritual, temporal and virtual, refers to a variety of interrelated environments that influence a child's performance (AOTA, 2002). When possible, the OTA observes family/caregiver interactions and routines to gain insight into occupational roles each child will be expected to learn, conform to, or ultimately perform. This information contributes to and becomes part of the evaluation process. In order to insure that the child's occupational roles that are facilitated through occupational therapy interventions are characteristic of a child's contextual background, the OTA must also develop an appreciation of the unique environments in which the child is growing and developing (Humphry, 2002).

The evaluation process is completed primarily by the OT, however the OTA may, depending on demonstrated competency level, gather preliminary information and complete an observation of a child's occupational performance. For instance, the OTA may observe and share information regarding a child's ability to maneuver a wheelchair and transfer to various surfaces within his/her environment. The OTA's involvement in the evaluation process may also include the administration of standardized evaluation tools such as the Developmental Test of Visual Perception-2 (Hammill, Pearson, & Voress, 1993), as long as the supervising OT has documented that the OTA is competent in the administration of a specific evaluation tool. The OT completes interpretation of evaluation results. The OT, in collaboration with the OTA, develops an intervention plan based on the evaluation results, and the individual needs and goals of the child and family/caregiver.

Interventions focus on the unique strengths and needs of the child. Occupational therapy intervention is based on consideration of the child's current status, his/her ability to adapt, and the environment or context within which a new occupational behavior can emerge. The OT practitioner serves as the catalyst to provide a just-right challenge for the child so that ongoing acquisition of new and more complex occupational behaviors might occur (Humphry, 2002). By *grading* an activity to make it a just-right challenge, a child can gain new skills and begin to feel the confidence that comes from successfully mastering an activity. Based on the premise that a just-right challenge is motivating for the child, reasonable outcomes of OT intervention with children should be:

Child centered:

- Provide higher levels of occupational performance.
- Support motivation (intrinsic or extrinsic).
- Offer self-organization opportunities allowing the child to adjust to changes within their skill levels.
- Allow for active participation in inclusive settings and natural contexts.

Team centered:

- Include family/caregiver (team) consultation and education.
- Validate feedback from child, family/caregiver, and team regarding the outcome of the child's occupational behavior source.
- Provide adaptation and/or modification of the environment or components of the environment (Case Smith, 2001).

Grading these choices or activities is the art of occupational therapy. Grading involves systematically increasing or decreasing the demands of the activity in order to promote successful performance (Lamport et al., 2001). Occupational therapy intervention is suboptimal if the child experiences frustration and failure during activity performance. A child should be given choices of increasingly complex activities to spark motivation and increase active participation in treatment.

OT intervention with children leads to a variety of outcomes, including emergence of completely new skills that result in occupational roles not previously observed. An example of this is when a child begins to combine *grasp* of a crayon with an arm and hand action, which leads to eventual scribbling on a surface, and ultimately results in acquisition of a new occupation: the drawer/artist.

Interventions may also help the child learn alternative strategies to produce an already existing occupation.

In this instance a child may learn several methods to don a coat. If increased muscle tone prevents the child from putting a coat on using the flip-over-the-head method, the child may, instead, use the dress-the effected-side method and maintain the occupational role of self-dresser.

Lastly, interventions may provide the child with the opportunity to generalize existing occupational behaviors to new environmental contexts.

For example, a child who has learned to request favorite foods from an employee behind a counter at a fast food restaurant may now successfully walk through a school cafeteria line and request food from the grill employee (Humphry, 2002).

REPORTING PROCEDURES

As suggested throughout this chapter, the level of autonomy an OTA assumes in terms of observation, assessment, goal writing, treatment planning and implementation, adaptation of treatment plans, documentation, and case reporting is determined through federal, state, and facility regulations, as well as ongoing assessment of service competency (AOTA, 1999b). Occupational therapy assistants also function on interdisciplinary teams in numerous settings, including rehabilitation teams, educational teams, early intervention teams, and habilitation or community support teams. In general, at these team meetings, the OT is ultimately responsible for reporting on a child's status and progress. However, if the OTA has been deemed competent in reporting progress and proposing treatment changes regarding a specific child, then he/she may be responsible for reporting at team meetings, as indicated. In collaboration with the OT, the OTA may also develop goals and objectives (i.e., short-term goals or benchmarks). Please refer to Chapter 6: Documentation.

Occupational Therapy Terminology

As previously discussed, the use of occupation as a therapeutic medium and as the focus of intervention historically has been, and continues to be, the focus of occupational therapy. In order to represent professional concepts and practice techniques, appropriate words are needed to describe them. These words reflect the OT and OTA's education and practice beliefs (Piersol, 2002). In occupational therapy there is an established vocabulary and set of terms that are used in documentation, and in verbal communication with occupational therapy practitioners, other health care professionals, clients, and caregivers/family members (Piersol, 2002).

Since 1979, the AOTA provided official documents that offer a uniform set of terms (AOTA, 1979; AOTA, 1989; AOTA, 1994), the last version being *Uniform Terminology for Occupational Therapy*, 3rd Edition, (UT-III, AOTA, 1994).

Most recently, and to replace the UT-III and its predecessors, the AOTA adopted the *Occupational Therapy Practice Framework: Domain and Process* (*Framework*), which delineates the "language and constructs that describe the profession's focus" (AOTA, 2002, p. 609) The *Framework* offers the OT and OTA a basis from which to describe and practice occupational therapy.

The *Framework* (AOTA, 2002) also provides practitioners with a common language and focus, which reflects the profession's foundation in occupation. The domain terms and process concepts established in the *Framework* (AOTA,

---

Engagement in Occupation to Support Participation in Context or Contexts

Performance in Areas of Occupation
Activities of Daily Living (ADL)
Instrumental Activities of Daily Living (IADL)
Education
Work
Play
Leisure
Social Participation

Performance Skills   Performance Patterns
Motor Skills   Habits
Process Skills   Routines
Communication/Interaction Skills   Roles

Context   Activity Demands   Client Factors
Cultural   Objects Used and Their Properties   Body Functions
Physical   Space Demands   Body Structures
Social   Social Demands
Personal   Sequencing and Timing
Spiritual   Required Actions
Temporal   Required Body Functions
Virtual   Required Body Structures

Figure 2-2. *Domain of Occupational Therapy*. Reprinted with permission from the American Occupational Therapy Association.

2002) foster communication between occupational therapy practitioners as well as with other professionals, and provide a common language for documentation. In creating this document, the AOTA sought to describe and explain the domain of occupational therapy and the process of evaluation, intervention and outcome in occupational therapy (AOTA, 2002). It is stated,

> The Framework *was developed in response to current practice needs—the need to more clearly affirm and articulate occupational therapy's unique focus on occupation and daily life activities and the application of an intervention process that facilitates engagement in occupation to support participation in life* (AOTA, 2002, p. 609).

The *Framework* (AOTA, 2002) is organized into two distinct sections: Domain and Process. "The domain of occupational therapy frames the areas in which occupational therapy evaluations and interventions occur" (AOTA, 2002,

p. 610). The domain section provides the practitioner with the language and terminology of the profession. These terms are used when communicating about a child's status through documentation and when discussing a child's progress during a team meeting. As is depicted in Figure 2-2, "engagement in occupation to support participation in context or contexts" (p. 610) is the overriding domain of concern for the OT practitioner (AOTA, 2002). Within this broad context, the practitioner attends to specific domains: areas of occupation, performance skills, performance patterns, context, activity demands, and client factors. In collaboration, the OT and OTA address these domains through the occupational therapy assessment and intervention process. Each of the six domains offers important information that assists the OT and OTA in designing intervention that meets the child's needs and abilities. Context, activity demands, and client factors influence the child's performance skills and performance patterns (AOTA, 2002).

Evaluation

Occupational profile—The initial step in the evaluation process that provides and understanding of the client's occupational history and experiences, patterns of daily living, interests, values, and needs. The client's problems and concerns about performing occupations and daily life activities are identified, and the client's priorities are determined.

Analysis of occupational performance—The step in the evaluation process during which the client's assets, problems, or potential problems are more specifically identified. Actual performance is often observed in context to identify what supports performance and what hinders performance. Performance skills, performance patterns, context or contexts, activity demands, and client factors are all considered, but only selected aspects may be specifically assessed. Targeted outcomes are identified.

Intervention

Intervention plan—A plan that will guide actions taken and that is developed in collaboration with the client. It is based on selected theories, frames of reference, and evidence. Outcomes to be targeted are confirmed.

Intervention implementation—Ongoing actions taken to influence and support improved client performance. Interventions are directed at identified outcomes. Client's response is monitored and documented.

Intervention review—A review of the implementation plan and process as well as its progress toward targeted outcomes.

Outcomes (Engagement in Occupation to Support Participation)

Outcomes—Determination of success in reaching desired targeted outcomes. Outcome assessment information is used to plan future actions with the client and to evaluate the service program (i.e., program evaluation).

Figure 2-3. *Framework* process of service delivery as applied within the profession's domain. Reprinted with permission from the American Occupational Therapy Association.

Performance skills and patterns are used to describe how the child actually performs specific areas of occupation (AOTA, 2002).

The *Framework* (AOTA, 2002) also offers the practitioner a method for describing and organizing the service delivery process. As depicted in Figure 2-3, the three broad components of the process portion of the *Framework* (AOTA, 2002) include Evaluation, Intervention, and Outcomes (Engagement in Occupation To Support Participation). The Evaluation process includes an occupational profile and an analysis of occupational performance (AOTA, 2002). The OT is primarily responsible for gathering information about the child and his or her contexts, and describing the problems he or she is having in performing occupations as well as the specific performance skills, patterns, and factors limiting his/her child's occupational performance. The OTA may assist the OT in gathering this important information. The Intervention process, in which the OTA is very involved and assumes responsibility under the supervision of the OT, includes the intervention plan, intervention implementation, and intervention review. As the child participates in the intervention process, specific activities and approaches are modified and graded in order to facilitate the child's success and attainment of goals. The Outcomes process involves "determination of success in reaching desired targeted outcomes" (AOTA, 2002, p. 614). The OT is responsible for assessing individual outcomes of each child as well as overall program outcomes. The OTA assists with this vital process. As a child is involved in occupational therapy services, the OT and OTA must systematically assess the efficacy of the services and make adjustments and recommendations as indicated.

Summary

As a profession, the foundation of occupational therapy practice involves the application of occupation as a therapeutic tool. The role of the OTA emerged in the late 1950s. Since that time OTAs and OTs have partnered to provide services in a variety of settings including medical, community, and school-based settings. When working in the area of pediatrics, the OTA plays an important role in the provision of occupational therapy services in a variety of practice settings. Working with children and families/caregivers presents a unique combination of challenges and joys to the OTA. Ongoing developmental, biomechanical, structural, and psychosocial changes within a child require constant monitoring and re-evaluation to insure the efficacy of occupational therapy services. The OTA, in partnership with an OT, must carefully and sensitively select and implement the best treatment approaches so as to meet the changing needs of the child and the family/caregiver.

The role of the OT practitioner in a pediatric setting is to develop a partnership with the child and the family/caregiver. Coupling this partnership with best practice guidelines facilitates trust, respect from the child and family/caregivers, and engenders professionalism within the OT practitioner. These traits develop from initial contact and interview, through the evaluation and intervention process, and into discharge planning. Occupational roles, environmental contexts, cultural and social values, and hopes and dreams of the family/caregivers are unique and integral components of occupational therapy service in pediatric practice.

Application Activities

1. Select an age and a diagnosis typically seen in the pediatric population and list up to 10 manifestations of that diagnosis (e.g., a 6-year-old girl with pervasive developmental disorder). Postulate how the manifestations of the disease/disability will affect the role performance of that child.

2. Visit a day care or preschool that services both typically developing and special needs children or view a brief videotape of a typically developing child in a play activity and list the various skills the child demonstrates. By comparison, view a child with special needs who is unable to play due to a cognitive/psychosocial or physical disability. Compare the similarities and differences in their occupational performance. Postulate why this is happening. Begin to generate a list of interfering factors and potential solutions to these factors.

3. Imagine you are an entry-level OTA assigned to work in an integrated preschool classroom of 3-year-olds. There are 12 children in the classroom; six are identified as special needs. Classroom staff includes a full-time teacher and a teacher's aide. A speech pathologist comes into the classroom 2 ½ days per week and runs "language groups". You are assigned to the classroom 2 days.

   Your OT supervisor wants to work with you to design an innovative method for your supervision and training. Generate a list of ways this could be accomplished considering the site and the staff.

   How would you implement the concept of occupation-based intervention in this setting?

4. Using the language and concepts described in the *Occupational Therapy Practice Framework: Domain and process*, answer the following: If a child had deficits in the performance skills of strength and effort, coordination and temporal organization, how might the following areas of occupation be impacted:

   • Dressing to go outside
   • Taking a tub bath
   • Going through a cafeteria line
   • Playing cooperatively in a sandbox with a friend.

Case Study

Melissa is a 6-year-old girl who attends her community public school. She is in a regular first grade classroom and has an *Individual Education Plan (IEP)* that addresses her special learning needs. She receives part-time learning support in addition to speech and language, occupational ther-apy, and adapted physical education (APE). Melissa likes school, especially computers. She is accepted by her teachers but does not have many friends at school. In her neighborhood, she enjoys playing with younger children after school and on the weekends. Melissa lives with her parents and younger brother, Daniel, who is in preschool. Both Melissa's parents work full-time, so Melissa attends an after school program. Her maternal grandmother watches Daniel in the afternoon, before the parents get home from work.

During her infancy, her parents reported that Melissa was a fussy, irritable baby who had irregular sleeping patterns and did not tolerate schedule changes or changes in diet. She had multiple ear infections; had bilateral ear tubes inserted twice, and subsequently has been diagnosed with a severe speech delay. Melissa was late to walk; she cruised around furniture up until 2 ½ years old, at which time she began to walk on her own. Her gait remains awkward; she loses her balance and falls frequently, and still has problems going up and down steps. In addition, she tires easily during physical activities. As Melissa began to express her opinions about clothing, she showed a strong preference toward soft, loose clothing without fasteners, which continues to this day.

Prior to attending public school she received early intervention services, first at home and then in a preschool, which her brother currently attends. The home-based services included physical therapy, occupational therapy, speech/language, and *early childhood* education. By preschool, her motor skills had sufficiently improved for her to navigate the classroom and playground, so that physical therapy was only provided on a consultative basis, while occupational therapy, speech, and educational services continued on a weekly basis. She remained at the preschool for full-day kindergarten.

In the spring, prior to her transition to public school, therapists from Melissa's home school district evaluated Melissa to determine her strengths and needs and to help plan for her successful transition to first grade. After the team members completed their evaluations, they met with Melissa's parents, the first grade teacher, and learning support teacher to formulate the IEP for the coming school year. The team identified the following strengths and needs:

AREAS OF STRENGTH

1. Melissa can attend to, initiate, and sequence age-appropriate tasks that would meet classroom expectations for classroom arrival, access and use of bathroom facilities, and transportation.

2. Melissa heeds 1 and 2 step verbal directions to complete goal-directed actions, when accompanied by an initial environmental cue (i.e., demonstration).

3. Melissa is able to walk, *reach*, and bend to adequately interact within the school environment.

AREAS OF NEED

1. Melissa appears fatigued by mid school day, so that she cannot persist and complete tasks commensurate with her classroom peers.

2. Melissa has difficulty with coordination and manipulation, evidenced by diminished fine dexterous finger and hand movements and limited use of both sides of her body to complete typical classroom activities such as cutting with scissors, coloring, and opening containers, e.g., glue stick, juice box, snack bags.

3. Melissa has difficulty articulating and asserting herself relative to personal needs and classroom activities. She uses gestures and facial expressions inconsistently with peers and adults.

4. Melissa has difficulty accommodating and adjusting to multiple transitions that are part of the classroom routine. She cannot adapt to new or different situations, such as using red-handled versus blue-handled scissors and changes in the routine daily schedule.

5. Melissa does not demonstrate an adequate understanding of classroom social *norms* such as waiting her turn or sharing materials, and as a result, other students do not like to be matched with her for small group activities.

On the first day of class, the OT and the OTA complete a 2-hour classroom observation together. The OT and OTA collaborate to identify the occupational therapy intervention approaches that would best address Melissa's need to participate and benefit from the educational program. The educational team works on an integrated therapy model, in which the OTA and speech and language therapist will each spend approximately 1 hour per week in the classroom consulting on Melissa's and another child's similar needs, and collaborating with the classroom teacher.

Learning Activities

1. Based on the information provided about Melissa and her performance skills complete the following:

   • List three areas that the occupational therapy services should address within the school environment.

   • Design age-appropriate, occupation-based activities that address each of the areas you identified above.

   • List strategies that the OTA could provide to the regular education and learning support teachers to be used in the classroom to help Melissa adapt and accommodate to classroom activities and routines.

2. What are some of the unique contributions the OTA can provide to Melissa and the team?

3. There is a change in Melissa's status and she appears to be declining in overall performance. The teacher asks the OTA for major adjustments to the type of intervention currently being provided. What should the OTA do?

4. This is the second year that the OTA has been practicing in this school. What would be the reasonable supervisory expectations from the OT?

5. Develop a professional development plan for the OTA to establish service competency.

References

American Occupational Therapy Association (1994). Uniform terminology for occupational therapy, 3rd ed. *American Journal of Occupational Therapy, 48*, 1047-1054.

American Occupational Therapy Association (1999a). Fortieth Anniversary timeline: OTA history. *OT Practice, 21*, July/August.

American Occupational Therapy Association (1999b). *Guide for supervision of occupational therapy personnel in the delivery of occupational therapy services*. Rockville, MD: AOTA.

Carr, S. H. (2001). The COTA heritage: Proud and dynamic. In K. Sladyk & S. E. Ryan (Eds.), *Ryan's occupational therapy assistant: Principles, practice Issues, and techniques*. Thorofare, NJ: SLACK Incorporated.

Case-Smith, J. (2001). An overview of occupational therapy for children. In J. Case-Smith (Ed.), *Occupational therapy for children* (4th ed.). (pp. 2-20). St. Louis, MO: Mosby.

Dunn, W. (2000). *Best practice occupational Therapy: In community service with children and families*. Thorofare, NJ: SLACK Incorporated.

Commission on Practice (2002). *Roles and responsibilities of the occupational therapist and the occupational therapy assistant during the delivery of occupational therapy services*. Self..

Dunst, C., Trivette, C. M., and Deal, A. (1988). *Enabling and empowering families: Principles and guidelines for practice*. Cambridge, MA: Brookline Books, Inc.

Hammill, D. D., Pearson, N. A., & Voress, J. K. (1993). *Developmental test of visual perception* (2nd ed.). Austin, TX: Pro-Ed.

Hinojosa, J., Sproat, C. T., Mankhetwit, S., & Anderson, J. (2002). Shifts in parent-therapist partnerships: Twelve years of change. *The American Journal of Occupational Therapy, 56*, 556-563.

Humphry, R. (2002). Young children's occupations: Explicating the dynamics of developmental processes. *The American Journal of Occupational Therapy, 56*, 171-179.

Lamport, N. K., Coffey, M. S., & Hersch, G. I. (2001). *Activity analysis & application*. Thorofare, NJ: SLACK Incorporated.

Law, M., Missiuna, C., Pollock, N., & Stewart, D. (2001). Foundations for occupational therapy practice with children. In J. Case-Smith (Ed.), *Occupational therapy for children* (4th ed.). (pp. 39-70). St. Louis, MO: Mosby.

Low, J. F. (1992). The reconstruction aides. *The American Journal of Occupational Therapy, 46*, 38-43.

Maruyama, E., Chandler, B., Frolek Clark, G., West Dick, R., Lawlor, M., & Lewis Jackson, L. (1999). *Occupational therapy services for children and youth under the individuals with disabilities act (IDEA)* (2nd ed.). Bethesda, MD: American Occupational Therapy Association.

Mayer, M. L., White, B. P., Ward, J. D., & Barney, E. M. (2002). Therapists' perceptions about making a difference in parent-child relationships in early intervention occupational therapy services. *The American Journal of Occupational Therapy, 56,* 411-421.

Parham, L. D., & Primeau, L. A. (1997). Play and occupational therapy. In L. Diane Parham & L. Fazio (Eds.), *Play in occupational therapy for children.* (pp. 2-21). St. Louis, MO: Mosby.

Rainville, E. B., Cermack, S. A., & Murray, E. A. (1996). Supervision and consultation for pediatric occupational therapists. *American Journal of Occupational Therapy, 50,* 725.

Salisbury, C., & Dunst, C. (1977). *Homes, schools and community partnerships: Building inclusive teams. Collaborative teams for students with severe disabilities.* Baltimore, MD: Paul H. Brookes.

A BRIEF OVERVIEW OF OCCUPATIONAL THERAPY THEORIES, MODELS, AND FRAMES OF REFERENCE

Michael Roberts, MS, OTR/L

Chapter Objectives

- Compare and contrast the frames of reference presented in this chapter.
- Describe the basic premises of each of the frames of reference provided in this chapter.
- Identify the foundational roots of the frames of reference presented in this chapter.

Introduction

As an occupational therapy assistant (OTA) working with children, it is important to understand the frame of reference(s) from which occupational therapy services are provided. A *frame of reference* is defined by Mosey (1986) as: "...a set of interrelated internally consistent concepts, definitions, and postulates that provide a systematic description of and prescription for a practitioner's interactions with a particular aspect of a profession's domain of concern" (p.129). The frame of reference represents the occupational therapy (OT) practitioner's definitions of function and dysfunction, the theoretical basis for clinical problem solving, and rationale for intervention and treatment planning. As the OTA may work closely with the OT in developing the occu-

pational therapy intervention plan and report, and/or recording information from data collection procedures, understanding and working within the frame(s) of reference through which occupational therapy services are provided is critical (AOTA, 1987). It is also important to understand the theories and reasoning behind interventions, because through interactions with families, clients, payers, and other healthcare professionals, the OTA must be able to effectively articulate the value and intent of the team's chosen intervention approaches (Jirikowic, 2001).

Occupational therapy practitioners actively guide their practice and develop clinical reasoning skills based on frames of reference (Kielhofner, 1992). Which frame of reference is implemented depends on a number of factors. A frame of reference is implemented if it is compatible with the needs and goals of a child, and/or if it is compatible with the OT practitioner's facility and personal frame of reference (Storch & Goldrich Eskow, 1996). Occupational therapy practitioners do not necessarily limit themselves to incorporating a single frame of reference in their treatment. Many OT practitioners use several frames of reference or different combinations of frames of reference as called for by the needs of the children and families or the setting in which they work (Lawlor & Henderson, 1989; Storch & Goldrich Eskow, 1996). There are many frames of reference that guide the OT practitioner's work. While the frames of reference explored in this chapter are not necessarily used by all OT practitioners, this chapter presents an overview of several frames of reference commonly associated with contemporary pediatric practice.

Psychosocial Frames of Reference

Frame of Reference: "Doing and Meaning" Psychosocial Frame of Reference

Theorist: Gail and Jay Fidler

Description: The benefits of occupational activity in a mental health treatment setting are augmented by therapeutically manipulating three factors: "first, those interpersonal events which occur between the therapist and the patient; second, the activities that go on between patients; and third, the effects produced by the relation between occupational therapy and the rest of the patient's treatment program" (Fidler & Fidler, 1954, p. 8). The Psychosocial Frame of Reference does not advocate using activities as the treatment per say, rather "the activity is the tool used in making treatment possible" (Fidler & Fidler, 1954, p. 9).

Application: Treatment focus is on the client's quality of performance of independent living skills and daily living skills of patients, as well as the message inherent in their performance rather than the quality of the end result of a task Instead, processing and activity participation help achieve the overall goals of mental health, quality of life, and independent function.

Frame of Reference: Cognitive-Behavioral Frame of Reference

Theorist: Claudia Kay Allen

Description: The Cognitive Behavioral frame of reference describes a person's cognitive disability as falling into one of six stable and for the most part, unchanging levels. While short-term changes may be seen as a result of medication usage or therapeutic intervention, the true capacity, or true cognitive disability is assumed to be a constant.

Application: The main focus is adaptation of the environment for maximal function. Therapeutic activities focus on achieving effective and appropriate communication, self-expression, and self-care, while using qualities of the environment to make up for absent cognitive function or psychological compensations (Allen, 1985).

Frame of Reference: Multicontextual Approach: A Cognitive-Perceptual Frame of Reference

Theorist: Joan Toglia

Description: Learning is defined as the interaction between personal and external (task and environmental) variables. Personal variables include metacognitive processes such as awareness of one's own cognitive processes and processing strategies. External variables refer to task param-

eters, or the demands of the occupational task, and environmental factors (Toglia, 1992).

Application: The Multicontextual Approach involves specifying strategies for more effective learning, using task analysis to inform the transfer of learned skill or behaviors, applying learned skills or strategies to different environments and tasks, developing self-monitoring for application and proper utilization of strategies, and using motivation or active participation and awareness to drive further learning (Toglia, 1996).

Occupational Therapy Performance Frames of Reference

Frame of Reference: Model of Human Occupation (MOHO)

Theorist: Gary Kielhofner

Description: The MOHO is an open-system model, in which a person's occupational performance dynamically affects and is affected by a constantly changing and developing environment. The environment encompasses the physical surroundings, the objects, tasks, social groups, and culture in which the performance occurs.

Application: In an effort to restore the organization of the "system," treatment focuses on the components of the person's performance, as well as on tools or objects in the environment.

Frame of Reference: Person-Environment-Occupation (P-E-O) Model

Theorist: Mary Law and Colleagues

Description: The P-E-O is based on a systems *theory* model, and presumes a transactional and interdependent relationship between a person, and his or her environments and occupations. In this model environments encompass "contexts and situations which occur outside an individual and [in turn] elicit a response [from the person]" (Stewart, et al., 2003, p. 227; Law, et al., 1996, p. 10). Occupations are activities that are done to meet "intrinsic needs… self maintenance, expression, and fulfillment" (Law, et al., 1996, p. 16).

Application: In the P-E-O model, treatment focuses on the complex relationship of performing occupations within a broad environmental context. It also supports a strong "collaborative relationship between the client, occupational therapy practitioners, and all others in the client's environment" (Stewart et al., 2003, p. 230). Working to change the environments and those factors that influence them rather than changing the person is the goal of the model. Occupational performance is achieved when there is a transaction between the person experiencing specific challenges, and his/her environment, and occupations.

Frame of Reference: Ecology of Human Performance Model

Theorist: Winnie Dunn and Colleagues

Description: Considers how the interaction between a person and his/her contexts, which include the "physical environment, social, cultural, and temporal factors" (Dunn, Brown, & McGuigan, 1994, p. 595) influences "task performance and human behavior" (p. 531). Four major assumptions of the Ecology of Human Performance Model include:

- Persons and their contexts are unique and dynamic.
- Contrived contexts are different from natural contexts.
- Occupational therapy practice involves promoting self-determination and inclusion of persons with disabilities in all contexts.
- Independence includes using contextual supports to meet client's needs and wants. (Dunn, Haney McClain, Brown, & Youngstrom, 2003, p.224).

Application: The scope of this model goes beyond variables that influence human performance and instead, takes into account the performance "in context", including the effects of the context and tasks on human performance and the person-context match (Dunn, Haney McClain, Brown, & Youngstrom, 2003, p. 226; Dunn, Brown, & McGuigan, 1994, p. 595).

Frame of Reference: Occupational Adaptation

Theorist: Janette Schkade and Sally Schultz

Description: The theory combines two main concepts relative to occupational therapy, "occupation and adaptation" (Schultz & Schkade, 2003, p. 220). It is derived from the concept that occupational adaptation is a normal process that enables people to "respond masterfully and adaptively" (Schkade & McClung, 2001, p. 2; Schkade & Schultz, 1992; Schultz & Schkade, 1992). to various life roles and situations. "Life roles" (Schkade & McClung, 2001, p. 2) provide the backdrop for competence, while occupational adaptation offers the "systems" to carry out these roles.

Application: The occupational adaptation process is most challenged when a person faces a "transitional" experience. In order to most adaptively respond to these challenges, treatment is client selected, centered, and collaborative (Schkade & McClung, 2001; Schkade, & Schultz, 1992; Schultz, & Schkade, 1992).

Developmental Frames of Reference

Frame of Reference: "Recapitulation of Ontogenesis" Developmental Frame of Reference

Theorist: Anne Cronin Mosey

Description: According to the Developmental Frame of Reference, maturity and development occurs as the result of the acquisition of adaptive skills. Adaptive skills are "learned patterns of behavior" which the mature individual uses to "adjust to his internal system of needs and impulses and to the external demands of the environment" (Mosey, 1968, p. 9) as well as "to satisfy the majority of his needs, to satisfy the needs of others, to manipulate the environment so as to gain personal goals, and to select those environmental demands he wishes to meet" (Mosey, 1968, p. 9).

Application: In order to focus on how interaction between adaptive skills and environmental elements influence timely achievement of performance of necessary occupations of childhood, the sequential aspect of the Developmental Frame of Reference translates from treatment planning and evaluation strategies to discussions of function and dysfunction. Activity planning is based on acquisition of skills and subskills.

Frame of Reference: Developmental Theory

Theorist: Lela A. Llorens

Description: Throughout the lifespan, there is notable development of physical and psychological skills. If psychosocial or physical trauma occurs, it can derail this process, creating a disparity between current behaviors and the skills or abilities needed to achieve the expected behavior for that developmental level. Treatment focuses on eliminating this disparity by using activities to increase the skills and abilities necessary to achieve typical developmental performance (Llorens, 1970).

Application: Through incorporation of activities, daily life tasks, and the therapeutic relationship to improve skills and prevent maladaptive behaviors, "gaps" in a child's development are addressed. (Llorens, 1976).

Sensory Integration

Frame of Reference: Sensory Integration Frame of Reference

Theorist: A. Jean Ayres

Description: The *sensory integration* theory frame of reference suggests that by and large, learning and function depends on efficient sensory integration. In turn, learning, functional skills, and behavioral issues are negatively influenced by sensory processing difficulties. Providing specific sensory experiences within the context of a meaningful activity, which requires an *adaptive response*, facilitates learning, skill, and behavior (Bundy & Murray, 2002).

Application: Sensory integration will be covered in depth in Chapter 12: Introduction to Sensory Integration.

Frame of Reference: Biomechanical Frame of Reference

Theorist: Bird T. Baldwin

Description: Structural and movement characteristics that deviate from the norm are targeted for remediation. The Biomechanical Frame of Reference presumes that while "treatment modalities may not be inherently meaningful to client" (Birge, 2003, p. 240); the restoration of occupational function is meaningful unto itself.

Application: In order to successfully engage in "functional skills" (Colangelo, 1999, p. 321) postural control and central stability must be enhanced. Developing and carrying out a treatment plan that intimately integrates *assistive devices* and other adaptive equipment into the treatment process accomplishes this.

Rehabilitative Frames of Reference

Frame of Reference: Rehabilitative Frame of Reference

Theorist: Based on early seminal works of Eleanor Slagle, William Rush Dunton, George Barton, Susan Cox Johnson, and Thomas Kidner (Trombly, 1995).

Description: Primary concern is for an individual to live as independently as possible despite any disease process or disability. The Rehabilitative Frame of Reference focuses on the teaching-learning process associated with learning and applying compensatory techniques as well as the skills necessary to effectively use adapted equipment to carry out ADL and IADL tasks (Seidel, 2003, p. 239).

Application: Restoration of function occurs through implementation of age appropriate activities of daily living (ADL) tasks, instrumental activities of daily living (IADL) tasks, adaptive equipment training, leisure or work activities, environmental assessment and modification, and work simplification/ energy conservation techniques.

Summary

Contemporary practice of occupational therapy is based on many theories and frames of reference that are used to develop new ideas and integrate modern research with the underpinnings of the profession. To most effectively help children achieve maximal functional independence and improve their quality of life, understanding and implementing applicable frames of references are an important part of sound pediatric practice.

Case Study

Alex is 14 years old and was diagnosed at birth with athetoid cerebral palsy. Alex lives in a rural area in which the elementary school houses grades K-8, and the high school, grades 9-12. Alex is in 8th grade this year, and will be going on to the community high school next year. How might OT and OTA team working within the MOHO frame of reference address the specific challenges that Alex may face when transitioning from grade school to high school? Keep the three subsystems (volitional, performance, and

habituation) of the MOHO in mind when discussing this case study.

1. What are the potential impacts of the three subsystems on Alex's transition to high school?
2. What specific issues, as oriented through a MOHO treatment approach might the OT/OTA team address as part of the transition process?

Application Activities

1. Discuss how a single frame of reference may be used effectively in clinical practice. How and why might this orientation be explained?
2. Break into small groups and discuss which of the frames of reference presented in this chapter is most comprehensive? Which is most specialized? Explain. Present your findings to the class. It may be fun to record this data on the chalkboard and determine if there is some kind of trend with regard to the responses.
3. Reflect on and prepare a short essay on which frame of reference most resembles your personal philosophy as an OTA student, and why? Which is least similar to your practice philosophy, and why?
4. Working in pairs or small groups, determine which subset of the pediatric patient/client population would most benefit most from each frame of reference described in this chapter. Present your findings to the class.

References

Allen, C. K. (1985). *Occupational therapy for psychiatric diseases: Measurement and management of cognitive disabilities*. Boston: Little Brown & Co.

American Occupational Therapy Association (1987). *Roles of occupational therapists and occupational therapy assistants in schools*. Rockville, MD: Author.

Birge J. A. (2003). Biomechanical frame of reference. In E. Blesedell Crepeau, E. S. Cohn, & B. A. Boyt Schell (Eds.), *Willard and Spackman's occupational therapy* (10th ed.). (pp. 240-243). Philadelphia: Lippincott, Williams, and Wilkins.

Bundy, A., & Murray, E. (2002). Sensory integration: A. Jean Ayres' theory revisited. In A. Bundy, S. Lane, & E. Murray (eds.). *Sensory integration: Theory and practice* (2nd ed.). Philadelphia: F. A. Davis.

Colangelo, C. A. (1999). Biomechanical frame of reference. In P. Kramer & J. Hinojosa (Eds.). *Frames of reference for pediatric occupational therapy* (2nd ed.). (pp. 257-323). Philadelphia: Lippincott, Williams, and Wilkins.

Dunn, W., Brown, C., & McGuigan, A. (1994). The ecology of human performance: A framework for considering the effect of context. *American Journal of Occupational Therapy, 48*, 595-607.

Dunn, W., Haney McClain, L., Brown, C., & Youngstrom, M. J. (2003). The ecology of human performance. In E. Blesedell Crepeau, E. S. Cohn, & B. A. Boyt Schell (Eds.), *Willard and Spackman's occupational therapy* (10th ed.). (pp. 223-227). Philadelphia: Lippincott, Williams, and Wilkins.

Fidler, G. & Fidler, J. (1954). *Introduction to psychiatric occupational therapy.* New York: The MacMillan Company.

Jirikowic, T., et al. (2001). Contemporary trends and practice strategies in pediatric occupational and physical therapy. *Physical and Occupational Therapy in Pediatrics, 20*(4), 45-62.

Kielhofner, G. (1992). *Conceptual foundations of occupational therapy.* Philadelphia: F. A. Davis Co.

Law, M., Cooper, B. A., Strong, S., Stewart, D., Rigby, P., & Letts, L. (1996). The Person-Environment-Occupation Model: A transactive approach to occupational performance. *Canadian Journal of Occupational Therapy, 63*(1), 9-23.

Lawlor, M. C., & Henderson, A. (1989). A descriptive study of the clinical practice patterns of occupational therapists working with infants and young children. *American Journal of Occupational Therapy, 43*(11), 755-764.

Llorens, L. A. (1970). Facilitating growth and development: The promise of occupational therapy. *American Journal of Occupational Therapy, 25,* 1-9.

Llorens, L. A. (1976). *Application of a developmental theory for health and rehabilitation.* Rockville, MD: American Occupational Therapy Association.

Mosey, A. C. (1968). *Occupational therapy: Theory and practice.* Medford, MA: Pothier Brothers, Printers, Inc.

Mosey, A. C. (1986). *Occupational therapy: Configuration of a profession.* New York: Raven Press.

Schkade, J. K., & McClung, M. (2001). *Occupational adaptation in practice: Concepts and case.* Thorofare, NJ: SLACK Incorporated.

Schkade, J. K., & Schultz, S. (1992). Occupational adaptation: Toward a holistic approach to contemporary practice, Part 1. *American Journal of Occupational Therapy, 46,* 829-837.

Schultz, S., & Schkade, J. K. (2003). Occupational adaptation. In E. Blesedell Crepeau, E. S. Cohn, & B. A. Boyt Schell (Eds.), *Willard and Spackman's occupational therapy* (10th ed.). (pp. 220-223). Philadelphia: Lippincott, Williams, and Wilkins.

Schultz, S., & Schkade, J. K. (1992). Occupational adaptation: Toward a holistic approach to contemporary practice, Part 2. *American Journal of Occupational Therapy, 46,* 917-925.

Seidel, A. C. (2003). Rehabilitative frame of reference. In E. B. Crepeau, E. S. Cohn, & B. A. Schell (Eds.), *Willard and Spackman's occupational therapy* (10th ed.). (pp. 238-240). Philadelphia: Lippincott, Williams and Wilkins.

Stewart, D., Letts, L., Law, M., Acheson Cooper, B., String, S., & Rigby, P. J. (2003). The Person-Environment-Occupation model. In E. Blesedell Crepeau, E. S. Cohn, & B. A. Boyt Schell (Eds.), *Willard and Spackman's occupational therapy* (10th ed.). (pp. 227-235). Philadelphia: Lippincott, Williams and Wilkins.

Storch, B., & Goldrich Eskow, K. (1996.) Theory application by school-based occupational therapists. *American Journal of Occupational Therapy, 50*(8), 662-668.

Toglia, J. P. (1992). A dynamic interactional approach to cognitive rehabilitation. In N. Katz (Ed.), *Cognitive rehabilitation: Models for intervention in occupational therapy.* Boston: Andover Medical Publishers.

Toglia, J. P. (1996). *A Multicontextual Approach to Cognitive Rehabilitation.* Supplemental manual to workshop conducted at New York Hospital–Cornell Medical Center, NY.

Trombly, C. A. (1995). Theoretical foundations for practice. In C. A. Trombly (Ed.), *Occupational therapy for physical dysfunction* (4th ed.). Baltimore: Williams and Wilkins.

COLLABORATIVE MODELS OF TREATMENT

Priscilla Hayden-Sloane, MHA, OTR/L, LEND Fellow

Chapter Objectives

- Describe intraprofessional and interprofessional collaboration and identify the characteristics of effective collaboration.

- Identify potential members of a collaborative team and briefly describe the services they might provide to children with disabilities and their families.

- Compare multidisciplinary, interdisciplinary, and transdisciplinary models of professional collaboration and explain the differences between these models.

- Describe the role of an OT practitioner within the family, medical, and educational systems of care.

The Meaning of Collaboration

Collaboration, as defined by Roberts (2000) is the ability "to work together, act jointly and cooperate" (p. 4). AOTA (2002) defines collaboration as "working together with a mutual sharing of thoughts and ideas" (p. 667). When examined within the context of the healthcare system, the meaning of collaboration is more complex. Simpson (et al., 2001) defined collaboration as "a partnership among different professionals for the purpose of providing quality health care to individuals and communities" (p. 5). Based on Perkins and Tryssenaar's 1994 work on providing effective interdisciplinary education for rehabilitative students, Paul and Peterson (2001) suggest,

Collaboration occurs when a group of individuals with diverse backgrounds work together as a unit to solve patient problems, set up mutual goals, work interdependently to define and treat patient problems, accept and capitalize on disciplinary differences, share leadership, and communicate effectively with each other (pp. 2-3).

In the past, the term *interdisciplinary* was most commonly used to describe collaboration between disciplines, but this model did not support the need for cooperation within professional disciplines when multiple providers were involved in a child's care (e.g., physician specialists, per diem/covering occupational, physical, or speech therapists, shift nurses). New terms have emerged to describe professional collaborations.

According to Roberts (2000), *intraprofessional* collaboration occurs between two or more professionals from the same discipline. *Interprofessional* collaboration occurs between two or more professionals from different disciplines. Characteristics of effective collaboration include a common purpose, professional competence, interpersonal skills, and a sense of humor. Trust, respect, and valuing each other's knowledge and skills reflect the interpersonal process.

Identifying Members of a Collaborative Team

According to Smith (2001), a child with disabilities benefits most from holistic intervention. She writes,

The collaborative efforts of a multidisciplinary team of professionals are needed to design and provide an intervention program. In medical, educational and

community-based settings where children are served, individualized plans of intervention are developed and child outcomes become the responsibility of a team of professionals (Smith, 2001, p. 21).

Once developed, the child's individualized plan identifies the specialized professionals who will make up the child's "team". The providers of service become responsible for implementing the plan (Table 4-1).

Members of the team are determined by the needs of the child, the severity of the disability, the child's age, support systems, and environment.

Example 1

A preschooler experiencing difficulty following directions, following classroom routines, and moving safely around the environment without tripping or bumping into others may be referred by her preschool program and/or her parent/caregiver for an Early Childhood Developmental Assessment. Team members asked to participate in this assessment may include a developmental educator, a speech pathologist, a physical therapist (PT), an occupational therapist (OT), and the child's parent/caregiver. If identified as having special needs, the child would be offered an appropriate preschool program placement (at no cost to the family) staffed with a special needs teacher and/or related services.

Example 2

An 18-month-old with a significant language delay is referred by his pediatrician to Early Intervention (EI). EI would assign the child a case manager, who then requests a speech and language evaluation.

The speech pathologist typically assesses the child in the home with the parent/caregiver present to facilitate interaction with the child, provide background and share caregiver concerns, and once instructed, implements the home program. The child may receive home visits from the case manager as well as possible speech therapy or participate in a language-based play group.

No single discipline poses all the skills and knowledge needed to address the medical and educational needs within the complex systems (Headrick, 2001). Because a team of professionals from multiple disciplines defines the context for almost all pediatric occupational therapy practice, it is essential that therapists develop collaborative skills. Effective teaming skills can be as important as the technical and professional skills that define one's profession (Smith, 2001).

Systems of Care in Pediatrics

FAMILY SYSTEM

Winton & Winton (2000) write, "Families have a significant environmental influence on a young child's development. The majority of a young child's time is spent with family members and caregivers" (p. 13). Family-centered practice involves family members/caretakers as essential members of the assessment and/or intervention team. It ensures that the needs, strengths, and priorities of the family drive the assessment and intervention process (Crais & Wilson, 1996).

Family Systems Theory (Hammer, 1998) assumes that:
- A child is part of a system that includes him/her as an individual, and as an interdependent member. Therefore, the child can only be understood in the context of this system or the context of the relationships that form the "family" in which the child resides.
- Patterns of behavior exhibited by one member, such as the child, may influence the other members or vice versa.
- Families go through changes, such as death, divorce, children leaving home, that may positively or negatively influence the relationships within the family.
- Each member of the family has a different perspective of the relationships that exist in his/her particular family system.

OT practitioners must observe and gather information about the daily routines of the child and the family. They must gather and share information with families about development and intervention strategies, and implement therapy in collaboration with parents/caregivers and team members (Winton & Winton, 2000). OT practitioners, as well as other professionals, are involved with a child and the family for a short period of time. If the caregivers are not convinced of the benefits of therapy or are unable to find time to carry out the plan, the child may not improve. When families/caregivers are involved in providing therapeutic activities at home, the model of service is typically considered to be interprofessional or transdisciplinary.

MEDICAL SYSTEM

Rapid, dramatic changes in the United States health care system were ushered in during the 1980s with the establishment of Diagnostic Related Groups (DRGs) and the growth of managed care (Health Maintenance Organizations or HMOs) in an effort to control health care spending. HMOs began to compete for members while health care providers competed for patients. In addition, nonreimbursable costs

Table 4-1

Members of a Collaborative Team

Discipline/Service Providers	Educational Requirements	Responsibilities
Family/Caregivers	None	Maintain health and well-being of child; implement health, education, & behavioral programs; ensure child's safety.
Physician/MD Family Practitioner, Pediatrician	Bachelor's degree, 4 yrs of medical school, residency and/or fellowship in area of specialty, exam and state licensure.	Mandated to identify developmental delays in addition to routine care. Manage diagnostic work-up, explore implications of disability, refer to specialists for evaluation and/or treatment. Prescribe & monitor medication.
Physician Assistant/PA	Advanced degree (2-3 yrs), exam and state licensure.	Implement physician-administered procedures under supervision of physician. Prescribe & monitor medication.
Pediatric Specialist: Neurology, Surgery, Orthopedics, Cardiology, Ophthalmology, Pulmonary, Developmental	Medical school, residency & fellowship in area of specialty, exam & state licensure.	Provide assessment, treatment, & consultation for acute, sub-acute, & long-term medical conditions and/or disabilities.
Nurse Registered Nurse/RN	Bachelor's degree, clinical internships, registration exam, & state licensure	Provide assessment, treatment & consultation for acute, sub-acute, & long-term medical conditions following physician's orders. Implement routine medical procedures in schools. Interdisciplinary/interagency coordination & care management.
Clinical Nurse Specialist/CNS	Advanced nursing degree (1 yr), exam & licensure	Implement physician-administered procedures under direct supervision of physician (ANA, 1990).
Pediatric Nurse Practitioner/PNP	Advanced nursing degree (2-3 yrs), exam & state licensure	Practice independently without direct supervision of physician (see MD responsibilities above).
Licensed Practical Nurse/LPN	2 yr program, exam & state licensure	Basic patient care, train children in health-care procedures. Work under supervision of RN.
Physical Therapist/RPT	As of 2002, Master's degree required, clinical internships, registration exam, & state licensure	Provide assessment, treatment, & consultation for developmental, muscular, orthopedic, neurological, balance/coordination, safety assessments (transfers, ambulation, home/school environment), ADLs/adaptive equipment, exercise/conditioning programs.
Physical Therapy Assistant/PTA	2 yr program, certification exam & state licensure.	Implement treatment programs, train children in exercises & ADLs. Work under supervision of RPT.
Occupational Therapist/OTR	As of 2004, Master's degree required, clinical internships, registration exam, & state licensure	Provide assessment, treatment, & consultation for developmental, sensorimotor, balance/coordination, neurological, orthopedic, fine motor, visual/perceptual, safety assessments (home/school environment), ADLs/adaptive equipment, exercise/conditioning programs.
Occupational Therapy Assistant/OTA	2 yr. program, certification exam, & state licensure	Implement treatment programs, train children to implement *accommodations* in exercises & ADLs. Work under supervision of OTR.

Table 4-1 (continued)

Members of a Collaborative Team

Discipline/Service Providers	Educational Requirements	Responsibilities
Speech & Language Pathologist/ CCC-SLP	Master's degree, 1 yr. clinical fellowship, certification exam, & state licensure	Provide assessment & treatment for receptive & expressive language delays, articulation & motor production disorders, hearing impairments, pragmatic language, *augmentative & alternative communication*, oral-motor/feeding/swallowing disorders (ASHA, 1999).
Audiologist/Aud, CCC-A	Master's degree, 1 yr. clinical fellowship, as of 2011 Doctoral degree required, certification exam, & state licensure	Provide assessment & treatment for hearing disorders, balance disorders, communication problems, augmentative hearing, & alternative communication systems. Education & consultation regarding prevention of hearing loss & psychosocial effects of hearing loss (ASHA, 2001).
Psychologist/LMLP or PhD	Master's or doctoral degree, 1 yr. clinical fellowship, certification exam, & state licensure	Provide multifactorial & *psychoeducational assessments*, identify educational disability & assist in determining level of inclusion, consultation & collaboration regarding behavioral & mental health issues (NASP, 1999).
Social Worker/MSW	Master's degree, 2 yrs. post-Master's supervised experience, licensure exam, state licensure	Provide counseling or therapy to children & families. Help establish financial & community support systems for parents/caregivers, coordinate interagency services (NASW, 2002).
Teacher	Bachelor's degree, teaching internship, certification exam, Master's degree earned within 10 yrs, certification exam.	Provide classroom-based education in core subject areas according to national and state curriculum guidelines.
Special Education Teacher/MEd	Master's degree, certification exam by grade (pre-K-8, 5-12) & specific student category (mild/moderate/ severe special needs, early childhood), & state licensure	Provide child assessment, implementation & IEP/ program planning. Establish & implement curriculum modification & accommodations, collaborate with classroom teachers, related service providers, & parents/caregivers (NCATE, 2001).
Complementary & Alternative/CAM Medical Providers Chiropractor, Acupuncturist, Massage Therapist, Homeopathy, Naturopathy, etc.	Consult "The Alternative Medicine Homepage" at http://www.pitt.edu/ cbw/altm.html	Prevent or treat illness, promote health & well-being. Not considered integral part of conventional allopathic medicine. Complementary–used in addition to conventional care treatments. Alternative–used instead of conventional treatment.
Palliative Care Providers Physician (internal medicine, oncology), RN/LPN, RPT/PTA, OTR/COTA, Psychologist/ Social Worker (Grief counselors), Volunteers	Refer to specific service provider education & responsibilities	Provide symptom control, prolonged quality of life, & preparedness for death, psychosocial support for child and family/caregivers.

Table 4-2	
Pediatric Medical Care System	
Setting	*Purpose of Setting*
Neonatal Intensive Care Unit (NICU)	Addresses acute or extremely severe symptoms or conditions (e.g., physiological, neurological, musculoskeletal) so that an infant can become physiologically stable (body temperature, heart rate, respiratory rate, etc.).
Progressive Care Unit (PICU)	Step-down nursery when ability to satisfactorily maintain physiological functions. Continue treatment for physiological, neurological, musculoskeletal conditions, etc. Begin to address self-regulatory, sensory/motor, developmental issues, etc.
Sub-acute	Home, residential or long-term care facility to maintain or maximize functional ability/independence. Access developmental, educational, outpatient/community programs.

Adapted from Oakley, D.,& Logan-Bauer, K. (2000). Medial Systems. In J. Solomon, *Pediatric Skills for Occupational Therapy Assistants*. St Louis, MO: Mosby.

for providing health care services were also being shifted to the providers. Hospitals, clinics, and home care agencies were forced to economize, reducing the size of their work force while maximizing the reimbursement for services provided.

Example 1

Providers (hospitals/clinics/home care agencies) laid off administrative and supervisory personnel while increasing the caseloads of direct service providers such as nurses, rehab therapists including OT, PT, Speech; hospitals laid off social workers while shifting the responsibility of case management to nursing.

This trend continued into the 1990s when hospital and home health care mergers strove to further reduce administrative costs. Facilities shared management costs or closed. The remaining health care professionals were forced to collaborate; prioritizing and sharing goals, and establishing complementary approaches to enable patients to meet discharge goals after a pre-established length of stay (LOS); the minimal number of days/visits of medical/therapeutic services covered by insurance.

Table 4-2 represents the progression of care in the medical model.

According to Paul and Peterson (2001), the 1998 O'Neil and Pew Health Professionals Commission document indicates, "the future of health care requires all health professionals including physicians, nurses, allied health professionals, and public health officials work closely together" (p. 10).

Because the multidisciplinary model is not cost effective, opportunities exist for OT practitioners to advance in knowledge and skills for effective practice, to enrich their education and practice experience, and to enhance patient care (Holmes & Osterweis, 1999).

EDUCATIONAL SYSTEM

With the reaffirmation of the Individuals with Disabilities Education Act (known as IDEA '97), federal law now ensures a free and appropriate education (FAPE) for eligible children and youth with disabilities, with emphasis on access to the general curriculum. This means, to the maximum extent appropriate, children are being educated in regular classes with nondisabled peers, participating in state and district-wide assessments, and achieving measurable goals on their Individualized Educational Programs (IEPs). This law ensures that students receive special education and related services within the classroom environment through interprofessional consultation, collaboration, and intervention (NICHCY, 1999).

Children (3 to 22 years) who are suspected of having or are identified as having developmental delays and/or other identified disabilities are served under IDEA Part B, and may be referred to a school system via the referral network that includes doctor's offices, outpatient clinics, early intervention services, parents, daycare providers, teachers, private preschools/schools or outside school district (referring a child moving into a new district). The child and the family/legal guardian must be a resident of the town where the assessment is requested.

The child may be screened or evaluated by members of the *early childhood* developmental evaluation team or the elementary, middle, or high school evaluation team at the school where the child is currently enrolled. The assessment process is child-centered, identifying the child's current level of development or educational performance, and the ways in which the disability affects the child's ability to access the general curriculum or age appropriate activities (Suchomel, 2000). If determined eligible for special needs, the child would receive special education and or related services as part of his/her school day, within the classroom environment, unless otherwise indicated in the IEP.

Occupational therapy practitioners may be involved with providing direct services, and/or instructing others in health-related procedures, such as feeding or positioning techniques, or educationally based interventions, such as sensory-motor techniques, visual and/or *fine motor* strategies, behavioral management techniques. Occupational therapy practitioners also serve as a resource for families and school personnel, providing consultation and collaborative problem solving. Please refer to Chapter 11: Positioning in Pediatrics; Chapter 12: Introduction to Sensory Integration; Chapter 13: Oral Motor Skills and Feeding; Chapter 16: Visual Perceptual Dysfunction and Low Vision Rehabilitation; Chapter 19 Early Intervention; Chapter 20: Preschool and School-Based Therapy; and Chapter 22: Pediatric Psychosocial Therapy.

COMMUNITY-BASED SYSTEMS

Early intervention is the largest community-based system serving children and their families/caregivers. In 1986, Congress established Part C (formerly Part H) of IDEA, known as the Early Intervention Programs for Infants and Toddlers with Disabilities. The intent of Part C Early Intervention programs was to facilitate statewide systems and coordinate payment of early intervention services for children under 3 years of age with a disability or at risk of manifesting substantial developmental delays without early intervention services (AMCHP, 2003). However, Part C and Part B preschool were not permanently authorized by Congress, therefore these programs must continue to fight to maintain the stature and the funding they have gained. Today, individual states are struggling with budget cuts and without the financial commitment from Congress, cannot continue to fund early intervention and preschool programming.

Families raising young children with disabilities have to navigate complex medical and educational systems and often fight long battles with each to acquire the services their children need to function within their natural and/or educational environment.

OT practitioners must respect a family's values, beliefs, and customs while providing services to children, especially in the home. As children mature, additional therapy services that might be needed and may be provided in an outpatient clinic or a community-based setting.

OT practitioners working in early childhood may be involved with providing direct services, and/or instructing others in health-related procedures, such as feeding or positioning techniques, or educationally based intervention, including sensorimotor techniques or behavioral management techniques. OT practitioners also serve as a resource for families and school personnel.

Models of Professional Collaboration

Young (1998) defines a team as "a group of professionals working toward a common purpose, in which a variety of disciplines may be represented" (p. S138). In order to achieve shared goals for children and families, a willingness to share knowledge, expertise, and the responsibility for organizing, planning and implementing health care/educational programs is required (Swensen, 2000). Interprofessional teams must be flexible. The membership of the team may change over time. Likewise, the model of collaboration may evolve or change as children age/mature, as the source of funding changes, or as respectful and trusting relationships develop between team members.

MULTIDISCIPLINARY MODEL

In a multidisciplinary model, multiple professionals individually assess the child and complete separate reports and treatment plans. Intervention is typically carried out separately by discipline. Professionals do not necessarily consult or interact with each other on a regular basis when working in a multidisciplinary model.

Instead, communication happens informally, such as via a quick phone call from physical therapy to occupational therapy to say a child is finished with transfers and ready for hand splints. A chart or medical record may serve as a primary form of formal communication. The focus of communication in a multidisciplinary model involves the essential elements of a child's care or the tasks that need to be accomplished to restore health, or meet functional goals that will lead to discharge. Communication often results in actions and leads to other immediate communication (Smith, 2001).

Example

A call to order lab work leads to a lab report. The test results indicate that the doctor can prescribe a new medication. This new treatment will require monitoring via additional lab work.

Within a multidisciplinary model, there is heavy dependency on a leader. Paul and Peterson (2001) refer to a hierarchy of authority, as in the medical system in which a physician heads the team, and a doctor's order is required for most interventions. The multidisciplinary model works best within settings where team membership is stable and team members perceive that they have equal status with one another. Hospitals, rehabilitation units, and specialty clinics typically operate within a multidisciplinary model.

Although parents/caregivers are the experts when it comes to their children, being an authority on health conditions, especially those with children who have been newly diagnosed with a serious illness or disability, is beyond the scope of most parents/caregivers. Therefore, the parent/caregivers' participation in the team process and their role as a member of a multidisciplinary team is usually limited. Because of their expertise and professional prestige, parents and caregivers typically defer to the physician or other health professional (Gilkerson, 1990).

INTERDISCIPLINARY MODEL

In an interdisciplinary model, professionals may choose to individually assess a child or collaborate with other evaluators to assess the child. Although they typically prepare separate reports, an integrated plan is formulated and goals are set with input from parents and professionals. In an interdisciplinary model, each professional discipline retains the responsibility for providing the services he/she recommended (Angelo, 1997). Treatment may occur as separate disciplines or professionals may choose to team up to provide joint treatment.

Within the interdisciplinary model, each professional as well as the parents/caregivers are viewed as respected members of the team, and each is perceived to contribute equally to the welfare of the child (Paul & Peterson, 2001). The leadership role in an interdisciplinary team may vary from child to child, depending on the service providers involved, and the focus of the intervention (Perkins & Tryssenaar, 1994).

Example 1

An elementary school student who is achieving academically at grade level but has difficulty navigating the school environment due to crutches may have a physical therapist as her team liaison.

Example 2

A preschool student with global developmental delays such as cognitive, speech and language, and *gross*/fine motor may have a special needs preschool teacher as his team liaison. The goal of an interdisciplinary team is to provide comprehensive, coordinated care (Oakley, 2000). Professionals interact directly and frequently, updating one another on a child's progress, as well as changes in the home and school environment that may impact a child's performance. Formal and informal meetings, and written progress reports provide opportunities for parents/caregivers and team members to share information. Communication and collaboration are the essential components for success for an interdisciplinary team (Roberts, 2000).

TRANSDISCIPLINARY

Idol, Paolucci-Whitcomb, and Nevin (1986) describe the transdisciplinary model as the model of collaboration. It involves the practice of multiple disciplines and caregivers collectively identifying and defining mutual problems, and cooperatively generating solutions to those problems. In a transdisciplinary model, all team members share the respon-

sibility for outcomes by expanding and exchanging knowledge with other team members (Linder, 1993; Prelock, Miller, & Reed, 1995).

As compared to other models, in the transdisciplinary model professional lines blur more often than multidisciplinary or interdisciplinary models. Assessments, treatment plans, and interventions are often carried out jointly. Role exchange may occur during the intervention stage when different professionals carry out a program recommended by another professional (Clay, Cummings, Mansfield, & Hallock, 1999).

Example

A feeding program developed through collaboration between a speech therapist and an occupational therapist may be implemented by the parents/caregivers at home and by the classroom staff (special education teacher, classroom aide, paraprofessional) at school.

Preparing for Collaboration

Collaborative teaming is essential to all service-delivery models. It combines the design of integrated therapy with the sharing of skills and information across disciplines. It creates a child-centered program, a program in which the child's goals are the center of decision making and program planning (Smith, 2001). Collaborative consultation emphasizes that the roles of consultant and consultee are equally important, regardless of the disciplines involved. Team members engaging in consultation agree on and work jointly toward common goals. However, members have different roles. These differing responsibilities necessitate that professionals develop complementary and interdependent working relationships as a part of the team process (Zins & Erchul, 1995).

This is particularly true when it comes to the relationship between occupational therapists (OTs) and occupational therapy assistants (OTAs). The document *Roles and Responsibilities of the Occupational Therapist and the Occupational Therapy Assistant During the Delivery of Occupational Therapy Services* provides a guide for role delineation and supervision parameters for OTs, COTAs and OTAs (AOTA, 2002). In addition to knowing the laws and practice guidelines, OTs and OTAs need to develop skills that support collaboration.

Hanft & Banks (1999) identified sensitivity to the needs of others, dependability, attentive listening, respect, the ability to work collaboratively, and reflective thinking as personal attributes that the support the development of successful supervisory relationships. AOTA (2002) defines supervision as a "cooperative process in which two or more people participate in a joint effort to establish, maintain/or to elevate a level of competence and performance" (p. 9). Therefore, the ability to discuss expectations for both/all persons participating in supervision was identified as a key factor in developing a collaborative OT/OTA partnership (Hanft & Banks, 1999).

A successful partnership requires that the partners respect the knowledge and skill they each bring to the relationship. The OT and OTA should work together to select the work assignments that match the skills and interests of the OTA. Depending on their level of experience and the ability to demonstrate service competency in delegated tasks, as well as state and facility guidelines, an OTA may assist the OT in almost all aspects of service delivery from referral and evaluation to intervention AOTA, 2002). The OT should be aware of the strengths and limitations of the OTA and delegate tasks accordingly.

Example

In preparation for an interdisciplinary early childhood assessment, the OTA might help by copying the EI report or other relevant assessments. He/she might schedule and attend an onsite program/preschool/daycare observation or home visit on behalf of the team to gather additional information about the child's level of function/performance in their natural environment. He/she might also assist with administering parts of an arena or occupational therapy assessment, or attend the meeting on behalf of OT to report the findings and recommendations. The OTA may also provide some/all of the direct service, reviewing progress with the OT, and assisting with reassessment. He/she may also be asked to help instruct the parents/caregivers in a home program.

Summary

Communication is the essential factor in successful partnerships. The OT should clearly communicate the roles, responsibilities, and the expectations he or she has for the OTA. In addition, the OTA needs to feel comfortable asking questions and letting the supervising therapist know when he or she feels unprepared for or uncomfortable taking on a particular responsibility. Scheduling time for supervision, including problem-solving sessions, joint therapy sessions and co-leading classroom/therapy groups, allows children to be served while simultaneously developing a supportive and collaborative relationship that offers opportunities for professional growth and development (Handley-Moore, 2003).

Intraprofessional collaboration and interprofessional collaboration (Roberts, 2000) are the hallmarks of successful teams and successful team relationships. Effective collaboration includes a common purpose, professional competence, interpersonal skills, and a sense of humor. Trust, respect, and valuing each other's knowledge and skills are a reflection of this interpersonal process, and serve to enhance professional relationships among collaborative team members, especially OTs and OTAs.

Case Study

Identify the professionals who might be involved in evaluating a 2-year-old who has had a cleft palate repair but continues to have difficulty eating and drinking and is significantly underweight. She lives with her grandmother. What might her "team" look like? Describe the roles of the OT/OTA as a member of this team.

Application Activities

1. Describe another cycle of communication that leads to a series of interventions that can be instituted without requiring direct contact between team members.

2. Identify the interdisciplinary team liaison for a teenager who has academic and behavioral problems secondary to a traumatic brain injury (TBI). He has difficulty reading and writing, yet he likes computer games.

3. Identify all the team members who might collaborate to develop a therapeutic gym program for a preschooler with Down syndrome. Identify which service providers might implement the program with the child.

4. If you were in charge of an occupational therapy department, what ways can you think of to cut costs and save money, without overburdening your staff?

5. Based on what you have read about IDEA '97 so far, if a first grader needed to improve his fine motor strength and coordination for developing his handwriting skills, would you provide your occupational therapy intervention via hand strengthening exercises in the therapy room or would you assist the child during art class and during journal writing in the classroom? What suggestions might you offer to the child's classroom teacher?

6. You are working with a preschooler who presents with significant sensory issues (tactile, visual, and auditory defensiveness). The parents/caregivers dress the child in crisply ironed party dresses, with elastic bows in her hair and little bell earrings on her ears. Recognizing that the family culture values cleanliness and a tidy appearance, what suggestions might you make to the caregivers, to lessen the child's discomfort? What explanations might you offer to help the family understand how the child might be feeling?

7. What can the OT and OTA do to develop their collaborative relationship? How do they determine which OT practitioner will be responsible for each task cited in the previous early childhood example? Are there any tasks the OTA should not be asked to do? If so, why?

References

American Speech-Hearing-Language Association (ASHA). (2001b). New audiology standards. Retrieved Dec 15, 2003 from:
   http://professional.asha.org/certification/aud_standards_new.cfn

Angelo, J. (1997). *Assistive technology for rehabilitative therapists.* Philadelphia, PA: F.A. Davis.

Association of Maternal and Child Health Programs (AMCHP). (2003). *Supporting early intervention services for young children with disabilities and developmental delays.* (Policy Recommendations). Washington, DC.

American Occupational Therapy Association. (2002). Glossary: Standards for an accredited educational program for the occupational therapist and the occupational therapy assistant. *American Journal of Occupational Therapy, 56,* 667-668.

American Occupational Therapy Association. (2002). New supervision and role documents. *OT Practice, 7,* 9-10.

Baldwin, D. (1996). Some historical notes on interdisciplinary and Interprofessional education and practice in health care in the USA. *Journal of Interprofessional Care, 10,* 173-187.

Berhinger, B., Bishop, W., Edwards, J., & Franks, R. (1999). A model for partnerships among communities, disciplines, and institutions. In D. Holmes & M. Osterweis (Eds.), *Catalysts in interdisciplinary education: Innovation by academic health centers* (pp. 25-41). Washington, DC: Association of Academic Health Centers.

Clay, M., Cummings, D., Mansfield, C., & Hallock, J. (1999). Retooling to meet the needs of a changing health care system. In D. Holmes & M. Osterweis (Eds.), *Catalysts in interdisciplinary education: Innovation by academic health centers.* Washington, DC: Association of Academic Health Centers.

Christiansen, C., & Baum, C. (1997). *Occupational therapy: Enabling function and well-being* (2nd ed). Thorofare, NJ: SLACK Incorporated.

Crais, E., & Wilson, L. (1996). The role of parents in child assessment: self-evaluation by practicing professionals. *Infant-Toddler Intervention, 6,* 125-147.

Donahue-Kilburg, G. (1992). *Family-centered early intervention for communication disorders: Prevention and treatment.* Gaithersburg, MD: Aspen.

Fisher, A., & Kielhofner, G. (1995). Skill in occupational performance. In G. Kielhofner, (Ed.), *A model of human occupation: Theory and application* (2nd ed), pp 113-128). Philadelphia, PA: Lippincott, Williams and Wilkins.

Foley, G. (1990). Portrait of the arena evaluation: Assessing the transdisciplinary approach. In E. Gibs & D. Teti (Eds.), *Interdisciplinary assessment of infants.* Baltimore, MD: Paul H. Brookes.

Gilkerson, L. (1990). Understanding institutional functioning style: A resource for hospital and early intervention collaboration. *Infants and Young Children, 2,* 22-30.

Hammer, C. (1998). Toward a "thick-description" of families: Using ethnography to overcome the obstacles to providing family-centered early intervention services. *American Journal of Speech-Language Pathology, 7,* 5-22.

Hamric, A., Spross, J., & Hansen, C. (1996). *Advanced nursing practice: An integrative approach.* Philadelphia, PA: W. B. Saunders.

Hanft, B., & Banks, B. (1999). Competent supervision: A collaborative process. *OT Practice, 4,* 31-34.

Handley-Moore, D. (2003, March). Supervising occupational therapy assistants in the schools. *School System Special Interest Section Quarterly, 10,* 1-4.

Headrick, L. (2001, January). Interdisciplinary education in the service of others: Benefits and challenges. Presentation to the National Advisory Committee on Interdisciplinary, Community-based Linkages, Washington, DC.

Holmes, D., & Osterweis, M. (1999). What is past is prologue: Interdisciplinary at the turn of the century. In D. Holmes & M. Osterweis (Eds.), *Catalysts in interdisciplinary education.* Washington, DC: Association of Academic Health Centers.

Hyter, Y., Atchison, J., Sloane, M., & Black-Pond, C. (2001). A response to traumatized children: Developing a best practices model. *Occupational Therapy in Health Care, 15,* 113-141.

Idol, L., Paolucci-Whitcomb, P., & Nevin, A. (1986). *Collaborative Consultation.* Rockville, MD: Aspen.

Koppel, I., Barr, H., Reeves, S., Freeth, D., & Hammick, M. (2001). Establishing a systematic approach to evaluating the effectiveness of Interprofessional education. *Issues in Interdisciplinary Care, 3,* 41-49.

Lawlor, M., & Cada, E. (1994). *The VIC therapeutic partnership project final report.* Chicago, IL: University of Illinois at Chicago.

Linder, T. (1993). *Transdisciplinary play-based intervention: Guidelines for developing a meaningful curriculum for young children.* Baltimore, MD: Paul H. Brookes.

McCormick, L., & Schiefelbusch, R. (1990). *Early language intervention: An introduction* (2nd ed.). Columbus, OH: Merrill.

Mullens, L., Balderson, B., & Chaney, J. (1999). Implementing team approaches in primary and tertiary care settings: Applications from the rehabilitation context. *Families, Systems and Health, 17,* 413-426.

National Association of Social Workers (NASW). (2001). http://www.socialworkers.org

National Council for Accreditation of Teacher Education (NCATE). (2001). http://www.ncate.org

National Information Center for Children and Youth with Disabilities (NICHCY). (1999). *Individualized education programs.* (Briefing Paper LG2, 4th ed.). Washington, DC.

Nochajski, S. (2001). Collaboration between team members in inclusive educational settings. *Occupational Therapy in Home Care, 15,* 101-112.

Oakley, D., & Logan-Bauer, K. (2000). Medical systems. In J. Solomon (Ed.), *Pediatric skills for occupational therapy assistants.* St Louis, MO: Mosby.

O'Neil, E. & Pew Health Professionals Commission. (1988). *Recreating health professional practice for a new century.* San Francisco, CA: Pew Health Professions Commission.

Paul, S., & Peterson, C. (2001). Interprofessional collaboration: Issues for practice and research. *Occupational Therapy in Home Care, 15,* 1-12.

Perkins, J., & Tryssenaar, J. (1994). Making interdisciplinary education effective for rehabilitative students. *Journal of Allied Health, 23,* 133-141.

Prelock, P., Miller, B., & Reed, N. (1995). Collaborative partnerships in a language-based classroom program. *Language, Speech, and Hearing Services in Schools, 26,* 286-292.

Rainforth, B., York, J., & Macdonald, C. (1992). *Collaborative teams for student with severe disabilities.* Baltimore, MD: Paul H. Brookes.

Roberts, K. (2002). Collaborative health care models and the common good. *Oates Journal, 3,* http://bsd.oates.org/journal/mbr/vol-03-2000/articles/k_roberts-01.html

Simpson, G., Rabin, D., Schmitt, M., Taylor, P., Urban, S., & Ball, J. (2001). Interprofessional health care practice: Recommendations of the national Academics of Practice Expert Panel on health care in the 21st century. *Issues of Interdisciplinary Care, 3,* 5-20.

Suchomel, S. (2000). Educational systems. In J. Solomon (Ed.), *Pediatric skills for occupational therapy assistants.* St Louis, MO: Mosby.

Winton, P., & Winton, R. (2000). Family systems. In J. Solomon (Ed.), *Pediatric skills for occupational therapy assistants.* St Louis, MO: Mosby.

World Health Organization (WHO). (1988). *Learning together to work together to work together for health.* (Technical Report No. 769). Geneva, Switzerland.

Young, C. (1998). Building a care and research team. *Journal of Neurological Sciences, 160*, 137-140.

Youngstrom, M. (2002). The OT Practice Framework: The evolution of our professional language. AJOT, 56, 607-639.

Zins, J. & Erchul, W. (1995). Best practice in school consultation. In A. Thomas & J. Grimes (Eds.), *Best practices in school psychology-III.* (pp. 651-660). Washington, DC: The National Association of School Psychologists.

LEGAL MANDATES

Lisa A. Dixon, PhD, JD

Chapter Objectives

- Describe the history of special education law.
- Understand the ethical basis of practice as set forth by the AOTA.
- Be able to identify and appropriately address ethical and legal issues in practice.

Introduction

This chapter presents an overview of the history of child protection laws, an introduction to ethics, and a summary of how to seek legal advice. It is not meant to be exhaustive in its scope, but rather to provide an introductory framework for understanding how the legal system works to protect people. In the context of this chapter, this protection is applicable to both patients and practitioners.

History of Education Laws

Today, thanks to the implementation of IDEA 97, all children regardless of disability are required by law to have access to an education. This has not always been the case. Significant improvements in access to education for children with disabilities have only been recognized since the 1970s. These improvements were brought about in part by parents advocating for their children, sometimes by bringing legal action (Murdick, Gartin, & Crabtree, 2002). The improvements were furthered by federal legislation stemming from

the realization in Congress that the educational needs of children with disabilities were not being met (Murdick, Gartin, & Crabtree, 2002).

In the United States, public schools were originally envisioned as a way to address potential problems associated with a diverse immigrant population (Wright & Wright, 1999). Immigrants from many backgrounds were often poor and did not speak English (Wright & Wright, 1999). It was thought that this diversity could lead to social problems such as "class hatreds" and religious intolerance (Wright & Wright, 1999, p. 7). Publicly funded schools were proposed as a way to foster acceptance and respect among children of all racial, ethnic, and cultural backgrounds (Wright & Wright, 1999). The public schools were also thought of as a vehicle to foster common values and improve socialization among children as well as improve "social conditions" (Wright & Wright, 1999, p. 7).

Special education programs were originally "delinquency prevention programs for 'at risk' children who lived in urban slums" (Wright & Wright, 1999, p. 7). In these programs, children had "manual training classes" in addition to their general education (Wright & Wright, 1999, p. 7). Although the goal of manual training was to teach children to be industrious and to improve their moral disposition, social values were also taught in these classes (Wright & Wright, 1999). As an additional benefit, it was thought that manual training "would attract children to school" (Wright & Wright, 1999, p. 7).

An important step forward in education law was to make public school attendance mandatory. Nevertheless, despite the development of education laws, children with disabling conditions were often excluded from school (Wright & Wright, 1999). This exclusion was based both on a misperception about their ability to learn and the negative effect that they allegedly had upon others (Hehir & Gamm, 1999). If allowed to attend, children with various disabilities were often placed all together in generic special education classes that did not meet their educational needs (Wright & Wright, 1999, p. 8).

This exclusion of children with disabilities from the regular classroom continued well into the 20th century (Hehir & Gamm, 1999). In 1919, Wisconsin representatives excluded a child named Bud Beattie from his fifth grade class. Beattie had cerebral palsy and speech difficulties, but he did not have learning disabilities. Beattie's parents filed suit to allow him to remain in school. The Wisconsin Supreme Court upheld his exclusion based on how he allegedly affected others (Hehir & Gamm, 1999). According to the court,

> [t]he rights of a child of school age to attend the public schools of this state cannot be insisted upon when its presence therein is harmful to the best interests of the school. This, like other individual rights, must be subordinated to the general welfare (Hehir & Gamm, 1999, p. 210 citing *Beattie v. Board of Education*, 1919).

As late as the 1950s and 1960s, children were still being excluded from schools because of their disabilities. For example, "[i]n 1958, the Illinois Supreme Court held that compulsory education laws did not apply to children with mental impairment" (Wright & Wright, 1999, p. 8). Similarly, in Ohio throughout the 1960s, classes did not have to be provided for children who would be "unable to profit substantially from an education" (Hehir & Gamm, 1999, p. 211 citing *Opinion of Attorney General of the State of Ohio, 69-040* 1969). This time period also saw an increase in concern with individual rights. Although this concern was mainly directed toward racial minorities, individuals with disabilities also benefited from the expanding civil rights movement. The landmark Supreme Court case, Brown v. Board of Education provided a basis for later arguments against excluding children with disabilities from public schools (Murdick, Gartin, & Crabtree, 2002). The Court disapproved of "segregation based on unalterable characteristics" (Murdick, Gartin, & Crabtree, 2002, p. 11). According to the Court,

> In these days, it is doubtful that any child may reasonably be expected to succeed in life if he is denied the opportunity of an education. Such an opportunity, where the state has undertaken to provide it, is a right which must be made available to all on equal terms. (Murdick, Gartin, & Crabtree, 2002, p. 10 citing *Brown v. Board of Education*, 1954).

The exclusion or segregation of children with disabilities led to many discrimination suits and ultimately to the creation of PL 94-142, the Education for All Handicapped Children Act of 1975 (EAHCA) (Murdick, Gartin, & Crabtree,

2002). Two lawsuits in particular paved the way for further cases and provided an outline for later legislation. The Pennsylvania Association for Retarded Children (PARC) brought the first case against Pennsylvania. The Court ordered Pennsylvania to stop excluding children with retardation from "educational opportunities" (Murdick, Gartin, & Crabtree, 2002, p. 12). According to the Court,

> [A] free, public program of education and training appropriate to the child's capacity within the context of the general educational policy that, among the alternative programs of education and training required by statute to be available, placement in a regular public school class is preferable to placement in a special public school class [i.e., a class for 'disabled children'] and placement in a special school class is preferable to placement in any other type of program of education and training (Murdick, Gartin, & Crabtree, 2002, p. 12, quoting PARC v. Commonwealth of Pennsylvania 1972).

The Court based the decision on the equal protection and due process clauses of the Constitution's 14th Amendment. In the context of special education, these clauses mean that children with disabilities are entitled to the same, or equal protections under the law. That is, children with disabilities are entitled to a public education as long as children without disabilities are entitled to a public education. Additionally, children with disabilities may not be denied access to public education without due process. In this context, due process has come to mean that notice must be given, usually to a parent, that a decision has been made to exclude a child from school and there must be an opportunity to contest the decision (Murdick, Gartin, & Crabtree, 2002).

A similar outcome occurred in a District of Columbia case involving "students who had been labeled as having behavioral problems, or being mentally retarded, emotionally disturbed, and/or hyperactive" (Murdick, Gartin, & Crabtree, 2002, p. 12). The outcome essentially expanded the PARC decision, involving mentally retarded children to "all children with disabilities" (Murdick, Gartin, & Crabtree, 2002, p. 12). In other words,

> [n]o child eligible for a publicly supported education in the District of Columbia public schools shall be excluded from a regular public school assignment by rule, policy, or practice of the Board or its agents ... The District of Columbia shall provide to each child of school age a free and suitable publicly supported education regardless of the degree of the child's mental, physical, or emotional disability or impairment. Insufficient resources may not be a basis for exclusion (Murdick, Gartin, & Crabtree, 2002, p. 12, quoting *Mills v. Board of Education of the District of Columbia* 1972).

The first major legislation taking into account the rights of children with disabilities was *Section 504* of the Rehabilitation Act of 1973 (Hehir & Gamm, 1999). Both PARC and Mills played a large role in this legislation, particularly in calling for children to be placed, if possible, in regular classrooms (Hehir & Gamm, 1999). This Act provided, therefore, the right of disabled children to participate in federally funded programs (Murdick, Gartin, & Crabtree, 2002). This right had previously been extended only "to persons of different races and ethnicity" (Murdick, Gartin, & Crabtree, 2002, p. 14).

The Rehabilitation Act was followed by the Education for All Handicapped Children Act of 1975 (EAHCA), also known as Public Law (PL) 94-142. Amendments followed in 1986 (Handicapped Children's Protection Act of 1986, P.L. 99-372, allowing attorneys' fees to be awarded in EAHCA lawsuits) and the Education of the Handicapped Act Amendments of 1986 (expanding EAHCA to include children from age 3 to 5) (Murdick, Gartin, & Crabtree, 2002).

The EAHCA embodies six fundamental principles:
1. Zero reject
2. Nondiscriminatory assessment
3. Procedural due process
4. Parental participation
5. Least restrictive environment
6. Individualized education program.

These principles continue in what is now known as the Individuals with Disabilities Education Act (IDEA). IDEA was enacted in 1997 (http://www.ideapractices.org/law/index.php). To benefit from the IDEA, a child must have a disability that negatively effects the child's education (Murdick, Gartin, & Crabtree, 2002). IDEA is a funding statute. That means that a state may decide to not comply with IDEA if it is willing to give up federal funding. Some of the protections of IDEA are, however, covered under other legislation.

As discussed above, the EAHCA (now a part of IDEA) embodies six fundamental principles. However, guiding the implementation of IDEA is the right to a free and public education (FAPE), which is embodied in the zero reject principle and the less restrictive environment requirement principle, discussed below.

The first principle of EAHCA is referred to as *zero reject* and is the core principle of the Act (Murdick, Gartin, & Crabtree, 2002, p. 22). This means that all children, regardless of "severity or type of their disability, are entitled to receive a free appropriate public education" (Murdick, Gartin, & Crabtree, 2002, p. 22). This component, referred to as FAPE, embodies "the belief that all children can learn and can be taught" (Murdick, Gartin, & Crabtree, 2002, p. 23). What constitutes FAPE may be open to conflicting views between parents/caregivers and local education administrations (LEA) and state education administrations (SEA), and

may ultimately need to be resolved through procedural due process.

The second principle is *nondiscriminatory assessment*. Obviously, some thought must go into placing a child with special needs in a public school. The first step in placement is to evaluate the child's needs. The EAHCA calls for an evaluation that is not "racially or culturally discriminatory" (Murdick, Gartin, & Crabtree, 2002, p. 23). This principle recognizes that any test or testing procedure may be biased. If bias is introduced into the assessment process, then the needs of a child may not be appropriately determined. In an effort to minimize bias, the IDEA sets forth guidelines for the evaluation process (Murdick, Gartin, & Crabtree, 2002).

The third principle is *procedural due process*. There are two types of due process—substantive due process and procedural due process. *Substantive* due process protects the basic rights of citizens and requires laws to be fair and reasonable. *Procedural* due process requires proper procedures to be followed when these basic rights are being infringed. Early case law as well as legislation clarified that excluding a child with disabilities from school is a violation of that child's substantive due process rights. The due process issues today involve mostly procedural due process.

Procedural due process requires notice and a fair hearing if any child is being denied access to school. IDEA sets forth guidelines for meeting the notice requirement. Various litigations have further defined the requirement (Murdick, Gartin, & Crabtree, 2002). The notice must be written, provide "all facets of possible" changes in the education program, and be in a format that the child's parents can understand (Murdick, Gartin, & Crabtree, 2002, p. 122).

The fourth principle is *parental participation*. A "parent" according to the statute is an actual parent or someone acting as the parent. Parents have always played an important role in advocating for their children. This role is required by IDEA. Under IDEA, parents must be informed about educational opportunities and are an integral part of decisions regarding a child's education.

The fifth principle is *least restrictive environment* (LRE). IDEA contains the same LRE provisions as EAHCA. However, the term "handicapped children" in EAHCA was replaced by "children with disabilities" in IDEA (Murdick, Gartin, & Crabtree, 2002, p. 98).

The LRE principle means that children with disabilities are ideally placed in a regular classroom with typically developing children. It does not mean, however, that children must always be placed in regular classrooms. IDEA recognized the need for a "continuum of alternative placements" (CPA) for children based on their disabilities (Murdick, Gartin, & Crabtree, 2002, p. 98). One end of continuum consists of regular classrooms with the other end of the continuum consisting of some type of institution or hospital. Children with the least restrictive disabilities should be placed in regular classrooms, with the use of "supplemental aids and services," as needed (Murdick, Gartin, & Crabtree, 2002, p. 99). As the intensity of disability increases, it is acceptable to move a child along the continuum to an appropriate alternate placement that meets the child's needs.

The sixth principle is *Individual Education Program* (IEP). Each child must have an IEP. The IEP sets forth an approach for educating the child and for following up throughout the education process. An IEP team consisting of the child's parents, "school personnel, and other service providers" develops the plan (Murdick, Gartin, & Crabtree, 2002, p. 77). The procedure for preparing the IEP is set by the IDEA and related regulations. The IEP addresses the special needs of children with disabilities. Merely placing such a child with disabilities in a regular classroom may not be sufficient to educate that child. The IEP ensures that the childrens' educational experiences will be appropriate to their needs.

The IDEA was amended in 1997 to emphasize "standards-based reform and success in the general curriculum" (Weckstein, 1999, p. 338). The most recent IDEA regulations were released in 2004. Today, thanks to the implementation of IDEA 97, all children regardless of disability are required by law to have access to an education. The IDEA continues to ensure "all children with disabilities access to a free and appropriate public education" in the least restrictive environment. Specific applications of the IDEA with regard to occupational therapy are discussed in Chapter 6: Documentation; Chapter 19: Early Intervention; Chapter 20: Preschool and School-Based Therapy; Chapter 22: Pediatric Psychosocial Therapy; and Chapter 23: An Overview of Assistive Technology.

Ethics

Ethics involves concepts such as "right versus wrong, justice, equality, free will, and responsibility" (Bloom, 1994, p. 52). Ethical standards of occupational therapy practice are governed by the AOTA's Standards and Ethics Committee (SEC), the Accreditation Council for Occupational Therapy Education (ACOTE), state regulatory boards, and the National Board for Certification in Occupational Therapy (NBCOT). These organizations set ethical standards and enforce acceptable practice of the standards. Breach of the standards may involve disciplinary actions. As health care professionals, occupational therapy assistants (OTAs) must also follow general biomedical ethical standards. Developing personal moral and ethical standards within the practice and scope of occupational therapy is important to analyze and justify one's actions and to meet the profession's highest standards of professional conduct.

OCCUPATIONAL THERAPY AND ETHICAL PRACTICE STANDARDS

The occupational therapy profession is guided by several important documents. Occupational therapy assistants must fully understand the *Occupational Therapy Code of Ethics* (AOTA, 2000), *Guidelines to the Occupational Therapy Code of Ethics* (Hansen, 1998), *Core Values and Attitudes of Occupational Therapy Practice* (Kanney, 1993), and the *Enforcement Procedures to the Occupational Therapy Code of Ethics* (2000b). While these documents set forth the ideal and ethical practices that every OTA should aspire to, they do not necessarily set forth legally required standards. In other words, every OTA should maintain AOTA's high standards, but it is not mandatory under the strict sense of the law. According to the AOTA, these documents "serve as moral and philosophical statements that encourage occupational therapy practitioners to attain a high level of professional behavior … [and] bind the profession to the singular purpose of assuring the public of high quality occupational therapy services" (Hansen, 1998, p. 881). As part of a best practice model, the OTA is encouraged to act as an ambassador or representative of the profession. Maintaining a high level of professional conduct, and above all striving to provide optimal services, form the basis of ethically sound practice.

In terms of ethical standards, the SEC does not handle certain disputes such as those of a general business or legal nature. Instead, the SEC is responsible for questions or issues of an ethical nature. Laws, as defined by the AOTA are "rules used by an authority to impose control over a system or humans" (AOTA, 2003). In contrast, ethics relate to morals-based decisions. It is therefore important to determine whether the situation you might be encountering involves ethical issues or legal issues. To aid this determination, the AOTA suggests considering the following questions:

1. *Have you already contacted your state regulatory board? Often the answer lies with them.*

2. *What type(s) of work environment are you in? Have you checked the policy or procedures within your work environment? Have you spoken confidentially with someone in authority?*

3. *Who have you already spoken to regarding this issue (supervisor, human resources department representative, lawyer, etc.).*

4. *What outcome are you expecting from your actions? (an answer, a new resource, the ability to file a complaint, just to 'vent', etc.).*

5. *Is your call a legal matter? AOTA does not have the resources to handle legal calls. Further, each state has different laws and regulations covering*

issues such as occupational therapy practice, employer and employee relations, and the obligation of health professionals to report possible harmful behaviors. You may wish to speak to an attorney who is knowledgeable in the subject matter of concern. Options for you to consider when seeking an attorney are calling your local bar association, a lawyer referral service, a local law school, or visiting www.findlaw.com (AOTA, 2003).

Within the AOTA, the SEC oversees ethics matters. Specifically, the SEC "serves to promote and maintain quality standards of professional conduct" (AOTA, 1996).

The SEC strives "to identify ethical trends, inform and educate members about current ethical issues, to uphold the practice and education standards, and to review all allegations of unethical conduct" (AOTA, 1996). The SEC has jurisdiction only over members of AOTA. The SEC relies on several documents to set forth and enforce practice standards.

Occupational Therapy Code of Ethics

The *Occupational Therapy Code of Ethics* (AOTA, 2000) is "a public statement of the values and principles that guide the behavior of members of the profession" (p. 614). The *Code of Ethics* applies to all levels of occupational therapy practice and any other conduct that may affect occupational therapy practice. The *Code* serves to protect the public, the AOTA, and occupational therapy practitioners by promoting and maintaining "high standards of behavior in occupational therapy" (AOTA, 2000, p. 614).

The *Code of Ethics* embodies seven principles that should be part of every occupational therapy practitioner's lifelong goals (http://www.aota.org/general/coe.asp). These seven principles are beneficence; nonmaleficence; autonomy, privacy, and confidentiality; duties; justice; veracity; and fidelity.

Principle 1: Beneficence

Beneficence is the "concern for the well-being of the recipients" of occupational therapy services (AOTA, 2000, p. 614). Occupational therapy (OT) practitioners should "provide services in a fair and equitable manner" and take into account the "cultural components of economics, geography, race, ethnicity, religious and political factors, marital status, sexual orientation, and disability" (AOTA, 2000, p. 614) of all recipient of services, which for this discussion refers to the child, and his/her family/caregivers (as indicated). When applicable, the fees for services charged to the child's family/caregivers should be "fair and reasonable and commensurate with services performed" (AOTA, 2000, p. 614). Fees should be set in line with the family/caregiver's ability to afford services, as well as applicable regulations These regulations refer to any fee structures as dictated by individual facility, state, or federally funded organization. Every effort should be made to help children and their fam-

ily/caregivers obtain any needed services. For example, if a family/caregiver is unable to afford services, they should be directed to appropriate agencies that can help offset the financial limitation of the family/caregiver. In situations such as this, the OTA must seek the advice of the supervising OT or other applicable supervisor.

Principle 2: Nonmaleficence

Nonmaleficence means basically that OT practitioners should do no harm. Specifically, OT practitioners should take "reasonable precautions to avoid imposing or inflicting harm upon the recipient of services or his or her property" (AOTA, 2000, p. 614). Practitioners must never exploit the recipient in any way, including "sexually, physically, emotionally, financially, or socially" (AOTA, 2000, p. 614). Occupational therapy practitioners should also "avoid relationships or activities that interfere with professional judgment and objectivity" (AOTA, 2000, p. 614).

Principle 3: Autonomy, Privacy, Confidentiality

Occupational therapy practitioners must always respect the child/family/caregiver and their rights. Children (when appropriate) and their family/caregivers must be consulted in setting goals and priorities during the entire course of treatment (please refer to Chapter 6: Documentation). Lines of communication should be kept open at all times, and children and their family/caregivers should be informed of the "nature, risks, and potential outcomes" (AOTA, 2000, p. 614) of any intervention. It is also important to understand that children and their families have a right to decline treated or participation in "research or educational activities" (AOTA, 2000, p. 615). The OT practitioner must *always* respect any such choice. Additionally, communications between an OT practitioner and a child may be privileged and confidential. These communications should be protected from disclosure "unless otherwise mandated by local, state, or federal regulations" (AOTA, 2000, p. 615). For example, based on the child's age, if the welfare of the child is at issue, the confidential nature of the communication may not be recognized.

Principle 4: Duties

Occupational therapy practitioners should strive to become highly competent professionals. As part of achieving competency as an OTA, appropriate national and state credentials should be maintained. Professional competency may come in the form of taking classes, working closely with the supervising OT, and keeping up to date with the currently accepted standards of practice. If a situation arises in which the OTA does not feel competent to work with a particular child, it is his/her duty to discuss this with the supervising OT in order to seek alternate care for the child.

Principle 5: Justice

Occupational therapy practitioners "shall comply with laws and Association policies guiding the profession of occupational therapy" (AOTA, 2000, p. 615) Occupational therapy practitioners should keep in mind that laws encompass federal, state, and local laws, as well as facility rules (i.e., workplace rules). In addition to being informed of all levels of law as applied to the practice of occupational therapy, OT practitioners have a duty to "take reasonable steps to ensure employers are aware of occupational therapy's ethical obligations" (AOTA, 2000, p. 615). Principle 5 also calls for practitioners to "record and report" their professional activities (AOTA, 2000, p. 615) (please refer to Chapter 6: Documentation).

Principle 6: Veracity

Principle 6 relates to truthfulness and accuracy. Occupational therapy practitioners must be truthful and accurate about all aspects of their ability to perform occupational therapy services. Furthermore, practitioners should not get involved in communications that are "false, fraudulent, deceptive, or unfair" (AOTA, 2000, p. 615). Any conflicts of interest should be disclosed to the employer before establishing any "professional, contractual, or other working relationship" (AOTA, 2000, p. 615). Finally, OT practitioners should accept responsibility for acts "which reduce the public's trust in occupational therapy services and those that perform those services" (AOTA, 2000, p. 614). In other words, being truthful, honest, and accurate are a vitally important part of upholding the high standards associated with the practice of occupational therapy.

Principle 7: Fidelity

Principle 7 calls for OT practitioners to "treat colleagues and other professionals with fairness, discretion, and integrity" (AOTA, 2000, p. 615). Occupational therapy practitioners should protect "confidential information about colleagues and staff" otherwise required by law (AOTA, 2000, p. 615). Information involving colleagues should never be misrepresented. Occupational therapy practitioners should endeavor to avoid any "breaches of the Code of Ethics" (AOTA, 2000, p. 615) and should "report any breaches to the appropriate authority" (AOTA, 2000, p. 615), which may include the supervising OT or other appropriate manager.

Guidelines to the Occupational Therapy Code of Ethics

The *Guidelines to the Occupational Therapy Code of Ethics* (Hansen, 1998) address some of the more common issues regarding ethics brought before the AOTA. The issues include "honesty, communication, ensuring the common good, competence, confidentiality, conflict of interest, the impaired practitioner, sexual relationships, and payment for services" (Hansen, 1998, p. 881-884). The *Guidelines to the Occupational Therapy Code of Ethics* (Hansen, 1998) are supported by the *Enforcement Procedures for Occupational Therapy Code of Ethics* (AOTA, 2004).

The *Enforcement Procedures for Occupational Therapy Code of Ethics* (AOTA, 2004) guide the SEC's disciplinary actions. The procedures are to protect both the AOTA as a professional organization and to protect members who have had complaints filed against them. Some complaints brought before the SEC may overlap with complaints brought before the NBCOT. These complaints include "fraudulent documentation, sexual misconduct, nonadherence to contracts and professional incompetence in providing direct service" (AOTA, 1996). In contrast, some complaints would be the exclusive domain of the SEC. These complaints include plagiarism, supervision of students or staff, misrepresentation of research findings, or incompetence in teaching. The SEC normally informs the NBCOT of disciplinary actions.

Upon filing of a complaint against an AOTA member, the SEC reviews the complaint and decides what action to take. The SEC decides whether to dismiss or investigate the complaint. If the SEC investigates the complaint, the final outcomes include a later dismissal, taking disciplinary action against the member, and writing an "educative letter" (AOTA, 2004).

At any point, the SEC may dismiss a complaint. Grounds for dismissal include the lack of an ethics violation or the lack of evidence of a violation. Furthermore, if a violation has been adequately corrected, the SEC may dismiss the complaint. The SEC may also dismiss a complaint for failure to comply with procedural requirements. For example, a violation must have occurred within 7 years of the date of the complaint and the AOTA must have the proper jurisdiction (i.e., must be the appropriate body to hear the complaint) (AOTA, 2004).

The SEC may also write what is called an "educative letter." Such a letter would be appropriate in a situation that may not rise to the level of an ethics violation, but, nevertheless, represent a situation that the SEC could address by educating the involved parties.

Disciplinary action comes in the form of reprimand, censure, suspension, revocation, or dismissal. To reprimand a practitioner, the SEC sends a private letter to the practitioner formally disapproving of the conduct in question. Censure also involves a "formal expression of disapproval" (AOTA, 2004) except that expression is public. Suspension involves removing temporarily the practitioner's membership in the AOTA. Dismissal involves the permanent expulsion of the practitioner from the AOTA (AOTA, 2004).

To aid compliance, the SEC also disseminates information about ethical standards of practice to AOTA members and to the public. The SEC makes documents such as the *Code*, the *Guidelines* and the *Enforcement Procedures* available on the AOTA website. The SEC also offers courses and lectures to members of AOTA in order to educate them about ethical matters.

Legal Advice

It is important to understand that the AOTA handles ethical issues, but does not handle legal issues. Examples of legal issues that may arise throughout the course of an OT practitioner's career include malpractice, employment disagreements, and harassment issues.

If any of these legal issues arise, it may be appropriate to seek legal counsel. It would be necessary first to determine the type of counsel needed. Many attorneys specialize in areas such as employment law, "medical malpractice, insurance law, criminal law, health care law, *Americans with Disabilities* (ADA) law, Individuals with Disabilities Education Act (IDEA) law, or local health care regulations" (Wagenfeld & Hsi, 2003, p. 52). Although attorneys may work in more than one of these fields, it is best to pick an attorney that has experience with your area of concern.

In certain situations, your employer may already have counsel. Be aware that your interests may not be the same as your employer's interests. If you are "concerned that your job, or reputation as a practitioner may be at risk because your actions conflict with the positions of your employer" you may need to seek advice from your own attorney (Wagenfeld & Hsi, 2003, p. 52).

Seeking the advice of an attorney should not be taken lightly. However, if you decide to do so, you may seek an appropriate attorney through local bar associations, referral services, local law schools, and www.findlaw.com.

An initial consultation with an attorney should be free of charge or involve only a small fee (Wagenfeld & Hsi, 2003). During the consultation, you should tell the attorney about "the facts surrounding your situation" (Wagenfeld & Hsi, 2003, p. 53). In turn, the attorney should then give you preliminary advice regarding your situation and explain your options for going forward. These consultations are both confidential and subject to attorney-client privilege. Attorney-client privilege means that a court may not force the attorney to disclose confidential communications between you and the attorney if the communication involves your "professional relationship" (Wagenfeld & Hsi, 2003). Confidentiality affords a broader protection than does attorney-client privilege. The attorney may not disclose or use "any information relating to" your representation unless you consent to such disclosure (Wagenfeld & Hsi, 2003, p. 53). Both protections apply even if you do not ultimately hire the attorney you have sought initial consultation with.

When seeking the advice of an attorney, it is important to be aware of conflict of interest issues. Conflicts may arise when your interests are not the same as one of the attorney's other clients. In fact, all "attorneys are under an ethical obligation to avoid representing clients where a conflict of interest may be present" (Wagenfeld & Hsi, 2003, p. 53). Nevertheless, if a conflict is possible, it may be wise to seek the advice of another attorney before telling this attorney about your specific situation.

Summary

This chapter provided an overview of child protection and advocacy laws. A discussion of ethical practice as directed by the AOTA was also shared. When and if the OTA should consider taking legal action and steps to determining the necessity of such action was also explored.

Case Study

Melinda has been a practicing COTA for 11 years, having spent the bulk of her career working for her local school district. In the past few months, Melinda has noticed that one of the preschool aged children she works with has become withdrawn. Not only that, when they were "warming up" by playing in the water table filled with water and toys, Melinda noticed a series of small, suspicious circular marks on the child's arms. Melinda felt uncomfortable questioning the child directly about these marks.

1. What advice would you offer to Melinda?

2. Do therapist–patient confidentiality rules apply in a situation like this?

3. What principle(s) of the *Code of Ethics* best applies to this situation?

Application Activities

1. Divide the class in half and role-play the seven principles of the *Code of Ethics*.

2. Prepare posters comparing and contrasting the governing principles of the AOTA and other international occupational therapy organizations.

References

American Occupational Therapy Association. June 1996. Scope of SEC disciplinary action program. Retrieved February 19, 2003 from:
http://www.aota.org/members/area2/links/link06.asp?PLACE=/members/area2/links/link06.asp .

American Occupational Therapy Association (2003). Frequently asked questions about ethics. Retrieved February 18, 2003.

American Occupational Therapy Association (2000). Occupational therapy code of ethics 2000. *American Journal of Occupational Therapy, 54,* 614-616.

American Occupational Therapy Association (2004). Enforcement procedures for occupational therapy code of ethics. *American Journal of Occupational Therapy, 58*(6), 655-662.

Bloom, G. M. (1994). Ethical issues in occupational therapy. In K. Jacobs, & M. K. Logigian (Eds.). *Functions of a manager in occupational therapy* (rev ed.) (pp. 52-66). Thorofare, NJ: SLACK Incorporated.

Federal Resource Center for Special Education. IDEA. Retrieved January 15, 2003 from: http://www.dssc.org/frc/idea.htm

Garner, B. A. (Ed.). (2000). *Black's law dictionary* (7th ed.). St. Paul, MN: West Group Publishing Co.

Hansen, R. A. (1998). Guidelines to the occupational therapy code of ethics. *American Journal of Occupational Therapy, 52*(10), 881-884.

Hehir, T., & Gamm, S., (1999). Special education: From legalism to collaboration. In J. P. Heubert (Ed.), *Law and school reform: Six strategies for promoting educational equity,* pp 205-243. New Haven, CT: Yale University Press.

IDEA Practices. IDEA '97. Retrieved January 27, 2003 from: http://www.ideapractices.org/law/index.php

Kanney, E. (1993). Core values and attitudes of occupational therapy practice. *American Journal of Occupational Therapy, 47*(12), 1085-1086.

Murdick, N., Gartin, B., & Crabtree, T. (2002). *Special education law.* Upper Saddle River, NJ: Merrill Prentice Hall.

Statsky, N. (1992). *Introduction to paralegalism: Perspective, problems, and skills* (4th ed.). St. Paul, MN: West Group Publishing Co.

Wagenfeld, A. E., & Hsi, J. D. (2003). Credentialing, ethics, and legalities of practice. In A. Solomon, & K. Jacobs (Eds.), *Management skills for the OTA,* pp. 39-58. Thorofare, NJ: SLACK Incorporated.

Weckstein, P. (1999). School reform and enforceable rights to quality education. In J. P. Heubert (Ed.), *Law and school reform: Six strategies for promoting educational equity,* pp 306-389. New Haven, CT: Yale University Press.

Wright, P. W. D., & Wright, P. D. (1999). *Wrightslaw: Special education law.* Hartfield, VA: Harbor House Law Press.

Chapter 6

DOCUMENTATION

Sue Berger, MS, OTR/L
Rachel B. Diamant, MS, OTR/L, BCP

Chapter Objectives

- Understand the purpose and types of documentation used in a variety of pediatric environments.
- Demonstrate ability to write a SOAP and/or DAP note for a specific pediatric setting.
- Be aware of the importance of functional, measurable, and objective goals for planning intervention.
- Recognize the laws governing OT and OTA roles with regard to documentation within different pediatric settings.
- Understand the different types of documentation needed for specific pediatric environments.

Introduction

A document is a printed record of something, such as an action, event, or behavior that occurred (Agnes, 2001). Occupational therapy practitioners often write documents, putting on paper information about assessments, interventions, and conversations that have occurred between client and practitioner. *Documentation* is a term used for this method of communicating information about a client (Robertson, 1998). Documentation requires time, thought, and skill. Once one becomes skilled at documentation, the time for completion will be greatly decreased. There are many advantages to written documentation. Writing down what has occurred gives the practitioner time to reflect on the assessments done and the interventions used. Documentation facilitates the clinical reasoning behind intervention choices. It encourages one to look at a child's status, to assess if progress has occurred, if outcomes have been achieved, or if a new strategy should be attempted. Though the purpose of documentation is primarily for communication with others, it also provides an opportunity for reflective practice (AOTA, 1995).

Documentation includes evaluations, both standardized and nonstandardized, goals and treatment plans, treatment notes, progress notes, and discharge notes (AOTA, 1995). Notes for physicians, justification of equipment, home programs, and home modification recommendations are other examples of documentation. This chapter will focus on treatment and progress notes, writing goals, and some basic information for writing home programs, whereas Chapter 8: An Overview of Developmental Assessments will address assessments. Formats for documenting other types of information vary, depending on the facility and the clients served.

Purpose of Documentation

It is important for the occupational therapy (OT) practitioner to be skilled at written communication. Documentation is one way to communicate with the many team members working with an individual. Though oral communication is effective during team meetings and informally when working with a child and family, finding time to discuss a child's case with practitioners from other disciplines may be difficult to schedule, and rarely the best use of time. Written documentation is one way to assure that all people involved with a child are receiving the same information. With written communication, team members can also review the information at their convenience, taking as much or as little time as necessary to review any or all parts of the occupational therapy program.

Insurance companies read occupational therapy documentation to review a child's status and ensure that guidelines for reimbursement are met. Third party payers are looking for functional improvements to assure that occupational therapy intervention is making a difference in the child's daily activities. If progress has not been made, but occupational therapy continues, justification for decline or no change in status must be clear in the documentation.

Schools, hospitals, long-term care facilities, and community programs all operate under different umbrella accrediting agencies. These agencies provide strict guidelines to ensure quality and consistent care. When a facility is reviewed for accreditation, the accrediting agency often uses written records as one way to monitor the quality of services provided.

Documentation must be accessible to families. Hospitals have patient and family "Bill of Rights" that assure this. School systems are required by law (IDEA '97) to make records available to the families upon request. Many families request records for personal files and to review information at their own pace.

To support the outcomes of occupational therapy, researchers may also use documentation. The quality of the documentation directly affects the quality of the research. For that reason, accurate, objective, concise, and easily accessible documentation is important.

There are times when documentation is called for in a court of law. It is extremely important to make sure all notes are timely, accurate, and complete. Often, only written notes are used to explain a situation. A practitioner is not always asked to provide additional input. Therefore, it is critical to make sure that what occurred during therapy is written down accurately in an easy to understand format.

Types of Medical Records

Medical records are source-oriented, problem-oriented, or integrated (Huffman, 1994). The *source-oriented chart* is organized by discipline in chronological order, with the most current information first. In this format, all occupational therapy notes are in one section and other disciplines each have their own section. This is advantageous if someone is looking to find out how a child is progressing in occupational therapy or what the goals are for a specific discipline. However, to get an overall picture of the child, one would need to spend an extensive amount of time looking through all sections of a source-oriented chart.

Lawrence L. Weed introduced the *problem-oriented chart* in the 1960s (Huffman, 1994). This type of chart is organized by the problems being addressed by the therapy team. Practitioners from all disciplines document in the same sec-

tion under the problem they are addressing. For example, if a child is learning to use a wheelchair, physical therapy (PT) practitioners may be working on sitting balance and positioning in the wheelchair while OT practitioners may be addressing safety issues such as remembering to lock brakes and attending to other people nearby while maneuvering the wheelchair. Both OT and PT practitioners document about the same problem, and in this charting system, the information is found in the same section. A problem list is kept in a separate section of the chart and used by all involved practitioners to add to or sign off on, as a problem is resolved. This type of documentation is easy for others to review and see if progress has been made or outcomes have been achieved. It facilitates team members working together toward a common goal. Unfortunately, using the problem-oriented medical record can take more time than other documentation methods for team members to learn and correctly implement .

An *integrated medical record* is one that is kept in chronological order, usually providing the most current information first. Though this format enables one to quickly find out the status of a child at any one time, it is difficult to follow changes on a specific issue. For example, the occupational therapy assessment may reveal decreased ability with toileting. The OT practitioner may address this issue over the course of 2 weeks, with the child making small but consistent gains. When looking through an integrated medical record, one might see that the child now requires moderate assistance with toileting. It would take time to review the chart to realize that this was significant progress.

Types of Documentation Procedures

The type of written documentation process is often determined by the facility. Some facilities have moved toward computerized documentation, as there are now many software programs available to facilitate the process. Most programs include specific forms containing a check-off format with space for comments and narrative. Computerization is one strategy to help practitioners meet the demands of providing timely, quality documentation. Though the move toward implementation of computerized documentation is to improve efficiency and consistency, due to cost, resistance to change, and software that does not meet the specific needs of the occupational therapist, facilities have been slow to transition to computerized documentation (Austin, 1998). This trend is slowly changing as computers are becoming as commonplace in the workplace as paper and pen.

Many OT practitioners use handwritten notes, which may be written in a variety of formats. When OT practitioners write progress notes, the straight narrative is sometimes

---

Table 6-1

SOAP Note

S. Child states, "My back still hurts at the end of the day."

O. Child seen for OT to address correct backpack use and to decrease complaints of back pain. Weighed child and the filled backpack. Filled backpack weighed 20% of body weight. Child was instructed in the following strategies to decrease weight of backpack: 1. Requesting duplicate books to leave one copy at home; 2. Sharing books with next-door neighbor; 3. Going through assignment book at end of day to make sure to only bring home needed books. Child stated that first option seems most realistic, and he would ask teachers for extra copies of books.

A. Child seems willing to decrease weight of backpack so that his pain will decrease. As backpack is 5% heavier than recommended, potential to decrease pain by decreasing weight of backpack is good.

P. Continue OT two more times to address strategies for backpack packing and monitor follow-through.

LTG: By discharge, child will have no complaints of back pain after packing backpack correctly and decreasing weight of backpack.

Table 6-2

DAP Note

D. Child seen for OT to address correct backpack use and to decrease complaints of back pain as child continues to state that "my back hurts me at the end of a school day". Weighed child and the filled backpack. Filled backpack weighed 20% of body weight. Child stated, "this is what I typically carry in my backpack each day". Child was instructed in the following strategies to decrease weight of backpack: 1. Requesting duplicate books to leave one copy at home; 2. Sharing books with next-door neighbor; 3. Going through assignment book at end of day to make sure to only bring home needed books. Child stated that first option seems most realistic, and he would ask teachers for extra copies of books.

A. Child seems willing to decrease weight of backpack so that his pain will decrease. As backpack is 5% heavier than recommended, potential to decrease pain by decreasing weight of backpack is good.

P. Continue OT two more times to address strategies for backpack packing and monitor follow-through.

LTG: By discharge, child will have no complaints of back pain after packing backpack correctly and decreasing weight of backpack.

---

used, though it is hard for others to quickly scan and pull out key information from this format. The *SOAP note* was introduced by Weed (Huffman, 1994) to use with a problem oriented charting system, as part of a more patient-centered approach to documentation. The SOAP note is a structured form of a narrative note that is commonly used today in many settings, with all types of medical records. The acronym SOAP stands for subjective, objective, assessment, and plan. The *S* contains information received from the client, including comments, perceptions, and ideas relevant to the occupational therapy intervention/outcomes. The *O* section includes observable and measurable information. Formal assessments and levels of function are included here. The *A* is the section where the OT practitioner's clinical reasoning is documented. The OT practitioner's interpretation and assessment of the situation, documentation of progress, lack of progress or potential for progress is written here. The *P* includes the plan for continued therapy, how many more sessions are indicated, the goals, and the plan to achieve these goals. Any plans to contact other professionals or fam-

ily members, assess or order equipment, or gather other resources are included in the plan section (Table 6-1).

Some practitioners have adapted the SOAP note to a *DAP note*. In this format, the S and O are combined into one data section (D). In the data section, both client/family perceptions and comments are included along with objective information gained from practitioner observation and assessment (Table 6-2).

The SOAP and DAP notes are types of narrative notes that are organized in a user-friendly manner. Anyone who reviews a note can quickly scan a specific section. For example, a PT practitioner working with the same child as the OT practitioner might review the data section to see if the child requires the same amount of assist with each discipline. A teacher might quickly look at the plan section to see how often a student is being seen by OT practitioners.

As an easy and consistent way to document change and a quick way to view the status of a child, many facilities prefer using charts and grids for documentation. A grid may be used each time the child is seen, and then periodically (such as weekly or monthly), a narrative note is written to summarize the child's status. At times when documentation is only required on an infrequent basis, an OT practitioner may keep a checklist for him/herself to remember what occurred at each session. In summary, the practice environment, the reimbursement agency and accrediting agency requirements, and the practitioner him/herself determine the format of documentation used.

No matter what the format of the note, all documentation should be either typed or written with nonerasable black ink. So that information cannot be added later, no spaces should be left between sections, and all errors should be crossed out with a single line, initialed, and dated. Never use white erase liquid or erase any information. All notes should be signed with official signature (name and professional initials), and dated and all notes by OT/OTA students must be cosigned by the supervising OT practitioner (Borcherding, 2000). Based on state licensure requirements, an OT cosignature may be required for all OTA notes.

WRITING GOALS

As part of the evaluation process, the OT is responsible for establishing goals in conjunction with the child and caregiver. The OTA might contribute to this process through information gained from implementing "specifically delegated assessments for which service competency has been established" (AOTA, 2002, p. 10). Although the OT writes the occupational therapy goals, it is important for the OTA to fully understand them, as the OTA will be working with the child to meet these goals. The OTA needs to know what the child and caregiver goals are in order to inform the supervising OT when the goal has been met or needs modification. Below is a brief discussion about types and components of goals.

OTs write two types of goals. *Long-term goals* (LTGs) are goals that once achieved, often indicate that the child is ready for discharge. However, in a school setting, long-term goals are usually written with a time frame for the entire school year. Though the hope is that the goal will be met by the end of the year, meeting the goal is not necessarily an indication to terminate therapy. In other settings, long-term goals might be written for 3 to 6 month periods, even though continued therapy after that time is anticipated. *Short-term goals* (STGs) are those small steps needed to reach the long-term goals. They have a shorter time frame for attainment. Sometimes short-term goals are written with the intent that they will be met after the next intervention session, in 1 week, or in 1 month. The time frame of both long-term and short-term goals depend on the facility, the type of program, the child, and the third party reimbursement. For example, in a school setting, as mentioned above, the time frame for LTGs are often the end of the school year, while the STG time frames are often the end of the quarter or grad-

ing period. For a medical environment, the LTG time frame is often discharge or a 1- or 2-month period, with STG timelines often set on a weekly basis. When working in early intervention, LTGs are often set for 6 months or yearly, with STGs set on a quarterly basis. These are guidelines only. As mentioned above, the facility, the reimbursement system, and the individual occupational therapy treatment program will all influence the timeline set for goal attainment.

All goals must have a time frame, be measurable, objective, and functional. "By August 1", "in 2 weeks", "by discharge", and "after 3 sessions" are all acceptable ways to set a time frame. Goals must always be framed by what the child or caregiver will achieve, not the therapist's treatment plan. For example, goals can begin with "child will", "mom will be able to", or "teacher will implement". Beginning a goal with "therapist will provide" is not acceptable, since this statement refers to the therapist's plan.

Goals must be written in functional terms. They should focus on areas of occupation rather than performance skills, body structure, or body function. While impairment in performance skill, body function, or body structure may be what is limiting the child from participating in an area of occupation, long-term goals must address what will functionally change. Short-term goals should also focus on function, but if necessary, the OT practitioner may address improvement in performance skills or client factors that will increase function. If a long-term goal states, "By the end of second grade, child will don his outerwear independently each day for recess and dismissal", one short-term goal might address the performance skill of identifying his/her outerwear, "By end of first quarter, child will independently identify his jacket, daily, before going outside for recess."

To assure that a goal is clear and measurable, the specific condition(s) required to perform the activity should be included. If a child is working towards self-feeding, a condition of "after set up" or feed self with "minimum assistance" might be added. Cues, physical assistance, and adaptive equipment are all examples of conditions that might be included in a goal. Goals that include statements such as "increase participation" or "decrease time needed" are not acceptable goals. The goal needs to clearly state how much time will be decreased or how one will measure increased participation. There must always be a way to objectively identify whether a goal has been achieved.

In summary, Borcherding (2000) reminds us about the following important facts when writing in any official client record:

- To assure accuracy, write in the chart as soon as possible after you see a client. It is difficult to be accurate if you don't remember what has occurred.
- A note is a reflection on the clinician, the department, and the OT profession. Therefore, accurate notes are important.

- In terms of fiscal and legal accountability, "If it isn't written, it didn't happen" (p. 10).

WRITING HOME PROGRAMS

Often seen as an extension of occupational therapy intervention, OT practitioners sometimes write activity and/or exercise programs for the child to do at home. To facilitate follow through with these activities, Berger (2002) suggests considering the following key points:

- Vision: Can the child (or parent/caregiver) see? When space permits, use a font size of 14 or greater for an individual with visual impairment (Osborne, 2001). Also, to ensure contrast, use white paper with black lettering.
- Literacy: Can the child read and at what grade level? If the recommendations are for the parent/caregiver, it is important to consider the adult's reading ability. To write something geared toward a low literacy level, use short sentences and words with only one or two syllables, whenever possible (Doak, Doak, & Root, 1996).
- Prioritize: Too much information is overwhelming and discourages someone from beginning the program. Limit exercises/activities to those that are most important.
- Format: Be sure to include white space so that the material appears "doable." Use a simple format, both upper and lower case lettering (all capitals slow down reading) and group material in an understandable manner, such as categorizing by strategies for meals, for self-care, for play; recommendations for school, for home, for outside.
- Pictures: A picture says a thousand words. When possible, use pictures to illustrate and emphasize a point.
- Age and culturally appropriate: Be sure to use age and culturally appropriate language and examples. When possible, use pictures that include children of the same age and culture of the child the handout is intended for.

A written home program is only useful if one can see it, read it, understand it, and use it. Keep the above suggestions in mind when using written handouts to facilitate follow through of occupational therapy recommendations.

OVERVIEW OF THE ROLE OF THE OTA IN GOAL WRITING AND DOCUMENTATION

Requirements for goal writing and documentation for OT practitioners vary depending on the state, facility, accrediting agencies, third party payers, practice arena, and the laws or regulations that govern that arena of practice. Although state occupational therapy licensing board practice guidelines and AOTA guidelines are usually similar, state occupa-tional therapy licensing board practice guidelines overrule AOTA guidelines. Therefore, both the OT and the OTA must be familiar with these requirements and regulations in order to write consistent and concise documentation. The next section provides an overview of goal writing and documentation procedures in different pediatric practice arenas and the roles of the OT and OTA in preparing them.

Early Intervention

Early Intervention (EI) in the pediatric practice arena refers to services provided to children (birth to 3 years) and their families. Children who participate in EI programming usually have an established condition that places them at risk for developmental delays, have a diagnosis of developmental delay, or have environmental or biological factors that place them at risk for developmental delays. Part C of the P.L.101-476 or Individuals with Disabilities in Education Act (IDEA) describes and defines the regulations and services for Early Intervention. Please refer to Chapter 5: Legal Mandates for regulations regarding evaluation and program development. Development of the *Individualized Family Service Plan (IFSP)* follows the completion of the evaluation. IDEA specifies that a multidisciplinary team must evaluate the child. The team must complete the evaluation process and develop an IFSP within 45 days after the referral. The professional identified as the service coordinator organizes the evaluation process and identifies the team members to be involved in the evaluation. Goals that are developed during the IFSP process are based on the priorities identified by the family. Whenever a new need or priority is identified, an updated IFSP can be written. In addition, Part C of IDEA identifies EI services that are to be provided by qualified personnel. These services include *assistive technology* devices and services, audiology, family training/counseling, health services, medical services for evaluation and diagnostics only, nursing, nutrition, occupational therapy, physical therapy, psychological services, service coordination, social work, special instruction, speech and language therapy, transportation, and vision services.

ROLE OF OT PRACTITIONERS IN EARLY INTERVENTION

The OT is responsible for evaluation and determining service needs of the child and family in the areas of *adaptive behavior* and play, sensory, motor, and postural development. The OT also makes recommendations for the IFSP regarding supports that may assist the child in his or her skill development. These supports may include recommendations for therapy services, adaptive equipment, physical environment adaptations, or caregiver assistance. Occupational therapy services can be listed on the IFSP as they relate to the family's identified desired outcomes, but the OT does not write specific occupational therapy program goals on the IFSP. Specific occupational therapy program goals are usually written on a separate document; usually a discipline-specific occupational therapy evaluation or re-evaluation document. The initial occupational therapy evaluation may be used as a record of the child's baseline skills, and subsequent reports may document the child's progress in occupational therapy programming. Time frames for long-term and short-term goals for early intervention programming vary between states and between agencies. Usually long-term goals are written in three to six month intervals, and short-term goals are written in one to three month intervals (quarterly). The OT practitioner needs to be familiar with the specific regulations of the state in which he/she works and the agency regarding documentation procedures.

Example of OT Goal for Early Intervention Program

Long-term goal example: When sitting in high chair, Mark will independently finger feed himself bite-size pieces of table foods and drink from a cup with a lid during meals in 3 months.

Short-term goal 1: When sitting in high chair, Mark will use pincer grasp to feed himself cereal pieces during snack, in one month.

Short-term goal 2: When sitting in high chair, Mark will use both hands to hold and drink from a cup with a lid, with minimal assist, in one month.

The role of the OTA in the area of early intervention is a limited one. Due to the constraints dictated by IDEA, Part C, it is the OT that is responsible for evaluation and goal documentation, as well as program development and service provision (please refer to Chapter 19: Early Intervention).

REFLECTIONS FOR THE OTA

Some states (Arizona, for instance) elected to define the personnel qualifications of professionals identified as "Early Interventionists" and "Early Intervention Assistants". In the Arizona Early Intervention Program Standards of Practice, the "Early Intervention Assistant" may independently carry out activities with children that are prescribed by an early intervention professional. The "Early Intervention Assistant" has limited authority to make decisions about program planning and must meet with the supervising professional at least weekly to discuss the child's progress and family issues. Occupational therapy assistants are identified as personnel who qualify as an "Early Intervention Assistant." However, the OTA would not be able to identify services as occupational therapy, but could identify services as "Special Instruction." Therefore, it is important for the OTA to be familiar

with the personnel qualifications of service provision for early intervention for the state in which he/she resides. If an OTA chooses to work in early intervention as an "Early Intervention Assistant," he or she would be responsible for documentation of services, child behavior, and recommendations for each family visit. The visitation notes can then be used as communication with supervisor and as documentation of the child's progress. Format of these visitation notes can be written in a SOAP or DAP note format. Often, specific early intervention agencies have standard forms that all the service providers use to document their services. Generally notes are hand written. A copy of the visitation note is given to the family at the end of the session, and the original is kept in the child's file. As an "Early Intervention Assistant," the OTA will need to notify his/her supervisor of family concerns or issues that could lead to an update of the IFSP.

School-Based Practice

The enactment of the Education of the Handicapped Act (EHA), Section 504 of the Rehabilitation Act of 1973, Americans with Disabilities Act (ADA), and the Individuals with Disabilities in Education Act (IDEA) have all had a significant influence on the role of occupational therapy in school-based practice (Case-Smith, 2001). School-based occupational therapy services incorporate an educational model that focuses on a student's ability to participate in school activities. In school-based practice, occupational therapy evaluations, goals, and services must be educationally relevant. Eligibility for school-based occupational therapy services is based on a number of factors.

If a student is eligible for special education, then that student is eligible for services through IDEA. All students who receive special education have an Individual Education Plan (IEP). An IEP is a document that is written during a formal meeting, which includes parents, teachers, school administrators, the student, and other team members. The entire team collaborates on development of goals and outcomes designed to be educationally relevant. The first IEP is written within 60 days after initial contact with the student, and includes evaluations and results by all team members. To determine continued need for special education and related services, IEPs are reviewed and updated by the team on a yearly basis. Complete reevaluations of student progress occur every 3 years. Please refer to Chapter 5: Legal Mandates for more information about IDEA.

IDEA AND ROLE OF OCCUPATIONAL THERAPY

The focus of occupational therapy in the schools is to maximize the child's ability to participate in school activities. The OT practitioner develops goals and programming to meet the needs of students as outlined by IDEA. Through use of observation of child's skills in the school environment, interview of classroom personnel, and standardized assessments, the OT and OTA assess the student 's ability to participate in the areas of occupation that relate to education and social participation. Performance skills within the areas of occupation that relate to education and social participation usually addressed in goals by the OT practitioner include the following.

Motor Skills

This area includes evaluation of a child's ability to use gross and fine motor skills to move about the classroom, between classrooms, and playground environments, manipulate classroom materials, and perform self-care skills relevant to the school environment such as self-toileting, clothing management and other hygiene and self-feeding skills (please refer to Chapter 15: Self-Care).

Process Skills

In this area, OT practitioners assess the child's behavioral ability to attend, organize and complete tasks, and transition between activities. A child 's ability to use sensory and perceptual functions to maintain attention and alertness to classroom activities are also evaluated within this domain. In addition, evaluation of perceptual processing, especially in the area of visual perception, is an important component of school function (Case-Smith, 2001) (please refer to Chapter 12: Introduction to Sensory Integration and Chapter 16: Visual Perceptual Dysfunction and Low Vision Rehabilitation).

Communication/Interaction Skills

This area addresses the child's ability to develop peer relationships, appropriately interact with peers and adults, and develop social behaviors appropriate for the education context (please refer to Chapter 22: Pediatric Psychosocial Therapy).

ROLE OF THE OT IN SCHOOL-BASED PRACTICE

The OT is responsible for initial evaluation and 3-year re-evaluation of the student. The OT writes the evaluation, prepares goals and occupational therapy service recommendations for the IEP. Specific IEP goals for occupational therapy are written during the IEP meeting.

ROLE OF THE OTA IN SCHOOL-BASED PRACTICE

An OTA's experience and competency level, as well as state regulations, will determine his/her role in school-based

practice. Therefore, it is important for the OTA to be familiar with the requirements of the state in which he/she practices. For instance, the role of the OTA in data gathering for the initial evaluation may vary state to state. It will, however, be the role of the OT to analyze the data and make occupational therapy program recommendations for the initial evaluation and the first IEP. At this point, the OTA may be assigned a more autonomous role and be responsible for his/her own caseload of students. After the first IEP, the OTA follows recommendations of the OT and meets regularly with the OT to discuss the student's program. The OTA documents student progress using SOAP note or DAP note format. When the annual review of the IEP is scheduled, the OTA may attend IEP meetings, make occupational therapy program recommendations, and assist in IEP goal writing, although the OT must countersign goals written on the IEP. In terms of daily management of students on his/her caseload, the OTA may be responsible for developing classroom activity programs and make activity recommendations to classroom personnel.

Example

Below is an example of an educational goal and short-term objectives written by an OT to be included in an IEP.

Educational goal example #1: Tom will independently manage cafeteria tray and food items, without assist, during lunch, by the end of the school year.

Short-term objective #1: After food items are placed on his tray, Tom will independently carry cafeteria tray from the lunch line to the table, with stay-by assist by the end of the quarter.

Short-term objective #2: While sitting at the lunch table with his tray in front of him, Tom will independently open milk carton or other food containers, with stand-by assist by the end of the quarter.

Short-term objective #3: After he is finished with his lunch, Tom, with verbal cues, will carry cafeteria tray to clean up area, throw his trash into refuse container, and place tray in cleaning bins, by the end of the quarter.

Educational goal example #2: Using appropriate grasp on pencil, Ellie will write, from memory, upper and lower case alphabet, using manuscript printing by the end of the school year.

Short-term objective #1: Ellie will grasp pencil using a dynamic tripod grasp during writing or coloring activities by the end of the first quarter.

Short-term objective #2: Ellie will use pencil and accurately copy upper case letters of the alphabet by the end of the first quarter.

Short-term objective #3: Ellie will use pencil and accurately copy lower case letters of the alphabet by the end of the second quarter.

Short-term objective #4: After dictation, Ellie will write upper and lower case letters of the alphabet by the end of the third quarter.

SECTION 504 OF THE REHABILITATION ACT & OCCUPATIONAL THERAPY

Section 504 of the Rehabilitation Act (P.L. 93–112, passed in 1973) forbids discrimination against any person with a disability (physical or mental) in programs that receive federal funding. This includes public schools, charter schools and some private schools (Smith & Patton, 1998). Students with disabilities who do not qualify for special education, may be able to receive occupational therapy services through Section 504, if that student's disability creates a barrier to full classroom participation. For example, a child with spastic hemiplegia, who can attend regular classroom programs without need of special instruction, but has difficulty manipulating and accessing classroom materials, could qualify for assistance from occupational therapy through Section 504. For a student to receive occupational therapy services based on Section 504, the OT practitioner needs to document reasons why the child would benefit from an occupational therapy program in the school. Although the OT practitioner is not required to write an IEP, the OT practitioner, along with appropriate school personnel, will need to develop a plan that outlines service and educational accommodations (Case-Smith, 2001). In this situation, the OT evaluates and makes program recommendations and goals specific to the child's needs relevant for inclusion in school programming. The OT or the OTA, under supervision of the OT, is responsible for carrying out the plan. Should an OTA be assigned to implement the occupational therapy program, then he/she is responsible to document the student's progress through SOAP or DAP note format. Depending on the experience and competency level of the OTA, he or she may assist in data collection for the re-evaluation and have input toward updated or revised goals (please refer to Chapter 20: Preschool and School-Based Therapy).

Hospitals (In- and Outpatient)

Based on the child's condition, and to address functional and psychosocial needs of the child and family, occupational therapy programming for children in hospital-based programs usually follows a medical model. Most often, occupational therapy services are initiated through a physician's order. Occupational therapy practitioners communicate with referring physicians if services need to expand beyond the initial referral. For example, a physician's initial referral was for hand splinting only. But, during the occupational therapy initial evaluation, the need for improved function in the area of oral-motor and self-feeding skills was identified. In order to expand occupational therapy services to include programming for oral-motor and self-feeding skills, the OT practitioner would contact the referring physi-

cian. The focus of evaluation for occupational therapists in pediatric hospital-based practice is to determine age-appropriate or developmentally appropriate levels of independence in areas of occupation including ADL function, play, and social-participation. Evaluation of client factors such as body functions and body structures as defined by the *OT Practice Framework* (AOTA, 2002) that may affect the performance of ADL function, play and social participation also need to be considered. Evaluation involves a chart review, clinical interview of nursing staff and/or physician, discussion with family, observation of child's function, and formal testing. A statement(s) of a child's functional abilities and areas of concern, along with outcomes of formal testing, including range of motion measurements or standardized test scores, are also reported in the initial evaluation. The goals of occupational therapy programming in hospital-based services center on restoration of skills, adaptation of activities, or use of adaptive equipment to promote function, and prevention of complications due to immobility, neuromuscular issues, and issues related to tissue healing. Format and frequency of occupational therapy programming, evaluations, goals, treatment plans, progress notes, discharge summaries, programming to be carried out by nursing, and home programming to be completed by the family are all documented and become part of the child's medical chart.

Format and frequency of documentation are usually dictated by the policies and procedures of the medical facility and the occupational therapy department. For both inpatient and outpatient hospital-based pediatric programming, documentation must meet the criteria established by accrediting and reimbursement agencies. Further, some sources of reimbursement, such as Medicare and Medicaid, may require specialized documentation and following a specific format. Goals are selected to target specific functional outcomes within the time frame allotted for hospitalization. For children receiving occupational therapy services in a hospital-based outpatient clinic, duration of occupational therapy services is usually dictated by the source of reimbursement (private insurance, Centers for Medicare and Medicaid, or other funding). Therefore, long-term goals must be written to reflect the time frame allotted by the source of reimbursement. If a child is an inpatient in an acute care hospital, then long-term goals may be written for a 1- or 2-week length of stay, with short-term goals written for a daily or weekly time period. For children who are inpatients in a rehabilitation hospital setting, long-term goals may be written for a month or more, and short-term goals may be written for a week, depending on the projected length of stay. As discussed, goals are to be written in a measurable, behavioral format that reflects functional skills. Reimbursement sources from the Department of Health and Human Services, Centers for Medicare and Medicaid Services (CMS) require use of specific forms for initial evaluation and reevaluation. These forms are developed by the CMS and are currently called CMS forms. CMS-700 forms are used for initial evaluation/plan of treatment and CMS-701 forms are used for reevaluation and updated plan of treatment. Like initial goals, updated goals are to be written in a measurable, behavioral format that reflects functional skills.

Below are examples of goals for hospital-based inpatient and outpatient OT program.

Long-term goal: Raul will independently feed himself using regular utensils by discharge.

Short-term goal #1: With use of hand splint, adapted spoon, and scoop dish, Raul will feed himself 50% of his lunch & dinner meal, independently, in 1 week.

ROLE OF THE OT IN HOSPITAL-BASED PRACTICE

For both inpatient and outpatient services, the OT is responsible for documentation of initial contact, initial evaluation, program development and treatment plan, progress notes, programming for nursing or families, and communication with referring physician regarding the occupational therapy program. The OT may implement the occupational therapy program or assign the case for an OTA to implement. The OT is responsible for reevaluation, discharge planning, and documentation.

ROLE OF THE OTA IN HOSPITAL-BASED PRACTICE

The OTA is responsible for implementing the OT treatment plan designed by the OT. The OTA documents each occupational therapy session using a SOAP or DAP note. The supervising OT may need to countersign these notes, depending on the state occupational therapy practice regulations and requirements. The child's progress and function are discussed on a regular basis with the OT. Under the supervision of the OT, the OTA may update goals and daily programming in the SOAP/DAP note. Depending on the experience and competency level of the OTA and the specific state licensing, the OTA may assist the OT in data collection for re-evaluations and discharge summaries (please refer to Chapter 21: Pediatric Service Delivery in Hospitals, Outpatient Clinics, Home Health, Hospice, and Private Clinical Practice).

Neonatal Intensive Care Unit

Occupational therapy programming in the Neonatal Intensive Care Unit (NICU) is considered an area of specialization that requires intervention be carried out by a qualified OT who has demonstrated advanced competency in this arena of practice. Therefore, OTAs rarely participate in this area of OT practice (please refer to Chapter 21: Pediatric Service Delivery in Hospitals, Outpatient Clinics, Home Health, Hospice, and Private Clinical Practice).

Home Health

Much like hospital-based outpatient practice, documentation of OT services in a pediatric home health program is determined by the policies and procedures of the reimbursement agency. The OT is responsible for initial evaluation, program planning, setting goals, and documentation. The OTA, if assigned the case, will be responsible to follow the plan designed by the OT and document each OT session using a SOAP or DAP note format. The OTA may provide input regarding goals as the child progresses and report skill changes to the supervising OT. OTAs can document changes in goals in the SOAP/DAP note, which may need to be countersigned by the supervising OT, depending on the state occupational therapy practice regulations and requirements. Depending on the experience and competency level of the OTA and the specific state licensing regulations, the OTA may be responsible for reevaluating the child and/or writing discharge summaries that are then countersigned by the supervising OT. Alternatively, the OT is responsible for completing the reevaluation, discharge plan, and documentation process (please refer to Chapter 21: Pediatric Service Delivery in Hospitals, Outpatient Clinics, Home Health, Hospice, and Private Clinical Practice).

Hospice Care

Children with chronic illnesses who become terminally ill are often cared for on an outpatient basis. Sometimes the child and his/her family choose to receive hospice care. Hospice care is an interdisciplinary program of palliative care and supportive services to address the physical, spiritual, and social needs of the terminally ill child and his or her family (Taber, 1997). Hospice services may occur in a hospital, in a specialized care center, or at home. The child and/or family must agree to terminate curative care to receive hospice services. The focus of occupational therapy programming in hospice care involves both the child and his/her family. The emphasis of occupational therapy hospice services is to provide developmentally appropriate psychosocial support directed towards maintaining quality of life. It is also the role of the OT in hospice service to evaluate and document the child's ADL and play function, interests of the child and family, and determine adaptations or adaptive equipment needs. Depending on the experience and competency of the OTA, the OTA, under the supervision of the OT, may, based on regulations that affect occupational therapy practice in the state where he or she practices, assist with evaluations of the child's functional skills and play interests, make recommendations for adaptations, and provide psychosocial supports for the family. As with other service delivery models, the OT has the primary responsibility to document the evaluations and occupational therapy programming. As previously discussed, documentation of occupational therapy program sessions can be recorded in SOAP or DAP note format, and must be in compliance of the policies and procedures of the hospice program (please refer to Chapter 21: Pediatric Service Delivery in Hospitals, Outpatient Clinics, Home Health, Hospice, and Private Clinical Practice).

Private Clinic

Along with the guidelines dictated by reimbursement agencies, documentation of occupational therapy services is regulated by the policies and procedures of each private clinic. The OT is responsible for the documentation of initial evaluation and program goals, and development of the therapy program. The OTA then follows the therapy program as designed by the supervising OT and is responsible for documentation of each occupational therapy session, using SOAP or DAP note format. If indicated, the OTA may develop a written home program, assist the supervising OT in data collection for re-evaluation, and update program goals as needed. Depending on the policies of the private clinic, the OTA may also be responsible for documentation of re-evaluation and discharge summaries. These documents may need to be co-signed by the supervising OT, depending on the state occupational therapy practice regulations, and requirements (please refer to Chapter 21: Pediatric Service Delivery in Hospitals, Outpatient Clinics, Home Health, Hospice, and Private Clinical Practice).

Summary

Documentation is an important component of best practice in occupational therapy. Documentation reflects upon the quality of occupational therapy services and programming. Therefore, it is important for OT practitioners to document accurately, clearly, and concisely, no matter what format is used, and have a clear understanding of regulations and requirements of the various settings in pediatric practice.

Goal Writing and SOAP Note Writing Case Study: Pediatric Outpatient Clinic

Fred is a 12-year-old boy who is recovering from recent surgery to remove a benign tumor that was pressing on C-5 and C-6 nerve roots. He has medical clearance to begin an occupational therapy program in the outpatient clinic where you are working. Fred demonstrates difficulty lifting right arm to put on a t-shirt and has trouble combing and washing his hair on the right side of his head. Fred enjoyed playing basketball and baseball before he began to develop weakness in his shoulder and he would like to be able to do those activities again. He also states that he does not want to rely on his parents to "help me do stuff". He is right hand dominant. His hand fatigues after about 5 minutes when doing writing activities. Fred's family has insurance coverage that capitates occupational therapy services at a 60-day limit. He presents with muscle weakness in his right arm. Strength and ROM of left upper extremity is within normal limits. In his right upper extremity, he demonstrates the following strength limitations:

- Shoulder flexion and abduction (deltoids) = fair minus (3-)
- Shoulder protraction (serratus anterior) = fair minus (3-)
- Shoulder external rotation = fair minus (3-)
- Shoulder horizontal adduction (pectoralis muscle group) = fair plus (3+)
- Elbow flexion (biceps) = fair plus (3+)
- Elbow extension (triceps) = fair plus (3+)
- Wrist extensors = fair (3)
- Thumb extensors = fair (3)
- Demonstrates weakness in grip strength on right when compared to left.

  Grip strength using hand-grip dynamometer: 80 lbs with left hand; 25 lbs with right hand

  3 jaw-chuck pinch strength using pinch meter: 12 lbs. with left hand; 5 lbs. with right hand

- Demonstrates no sensory loss.

- Write 2 possible long-term goals for outpatient clinic.
- Write 2 possible short-term goals (one for each long-term goal).

SCENARIO

Fred participates in an outpatient occupational therapy program twice a week, and completes a daily home exercise program. He has been involved in an occupational therapy program for 2 weeks out of a 2-month program. The OT designed a program to improve strength and range of motion of his right arm so that Fred can be independent in ADLs, participate in his favorite sports, and complete writing assignments for school. The OTA has been implementing the program. Fred arrives to his occupational therapy session with his mother.

OTA: Hi Fred and Mrs. Jones! How has everything been going at home and at school?

Fred: OK, I guess. My arm sure feels tired at the end of the school day. It's tough trying to carry all of my stuff all day long.

Mrs. Jones: Fred tends to put way too much stuff in his backpack.

OTA: Do you have your backpack with you today? Maybe I can take a look at it.

Fred: Nope, it's at home.

OTA: Bring it next time and also bring a copy of your school schedule. We can then both figure out a way to maybe lighten your load.

Fred: Hey, guess what! I can raise my right arm high enough that I can comb my hair with a regular comb and I don't need to use that long-handed thing anymore!

OTA: Great! How's the hair washing going?

Fred: Ok. The pump bottles for the shampoo and soap work great. It's still a little hard to keep my right arm up to my head for very long to wash my hair. But I'm getting better at using my left hand instead.

OTA: All right, let's get started. How about we go out into the courtyard and try shooting a few baskets before we come inside to do the hand & writing exercises?

Fred: Ok.

Fred & the OTA go out into the courtyard where the OTA has a basketball game set up using 3 types of balls that include a lightweight beach ball, a rubber playground ball and a regular weight basketball. The hoop is attached to an adjustable pole, about 10 feet off the ground. Fred can raise his right arm over his head to about 120 degrees of shoulder flexion to make shots with the light ball and the rubber ball. He could lift the basketball with his right arm to about 90 degrees of shoulder flexion, which was better than last week when he couldn't lift it at all without help. Next, Fred practices his ability to swing a bat by using a t-ball set up and using a foam bat.

Fred: I can't wait until I'll be able to hold a real wooden bat again. I hope I'll be strong enough to be ready for baseball tryouts. Tryouts are next month.

OTA: Keep working hard at your home exercise program. If you want, we'll try a real bat the next time you come.

Next, Fred and the OTA return to the occupational therapy gym for hand strengthening activities by playing a target game where he squeezes different kinds of squirt guns and squirt bottles filled with water. Fred is able to use his right hand to squeeze out a stream of water to hit a target that is 18 inches away (compared to 8 to 10 inches away at last session). Then Fred practices some writing activities using dry erase markers on the white board that is mounted on the wall. Fred is able to complete 10 six-word sentences on the white board (five more than last week), before he complains of his hand being tired.

OTA: How are you doing with all of the writing activities that you need to do for school?

Fred: Fortunately, so far, the teachers are letting me have more time to finish my work.

OTA: Well, our time is up! See you in a couple days. Don't forget to bring your backpack and school schedule, and I'll remember to bring a real baseball bat. Let me know how the home exercise program is going. If the exercises are too easy now, then next time we'll talk about some different ones. Bye!

Application Activities

1. Write a SOAP note about the session above.
2. Write a possible daily home program for Fred.
3. Prepare a case study for hospital-based outpatient practice.
4. Practice writing SOAP notes.
5. Given specific information about a child, practice writing home activity programs
6. Given specific information about a child, practice writing a DAP note.
7. Given specific information about a child, practice writing goals using measurable, behavioral objectives that could be incorporated into an IEP.
8. Given specific information about a child, practice writing a classroom program.

References

Agnes, M. (Ed.). (2001). *Webster's New World College Dictionary* (4th ed.). Foster City, CA: IDG Books Worldwide, Inc.

Allen, C., Foto, M., Moon-Sperling, T., Wilson, D. (1989). A medical review approach to Medicare outpatient documentation. *American Journal of Occupational Therapy, 43*(12), 793-800.

Americans with Disabilities Act of 1990, 42 U.S.C. #12134. (1990)

American Occupational Therapy Association (1995a). Elements of clinical documentation (revision). *American Journal of Occupational Therapy, 49*(10), 1032-1035.

American Occupational Therapy Association (1999). *Occupational therapy services for children and youth under the individuals with disabilities in education act* (2nd ed.). Bethesda, MD: Author.

American Occupational Therapy Association (2002). Occupational therapy practice framework: Domain and process. *American Journal of Occupational Therapy, 56,* 609-639.

American Occupational Therapy Association (2002). Roles and responsibilities of the occupational therapist and occupational therapy assistant during the delivery of occupational therapy services. *OT Practice, 7* (15), 9-10.

Assistance to States for the Education of Children with Disabilities. 34 C.F.R., Part 300.

Austin, J. (1998). Computerized documentation. In J. D. Acquaviva (Ed.), *Effective documentation for occupational therapy*. Rockville, MD: American Occupational Therapy Association.

Berger, S. (2002). Making written education materials user friendly. *OT Practice, 7*(4), 19-20.

Borcherding, S. (2000). *Documentation manual for writing SOAP notes in occupational therapy*. Thorofare, NJ: SLACK Incorporated.

Case-Smith, J. (2001). *Occupational therapy for children* (4th ed.) St. Louis, MO: Mosby.

Chandler, B. E. (1998). Special considerations I: Pediatrics. In J. D. Acquaviva (Ed.), *Effective documentation for occupational therapy*. Rockville, MD: American Occupational Therapy Association.

Doak, C. C., Doak, L. G., & Root, J. H. (1996). *Teaching patients with low literacy skills* (2nd ed.). Philadelphia: Lippincott.

Dunn, W. (2000). *Best practice occupational therapy: In community service with children and families*. Thorofare, NJ: SLACK Incorporated.

Huffman, E. K. (1994). *Health information management* (10th ed.). Berwyn, IL: Physicians' Record Company.

Individuals with Disabilities Education Act Amendments of 1990. 20 U.S.C. #1400-1485.

McGuire, M. J. (1997). Documenting progress in home care. *American Journal of Occupational Therapy, 51*(6), 436-445.

Osborne, H. (2001). *Overcoming communication barriers in patient education*. Gaithersburg, MD: Aspen.

Robertson, S. C. (1998). Why we document. In J. D. Acquaviva (Ed.), *Effective documentation for occupational therapy*. Rockville, MD: American Occupational Therapy Association.

Ryan, S. (1993). *Practice issues in occupational Therapy: Intraprofessional team building*. Thorofare, NJ: SLACK Incorporated.

Smith, T. & Patton, J. (1998). *Section 504 and the public schools: A practice guide for determining eligibility, developing accommodation plans and documenting compliance*. Austin, TX: Pro-Ed, Inc.

Thomas, C., (Ed.). (1997). *Taber's Cyclopedic Medical Dictionary* (18th ed). Philadelphia, PA: F.A. Davis Company.

Wolf, S. C. (1987). Administration: Computerized care plans a strong management tool. *Provider*, 39-40.

Chapter 7

AN OVERVIEW OF EARLY DEVELOPMENT

Amy Wagenfeld, PhD, OTR/L

Chapter Objectives

- Recognize and identify the basic premises of psycho-analytical, social-cognitive, ecological, information processing, learning, and humanistic theories of development.
- Identify the nature of normal development.
- Understand basic principles of motor, cognitive, and social emotional development.
- Recognize the contexts and role of the Occupational Therapy Assistant in the facilitation of developmental skills with young children.

Introduction

Recognizing and embracing each child's individuality is one of the most exciting aspects of pediatric practice. While developmental theories and occupational therapy treatment modalities provide the basic framework for pediatric service delivery, respecting a child's unique and diverse qualities is also a crucial part of successful treatment. In essence, there is no (and should be no) "cookie cutter" approach to working with children and their families. In order to best adapt to the ever-changing, unique, and rewarding challenges presented by all children, understanding developmental processes is vital. However, equally as important in pediatric practice, is the ability to integrate and infuse foundational knowledge with practical application while maintaining an ongoing sense of flexibility when working with each child.

Pediatric occupational therapy is based, in part, on fundamental theories of development. In fact, theories of Occupational Performance (Law, Cooper, Strong, et al., 1996; Merrill, Slavik, Holloway, Richter, & David, 1990; Pedretti, 1996; Stewart, Letts, Law, et al., 2003), Human Occupation (Kielhofner, 1995), Neuro-Developmental Treatment (D'Ambrogio, 1997; Dutton; 1998; Law, Missiuna, Pollock, & Stewart, 2001), and Sensory Integration (Ayres, 1994; Merrill, Slavik, Holloway, Richter, & David, 1990) (please refer to Chapter 3: A Brief Overview of Occupational Therapy Theories, Models, and Frames of Reference) are validated and supported by the broad based underpinnings of developmental theory. What is known about child development is perhaps still in its "toddler stage," yet with each passing year, and thanks to technological advances and enhanced research methods, our understanding of how children develop continues to increase.

Learning about development leads to a greater appreciation of how children become who they are to be. To foster this appreciation, a brief overview of early developmental processes, which include gross and fine *motor development*, as well as cognitive, and *social emotional development* and the contexts or environments in which they occur, are discussed in this chapter. A discussion of several theories of development that align themselves with the practice of occupational therapy is also presented. These theories lend themselves to a fascinating discussion of the age-old question posed by children everywhere, "why"; which in this case may well be, "why" do children develop the way that they do? As this chapter addresses only an overview of developmental issues associated with childhood, the interested reader is encouraged to pursue further study into child development.

Foundational Theories of Learning and Development

The study of early development is based on many theories. To quickly review, a theory is a set of related ideas that explain, describe, and make predictions about specific phenomena. Ideally, a theory should offer an explanation for new or existing ideas. To support or reject a theory, and as part of the research process, investigators develop *hypotheses*, which are testable assumptions or predictions. It is important to understand that based on current available investigative methods, developmental research seeks to find relationships, rather than causality to explain developmentally oriented research outcomes (Collins, 1996).

On the surface, it may seem that some theories of development are more applicable to pediatric practice than others (please refer to Chapter 14: Childhood Occupations). Whether aligning with one or a combination of theories of learning and development, in terms of pediatric treatment there is much to be gained from each of these theories. Table 7-1 provides an overview of several theories of development and their application to the occupational therapy assistant (OTA). In other words, although what is done in treatment is very important, so too is how and why it is done. Theories of development help, in part, to frame the "how and why" pieces of treatment. To provide the most comprehensive and relevant therapy possible it is important to keep this concept in mind when working with children, as best practice (Dunn, 2000) extracts and applies the "best" from each discipline or theory.

THE NATURE VS. NURTURE DEBATE

The *nature vs. nurture* argument remains one of the long-standing debates in developmental research. Simply stated, nature refers to our individual biological make up, while nurture refers to external or outside environmental forces that influence us. The debate exists over what makes us who we are; is it forces of nature, or is it forces of nurture? Currently, the most widely accepted view is a middle ground view; that the relationship between internal biology (nature) and environmental (nurture) factors influences who we are to become. In other words, we are products of both our nature and our nurture. In fact, research suggests that the ongoing influence and interaction between nature and nurture shapes our past, present, and future individuality. As practitioners, it is important to keep in mind that it is not possible to change the actual biology or genetic predispositions of children. Instead, we can help to shape, facilitate, and nurture the environment of the children we treat. An occupational therapist (OT) or OTA cannot reverse the genetics or internal biologies of children, but can and must provide compensatory or facility techniques to optimize function.

REFLECTIONS FOR THE OTA

Instruction in, and consistent use of, developmentally appropriate adapted equipment (nurture) designed to help a child with limited range of motion (nature) may enhance his environment, as well as create a healthy feedback loop for overall development. Fostering a greater sense of physical independence through cognitively oriented problem solving and learning (such as successfully learning to use adapted equipment) invariably leads to a greater sense of social emotional health. In other words, as nature and nurture interact, enhanced physical function in turn often facilitates social emotional and cognitive health.

MODELS OF DISCONTINUITY AND CONTINUITY

From conception and throughout life, children undergo ongoing physical, cognitive, and social emotional developmental and maturational changes. The ways in which these changes occur is another debated issue in developmental research (Shaffer, 2002). A theorist or practitioner ascribing to the discontinuity model of development considers growth and development to occur in stages, or orderly and sequential patterns of change that usually follow a set timetable. Looking at growth as a "series of steps" necessary to climb in order to reach adulthood is another way to frame the discontinuity model of development (Charlesworth, 1992). Each developmental stage builds on the previous one and leads to more refined and complex behaviors and actions. In turn, with each progressive stage, children are better able to engage in more complex and challenging activities (Miller, 1989). Unlike discontinuity theorists, continuity theorists believe that development occurs in a gradual and ongoing fashion. Development, for a continuity theorist, is understood to progress in "degrees" rather than steps. Certainly there is common ground between the discontinuity and continuity oriented theorists. Like discontinuity theorists, continuity theorists believe that as development proceeds, children are better prepared to improve and refine existing skills, as well as undertake new and more challenging experiences.

REFLECTIONS FOR THE OTA

Which theoretical model, continuity or discontinuity, best exemplifies pediatric OT practice? Do you believe there is a middle ground between the two perspectives?

Growth and Development

Developmental norms or milestones provide important information to researchers and clinicians. Developmental norms are a guide and tool used by professionals and caregivers to monitor a child's development as compared to the

Table 7-1

Theories of Development and Their Primary Application to the Occupational Therapy Assistant

The following organizer provides a working overview of several theories of development, as well as their general application to the occupational therapy practitioner.

Theorist	Theoretical Orientation	Basic Premise	Application to the OT Practitioner
Jean Piaget (1896-1980)	Social Cognition (construction)	Thinking and development in general are a result of internal processes. Children are at their best to develop when provided with many hands on and observational experiences (Kamii, 1973; Piaget & Inhelder, 1969).	The OTA provides children with hands on experiences as a means to optimize performance and function.
Lev Vygotsky (1896-1934)	Social Construction	Children learn through social experiences. In most cases, given time and support, a child will achieve a desired skill or action (Vygotsky, 1978).	The OTA acts as a capable guide to provide mediation and support for development of more functional and increasingly complex skills.
Robert Siegler (1949-)	Information Processing	Proposes that the mind is like a computer, the brain is the hardware, and cognition is the software. Thinking skills such as memory, coding, and encoding are equated with information processing (Shaffer, 2002).	The OTA works to improve cognitive skills through enhancing learning strategies.
Sigmund Freud (1856-1939)	Psychoanalytic (psychosexual)	Personality development is, for the most part, an unconscious process that is influenced by emotions (Santrock, 2003).	The OTA may use projective and creative techniques such as art activities and journal writing to support personality development (Cole, 1998).
Erik Erikson (1902-1994)	Psychoanalytic (psychosocial)	A psychosocial explanation for sequential, lifelong development of personality. Each stage has specific tasks that must be accomplished to achieve a well adjusted or maladjusted sense of self (Erikson, 1982; Erikson, 1963).	To insure future healthy growth and development, and through specific tasks associated with each life stage, the OTA helps foster a positive sense of meaning in a child's life.

Table 7-1 (continued)

Theories of Development and Their Primary Application to the Occupational Therapy Assistant

Theorist	Theoretical Orientation	Basic Premise	Application to the OT Practitioner
Abraham Maslow (1908-1979)	Humanistic	Progressing through the Hierarchy of Needs, every person is motivated to mature and develop to his or her greatest potential, and ultimately, the most self-fulfilled person possible (Maslow, 1970; Maslow, 1968).	The most basic needs must be met prior to moving up the hierarchy, and like the principles and practice of occupational therapy, until fundamental skills are integrated, further progress towards goal acquisition may be impeded.
Urie Bronfenbrenner (1917-)	Human Ecology, Social Systems	A systems based theory proposing that a child develops as a result of the interactions of all parts of the ecosystem (environment) (Bronfenbrenner, 1986; Bronfenbrenner, 1979).	The OTA provides intervention at all levels of a child's environments to adapt, modify, and facilitate functional abilities.
B.F. Skinner (1904-1990)	Classical Learning	Learning is a change in behavior that results from experiences. Humans are capable of being "shaped" by predictable patterns of learning known as reinforcement and punishment techniques (Skinner, 1974).	Reinforcement schedules are frequently used by the OTA to support and encourage learning of new and desired skills and behaviors, or to extinguish undesired skills or behaviors.
Albert Bandura (1925-)	Classical Learning	Learning or cognition develops through observation or modeling, rather than direct reinforcement (Santrock, 2003).	When working with children, modeling and observation are useful tools for the OTA. Modeling might also be used to support abstract concepts such as modeling a kind action.
Konrad Lorenz (1903-1989)	Ethology	Looks at the biological relationship between critical or sensitive periods in development, and the importance they play in later growth. Attachment theory is based on ethology (Miller, 1989).	The OTA supports facilitation of critical periods of development, as well as helps to foster nurturing relationships between child and primary caregiver.

normally developing population (Ramey, & Ramey 1999). Based on these norms, developmental researchers and practitioners from many disciplines prepare guidelines and charts illustrating how typical development occurs. With regard to therapy services, norms may be helpful in determining a child's strengths and weaknesses. It is important to remember that although norms provide a suggested age range for when skills or milestones are expected to emerge, within that range, there is variation from child to child, especially a child with disabilities. Keep in mind that when developmental milestones emerge is important, and so too are how they emerge.

The three major areas of development studied by researchers are *cognitive, motor,* and *social emotional* development (Miller, 1989; Ramey, & Ramey 1999; Shaffer, 2002). Cognitive development refers to the way thinking develops. In terms of cognitive development, as thought processes unfold, a child's ability to better understand the world expands (Miller, 1989). Social emotional development pertains to the ways that children learn to actively participate in, and interpret, interpersonal relationships. Motor development, including reflex integration, postural control, and fine and gross motor development encompasses the way that movement skills develop in the body (please refer to Chapter 11: Positioning in Pediatrics, Chapter 17: Hand Development, the Developmental Milestones Chart, and the Major Infant Reflexes Chart). Motor development depends upon cognitive and social emotional development, and likewise, cognitive, and social emotional development is inextricably intertwined with motor development.

In addition to motor, cognitive, and social emotional development, there are also specific contexts or environments that play a significant role in both the development of patterns and skills associated with performance (AOTA, 2002). A *context* refers to multifaceted situations affecting function that may be externally or internally oriented and involve both human and nonhuman aspects of a person's life (AOTA, 2002).

Contexts may also encompass time and space dimensions (AOTA, 2002). These contexts include, the physical, cultural, social, personal, spiritual, temporal, and virtual context or environments (AOTA, 2002). While not all contexts may be applicable to all children at all times, it is important to note that the contexts in which therapy takes place does in fact, play a role in influencing growth and development. Because it may be presumed that children participate or engage in occupations of childhood (Christianson & Baum, 2004) within these seven contexts, understanding what each context represents is important.

The *physical context* includes the actual space and any potential barriers and limitations that children encounter. The physical context may be thought of as all parts of the environment that are not human, including natural geographical phenomenon as well as man-made structures (AOTA, 2002). Not only does the physical context encompass home and school, but also public accesses such as shops, restaurants, museums, and transportation issues. With the current influences of the Americans with Disabilities Act (Public Law 101-336, 1990), awareness and support for equality of access and domain has improved. The OTA must act as a strong advocate in assuring that children not be limited due to the physical context.

Consideration of *cultural context* has always been of importance and value to occupational therapy. Recognizing, expecting, and respecting diversity is a keystone of our practice. This is particularly true in pediatric practice, where the individuality of each child's development is not only explored, but also embraced. Cultural contexts take into account religious, sexual, and familial patterns of behavior that are, in part, based on customs, beliefs, rituals, and societal expectations (AOTA, 2002). Cultural mores also play a role in how children respond to their bodies, and associatively, their strengths and limitations (Zborowksi, 1969). For ethical reasons, making a strong commitment to understanding the different values and customs of children under your care is important, and in fact, failure to do so may impede the progress an OTA makes when working with children. This respect creates a positive and healthy milieu for children to receive therapy. Validating and respecting cultural diversity also helps to strengthen the relationship between practitioner, child, and family.

The *social context* refers to the relationships and routines that children forge with others (AOTA, 2002). Early in life, development of secure relationships with a primary caregiver is an important predictor for fostering future healthy relationship connections (Ainsworth, Blehar, Waters, & Wall, 1978; Bowlby; 1988). Working with families to help nurture these early connections may have lasting influence on a child's overall development and well-being. Not only does the social environment provide cues about early interpersonal interactions, it also influences behaviors in new or related settings.

The *personal context* refers to demographic features specific to each child, such as gender, age, socioeconomic, and educational status (AOTA, 2002). It is critically important to understand that a child has no control over personal context, and as such, the OTA must be cautioned to avoid any preconceived biases (Gardner, 2002) when working with children presenting with a wide range of demographic characteristics.

The *spiritual context* encompasses the inner resources that motivate and encourage a child attain goals and provide a sense of purpose (AOTA, 2002). As with most adults, the spiritual context is an ever-evolving aspect of development, and is inextricably linked with all other contexts. Working to nurture the spiritual context is an important part of pediatric practice.

The *temporal context* refers to the aspects of time and place, and their influence on performance, and subsequently, development (AOTA, 2002). The temporal context is dynamic and ever changing, such that the OTA must be ready and willing to accept that at any given time, temporal influences may either positively influence a child's performance.

The *virtual context* refers to the technological means through which children communicate (AOTA, 2002). As technology continues to forge ahead at a rapid pace, OTA must strive to stay abreast of new advances that may positively influence a child's performance, and apply them to successful pediatric practice.

Collectively, these seven contexts strongly effect developmental skill acquisition. *Deprivation* or lack of participation in any context may negatively impact a child's rate of development and maturation. The role of the OTA is not only to facilitate developmental skills, but also to support growth through nurturing of healthy contextual situations. In other words, for the OTA, the contexts in which development proceeds are of equal importance to the actual physical, cognitive, and social emotional developmental skills facilitation.

Developmental Stages

Based on existing knowledge of development, it is recognized that there are *critical and sensitive periods* in a child's life (Charlesworth, 1992; Ramey, & Ramey, 1999; Shaffer, 2002). A *sensitive* period of development refers to a time when a child is most vulnerable to outside influences. For instance, research indicates that certain *teratogens*, or outside forces such as disease or other negative factors are most harmful during sensitive periods of prenatal development (Charlesworth, 1992; Shaffer, 2002). The harmful effects of teratogen exposure may appear later in life as developmental delays in the areas of motor, cognitive, and social emotional competence (Charlesworth, 1992). When a child is most ready and available to learn and acquire new skills, he or she is in a critical period of development (Ramey, & Ramey, 1999). Lack of or limited opportunity to fully participate in critical periods of physical, cognitive, or social emotional developmental experiences may lead to negative long-term effects on a child and her family. Helping and nurturing children during sensitive and critical periods of development is important for all who work in pediatric settings.

As developmental scholars strive to understand and explain how a child develops into the most fully functioning adult possible, the supportive role of the OTA, to carry out and provide thoughtfully planned developmentally appropriate treatment is very important. So as to provide children with the most suitable therapy possible, the OTA working with children must, then, possess a working understanding of development and developmental influences and apply it to the treatment process.

STAGES OF DEVELOPMENT

Childhood is generally divided into five developmental stages or periods; *prenatal, infancy, early and middle childhood,* and *adolescence* (Charlesworth, 1992; Miller, 1989; Santrock, 2003). Taking into account developmental theory and research, the following is understood to occur in each developmental stage.

The prenatal period includes the time from conception until birth. A full term baby is considered to be one born at 38-42 weeks of gestation. During the prenatal period, the developing fetus undergoes many rapid changes, proceeding from a fertilized egg or zygote to a 7-pound, 20-inch long (average birth weight and length in the US) baby. At no other time in development does systemic growth occur so swiftly, nor is the fetus as predisposed to outside influences. During the prenatal period, ongoing medical management is critical as exposure to maternal teratogens may negatively impact later development.

Infancy is the time period from birth to about 18 months. During the first 18 months, infants acquire the skills to walk, use their hands, begin to communicate, and relate to others in their environment. This is a period of rapid growth and development. Infants learn about their world through sensory motor experiences, but are also significantly impacted by social emotional, cultural, and cognitive influences.

Early Childhood refers to the period from about 18 months until about 5-6 years of age. During these early years, children are learning to develop peer relationships and may begin to experience a sense of independence from their primary caregivers as they attend preschool. Along with relationship building, motor skills and cognitive skills-especially language skills, are rapidly expanding during early childhood.

Middle Childhood is the time period from about 6 to 12 years of age. Throughout this stage, children are refining motor skills, focusing on academic, school related tasks, and continuing to establish peer relationships.

Adolescence is the time period from about 12 to 18 years of age. During adolescence, boys and girls undergo significant physical and emotional changes in preparation for adulthood. Some of the tasks and challenges of adolescence include grappling with self-defined individuality and autonomy.

In order for the OTA to provide effective and efficacious intervention, it is important to be sensitive to the various stages of development, the environmental contexts in which they occur, and in turn, to provide developmentally appropriate treatment for children.

Motor Development

Many factors influence motor development (Miller, 1989; Santrock, 2003). The long "list" includes *genetics, nutritional status, pre- and perinatal care, social class, ethnicity, birth order,* and *maternal physical, cognitive,* and *social emotional status.* When taking these factors into account during treatment, working on motor skill deficits becomes more enriched because collectively, a child's biological, nutritional, environmental, cognitive, and social emotional status influences the way that motor movements are executed. Best practice (Dunn, 2000) dictates that in conjunction with a team of professionals, a holistic treatment approach be carried out to insure the most developmentally appropriate care for children possible.

GROSS MOTOR SKILLS

Motor development refers to the acquisition of new and increasingly complex patterns of movements and movement related skills. Motor skills (both gross and fine) typically develop in an orderly sequence and proceed from head to toe (cephalocaudal), and from *proximal* to *distal* (midline-outward) regions of the body (Exner, 1992; Gesell & Amatruda, 1947; Santrock, 2003). Typically, gross motor skill development precedes fine motor skill development (Exner, 1992). The "large" gross motor movements of childhood such as rolling, *crawling,* sitting, walking, throwing, and so forth are governed by the larger muscles of the body (Kagan, 1998). These muscle groups are located in the proximal regions of the body, such as the shoulders and upper arms, and the hips and upper legs. Without good control and stability associated with gross motor movements, fine motor skills are often challenged.

REFLECTIONS FOR THE OTA

If a child has limited proximal shoulder range of motion, yet has intact distal (wrist, hand, and finger) movements and wants to play catch, the practitioner and child, functioning as a therapeutic team, must work together to compensate for loss of gross motor function, while engaging in the pleasurable childhood occupation of playing catch.

FINE MOTOR SKILLS

Facilitating fine motor skills is one of the cornerstones of the practice of occupational therapy (Pedretti, 1996; Wilson, 1998). Like gross motor skills, fine motor skills involve movement, but instead refer to the small and refined movements of the arms, hands, and fingers. The fine motor skills associated with childhood include self-feeding, grooming, manipulative play, writing, and using scissors (Brook & Wagenfeld, in press; Exner, 1992; Exner, 2001; Wilson, 1998). Similar to gross motor skills, fine motor skills develop in an orderly sequence, beginning with the larger and more uncoordinated movements of the entire wrist and hand, and ultimately, to refined, and controlled use of the fingers (Brook & Wagenfeld, in press; Exner, 1992; Exner, 2001). Generally, fine motor skills are divided into three categories: *grasp, reach,* and *release* (Exner, 1992; Exner, 2001). The development of good fine motor skills is a critical part of motor, cognitive, and social emotional development, as hands are used to touch, feel, communicate, and care for ourselves. For further information on specific motor milestones, please refer to the Developmental Milestones Chart at the end of this book.

Cognitive Development

Broadly speaking, cognitive development can be equated to the development of thinking. *Cognition* refers to the way thought and information is processed and is characterized by perception, reasoning, judgment, intuition, and memory (Flavell, 1999; Pruitt, 1998). Like motor development, cognitive development is dependent on a number of inborn genetic and environmental factors, and is generally believed to follow an orderly sequence. While intact motor function provides the child with the ability to explore his environment, the role of cognitive development is to learn about the environment and make predictions and assumptions about what is being experienced. Cognitive skill development is influenced by a child's genetic make-up, his social emotional and motor development, as well as environmental contexts. For further information on specific motor milestones, please refer to the Developmental Milestones Chart at the end of this book.

Social Emotional Development

Social emotional development encompasses the ways in which a child learns to interpret, internalize, and use information and cues gleaned from relationship contexts (Lyons, 1984). Through the influence of social emotional development, a child learns to interact and relate with family, peers, and others in preparation to participate as a member of society. The degree of success to which a child masters relational skills is referred to as *social* or *emotional competency* (Saarni, 1999). The level of social competency varies from person to person, and is dependent, in part, on developmental and relational contexts. Social emotional development also encompasses how a child acquires self-esteem, as well as a sense of self (Denham, 1998), and is also influenced by cognitive and motor development. For further information on specific motor milestones, please refer to the Developmental Milestones Chart at the end of this book.

In sum, a child with motoric challenges will face greater limitations relative to environmental exploration, yet from a holistic perspective will likely benefit most from specific interventions to address overall motor, cognitive, and social emotional experiences. Once again, the importance of treating the whole child, and not simply the presenting limitations cannot be overemphasized. Understanding and applying the foundations of typical development to the therapy process strengthens the quality of treatment provided to a child and family. In conjunction with an entire team of professionals, the OTAs role in implementing an individualized treatment plan that best addresses the child's global functioning is a critically important part of therapeutic intervention.

Summary

In this chapter, an overview of child development, such as how and when developmental milestones are most likely to occur, and factors that may impede normal development, were explored. Several theories that form the foundation of the study of child development and influence pediatric occupational therapy practice were also presented, compared, and contrasted. To further build on this developmental foundation, in-depth study of the many available resources on child development is highly recommended. The following chapters will support the fundamental concepts that have been presented in this chapter and align them to the practice of the OTA working with children.

Case Study

A baby needs to feel warm and secure, and generally take comfort in being held close and snugly to her mother. In turn, the mother may also derive great pleasure in this early connection. At birth, a baby's visual range is only about 18 inches, the distance between the mother's breast and her eyes.

Based on ecological, psychosocial, and ethological theory, list and explain five ways that a mother might hold or position her baby in order to be able to facilitate this visual range and derive a mutual sense of comfort.

Application Activities

1. Complete observations of children at different ages and of different social class, and share these findings with your classmates.

2. Make or design toys that are designed to facilitate specific developmental skills.

3. Find photos or magazine pictures of babies engaging in specific developmental milestones and create your own developmental charts.

4. Design a fine motor developmental activity booklet for different age ranges.

5. Create collages of developmental theorists and of developmental stages.

6. Make a video of a child engaging in a specific task for classmates to view.

7. Interview (your) parents to find out about your developmental histories, compare and contrast with classmates, and observe the wide range of time at which skills were acquired.

8. Role-play situations such as helping a parent work with a baby who does not bring toys to her mouth, roll, etc.

References

Ainsworth, M. D., Blehar, M. C., Waters, E., & Wall, S. (1978). *Patterns of attachment: A psychological study of the strange situation*. Hillsdale, NJ: Lawrence Erlbaum Associates.

American Occupational Therapy Association. (2002). Occupational therapy practice framework: Domain and process. *American Journal of Occupational Therapy, 56,* 609-639.

Americans with Disabilities Act (1990). Public Law 101-336. Retrieved December 1, 2002 from http://www.usdoj.gov/crt/ada/pubs/ada.txt

Ayres, A. J. (1994). *Sensory integration and the child*. Los Angeles: Western Psychological Services.

Bowlby, J., (1988). *A secure base: Parent-child attachment and healthy human development*. New York: Basic Books.

Bronfenbrenner, U. (1979). *Ecology of human development*. Cambridge, MA: Harvard University Press.

Bronfenbrenner, U. (1986). Ecology of the family as a context for human development: Research perspectives. *Developmental Psychology, 22,* 6, 723-742.

Brook, G., & Wagenfeld, A. (In press). *Focus on fine motor skills program*. Bowen Hills, QLD, Australia: Australian Academic Press.

Charlesworth, R. (1992). *Understanding child development: For adults who work with young children* (3rd Ed.). Albany, NY: Delmar.

Christianson, C., & Baum. C. (2004). Enabling function and well-being (3rd ed.). Thorofare, NJ: SLACK Incorporated.

Cole, M. B. (1998). *Group dynamics in occupational therapy: The theoretical basis and practice application of group treatment* (2nd ed.). Thorofare, NJ: SLACK Incorporated.

Collins, N. L. (1996). Working models of attachment: Implications for explanation, emotion, and behavior. *Journal of Personality and Social Psychology, 71*(4), 810-832. Retrieved January 11, 2001, from PsycArticles database.

D'Ambrogio, K. J. (1997). *Positional release therapy: Assessment and treatment of musculoskeletal dysfunction*. St. Louis, MO: Mosby.

Denham, S. A. (1998). *Emotional development in young children*. New York: Guilford Press.

Dunn, W. (2000). *Best practice occupational therapy in community service with children and families*. Thorofare, NJ: SLACK Incorporated.

Dutton, R. (1998). Neurodevelopmental theory. In M. E. Neistadt & E. B. Crepeau (Eds.), *Willard and Spackman's occupational therapy* (9th ed.). Philadelphia: Lippincott.

Erikson, E. (1963). *Childhood and society.* New York: W.W. Norton Company.

Erikson, E. (1982). *The life cycle completed.* New York: W.W. Norton Company.

Exner, C. E. (1992). In-hand manipulation skills. In J. Case-Smith & C. Pehoski (Eds.), *Development of hand skills in the child* (pp. 35-46). Rockville, MD: American Occupational Therapy Association.

Exner, C. E. (2001). Development of hand skills. In J. Case-Smith (Ed.). *Occupational therapy for children* (pp. 289-328). St Louis, MO: Mosby.

Flavell, J. H. (1999). Cognitive development: Children's knowledge about the mind. *Annual Review of Psychology, 50,* 21-45.

Gesell, A., & Amatruda, C. S. (1947). *Developmental diagnosis* (2nd ed). New York: Harper and Row.

Gardner, R. (2002). *Psychology applied to everyday life.* New York: Wadsworth.

Kagan, J (Ed.) (1998). *Gale Encyclopedia of Childhood & Adolescence.* Detroit: Gale.

Kamii, C. (1973). Pedagogical principles derived from Piaget's theory: Relevance for educational practice. In M. Schwebel & J. Raph (Eds.), *Piaget in the classroom* (pp.199-215). New York: Basic Books.

Kielhofner, G. (1995). *A model of human occupation: Theory and application* (2nd ed.). Philadelphia: Williams and Wilkins.

Law, M., Cooper, B. A., Strong, S., Stewart, D., Rigby, P., & Letts, L. (1996). The Person-Environment-Occupation model: A transactive approach to occupational performance. *Canadian Journal of Occupational Therapy, 63*(1), 9-23.

Law, M., Missiuna, C., Pollock, N., & Stewart, D. (2001). Foundations for occupational therapy practice with children. In J. Case-Smith (Ed.), *Occupational therapy for children* (4th ed.) (pp. 39-70). St. Louis, MO: Mosby.

Lyons, B. G. (1984). Defining a child's zone of proximal development: Evaluation process for treatment planning. *American Journal of Occupational Therapy, 38,* 446-451.

Maslow, A. (1968). *Toward a psychology of being* (2nd ed.). New York: Van Nostrand Reinhold.

Maslow, A. (1970). *Motivation and personality* (2nd ed.). New York: Harper and Row.

Merrill, S. C., Slavik, B., Holloway, E., Richter, E., & David, S. (Eds.). (1990). *Environment: Implications for occupational therapy Practice: A sensory integrative perspective.* Rockville, MD: American Occupational Therapy Association.

Miller, P. H. (1989). *Theories of developmental psychology* (2nd ed.) New York: W. H. Freeman and Company.

Pedretti, L. W. (1996). Occupational performance: A model for practice in physical dysfunction. In L. W. Pedretti (Ed.), *Occupational therapy: Practice skills for physical dysfunction* (4th ed.). St. Louis, MO: Mosby.

Piaget, J., & Inhelder, B. (1969). *The psychology of the child.* New York: Basic Books.

Pruitt, D. B. (Ed.) (1998). *Your child: Emotional, behavioral, and cognitive development from birth through preadolescence.* New York: Harper Resource.

Ramey, C. T., & Ramey, S. L. (1999). *Right from birth: Building your child's foundation for life–birth to 18 months.* New York: Goddard Press.

Saarni, C. (1999). *The development of emotional competence.* New York: Guilford Press.

Santrock, J. W. (2003). *Children* (7th ed.). Boston: McGraw Hill.

Shaffer, D. (2002). *Developmental psychology: Childhood & adolescence.* (6th ed.). Belmont, CA: Wadsworth.

Skinner, B. F. (1974). *About behaviorism.* New York: Alfred A. Knopf.

Stewart, D., Letts, L., Law, M., Acheson Cooper, B., Strong, S., & Rigby, P. J. (2003). The Person-Environment-Occupation model. In E. Blesedell Crepeau, E. S. Cohn, & B. A. Boyt-Schell (Eds.). *Willard and Spackman's occupational therapy* (10th ed.). Philadelphia: Lippincott Williams & Wilkins.

Vygotsky, L. (1978). *Mind in society.* Cambridge, MA: Harvard University Press.

Wilson, E. B. (1998). *Occupational therapy for children with special needs.* London: Whurr.

Zborowksi, M. (1969). *People in pain.* San Francisco: Jossey-Bass.

Chapter 8

AN OVERVIEW OF DEVELOPMENTAL ASSESSMENTS

Cindee Quake-Rapp, PhD, OTR

Chapter Objectives

- Explain the importance of developmental assessment.
- Define the role of the occupational therapy assistant in developmental assessment.
- Describe the process of developmental assessment using the *Occupational Therapy Practice Framework*.

Historical Overview of Developmental Assessment

Prior to the 18th century, children were regarded as chattels, inherently good or bad, and had no independent rights. Conflicting beliefs emerged, comparing the economic value of children with economic dependency, whether children should be trained or permitted to develop, and whether children needed restrictions or advocacy. Childhood was not recognized as a stage in human development (Grotberg, 1977).

The first attempts to observe and record developmental sequence in children occurred in the 18th century by Johann Heinrick Pestalozzi (1746-1827), a Swiss educator. Through observation of his son, Pestalozzi identified childhood as a separate developmental phase. Friedrich Froebel (1837), a successor of Pestalozzi, founded the world's first kindergarten ("children's garden") in Blankenburg, Switzerland and developed a series of educational games for pre-school children. Froebel saw "play" as essential in developing the imagination and spiritual development of children (Bel Geddes, 1997).

The 19th century brought forth biologically based Darwinian theories of evolution. To support his work, Darwin kept a diary of the development of his infant son and published his findings in 1877. Darwin's research influenced scholars such as Sigmund Freud who were interested in biology related to personality development and human behavior. Freud was the first scholar to identify stages of development as occurring in a sequential and biologically predetermined order. Freud introduced one of the first conceptual developmental frameworks when he published "Infantile Sexuality" in 1910 (Grotberg, 1977).

Arnold Gesell was the first scientist to conduct research on the "ages and stages" of child development. He categorized growth and development in the physical, intellectual, social, and emotional realms, and identified the variability of age-related behavior among children. In 1907, Frenchman Alfred Binet developed a breakthrough in the measurement of age-related behaviors. Binet identified the method of "age scaling" in which he compared chronological age with cognitive functioning. The idea of chronological "age norms" can be attributed to Alfred Binet (Grotberg, 1977).

Jean Piaget (1896-1980) was the most influential developmental psychologist of the 20th century. His cognitive-developmental theory tied together maturation and experience with cognitive and social development. Piaget developed his theoretical stages by observing his own children and also by testing larger populations. He continues to be one of the most researched theorists on child development (Grotberg, 1977; Kail & Cavanaugh, 2000).

The Purpose of Developmental Assessments

Assessment is the process of gathering information for the purpose of making evaluative decisions. The assessment or tool used in evaluation is dependent on the type of decisions that need to be made. Developmental assessment is a process designed to understand a child's performance in areas of occupation specific to activities of daily living (ADLs), education, play, and social participation. Age–appropriate developmental milestones have been established to compare a child's competencies and resources in performance skills such as motor and cognitive processing skills, communication/interaction skills and performance patterns that are the habits, routines, and roles most likely to help a child make full use of his or her developmental potential.

The caregiving and learning environments that the child is exposed to also influence the context or interrelated conditions that promotes performance (AOTA, 2002). Developmental milestones give general ideas about how a child is functioning, but there is variability among children. Walking can begin as early as 9 months or be as late as 15 months and both milestones are considered age appropriate. While developmental guidelines should be used as a general rule, it is also important to understand that and early or faster development is not necessarily considered better development (Oesterreich, 1995).

According to Katz, (1997), an early childhood educator, developmental assessment serves the following purposes:

- To determine progress on significant developmental achievements.
- To make placement or promotion decisions.
- To diagnose learning and teaching problems.
- To help in instruction and curriculum decisions.
- To serve as a basis for reporting to parents.
- To assist a child with assessing his or her own progress.

The Zero to Three National Center for Clinical Infant Programs (1994), a health model, identifies that developmental assessments may be performed in order to:

- Identify children who are likely to be members of groups at risk for health or developmental problems (screenings).
- Confirm the presence and extent of a disability by a physician (diagnosis).
- Determine appropriate remediation (program planning or intervention).
- Ascertain a child's relative knowledge of specific skills and information (readiness tests).
- Demonstrate the extent of a child's previous accomplishments (achievement tests).

According to the *Occupational Therapy Practice Framework*, the extent to which an occupational therapy assistant (OTA), working under the supervision of an occupational therapist (OT), participates in an evaluation situation is based on established service competencies (AOTA, 2002). In determining competencies needed to evaluate the development of children, the OT and OTA should understand how development transpires, should recognize that child development is complex, and how biological and environmental influences can facilitate or impede the development of infants and young children (Zero to Three, 1994).

Introduction to Various Developmental Assessments

It is important to address the purpose of the developmental assessment when selecting an instrument or tool. The items or behaviors assessed should have demonstrable relationships to significant human functioning and personal meaning (Katz & Chard, 1996). Assessment of child development should be an ongoing collaborative process of systematic observations and analysis. Assessment of child development can occur in two stages, gathering an occupational profile, and analyzing occupational performance (AOTA, 2002).

The first step in the evaluative process is to develop an Occupational Profile, which describes the child's occupational history, patterns of living, interests, values, and needs. In determining the Occupational Profile of a young child, one must also identify the child's needs, wants and concerns regarding his/her engagement in occupations (Youngstrom, 2002). Since young children cannot always reliably articulate their needs, interests, and values, it is important for the OTA, under the supervision of an OT to observe the child's selection of occupations through play. It is also important to interview the parent or primary caregiver to interpret the needs and wants of the child. Table 8-1 provides examples of how to obtain information for an Occupational Profile.

The next step in the evaluation process is to analyze Occupational Performance. It is important to identify underlying factors that support and hinder performance.

- Observe performance.
- Perform selected specific assessments as needed.
- Consider context, activity demands and client factors.
- Identify child's strengths and weaknesses (Youngstrom, 2002; AOTA, 2002).

Table 8-2 provides examples of specific assessments for analysis of Occupational Performance in children 0 to 5 years.

Decisions related to the selection and purpose of assessments should begin with discussions on information gathering (Occupational Profile) among all stakeholders such as

Table 8-1

Examples of Information Gathering for an Occupational Profile

Occupational History	Interview parent/caregiver using a baby book to gather information on: • developmental milestones • medical history • favorite occupations (play behavior) • favorite toys
Patterns of Living	Interview parent/caregiver about daily routines: • bedtime • eating habits • toileting • dressing behavior • personal hygiene • socialization behavior with siblings, peers, and adults • response to stimulation
Interests	Interview parent/caregiver about • preferred occupations • time spent engaging with occupations • interests in toys or play objects • interest in activities of daily living (ADLs) • interest in socializing with others
Needs	Interview parent/caregiver about concerns and issues regarding his or her interpretation of child's needs. • nurturing needs • security needs • activity level needs
Priorities	Interview parent/caregiver to determine what his or her priorities are for the child's development.
Concerns	Interview the parent/caregiver to determine what concerns he or she has regarding the child's development.

parents, physicians, therapists, educators, and other members of the community.

ADMINISTRATION AND INTERPRETATION OF DEVELOPMENTAL ASSESSMENTS

Developmental assessment is an ongoing process in which qualified professionals, including families, use standardized tests and observations to address a child's development. Areas addressed by developmental assessment include motor, cognitive processing, communication/interaction skills and self-help skills. Qualified professionals identify areas of strength and areas requiring support and intervention following a developmental assessment. Qualified professionals who provide developmental assessments include the following.

An Audiologist is a professional trained in assessing a child's hearing. An audiologist would identify any hearing impairment or loss by placing earphones on a child and transmitting sounds and frequencies. Audiologists work closely with speech pathologists on communication problems.

A Child Psychologist is a psychologist who has specialized training in developmental assessment of infants and toddlers. A child psychologist would administer standardized tests that address social, emotional, and cognitive development. A child psychologist may observe the child during free play (play-based assessment) and involve the caregiver or family as part of the assessment.

A Child Development Specialist is a professional that is trained in infant/toddler development and in identifying developmental delays and disabilities. A child developmental specialist would identify strengths and weaknesses and develop strategies to promote optimal social, emotional, and cognitive development.

An Early Childhood Special Educator is a professional trained in young children's typical and atypical development. An early childhood special educator assists in developing plans and implementing intervention services based on outcomes of the evaluation/assessment.

An Early Interventionist is a person who works with infants and young children who have demonstrated developmental delays, disabilities, or are at risk of developmental problems. Early interventionists may have different kinds of

Table 8-2

Examples of Developmental Assessments for Analysis of Occupational Performance, Ages 0-14

Assessment Measured	Performance Skills	Activity Demands	Age Range
Ages & Stages Questionnaires, Western Psychological Corporation	Interview of parent or caregiver on: Communication skills Gross motor Fine motor Problem solving Personal-Social	None	0-5 and completed by parent at 2- to 6-month intervals
HELP (Hawaii Early Learning Profile), VORT Corporation	Cognitive Language Gross motor Fine motor Self-help	Space Demands Social Demands Sequencing and Timing Body Demands	0-3 years
Peabody Developmental Motor Scales (PDMS-2) (Folio and Fewell, 2000)	Reflexes Stationary (static) Locomotion (dynamic) Object Manipulation Grasping Visual-Motor Integration	Space Demands Social Demands Sequencing and Timing Body Demands	0-5 years
Southern California Ordinal Scales of Development (1985) Western Psychological Services	Cognition Communication Social Affective/Behavior Practical/Abilities Gross Motor Fine Motor	Space Demands Social Demands Sequencing and Timing Body Demands	0-5 years
Bayley Scales of Infant Development (Bayley, 1993)	Mental Scale Motor Scale Behavior Scale	Space Demands Social Demands Sequencing and Timing Body Demands	1-42 months
Mullen Scales of Early Learning (1997) Western Psychological Corporation	Cognitive Motor Language Visual Perception	Space Demands Social Demands Sequencing and Timing Body Demands	1-5 years
Early Coping Inventory (1988) Scholastic Testing Service, Inc.	Observation of Coping Behavior in Everyday Living - sensorimotor organization - reactive behavior - self-initiated behavior	Space Demands Social Demands Sequencing and Timing Body Demands	4-36 months
Test of Sensory Functions in Infants (TSFI) (1991) Western Psychological Corporation	Adaptive Motor Functioning Visual Tactile Integration Ocular Motor Control Reactivity to Vestibular Stimulation Reactivity to Deep Tactile Pressure	Space Demands Sequencing and Timing Body Demands	4-18 months
Miller Assessment for Preschoolers (1982) Western Psychological Corporation	Sensory and Motor Cognitive Complex Tasks Language	Space Demands Social Demands Sequencing and Timing Body Demands	2-5 years

Table 8-2 (continued)

Examples of Developmental Assessments for Analysis of Occupational Performance, Ages 0-14

Assessment Measured	Performance Skills	Activity Demands	Age Range
Developmental Profile II (DP II) Western Psychological Corporation	Physical Age Self-Help Age Social Age Academic Age Communication Age	Parent or Therapist Report	0-9 years
Bruininks-Oseretsky Test of Motor Proficiency Western Psychological Services	Gross Motor Fine Motor Visual Motor	Space Demands Social Demands Sequencing and Timing Body Demands	4.5-14.5 years
Developmental Test of Visual Perception (DVPT-2) Western Psychological Corporation	Eye-Hand Coordination Spatial Relations Figure Ground Visual Motor Speed Position in Space Copying Visual Closure Form Constancy	Social Demands Sequencing and Timing	4-9 years

professional training such as occupational therapy, speech pathology, or nursing, but have special training in helping children and their families.

An Occupational Therapist/Occupational Therapy Assistant is a professional who has specialized training in evaluating a child's age-appropriate development in motor skills, process skills, or communication/interaction skills that aid in occupational performance. Occupational performance for young children involves "activities of everyday life" such as self-help, education, play, and social interaction skills (Youngstrom, 2002). An occupational therapist/assistant would also observe how a child responds to sensory feedback from the environment (sensory integration).

A Pediatric Nurse Practitioner is a registered nurse with specialized post-graduate training in providing ongoing care for the child in both health (well-child visits) and illness. Their training often includes significant attention to child behavior and development.

A Pediatrician is a medical doctor who has specialized training in caring for the physical health and development of children.

A Physical Therapist is a professional trained to assess the ability and quality of the child's use of their legs, arms, and complete body by encouraging the display of specific motor tasks as well as observing the child at play.

A Public Health Nurse is a nurse who is specially trained to provide care, usually in the home, to families. They often have a strong background in social work skills and child and family development.

A Speech and Language Pathologist is a professional who is trained in assessing and treating problems in communica-

tion including expressive and receptive language (Zero to Three, 2003).

THE ROLE OF THE OT AND OTA IN DEVELOPMENTAL ASSESSMENT

Young children are notoriously poor test-takers (Katz, 1997) and there is evidence that the younger the child being assessed, the more errors are made (Shepard, 1994). Since younger children make more performance errors, they are at risk for being assigned false labels. Once labels have been assigned for academic placement purposes, it is very difficult to remove them. Awareness of potential errors of each evaluation can minimize errors in interpretation.

Young children are difficult to assess because of their activity level, distractibility, attention span, and inconsistent performance in unfamiliar environments (Vacc & Ritter, 1995). Current trends in assessment of young children are moving away from a "single-assessment" model to test environments in more naturalistic settings with family members present. The "Context" of the surrounding environment that the child is tested in influences performance. "Context", according the Occupational Therapy Practice Framework, (2002) includes the cultural, physical, social, personal, spiritual, temporal, and virtual environment that impacts the child during the assessment process.

The role of the OT, and OTA, depending on established service competency, state, and facility guidelines in developmental assessment is to identify underlying factors that support and hinder occupational performance. Following attainment of data on an Occupational Profile, the OT analyzes occupational performance. The first step in the analysis of occupational performance is to "observe performance." Informal, relaxed settings where the child can be at ease are recommended when conducting an informal observation. Parents or caregivers should be present to address factors that could affect a child's performance such as cultural differences, language barriers, accessibility to books and toys, and the child's opportunity to interact with other children. Assessing a child within the context of his or her community and the interacting social systems, and taking into account the families needs, resources, and concerns affect both the evaluation and possible interventions. One of the most effective ways to assess a child in a naturalistic environment is play-based assessment (Linder, 1993). The combination of informal play-based assessment and more directed and structured activities provide a greater opportunity to observe a high level of performance (Bagnato & Neisworth, 1994).

Following observation of motor, cognitive processing, and communication/interaction skills, the OTA may perform specific assessments if merited under the supervision of an OT.

Current trends in the assessment of young children include a move from norm-referenced to criterion-referenced tests. An ideal developmental evaluation of a child includes tests of cognitive processing with other measures such as assessment of social and motor skill development.

Criterion-references tests allow each child to be assessed as an individual and compared to developmental milestones, thus allowing the OT to select areas to reinforce through interventions specifically tailored to the child. Several of the developmental assessments highlighted on Table 8-2 are criterion-referenced tests.

Concurrent with determining the "context" in which the test will be administered, the test selection should address the activity demands and client factors that may impact the outcome of the evaluation. The "activity demands" of an assessment include the objects, space, social demands, sequencing or timing, required actions, and required underlying body functions and structures needed to perform the assessment (AOTA, 2002). Norm-referenced or standardized tests often ignore the activity demands related to testing and neglect to consider the variability among children's performance. Some children may need a longer period of time to complete an assessment activity while others may need more verbal feedback from the OT practitioner. Standardized tests follow strict administrative protocols that typically do not accommodate for the activity demands of an assessment.

"Client factors" must also be considered when performing developmental assessments. Client factors include body functions and structures needed when carrying out an activity/occupation. Body functions and structures encompass mental, sensory, movement, communication, and physiological systems. Body functions and structures are the underlying supports for engagement in occupation to support participation (AOTA, 2002). A primary goal of developmental assessment is to determine a client's strengths and weaknesses based on developmental milestones attained in mental functioning, sensory processing, communication skills, and movement-related abilities. Age-appropriate skills performance is a result of the successful transactions between the child's body functions/structure, the demands of the activity, and the context in which the performance occurs (Youngstrom, 2002).

Summary

The role of the OT and OTA in developmental assessment is to determine how to facilitate engagement in occupation to support participation in meaningful life activities/occupations. Based on a best practice model, synthesis of information gained from the "Occupational Profile," observation of the child's behavior in a naturalistic environment, and appropriate test selection to analyze occupational performance should lead to delineation of intervention plans.

Case Study

Jane is 12 months old and was referred for an occupational therapy assessment due to concerns regarding her motor, social, and cognitive skills. Jane's mother has indicated that she does not grasp objects well and drops them. She cannot sit unsupported for very long without falling over. She does not laugh, gurgle, or imitate sounds. Jane does not seem to know her own name and does not explore her environment. Jane's mother has two older children and she identified concerns that Jane's development does not seem the same as what she experienced in her older children.

- Organize a method for obtaining an Occupational Profile on Jane.

- Identify how you would set up a structured play environment to obtain information about age-appropriate performance through observation.

- Identify assessment/s that would provide a vehicle to analyze occupational performance. Consider the "activity demands" of the assessment and determine if Jane will be able to overcome the "activity demands" of the assessment.

Application Activities

1. Select a common developmental assessment used in occupational therapy practice (see Table 8-2). Identify what "Client Factors" (body functions and structures) a child would need to successfully complete the assessment. (Refer to the AOTA Practice Framework).

2. Interview a parent of a young child to obtain an occupational history (life experiences, values, interests, previous patterns of engagement in occupations and daily life activities (refer to Table 8-1).

3. Observe a child at play and identify the child's performance in desired occupations noting effectiveness in performance skills (refer to the AOTA Practice Framework).

4. Compare a norm-referenced evaluation with a criterion referenced tool. Identify the "Activity Demands" for each assessment and how they would impact test performance (refer to the AOTA Practice Framework).

5. Identify the perfect "Context" for testing a child who is withdrawn and insecure, a child with a high activity level, and a child who does not tolerate environmental sensory stimulation such as noise and visual stimulation (refer to the AOTA Practice Framework).

6. Assessment Hunt: Investigate various developmental assessments and determine which would be the most comprehensive in identifying strengths and weaknesses in motor, cognitive processing, and communication/interaction skills.

References

American Occupational Therapy Association. (2002). Occupational therapy practice framework: Domain and process. *American Journal of Occupational Therapy, 56*, 609-639.

Bagnato, S. J. & Neisworth, J. J. (1994). A national study of the social and treatment "invalidity" of intelligence testing for early intervention. *School Psychology Quarterly, 9*, 81-102.

Bel Geddes, J. (1997). *Childhood and children: A compendium of customs, superstitions, theories, profiles, and facts*. Phoenix, AZ: Oryx Press.

Greenspan, S. I., & Meisels, S. (1994). *Toward a new vision for developmental assessment of infants and young children*. Arlington, VA: Zero to Three National Center for Clinical Infant Programs.

Grotberg, E. (1977). *200 years of children*. Washington, DC: U.S. Department of Health, Education, and Welfare, Office of Human Development, Office of Child Development.

Kail, R. V., & Cavanaugh, J.C. (2000). *Human development: A lifespan view*. Belmont, CA: Wadsworth /Thompson Learning.

Katz, L. G. (1997) A developmental approach to assessment of young children. ERIC.EECE Clearinghouse on Elementary and Early Childhood Education. Retrieved from:
http://ericps.ed.uiuc/eece/pubs/digests/1997/katz97.html

Katz, L. G., & Chard, S. C. (1996). *The contribution of documentation to the quality of early childhood education*. ERIC Digest. Urbana, IL: ERIC Clearinghouse on Elementary and Early Childhood Education. ED 3293 608.

Linder, T. W. (1993). *Transdisciplinary play-based assessment: A functional approach to working with young children*. Baltimore, MD: Paul H. Brookes.

National Network for Child Care-NNCC (1995). Ages and stages: Individual differences. In L. Oesterreich, B. Holt, & S. Karas (Eds.), *Iowa family child care handbook* (pp.191-192.) Ames, IA: Iowa State University Extension.

Ratcliff, N. (1995). The need for alternative techniques for assessing young children's emerging literacy skills. *Contemporary Education, 66*, 169-171.

Shepard, L. A. (1994). The challenges of assessing young children appropriately. *Phi Delta Kappan, 76*, 206-212.

Youngstrom, M. J. (2002). *The occupational therapy practice framework: Domain & process*. Presentation by the American Occupational Therapy Association Commission on Practice.

Vacc, N. A., & Ritter, S. H. (2002). ERIC Digests. Assessment of preschool children. Retrieved January 14, 2002, from http://www.ericfacility.net/ericdigests/ed389964.html.

The Zero National Center for Clinical Infant Programs: Three New Visions for Parents Work Group, Frequently used terms in developmental assessment. Retrieved January 14, 2003. from:
http://www.zerotothree.org/glossary.htm.

Chapter 9

INTERACTING WITH FAMILIES

Darragh Callahan, EdD

Chapter Objectives

- Gain an understanding of a variety of the family situations and living arrangements an occupational therapy assistant may encounter in his/her work with young children.
- Recognize the contexts and role of the occupational therapy assistant in the facilitation of developmental skills with young children.
- Understand the impact attachment has on an individual as it develops in his/her earliest life experiences.
- Recognize varying styles of parenting that can affect the dynamics between parents and the children an occupational therapy assistant may encounter in his/her work.
- Obtain ideas for strategies to use in working with families and their child(ren).

Introduction

As an Occupational Therapy Assistant (OTA) working with young children, you will be interacting with families as well as individual children. This chapter will provide information that reinforces and expands your knowledge base for working with families and their young child(ren). To guide and support you in your work with families it is useful to have some knowledge of the contexts (AOTA, 2002) that influence the family system. These contexts also have a profound influence upon the child's behavior and performance outcomes.

Coming into the world presents many challenges for the newborn child who has previously enjoyed the comfort and protection of its mother's womb. One needs to understand the complexities involved between a young child and his/her primary caregiver upon the child's entry into the vast environment outside the womb and the bond that begins to build between the caregiver and child. Once entry is made into the world there are a multitude of environments and family types into which a child is born or placed. Your role as an OTA will put you into encounters with children who may or may not be accepting of new and unfamiliar situations in their environment. This chapter will provide a focus on the connection that begins to build between the caregiver and the child regardless of living environments and caring arrangements.

Parenting style is an element to consider when you meet new families. The parenting styles individuals implement are usually those with which they are most comfortable or familiar. In your work with families, one approach to parenting may appear to be better than another. However, you should be concerned with understanding the dynamics of the family rather than judging the situation (Bruch, 1974). If your style of working with a child contradicts with an existing situation, you may have to make adjustments in your treatment approach. Understanding and respecting various parenting styles is necessary for implementing effective treatment strategies for parents to use in order to provide carry-over in your absence.

A sampling of family types (Fields & Casper, 2000) is provided in this chapter to enable you, as an OTA, to develop strategies to support your work with young children. Understanding familial and parenting style differences are essential for effective treatment. This understanding also

Table 9-1

Bowlby's Phases of Infants' Experience in Developing Attachment

Phase	Age	Description
I	Birth to 1-2 months	Babies do not distinguish between attachment figures and others
II	1-2 months to 6-7 months	Babies can visually distinguish different attachment figures
III	6-7 months to 2-3 years	Attachment figure(s) are specific and lasting
IV	2-3 years and older	Two directional attachment exists

supports objectivity and tolerance of the range of diversity found within any society.

Your verbal and nonverbal interactions with parents, family members, and children can help to encourage a healthy and supportive therapy milieu. These interactions are the base upon which you build your therapeutic relationship. The final section of this chapter provides some information to reflect upon when you are visiting with a family and its child(ren). We begin by discussing a child's first relationship experience, the attachment connection.

Attachment

Attachment is a potent factor in an infant's development. It occurs not only with the primary giver, usually the mother, but also with other primary important care-giving people in the newborn's world such as the father, grandparent, or child care provider. Honig (2002) refers to attachment as a term that "…describes a strong emotional bond between a baby or young child and a caring adult who is part of the child's everyday life…" (p. 2). A baby is not born with a strong attachment to its mother; rather it develops later on during the baby's early life as a result of consistent caregiving. There are critical times when attachment develops and it is beneficial to know how you, as an OTA working with young children, fit into that developmental progression (Table 9-1). Attachment behavior and the development of attachment connections continue throughout a child's development into adulthood. To better understand the importance of attachment, it is useful to study the history and developmental progression of the theory.

John Bowlby developed the *Theory of Attachment* (Bowlby, 1958) during a time when theories put forward by ethologists (Charles Darwin and followers) and psychoanalysts (Sigmund Freud and followers) were being hotly debated (please refer to Chapter 7: An Overview of Early Development). Born in 1907 in England, Bowlby studied medicine but changed his focus to ethology (the study of animal behavior) after working in an institution and observing some 24 maladjusted children (Holmes, 1993). The difficulties these children faced were being addressed under a

psychoanalytic frame of reference with minimal impact. Instead, Bowlby recognized the importance of the early experiences of very young children and believed that direct and introspective observation was key to understanding behavior. Through observation and theorization, he recognized the impact that the surrounding environment had on a child and the reciprocal interaction that the two had on one another.

Bowlby supported the idea that the effects of separation of an infant from the environment of its mother's womb at birth needed to be studied more closely. He also recognized that studying and becoming familiar with ethology helped him to better understand the nature of the mother/child connection. Bowlby described certain behaviors naturally endowed to babies presumed to support their survival—behaviors such as crying, smiling, clinging to a caregiver, lifting arms in an effort to be picked up, and crawling——as an attempt to "train" their caregivers to be responsive to their needs. Bowlby's work focused on the strong attachment to the primary caregiver and the child's intense response to separation in which he/she grieves and mourns the mother's separation for as long as the mother is unavailable.

Mary Ainsworth (1973) used Bowlby's theory as a means to study and classify types of attachment connections between mother and baby. Her work with Ugandan mothers led her to observe two broad types of attachment: secure and insecure. She collaborated with Bowlby in providing an outline of modern attachment theory that consolidated her findings and his theory. Ainsworth is perhaps best known for her work in assessing the security of a child's attachment in which she observed the response of infants to an unfamiliar environment with and without the mother present. This procedure, referred to as the Strange Situation (Ainsworth, Blehar, Waters, & Wall, 1978), led Ainsworth to identify three patterns of attachment. In the 1980s, Mary Main and Judy Solomon (1986) identified another pattern of insecure attachment called disorganized. The four patterns of infant/child attachment are outlined in Table 9-2.

When you are working with children in their home, early intervention facility, school, or in a clinical setting, initially you will be the unfamiliar person in the child's environment.

Table 9-2
Ainsworth's Patterns of Attachment

Pattern	Description
Secure attachment	Baby may or may not show distress when attachment figures leaves, responds to comforting, but is happy to see attachment figure return.
Avoidant	Baby shows no distress when attachment figure leaves and is indifferent when attachment figure returns—a form of an insecure attachment.
Resistant or ambivalent	Baby shows great distress in anticipation of attachment figure leaving, continues distress when attachment figure leaves, and wants to be picked up when attachment figure returns but continues distress behavior—a form of an insecure attachment.
Disorganized	Baby does not fit into any of the above insecure patterns. These babies act in unpredictable ways and do not seem to have any consistent strategy for dealing with stress and attachment.

Being aware of the difficulties a child may be encountering due to attachment issues is important when working with children and their families/caregivers.

Parenting Styles

It will be helpful in your work with children and their parents/caregivers and to be aware of parenting styles, as these have a direct impact on the dynamics that exist within a family. In her research on parenting, Baumrind (1968; 1971; 1992) identified several parenting styles, some considered more effective than others. However, not all parents choose the style of parenting they implement. Many individuals parent in the way they were parented. In some families those participating in the parenting of a child display different parenting styles. A child may adapt accordingly or the inconsistencies may cause many difficulties within the family structure. General parenting styles, as well as inconsistent parenting styles within the family unit may directly or indirectly effect your work with children.

Baumrind (1968; 1971; 1992) discusses four types of parenting styles: authoritarian; authoritative indulgent (also referred to as permissive and nondirective); and uninvolved. Within each category there is a normal range of actions that parents exhibit to control their children and promote social competence. The styles outlined here do not include parenting that is outside the range of normalcy. An extreme in any case extends beyond the boundaries of normal behavior and may be an indicator of dysfunction. Indicators that suggest dysfunction within a family can be a red flag that signals necessary additional help that you are not trained to provide. In such a case you should immediately request support from your supervisor and you should in no way try to address such a situation. Remember that your role is to pro-

vide occupational therapeutic support based upon your professional OTA training.

The *authoritarian* parent is highly demanding of his/her child(ren) S/he expects obedience—often blind obedience, as explanations are not always provided—although clarity of expectations and rules is present. Children are to do something simply because a parent tells them. This parent tends not to be responsive to their child(ren). This parent is also punitive when expectations are not met.

The *authoritative* parent is demanding of his/her child(ren) but sets clear standards supported with explanations. This parent is responsive to the child and open for negotiation. Responsiveness is evident with the authoritative parent. Discipline methods are reasonable and supportive of the child(ren). Appropriate choices are available. Baumrind found that children who experience this parenting style exhibit more positive outcomes in terms of their social interactions, acceptable behavior, confidence level, and emotional regulations.

The *indulgent* parent does not make demands of the child. This parent is responsive but sometimes to a fault. The parent avoids confrontations, often giving in to the demands of the child. Permissiveness is observed in this parenting style. Indulgent parents are often immature and lack parenting skills in general.

The *uninvolved* parent has low demands of their child(ren) and exhibits little responsiveness. This parent is often simply neglectful.

A young child constantly tests boundaries with surrounding adults and learns quickly where these are. These boundaries are, in part, established by parenting styles. Knowing the complexities that can arise as a result of the parenting style a child experiences may help expand your understanding of the family situation and is contributive to fine tuning the therapy for a particular child.

Families

Asked to provide a description of the typical family today, several things may come to mind. The reflection of one's own family provides a filtered lens for an initial response. The contexts that influence the family system discussed earlier is one frame of reference to consider. In fact there may be as many descriptions of the family system as the number of individuals who are asked the question. Everyone has a different perspective. However, there is specific information about families that is helpful to know if your work requires you to interact with a variety of families and their children. While the following information will not provide you with a description of every type of family, it will offer some ideas of the variety of models that exist in today's society.

All family members sharing the young child's home contribute directly and indirectly to the social, emotional, physical, and cognitive development of that child. When working with families it is also important to be aware of the contexts or environments that affect development, as your work will be influenced by each of the contexts that apply to the child and his family at any given time and in any given situation. There are seven contexts that have been identified by occupational therapy practitioners (AOTA, 2002). They include the physical, cultural, social, personal, spiritual, temporal, and virtual contexts or environments. Detailed information on contexts may be found in Chapter 7: An Overview of Early Development. A short summary of each follows:

- The *physical context* refers to those things the child encounters through the five senses—touch, smell, taste, sound, or sight (AOTA, 2002).

- *Cultural context* includes patterns of group behavior based, in part, on customs, beliefs, rituals and societal expectations (AOTA, 2002).

- *Social context* includes the connections and routines that children develop with other people (AOTA, 2002).

- *Personal context* encompasses demographic specific factors such as a child's gender, age, socioeconomic, and educational status (AOTA, 2002).

- *Spiritual context* encompasses the inner resources that motivate and encourage a child to attain goals and offer a sense of purpose (AOTA, 2002).

- *Temporal context* refers to the aspects of time and place, and their influence on performance and development (AOTA, 2002).

- *Virtual context* refers to the technological avenues that children may use to communicate (AOTA, 2002).

Collectively, these seven contexts strongly influence a child and his/her family/caregivers' lives and impact the way that therapy services are provided.

Dramatic changes that have occurred within the American family over the past 40 or 50 years serve as an example of changing societies throughout the world. Changes in the American family may be more or less rapid and dramatic than in other nations because of a variety of factors including economic opportunities, family ties, political tensions, and war. While the ever-increasing global community may result in more dramatic change, and conversely, less difference among nations in the future, the variety of family types that occur and will evolve continues.

Reflecting back to American society five decades ago, the chances that an individual was raised in a two-parent family were over 85% and the majority of two-parent families consisted of the child's two biological parents. Today the percentage of two-parent families has been reduced to just over 55% (Fields & Casper, 2000). In addition, growing numbers of other family types—such as single parent, blended, foster, and extended families—are contributing to the changing picture of the American family. Added to the structure of the family is the complexity diversity brings, such as interracial marriages, and the mixing of cultures.

The family picture from a half-century ago reflects that families are doing different things today. Many children live in households where both parents work, and these children spend many of their waking hours in a child care situation outside of their home. The advance of technology is another factor that has had an enormous influence on the American family. Children have access to television, computers, and other electronic devices never before imagined. While today there are many more opportunities for children to learn in ways previously unavailable to them, there are also more and more restrictions placed upon them. For example, the advancement in computer and other technologies puts information into our homes and environment with great rapidity while putting individuals at risk in terms of their own identity and subjecting them to unwanted or offensive information. The fears and pressures from outside the family and its community, for example, increased crime, abductions, and terrorism, have contributed to yet other changes in the way the family does business.

A good place to begin a discussion about specific family types is to look at one country's demographics, in this case the United States, as demographic data provides a helpful source of information regarding the diversity of families that exist, the situations from whence they come, and where they are located. Hodgkinson (2003) has been looking at demographic trends in the United States and presents the following information. Looking at the economic demographics we find that one American child in five grows up in poverty. Further, today, one's economic status is often the predictor of success or failure in schools. Interestingly, with the exception of two-parent families, different types of families in each economic strata are growing, which, in turn, may influence a child's educational outcomes. In contrast, fifty years ago, ethnic background was the prominent factor for determining success or failure in American schools. (Hodgkinson, 2003). Based on this demographic information, the following section examines several types of families identified in today's society.

DUAL PARENT FAMILIES

In the 1970s, approximately 85% of the family types were identified as two-parent families as compared to just over 70% today. Of this 70%, today about 56% are family types represented by the presence of two biological parents. The balance (of the 70%) consists of blended and adoptive parent families (Hodgkinson, 2003).

Blended families are growing in number as the divorce rate increases and as the number of single, divorced, and widowed parents remarry. Adopted children are included in the characterization of blended families. Gay and lesbian couples are also joining the group of blended and adoptive families. The new combination of families often brings together new siblings. While the economic situation may improve as a result of joining incomes, there are many other difficult adjustments children face: a new household, a new neighborhood, different schools or child care arrangements, a requirement to share space they once had to themselves, and sharing the attention of their parent with a new spouse and/or other children.

Children are not always able to understand these new situations and may perceive one parent favoring the new siblings more. Children are not always able to understand why they have to leave their old surroundings or permit others into theirs on a permanent basis. In a situation of divorce or death, young children may see themselves as being the reason for the separation or loss. It becomes imperative that both parents in a blended family clarify their roles with their new and existing children. While there can be many benefits of the new situation, there can also be many difficulties which may negatively influence a child's communication, interaction and process skills (AOTA, 2002).

SINGLE PARENT FAMILIES

Reports of single parent families have doubled in the past three decades (Fields & Casper, 2000). Approximately 25% of all children in America now fall into this category (Fields & Casper, 2000). Single parenthood often results in additional stress placed on the custodial parent. If the parent is single as a result of divorce, there often was a period of additional emotional turmoil present in the family and consequent unresolved issues among all involved. Parental stresses may directly or indirectly influence children involved in a family system change from dual parent to single parent status.

In single parent homes, many of the responsibilities assumed by two are rolled into one job description. This creates a heavy burden for the single parent and can be complicated by the fact that a situation that was once supported by two incomes is now left to only one. While in some cases child support may be available, in many situations that simply does not make up for the additional responsibilities assumed by the remaining parent.

MULTIGENERATIONAL OR EXTENDED FAMILIES

Today, multigenerational families are becoming more common. These are families where more than two generations of the family live together. It includes grandparents, aunts, uncles, and cousins. In these situations everyone contributes to raising the child.

Some Native Americans have long enjoyed a multigenerational family model. In a Native American Pueblo community it is not unusual to have all family and related community members participating in a child's upbringing. Unlike some situations today, this family type did not evolve based solely on economic considerations, but rather from traditional practices and survival. Some multigenerational families do, however, live together for economic reasons. For example, coming to America from another country, some immigrants may find it necessary to live with relatives until the family obtains work, housing, and the social confidence to live in a strange and new world. This situation has potential for stress especially if there are a lot of children involved. Grandparents, aunts, uncles and cousins often provide both welcome and unwelcome advice as to how to raise a child. Old traditions mix with new ideas—some are a good recipe, others are not.

INTERRACIAL AND INTERCULTURAL FAMILIES

Interracial and intercultural families are situations where parents are from different racial, cultural, and/or ethnic groups. Going back to the discussion of demographics, Hodgkinson (2003) finds "two major shifts in our thinking about race brought about by changes in Census 2000 – first, the blurring of racial lines... second, ...the increased preference for national origin over race..." (p. 5) as evidenced in the clustering of cultural groups, such as the Chinese, the Japanese, and the Koreans. Although cultural clustering occurs, more and more interracial marriages occur today. This is in contrast to the turn of the 19th century when European groups clustered as cultural groups and as the century moved on, their cultural groups intermarried. For instance, Italians married Irish, and Germans married Polish. Today roughly 15% of those early European immigrants are Irish/Irish, German/German, Polish/Polish (Hodgkinson, 2003). The remaining generations of European Americans are of mixed cultural ancestry. Although it was uncommon during a good part of the 19th century that a European American would marry a person of African or Asian ancestry and vice-versa, today more and more are joining the ranks of mixed racial ancestry (Hodgkinson, 2003). The challenges and joys experienced by these families are an interesting one as a true blending occurs by bringing together race, culture, and ethnicity.

HOMELESS FAMILIES

Currently, the number of homeless families with children is on the rise (U.S. Conference of Mayors, 1998). Poverty, coupled with lack of affordable housing, is the primary cause of homelessness. Changes in welfare programs have also forced families into homelessness. The added problems of alcohol, drugs, and abuse that create dysfunctional situations overwhelming one's ability to responsibly maintain a job or home may also cause one to become homeless. Approximately one third of homeless people work, but at minimum wage, do not bring in enough salary for rent. Ironically, many families who leave the welfare rolls by obtaining work lose housing subsidies and become homeless as a result (Children's Defense Fund, 1998; National Coalition for the Homeless, 2001). Abusive home situations also cause a number of spouses to leave the living situation with their children, thus forcing them to look for alternative housing. These single parent families frequently join the ranks of the homeless.

The wait for public housing is approximately 28 months, forcing more families to "remain in shelters or inadequate housing arrangements longer. Consequently, there is less shelter space available for other homeless families, who must find shelter elsewhere or live on the streets" (National Coalition for the Homeless, 2001).

The consequences of being homeless have a negative impact on all involved. Children in these situations are especially vulnerable. The unhealthy situations put children at a high risk for a variety of global developmental delays, including physical, cognitive, and social emotional difficulties.

TEENAGE PARENTS

Teenage parents experience a number of difficulties relating to immaturity, they themselves are still children, often unable to finish high school and unable to obtain adequate wages to properly care for themselves and their children. The children in these families are also put at risk as the young parents grip with the realities of growing up themselves. While parents of the teenage parents may step in to help and provide assistance, there are emotional difficulties and other problems, such as economic ones that surface due to the overwhelming responsibility required for raising a child. Pregnancy creates an increased health risk for the teen carrying the baby and often confounds things with adolescent behavior associated with poor nutritional habits. In addition, it is also found that with teen pregnancy less atten-

tion is given to prenatal and postnatal care (National Institutes of Health, 2002).

ADOPTIVE FAMILIES/FOSTER FAMILIES

Children adopted at birth or very shortly thereafter often achieve the developmental milestones at the same rate as children raised by their biological families. However, there can be difficulties if the adopted child has not had the opportunity to experience a healthy attachment connection with the primary caregiver or has not had extensive experiences at a critical stage of development (please refer to Chapter 7: An Overview of Early Development) when living in a dysfunctional home situation. In such cases problems may be evident at the time of adoption or may show up at a later stage of development dependent on previously acquired social, emotional, cognitive, or physical development skills. Further, and when there is little medical history available to document any potential problems, adoptive children may have heredity conditions that are not present at the time of adoption, which may develop into unexpected problems later in life.

Children in foster homes are already in a difficult situation as this is a temporary condition and may not be under the best of circumstances. Temporary families are recruited by social service agencies for placement of a child while a home situation is being resolved or adoptive parents are being sought. Often children are placed into foster homes over and over again and may grow to adulthood in one or a variety of foster homes. In these situations the child is never a permanent family member. While the rate of adoptions of foster children has been increasing during the past decade (Children's Defense Fund, 2001), many remain without permanent homes.

IMMIGRANT FAMILIES

Families leave their native country to relocate in foreign countries for a variety of reasons including: war, economics, education, job relocation, and political asylum. Many of these families arrive in a foreign country knowing very little about their new surroundings. There are clusters of immigrant families throughout the United States. The values and traditions of immigrant families provide meaning for them and can be difficult to maintain in a new country. For instance, acquiring the language of the surrounding society is necessary for comfortable entry into social systems such as schools, jobs, and medical facilities. There can be resistance or lack of acceptance of immigrant families for a variety of reasons that may not be recognized by 'native' (less recent immigrants) individuals and, consequently, discussed or addressed in inappropriate ways. A number of factors lead to resentment on the part of 'native' populations towards immigrants. These factors may include miscommunication due to language barriers, perceived loss of job opportunities, and/or intolerance or lack of understanding of religious differences. This creates an undue amount of stress for immigrant families. It is important to recognize the effect of this divisiveness on parents and their children. Socially, intellectually, emotionally, and physically, school may prove to be a particularly difficult environment for immigrant children.

Caregiver-Child Relationship

In your role as an OTA, you will be interacting with a wide range of family types. Parenting styles, attachment issues, the family type, and the contexts that influence the child's behavior may support or interfere with your work. It is important to understand the many factors that influence the variety of situations you will encounter in your work with children. However, it is more important to recognize the fact that you are not in your field to change the family structure to represent what you think should be the ideal family. Rather, you are there to help a family and child cope with their situation and support them through appropriate necessary therapeutic interventions.

When you meet with a family, some ideas and perceptions will be unconsciously formed by both verbal and the often more potent non-verbal behavior patterns that each one of us displays. It is important to reflect upon your interpretations of both the verbal and non-verbal cues and recognize the subtle influences they have on you as a person, as well as an OTA. Some perceptions you may identify as arousing a sense of concern about the situation you find yourself in when working with a child and his/her family/caregiver should not be dismissed. Should these concerns arise, you need to discuss this with your immediate supervisor in a timely manner, especially if there are indicators of abuse or neglect present. In a situation such as this you are required to advocate for the child through appropriate reporting of the situation.

It is also important to recognize a child's strengths in those areas where no therapeutic intervention is indicated. One can use these strengths to help scaffold the assistance the child needs.

Communication

The children you will be working with will range in ability and temperament. Many children may be frustrated, some angry. Parents will also have their agendas. You need to remember that you are there to support the child regardless of the cooperation you obtain. Based on a Family Centered model (please refer to Chapter 2: Foundations of Occupational Therapy and Chapter 4: Collaborative Models of Treatment), learning about the expectations the family and child have before beginning your work can positively influence treatment outcomes. The family/caregivers expectations may be quite different from the goals developed by the OT, or collaboratively by the OT/OTA, so you need to be able to clearly articulate the focus of your work and the potential outcomes for the child. You will also want to provide guidance on how the family can reinforce the work that you do with the child. Remember that your work does not begin and end during one treatment session.

When you first encounter a family, it is helpful to find out a bit about how they like to be addressed (the adults and child involved). Depending upon the age of the child, it can be useful to talk with the child a bit about his/her likes and dislikes. This can put the child at ease and provide you with information about the child. Such inquiries must be sincere, reflect a genuine interest in knowing more about the child, and not be intrusive.

Nonverbal communication during your initial contacts with the family and child are important for both gaining information as well as sending messages to those involved. Become aware of yourself and the information you give nonverbally when talking with others you encounter in your role as OTA. Reflect and think about whether or not this information is consistent with the words you speak.

When possible, observe the family-child interactions during the course of your work. Observation provides information that may be helpful for optimizing the quality of your work. If the family/child interactions are counter-productive to the therapy, you may want to strategize during your reflections and discussions with your supervisor and develop a plan of action that can alter such behavior to more positively influence treatment outcomes.

Summary

This chapter has provided brief snapshots of the myriad of factors that may have an impact on the lives of the children you will be working with. Understanding the complexities involved outside the realm of the skills you develop purely for occupational therapy practice provides a platform to work comfortably and more effectively with families and children you serve.

Your role as an OTA is crucial in helping a child and his/her family work through many difficult issues. While you are not there to resolve everything, the quality of your work contributes to the overall help and support the family receives. You are one of the child's most important advocates.

Case Study

You enter a home to provide therapy to a young child seven years of age. Both parents work full-time and often do not arrive home until seven in the evening. The child's primary caregiver before and after school hours is his grand-mother. The grandmother welcomes you into the home and you explain to her what therapy you will be providing. As you begin your work with the child, the grandmother constantly interferes providing her advice, contrary to what you are doing, and believes you are doing harm to the child. She is from another country and, while she uses English to address you, it is difficult to know how well she understands your explanations. You are also a bit intimidated by her expressions while she takes notes while you are working with the child.

Discuss how this situation could be handled. You need this woman's support but she is adamant that you are not doing anything to help the child. As a future OTA, reflect upon how this can be handled diplomatically.

Application Activities

1. Consider the situation where there are conflicting parenting styles. The mother is authoritative and the father is authoritarian. You want to develop an appropriate course of therapy for the child to be continued when you are not present. Progress towards reaching therapeutic goals is clear but requires patience and time. However, the father feels the child can be "pushed" in order to reach the goals of the therapy whereas the mother feels that the child must be ready to move ahead based upon a pace determined by the child. Discuss your approach and support your choices.

2. The family situation appears dysfunctional and there is a possibility that abusive behavior exists within the environment. You notice that the child has a bruise on his forehead and another on the back side of his hand. Both parents are very defensive of the child's bruises stating that he is clumsy and falls often or bumps into things. When you start working with the child you find that he squints when you begin the therapy. Do you think there is a problem? How would you continue your work?

References

Ainsworth, M. (1973). The development of infant-mother attachment. In B. M. Caldwell & H. N. Riccuiti (Eds.), *Review of child development research*. (Vol. III). Chicago: University of Chicago Press.

Ainsworth, M., Blehar, M., Waters, E., & Wall, S. (1978). *Patterns of attachment*. Hillside, NJ: Lawrence Erlbaum Associates.

Baumrind, D. (1968). Child care practices anteceding three patterns of preschool behavior. *Benetic Psychology Monograph, 75*, 43-88.

Baumrind, D. (1971). Current patterns of parental authority. *Developmental Psychology, 4* (Monograph 1), 1-103.

Baumrind, D (1992). The influence of parenting style on adolescent competence and Substance use. *Journal of Early Adolescence, 11*(1), 56-95.

Bruch, H. (1974). *Learning psychotherapy*. Cambridge, MA: Harvard University Press.

Children's Defense Fund. (2001). *The state of America's children – Yearbook*. Washington, DC: Children's Defense Fund.

Children's Defense Fund and National Coalition for the Homeless. (1998). *Welfare to what: Early findings on family hardship and well-being*. Washington, DC: National Coalition for the Homeless.

Casper, L., & Bryson, K. (1998). *Household and family characteristics: March 1998 (Update), Current population reports*. p. 20-515. Washington, DC: U.S. Census Bureau.

Fields, J., & Casper, L. M. (2001). *America's families and living arrangements. March 2000. Current Population Reports*. p. 20-537. Washington, DC: U.S. Census Bureau.

Hodgkinson, H. (2002). Changing demographics: A call for leadership. In W. Owens & L. Kaplan (Eds.), *Best practices, best thinking, and emerging issues in school leadership*. pp. 3-14. Thousand Oaks, CA: Sage.

Holmes, J. (1993). *John Bowlby and attachment theory: Makers of modern psychotherapy*. Routledge: London.

Honig, A. S. (2002). *Secure relationships: Nurturing infant/toddler attachment in early care settings*. Washington, DC: National Association for the Education of Young Children.

Main, M., & Solomon, J. (1986). Discovery of an insecure disorganized/disoriented attachment pattern: Procedures, findings and implications for classification of behavior. In M. Yogman & T. B. Brazelton (Eds.), *Affective development in infancy*. Norwood, NJ: Ablex, pp. 95-124.

National Coalition for the Homeless. June 2001. Fact Sheet #7. Retrieved November, 2, 2002 from http://www.nationalhomeless.org/families.html

U.S. Conference of Mayors. A Status Report on Hunger and Homelessness in America's Cities: 1998. Washington, DC: U.S. Conference of Mayors. Retrieved October 15, 2002 from http://www.usmayors.org

DIAGNOSES COMMONLY ASSOCIATED WITH CHILDHOOD

Sidney Michael Trantham, PhD

Chapter Objectives

- Introduce major psychological disorders and conditions of childhood.
- Enhance knowledge of normal and abnormal child behavior.
- Increase knowledge of methods of assessing child behavior.

Introduction

The last two decades have shown an increased understanding of the relationship between the brain and behavior. Despite these advances in understanding the brain and behavior, one constant in the field of psychology, and as has been applied to the allied health professions, has been that the earlier a problem is assessed and diagnosed, the greater the opportunity for a healthy adjustment and outcome. Occupational therapy assistants (OTAs) working with the pediatric population are in a unique position of encountering children who may either be diagnosed with a common childhood disorder or are undergoing a psychological evaluation process where *collateral information* and observations may help clarify diagnostic questions. This chapter will briefly review a handful of the most common *neurocognitive*, *neurodevelopmental*, genetic, physical and orthopedic, and acquired diseases, disorders, and syndromes associated with childhood.

Before proceeding to a discussion of diagnoses commonly associated with childhood, it is important to note a valuable tool for OTAs: the *Diagnostic and Statistical Manual of*

Mental Disorders – Fourth Edition, Text Revision, or *DSM-IV-TR*. This text is the diagnostic classification system currently used by most mental health clinicians in the United States, including psychologists, psychiatrists, social workers, and licensed mental health workers. One important aspect of this classification system is the use of a multiaxial assessment approach; that is, examining an individual's functioning in several domains. The DSM-IV-TR's multiaxial approach includes five axis. Axis I is where clinical disorders and other conditions that may be the focus of clinical attention are classified. Axis I might include such disorders as depression, anxiety, or attention based problems. Axis II is where personality disorders are noted. Axis III is where general medical conditions would be listed, such as diabetes, hypothyroidism, or arthritis. Axis IV is where psychosocial and environmental problems are listed; this might include homelessness, unemployment, or discrimination. Finally, Axis V is where a global assessment of functioning occurs. This subjective rating scale ranges from 0 to 100, in which the higher the number the greater the adaptive living abilities and functionality of the individual. While the DSM-IV-TR is not the only way to classify and diagnose behavior and symptoms commonly related to disorders, it is one of the most widely reviewed and researched systems.

It is a unique challenge to have the opportunity to work with children and their family/caregivers who have learned that their child has been diagnosed with a disease, disorder, or syndrome. Part of providing good services involves developing a sense of *empathy* for what children and their parents/caregivers are not only going through now, but also where they have been, and what may lie ahead for them. This chapter provides a brief overview of diagnoses commonly associated with childhood, and ways in which the OTA may support the child and his or her family/caregivers.

Table 10-1

Core Cognitive Areas Disrupted in ADD/ADHD

Inattention

Difficulty focusing, sustaining, shifting; hard time keeping mind on one thing and easily bored after a short time-serious problem focusing deliberate, conscious attention to organizing and completing a task or learning something new is difficult.
Children with primary problems in this area will:
• Be easily distracted
• Fail to attend to details and making careless mistakes
• Not follow instructions carefully and completely
• Frequently lose or forget common things needed regularly (e.g., keys, coat, money, etc.)

Hyperactivity

Constant motion, fidget, excessive talking and *loose associations*, pattern of starting projects but not finishing it.
Children with primary problems in this area will:
• Appear restless, fidgety, squirmy
• Frequently run or climb objects at inappropriate times or without regard to safety, or in a classroom setting leave their seats in situations when asked to sit and be quiet

Impulsivity

Inability to curb immediate reactions, difficulty thinking before acting-may blurt things out inappropriately, do things without thinking of the consequences, trouble delaying gratification (e.g, having trouble waiting when playing games, grabbing toys from other children, etc.). .
Children with primary problems in this area will:
• Blurt out answers before hearing the whole question
• Have difficulty waiting in line or for a turn

Know what areas

Neurocognitive Disorders

ATTENTION DEFICIT DISORDER (ADD) AND ATTENTION DEFICIT HYPERACTIVITY DISORDER (ADHD)

Attention deficit disorder (ADD) and attention deficit hyperactivity disorder (ADHD) are two of the most common neurocognitive problems affecting children and their families/caregivers. ADHD, once referred to as hyperkinesis or minimal brain dysfunction (MBD), has been termed ADHD since the DSM-III-R was published in 1987. Estimates suggest that 3 to 5% of all children (upwards of 2 million) in the United States meet the criteria for this disorder (NIMH, 1994). Research consistently finds that boys are two to three times more likely to be affected by this disorder than girls, and to be diagnosed with ADHD (NIMH, 1994).

It is important to the recognize symptoms of ADD and ADHD and treat them early; *cross-sectional* and *retrospective studies* have consistently found that these symptoms continue into adulthood and that children with these disorders are at greater risk for developing other psychiatric disorders later in life (Doyle, Biederman, Seidman, et al., 2000; NIMH, 1994). The nature of these disorders interferes with a child's ability to adapt and adjust to the myriad of develop-

mental challenges that face all children (Doyle, Biederman, Seidman, et al., 2000; NIMH, 1994).

Children with ADD or ADHD typically exhibit impairments in attention and what are referred to as executive functions; that is, judgment, reasoning, and coordination of complex problem-solving behavior. It is important to note that attention is a complex cognitive skill that involves, for instance, an 11-year-old girl focusing her cognitive abilities on a task such as journal writing, sustaining her cognitive abilities on that task, and being able to shift her cognitive abilities to other tasks. Additionally, given the deficits in these three primary cognitive areas, children with ADD and ADHD often have secondary problems in learning and memory (Table 10-1).

ADHD is diagnosed not just when caregivers and professionals observe the symptoms or document them, but when it is established that the symptoms are excessive (e.g., developmentally inappropriate), long-term (e.g., longer than six months), and pervasive (e.g., a pattern of behaviors that happen inside and outside the home environment, at school and with peers). A thorough assessment should involve multiple sources of information, including psychological testing, neuropsychological evaluation, *behavioral assessment*, review of the child's pattern of academic performance, and history gathering from adults who have regular contact with the child.

Some researchers are beginning to note the limited knowledge about girls with ADHD (Crawford, 2003). This may be due in part to gender-bias involved in referral patterns by parents and teachers as well as the diagnostic criteria for ADHD (Crawford, 2003).

Working under the supervision of an occupational therapist (OT), and within state and facility guidelines, the role of the OTA in working with children with ADD/ADHD may include providing direct services to address attentional issues, and consulting with teachers and parents/caregivers on strategies to structure an effective learning or home environment. Structuring an effective learning environment may include suggestions such as providing multisensory experiences to enhance attention, and suggesting alternative seating options for the child in the classroom. For additional information about ADHD, please refer to Chapter 22: Pediatric Psychosocial Therapy.

Learning Disorders

The neuropsychological study of learning disorders has a relatively brief history dating back to the 1960s (Snyder & Nussbaum, 1998). Learning disorders are often seen as discrete disorders; that is, a specific problem in one area relevant to academic progress such as reading, math or written expression (Rains, 2002). Approximately 20% of the general population experiences some academic difficulties at one time or another, but an estimated 3% to 7% have impairments in learning so significant that learning is seriously compromised (Snyder & Nussbaum, 1998). Estimates suggest 5% to 10% of vocational rehabilitation caseloads include persons with learning disabilities (Snyder & Nussbaum, 1998). While learning disorders have specific areas of deficit and can be traced to central nervous system dysfunction, the cause of the dysfunction is often unknown (Rains, 2002).

Common features that must be present to warrant a classification of learning disorder (as defined by the DSM-IV-TR) include:

1. Failure to achieve in one or more areas of academic proficiency.

2. A documented and severe discrepancy between aptitude and achievement.

3. The presence of associated psychological process disorder.

4. The exclusion of other environmental factors that could affect normal development and thus influence a medical condition such as diabetes, or an emotional problem such as depression.

Three major components comprise a good assessment for learning disorders. They include: *psychoeducational assessment, behavioral assessment,* and *neuropsychological assessment* (Snyder & Nussbaum, 1998, p.143-144). It is important to note that the diagnosis of a learning disorder requires elimination of other possible explanations such as deficient *intellectual functioning*, lack of opportunity to learn, inadequate home environment, poor motivation, or the presence of a sensory deficit (Rains, 2002).

Working under the supervision of an OT, and within state and facility guidelines, the role of the OTA in working with children with learning disabilities may include providing direct services to address visual perceptual or motor challenges, and consulting with teachers and parents/caregivers on strategies to structure an effective learning or home environment. Structuring an effective learning environment may include suggestions such as providing multisensory experiences to support handwriting instruction, developing and implementing a fine motor strengthening program, and suggesting alternative seating options for the child in the classroom. Please refer to Chapter 23: Pediatric Psychosocial Therapy for further review of treatment approaches for learning disorders.

Autism

Diagnoses of autism and the autism spectrum disorders are often very emotionally charged for parents/caregivers. Many will grieve for what might have been in terms of hopes and dreams for their child. It is for this reason that it is particularly important for OTAs to provide feedback (when appropriate) to parents/caregivers that involves realistic report of the child's functioning.

Kanner first described the syndrome that we now refer to as autism in 1943, but Asperger also independently described a cluster of behavioral and relational problems that was also consistent with autism (Rains, 2002; Yirmiya, Erel, Shaked, & Solomonica-Levi, 1998). Autism is not commonly diagnosed until the age of 3, but symptoms almost always begin before 30 months of age (Charman, Swettenham, Baron-Cohen, et al., 1997; Rains, 2002). Some research suggests that as early as 20 months infants with autism display marked impairment in *empathy, joint attention,* and *imitation* as compared to other children (with and without neurocognitive disorders) (Charman et al., 1997). These problems are linked to later developmental problems in social understanding and reciprocal social communication (the characteristic features of autism) (Charman et al., 1997). Charman et al.'s (1997) research suggest that by the end of infancy there are notable differences between children with autism and other developmentally delayed children, including:

- Children with autism do not switch gaze between interesting objects and an adult's face.

- Children with autism do not coordinate emotional responses and gaze in response to an emotional display by an adult.

- Children with autism exhibit impaired imitation ability.

In the second year of life, children develop the nonsocial use of gaze to obtain information about the physical world and production of goal directed play. Infants with autism may exhibit the developmentally appropriate behaviors that go along with functional play, such as goal directed play; which may explain why the disorder may not be discerned earlier in childhood. However, from an eerily early time children with autism show poor coordination of affective response and difficulty with relational play (Charman et al., 1997). For example, they are less likely to combine smiles with eye contact, less likely to smile in response to smiles, and exhibit impaired empathic response.

Autism involves impairment in three areas. These include severe impairment in language (both verbal and nonverbal), failure to develop social relationships, and exhibition of stereotyped or repetitive behaviors, interests, and activities (Rains, 2002). Some research suggests that another significant problem for persons with autism is coordinating affect and attention (Charman et al., 1997). Rains (2002) states that "many children with autism are retarded, and 75% have an IQ below 50" (p. 438). It is important to note, however, that it would be unwise to characterize all children with autism as mentally retarded. Some children (and adults) with autism have normal intelligence or may exhibit a highly specific talent or skill, such as being able to play a song on a musical instrument after hearing it just once, or being able to perform highly complex calculations without paper or pencil. These individuals are often referred to as autistic savants. In the past, the more derogatory and inaccurate term "idiot savant" was used.

It is important to recognize that there is a range or spectrum of autistic and autistic-like behaviors. The problems associated with autism usually last a lifetime; many autistic children grow into severely impaired adults (Rains, 2002). However, some do exhibit improvement in ability to communicate and relate with others. The most current version of the Diagnostic and Statistical Manual (DSM-IV-TR, APA, 2000) categorizes five distinct developmental disorders that involve disruption in language, emotion, and social relational abilities. Those five diagnoses include autism, Rett's disorder, childhood disintegrative disorder, Asperger's syndrome and pervasive developmental disorder not otherwise specified. Children exhibiting higher abilities to communicate (such as adequate language, good ability to observe and respond to nonverbal social cues), minimal social skills, and normal or above normal intellectual functioning are frequently diagnosed as having Asperger's syndrome.

A variety of theories attempting to explain the cause of autism have been proposed. The psychogenic theories were an early attempt at understanding the disorder; these theories often identified the child's parents or some environmental stress as the root cause of the autistic behavior (Rains, 2002). However, after more careful research and evaluation of these theories, there was little evidence found to support them. Current theories suggest the cause of autism to be bio-

logically based (Rains, 2002). There is strong evidence that some forms of autism are inherited; between 2% to 3% of siblings of people with autism are autistic themselves. The concordance rate for monozygotic (identical) twins has been reported as high as 96%, while the concordance rate for dizygotic (fraternal) twins is no higher than that for non-twin siblings (Rains, 2002).

Working within state and facility guidelines and under the supervision of an OT, the role of the OTA in working with children with autism spectrum disorders may include providing direct services to address relevant self-care, work and play skills, as well as providing consultative services to teachers, and families/caregivers to maximize a child's functioning with his/her environment (please refer to Chapter 22: Pediatric Psychosocial Therapy).

MENTAL RETARDATION

Working with families that have a child with mental retardation requires an understanding of not only the child's cognitive limitations but also the parental expectations. Early after learning a child's diagnosis of mental retardation, many parents grieve about what the child might have been and begin the process of accepting the child who is. In addition, while a good psychological evaluation is one in which the child's cognitive strengths and weaknesses are assessed, psychologists often focus on helping parents understand their child's cognitive limitations and related behavior in order to make appropriate plans for the child's future. This is often to the detriment of examining the functional skills of the child. Working within state and facility guidelines and under the supervision of an OT, the OTA may be helpful to families with a child diagnosed with mental retardation by addressing and working with the functional strengths of the child.

To diagnose mental retardation there are two core areas that must be evaluated. Generally, a qualified psychologist carries out an evaluation of this nature. The American Association on Mental Deficiency has established guidelines that require an individual to evidence below average functioning in both intellectual functioning and adaptive behavior in multiple settings in order to be diagnosed with mental retardation (Wechsler, 1991).

The first area that is often evaluated to determine the presence of mental retardation is *intellectual functioning*. While theories of intelligence have varied over the years, many contemporary theories suggest that intelligence should not be defined by just one skill, but by the combination of many different abilities. Currently, the most widely used instrument to measure intellectual functioning is the Wechsler Intelligence Scale for Children, 3rd Edition (WISC-III). Wechsler (1944) put forth the idea that intelligence is "capacity of the individual to act purposefully, to think rationally, and to deal effectively with his or her environment" (p. 3). Thus, this test is primarily a measurement of various aspects of a child's cognitive abilities such as attention, memory, visualspatial and visuomotor skills, perceptual skills, and reasoning. As measured and defined by the WISC-III, *IQ* scores that fall below 70 are classified as "intellectually deficient" (p. 32). It is important to recognize that within this category is a range of intellectual ability.

However, a score below 70 on an intelligence test does not necessarily mean low intellectual functioning (Wechsler, 1991). Low IQ scores may result from extreme cultural impoverishment (such as poor school environment), emotional state at time of testing (including a high level of distractibility, anxiety or depression), or sensory impairments (such as deafness). Such factors must be accounted for prior to diagnosing a child with mental retardation.

The second area evaluated to determine the presence of mental retardation is *adaptive behavior* and *functional skills*. This includes such skills as being able to problem solve everyday dilemmas such as knowing the order of how to put on your sneakers (e.g., first put on socks, then pants, then sneakers, not sneakers then socks then pants). It is the realm of adaptive behavior and functional skills that the OTA addresses most closely when working with children with mental retardation.

FETAL ALCOHOL SYNDROME

One completely preventable childhood disorder is Fetal Alcohol Syndrome (FAS). Fetal Alcohol Syndrome is a disorder that begins during the perinatal phase of fetal developmental. This disorder is seen in children of alcoholic mothers who use alcohol during pregnancy. At birth, these children evidence significant behavioral dysfunction including decreased sleep, body tremors, and decreased physical activity (Rains, 2002). As these children grow older, they exhibit a constellation of significant developmental, physical, and behavioral disorders. FAS is characterized by facial malformations, affective instability, and neurocognitive deficiencies including attention deficits, impulse control problems, and mental retardation (Rains, 2002). Such children can be expected to require a lifetime of intensive caretaking and supervision. Working within state and facility guidelines and under the supervision of an OT, the OTA works with children and family caregivers to support adaptive behavior and functional skills for children with FAS.

Neurodevelopmental Disorders

CEREBRAL PALSY

Cerebral palsy (CP) is a commonly occurring chronic physical disorder (Wannamaker & Glenwick, 1998) whose onset begins in infancy or early childhood. A diagnosis of CP is generally made within a child's first five years of life. Cerebral palsy affects approximately 2 of every 100 live births (Bennett, 2002; Ferreri, 1995). According to Bennett (1999), "cerebral palsy is a nonprogressive disorder of movement and posture" (p. 65) and is "caused by irreversible brain lesions occurring before, during or shortly after birth" (Ferreri, 1995, p. 22). As there is no cure for CP, nor are there prenatal tests available to detect CP, in order to lay the foundation for maximal functional outcomes, early diagnosis and treatment are critical for both the child and his/her family/caregiver.

There are several classifications that describe the associated motor limitations that a child with CP may have. They include the athetoid spectrum which are characterized by fluctuating tone (low to high), the spastic spectrum which describes gradations of high tone, ataxia which refers to slightly elevated tone, and flaccid, which refers to low tone. It is important to note that an infant diagnosed with flaccid CP will later (generally in the toddler or preschool years) develop spastic, athetoid, or ataxic CP. Because CP is a disorder of movement and posture, one of its key characteristics is loss of, or impaired movement patterns and postural mechanisms. Secondarily, children with CP may present with limitations in cognitive skills, social emotional skills, as well as self care skills.

Working within state and facility guidelines and under the supervision of an OT, the role of the OTA in working with children with CP involves a team-oriented approach to providing direct and indirect services to maximize function in the areas of work, play, and leisure, to recommend and implement adapted strategies and appropriate assistive technologies, assist with positioning needs, and provide ongoing family/caregiver education.

SPINA BIFIDA

Spina bifida literally means divided spine. It has been identified as the most common birth defect of childhood that leads to some kind of permanent disability (Barker, Saulino, & Caristo, 2002; Honein, Paulozzi, & Mathews, 2001). Spina bifida is a defect of the neural tube in which one or more vertebrae of the spine do not form properly, causing a gap or opening to occur in the spine. This gap or opening leads to damage to the central nervous system. Damage to the spine leads to loss of function below the level of the lesion, often resulting in paralysis and loss of motor and sensory function, bowel and bladder dysfunction, and for some children, learning and cognitive challenges (Sandler, 1997). In an effort to minimize the damage to the nervous system (and functional capacity), within a day after birth, most infants undergo surgery to close the gap or split (Barker, Saulino, & Caristo, 2002).

The incidence of spina bifida is 1 in 1,000 births. Within the past few decades incredible strides have been made to both reduce the incidence of spina bifida and to increase the length and quality of a child's life. With advances in medicine has come the recognition that lack of folic acid in a mother's diet is directly correlated to an increased incidence of children born with neural tubes defects. Today, not only has the Food and Drug Administration mandated that all enriched grain products be enriched with folic acid, pregnant women, or women who are trying to become pregnant are strongly advised to take a folic acid supplement (Pace, 2001).

There are three forms of spina bifida and the impact of each form is dependent upon the size, location, and type of lesion (Barker, Saulino, & Caristo, 2002). They are spina bifida occulta, meningocele, and mylomeningocele. Spina bifida occulta is the mildest form and usually involves an incomplete closure of the laminae of the spinal vertebrae. Often it is so mild that people do not even know they have it. Meningocele involves the protrusion of the meninges through the defective vertebrae into a sac like cyst outside the spine. This cyst is filled with cerebral spinal fluid. The most serious form of spina bifida is called mylomeningocele in which a sac like protrusion containing both cerebral spinal fluid and neural tissues protrudes. Both meningocele and mylomeningocele require immediate surgical intervention.

Children with spina bifida often experience physical limitations including motor movement and bowel and bladder control. A majority of children with spina bifida have normal range IQs, and today, most survive well into adulthood. Because of the relationship between normal IQ function and physical limitations, many children with spina bifida may experience psychosocial difficulties when reaching adolescence (Barker, Saulino, & Caristo, 2002). That is, an increased awareness of physical limitations may bring on feelings of anger and resentment at a time when differences are difficult under normal circumstances.

Working within state and facility guidelines and under the supervision of an OT, the role of the OTA in working with children with spina bifida will involve adapting environments, instruction in use of adapted self care devices, addressing positioning issues, supporting psychosocial needs, and ongoing family/caregiver education.

HYDROCEPHALUS

Hydrocephalus is a condition that occurs as a result of increased cerebral ventricular pressure because of a disturbance in the balance of cerebral spinal fluid (CSF) production (Scott et al., 1998; Snyder & Nussbaum, 1998). The cause of this condition can be either a structural anomaly that develops during gestation, or the result of some structural damage caused by head injury. Two of the most common prenatal causes of hydrocephalus are *aqueductal stenosis* and *spina bifida* (Scott et al., 1998).

Children with hydrocephalus often exhibit nonverbal cognitive and motor skill deficits such as fine and gross motor coordination problems, psychomotor problems, and visualspatial deficits. Because of the varying ventricular

pressure, fluctuating attention is a persistent problem for child with this disorder. Working within state and facility guidelines and under the supervision of an OT, the OTA works with children diagnosed with hydrocephalus to improve motor and visual perceptual skills in order to maximize function in all contexts of the environment.

Genetic Disorders or Syndromes

DOWN SYNDROME

Down syndrome is a genetic disorder that was first identified in 1887 by a physician named John Langdon-Down (Davies & Hollman, 2001). At the time of his work, Langdon-Down was training in a hospital for the mentally retarded. Based on observation of common facial features that resemble those of Asian people, Langdon-Down called these children Mongoloids. In response to outcry from the Mongolian People's Republic, in 1965, the syndrome was renamed Down syndrome (Davies & Hollman, 2001). Down syndrome is considered to be the most common genetic disorder, occurring in approximately 1 of every 800 live births (Finesilver, 2002). Down syndrome is now recognized as being caused by the presence of three, rather than two chromosome number 21s. This extra chromosome leads to widespread developmental disabilities, including physical and cognitive limitations. Children with Down syndrome are also frequently (30-60%) identified as having cardiac problems requiring surgical correction within the first year of life (Finesilver, 2002). Less than 35 years ago the average life expectancy for a child with Down syndrome was a year, but due to advances in medical care as well as allied health and psychological care, today the average life expectancy for a person with Down syndrome is about 55 years. The incidence of Down syndrome positively correlates with a mother's age. That is, women over the age of 40 are at greater risk for delivering a baby with Down syndrome. Through prenatal testing such as amniocentesis and chorionic villi sampling, early identification of Down syndrome is now possible.

Working within state and facility guidelines and under the supervision of an OT, the role of the OTA in working with children with Down syndrome will be to work within a team to maximize age appropriate self care, functional, academic, and leisure skills as well as to prepare the child for a full and enriched life.

MUSCULAR DYSTROPHY

Muscular dystrophy is an inherited genetic disease that affects muscle groups throughout the body. Muscular dystrophy (MD) tends to follow a familial pattern, that is, if a family member (especially one in your immediate family) has been diagnosed with muscular dystrophy, the chances are higher that you may have it, as compared to someone who has no family history of it. There are several types of muscular dystrophies, with the common feature being progressive muscle wasting and weakening over time (Emery, 2002). A child with muscular dystrophy often presents with hypotonia and overall weakness either at birth or shortly thereafter. If there is a family history of muscular dystrophy, the family physician carefully monitors the baby for such symptoms.

Although specific genetic markers and proteins have been identified as causing MD, there is no cure for this progressive disease.

The most common form of muscular dystrophy is called Duchenne's and affects only boys. Edward Meryon, an English physician first identified Duchenne's in 1851 (Henry, 2002). Duchenne's MD is characterized by progressive muscle weakness and overall deterioration beginning in childhood, and ultimately, leading to death by the later stages of adolescence (Emery, 2002). Children with Duchenne's MD may experience difficulties with gross motor activities such as running, skipping, and stair climbing. Mental retardation is common, although about 80% of boys with Duchenne's have IQ scores above 70.

Becker's, another common form of MD, is also characterized by muscle wasting and deterioration and mental impairment. Becker's is not usually diagnosed until early adolescence and affects both boys and girls. Those with Becker's usually live through their mid 40s. Other forms of MD include Congential MD, Emery-Dreifuss MD, Distal MD, Fascioscapulohumeral MD, and Limb-Girdle MD. Like Duchenne's and Becker's, their common characteristics include progressive muscle wasting and deterioration over time.

Working within state and facility guidelines and under the supervision of an OT, the role of the OTA in working with children with muscular dystrophy is to work closely with the rest of the professional team to maintain and maximize the child's function and to develop and implement adapted strategies for self care, school, and leisure pursuits.

Physical and Other Orthopedic Disabilities

Although you may encounter children with many different types of physical and orthopedic disabilities, it is beyond the scope of this chapter to discuss more than a few of the more common ones. This section will focus on juvenile rheumatoid arthritis and amputations.

JUVENILE RHEUMATOID ARTHRITIS

Juvenile rheumatoid arthritis is a form of rheumatoid arthritis that affects children under the age of 16 (Mosby,

1998). Juvenile rheumatoid arthritis impacts the larger joints of the body and is a chronic condition. The symptoms of JRA are usually medically managed, yet the role of the OT practitioner is very important in helping a child with JRA function to his/her maximal capacity.

Working within state and facility guidelines and under the supervision of an OT, the role of the OTA in working with children with JRA involves teaching compensatory strategies to accommodate for joint limitations, pain management strategies, as well as range of motion, energy conservation, and joint protection techniques.

AMPUTATIONS

Amputations may occur congenitally (spontaneously, or as a result of medication complications) or as the result of accidents. Many years ago, mothers were given a drug called thalidomide to combat the symptoms of morning sickness in the first trimester of pregnancy. Unbeknownst to physicians, the drug caused infants to be born with malformed arms and legs. Amputations caused by accidents may occur from attacks from animals, from power tools or lawn equipment, burns, and car or bike accidents.

Working within state and facility guidelines and under the supervision of an OT, the role of the OTA in working with children with amputations will be to assist with instruction in use of prosthetic devices and to develop compensatory techniques to accommodate for loss of limb.

Pediatric Cancers

A diagnosis of childhood cancer is a "traumatic life event" (Hoekstra–Weebers, Jaspers, & Kamps, 1999, p. 1526) that evokes intense anxiety and concern on the part of family/caregivers, as well as (if developmentally germane) the child him/herself.

Although cancer is generally thought of as a single disease, Bracken (1986) indicates that that are over 100 forms of the disease. What sets cancer apart from other diseases is that it refers to "uncontrolled growth of abnormal cells" (Bracken, 1986, p. 3). Cancer cells block or interfere with normal cell functioning and make form masses or tumors (Bracken, 1986). There are two types of tumors; benign and malignant. Benign tumors are slow growing and localized masses that do not spread to other tissues or regions of the body. On the other hand, malignant tumors are fast growing and often invasive. While the treatment plans for children with cancer are analogous to treatment plans for children with other diseases, syndromes, or trauma affecting similar structures of the body, additional attention must be paid to cancer-specific issues which may affect treatment success. As a critical component of effective informed treatment, OT practitioners should make use of the free services, educational materials, and information resources available (especially those available through the National Cancer Institute, American Cancer Society, and other community resources) to consumers. These resources can provide important information to the family and the child, as well as to members of the clinical team. When taking advantage of these resources, it is important to remember that cancers and recovery outcomes differ for children and adults. For example, the morbidity and mortality rates are significantly higher for adults with leukemia as compared to children with the same medical diagnosis.

Responsible OT practitioners should be familiar with not only the physical effects of cancer and its treatment, but also the psychological impact of the physiological changes related to the disease as well as its treatments and resultant social effects. Also, OT practitioners should appreciate the impact of the disease and/or treatment on family and caregivers of the child, and how their ability to provide care and support may be affected by their psychological state. Working within state and facility guidelines, the role of the OTA in treating children with cancer is to be an active member of the rehabilitation team, and work closely with the child and his/her family/caregivers to regain and maintain self care, work, and leisure skills.

Acquired Injuries

TRAUMATIC BRAIN INJURY

Research indicates that traumatic brain injury (TBI) is the leading cause of death for children (McMahon, Noll, Michaud, & Johnson, 2001). In the United States alone, "almost 1.5 million people experience a TBI every year, and 13,000 children receive services for TBI in the public schools" (Youse, Le, Cannazzaro, & Coelho, 2002, p. 4). The highest risk age group for TBI is the 15-24 year old age group. Adolescents and young adults are most at risk for incurring a TBI because of a high rate of automobile accidents, as well as a tendency to engage in a greater incidence of other risky behaviors associated with this age group (Youse, Le, Cannazzaro, & Coelho, 2002). Those above 65 and below age 5 are the next age groups most likely to experience TBI because of increased risk for falls. Demographically males are twice as likely to experience a TBI (Youse, Le, Cannazzaro, & Coelho, 2002).

Although the most common cause of TBI is automobile accidents, other causes include falls, gunshot wounds, diving accidents, rapid acceleration and deceleration of the brain such as shaking a baby, or other wounds to the head (McMahon, Noll, Michaud, & Johnson, 2001; Youse, Le, Cannazzaro, & Coelho, 2002).

A TBI may be classified as either open or closed. An open TBI indicates that something penetrated the scalp, skull, and meninges of the brain. An open TBI may be the result of a gunshot wound. A closed head injury suggests that the meninges remain intact. A closed TBI may be the result of a fall involving the head hitting a hard surface, or rapid acceleration and deceleration of the brain seen when a baby is repeatedly and violently shaken. No matter the cause of the TBI, no two are alike, nor do the presenting symptoms or the recovery processes follow the same course.

Although there are several standardized assessments that measures a person's overall status following and throughout the rehabilitation process, the Rancho Los Amigos Scale is one that OT and PT practitioners frequently use when working with children with traumatic brain injuries. Results of the Rancho Los Amigos Scale provide family members and healthcare providers with information about a child's behavior and the progression of recovery throughout the rehabilitation process. The Rancho Los Amigos Scale does not measure progress over the long term, but rather for the first several months after the injury. Table 10-2 presents the Levels of Cognitive Functioning (RLA-R) as associated with early recovery from a TBI.

A TBI, depending on the location of the insult, may affect cognitive, motor, and/or emotional function (Bond, 2002; McMahon, Noll, Michaud, & Johnson, 2001). Not only does a TBI have significant impact on the life of the child, it also has a tremendous impact on the child's family/caregivers (McMahon, Noll, Michaud, & Johnson, 2001). Active family involvement at all phases of recovery is critically important for the child who has suffered a TBI.

Working within state and facility guidelines and under the supervision of an OT, the role of the OTA in working with children with TBI is critically important. Acting as a member of the rehabilitation team, the OTA works closely with the child and his/her family/caregivers to regain self care, work, and leisure skills.

SPINAL CORD INJURY

A spinal cord injury (SCI) drastically changes the life of the person sustaining the injury, as well as the lives of his/her family/caregivers. A spinal cord injury is both life threatening, and in most cases permanent. There are two types of spinal cord injuries, spinal cord concussion and spinal cord contusion. Spinal cord concussion, representing about 5% of all SCIs, impairs function for less than 48 hours and leaves no residual effects (Metules, & Unkle, 2000). On the other hand, spinal cord contusion is an injury that impairs function for a longer duration than 48 hours or leads to permanent loss of function (Metules, & Unkle, 2000; O'Hare, & Hall, 1997). Depending on where the level of injury occurs within the 33 vertebrae of the spine (which is divided into the cervical, thoracic, lumbar, or sacral vertebral regions), nerve innervation (sensory and/or motor) will be either limited or absent below the level of injury or lesion (Waters, Sie, Adkins, & Yakura, 1996). For instance, if a SCI occurs in the cervical or neck region, motor and/or sensory

Table 10-2

Rancho Los Amigos Levels of Cognitive Functioning, Revised

Level of Function	*Behavioral Characteristics*
Level 1 No Response Total Assistance	Complete absence of observable change in behavior when presented visual, auditory, tactile, proprioceptive, vestibular, or painful stimuli.
Level 2 Generalized Response Total Assistance	Demonstrates generalized reflex response to painful stimuli. Responds to repeated auditory stimuli with increased or decreased activity. Responds to external stimuli with physiological changes, generalized gross body movement and/or nonpurposeful vocalization. Responses noted may be same regardless of type and location of stimulation. Responses may be significantly delayed.
Level 3 Localized Response Total Assistance	Demonstrates withdrawal of vocalization to painful stimulation. Turns toward or away from auditory stimuli. Blinks when strong light crosses visual field. Follows moving objects passed within visual field. Responds to discomfort by pulling tubes or restraints. Responds inconsistently to simple commands. Responses directly related to type of stimulus. May respond to some persons (especially family and friends) but not to others.
Level 4 Confused-Agitated Maximal Assistance	Alert and in heightened state of activity. Purposeful attempts to remove restraints or tubes or crawl out of bed. May perform motor activities such as sitting, reaching, and walking but without an apparent purpose or upon another's request. Very brief and usually nonpurposeful moments of sustained attention. Absent short-term memory. Absent goal-directed, problem-solving, self-monitoring behavior. May cry out or scream out of proportion to stimulus even after its removal. May exhibit aggressive or flight behavior. Mood may swing from euphoric to hostile with no apparent relationship to environmental events. Unable to cooperate with treatment efforts. Verbalizations are frequently incoherent and/or inappropriate to activity or environment.
Level 5 Confused- Inappropriate Nonagitated Maximal Assistance	Alert, not agitated but may wander randomly or with a vague intention of going home. May become agitated in response to external stimulation and/or lack of environmental structure. Not oriented to place or time. Frequent brief periods of nonpurposeful sustained attention. Severely impaired recent memory with confusion of past and present in reaction to ongoing activity. Absent goal-directed, problem-solving, self-monitoring behavior. Often demonstrates inappropriate use of objects without external direction. May be able to perform previously learned tasks when structured and cues provided. Unable to learn new information. Able to respond appropriately to simple commands fairly consistently with external structure and cues. Responses to simple commands without external structure are random and non-purposeful in relation to the command. Able to converse on a social, automatic level for brief periods of time when provided external structure and cues. Verbalizations about present events become inappropriate and confabulatory when external structure and cues are not provided.
Level 6 Confused- Appropriate Moderate Assistance	Inconsistently oriented to place and time. Able to attend to highly familiar tasks in nondistracting environment for 30 minutes with moderate redirection. Remote memory has more depth and detail than recent memory. Vague recognition of some staff. Able to use assistive memory aid with maximal assistance. Emerging awareness of appropriate response to self, family, and basic needs. Emerging goal-directed behavior related to meeting basic personal needs. Moderate assistance to problem-solve barriers to task completion. Supervised for old learning (e.g., self-care). Shows carryover for relearned familiar tasks (e.g., self-care). Maximal assistance for new learning with little or no carryover. Unaware of impairments, disabilities, and safety risks. Consistently follows simple directions. Verbal expressions are appropriate in highly familiar and structured situations.
Level 7 Automatic- Appropriate Minimal Assistance For Routine Daily Living Skills	Consistently oriented to person and place, within highly familiar environments. Minimal assistance for orientation to time. Able to attend to highly familiar tasks in a nondistraction environment for at least 30 minutes with minimal assistance to complete tasks. Able to use assistive memory devices with minimal assistance. Minimal supervision for new learning. Demonstrates carryover of new learning. Initiates and carries out steps to complete familiar personal and household routine but has shallow recall of what he/she has been doing. Able to monitor accuracy and completeness of each step in routine personal and household ADLs and modified plan with minimal assistance. Superficial awareness of his/her condition but unaware of specific impairments and disabilities and the limits they place on his/her ability to safely, accurately, and completely carry out his/her household, community, work and

Table 10-2 (continued)

Rancho Los Amigos Levels of Cognitive Functioning, Revised

Level of Function	Behavioral Characteristics
(Level 7)	leisure ADLs. Minimal supervision for safety in routine home and community activities. Unrealistic planning for the future. Unable to think about consequences of a decision or action. Overestimates abilities. Unaware of others' needs and feelings. Oppositional/uncooperative. Unable to recognize inappropriate social interaction behavior.
Level 8 Purposeful and Appropriate Standby Assistance	Consistently oriented to person, place, and time. Independently attends to and completes familiar tasks for 1 hour in a distracting environment. Able to recall and integrate past and recent events. Uses assistive memory devices to recall daily schedule and "to do" lists and record critical information for later use with standby assistance. Initiates and carries out steps to complete familiar personal, household, community, work, and leisure routines with standby assistance and can modify the plan when needed with minimal assistance. Requires no assistance once new tasks/activities are learned. Aware of and acknowledges impairments and disabilities when they interfere with task completion but requires standby assistance to take appropriate corrective action. Thinks about consequences of a decision or action with minimal assistance. Overestimates or underestimates abilities. Acknowledges others' needs and feelings and responds appropriately with minimal assistance. Depressed. Irritable. Low frustration tolerance/easily angered. Argumentative. Self-centered. Uncharacteristically dependent/independent. Able to recognize and acknowledge inappropriate social interaction behavior while it is occurring and takes corrective action with minimal assistance.
Level 9 Purposeful and Appropriate Standby Assistance On Request	Independently shifts back and forth between tasks and completes them accurately for at least 2 consecutive hours. Uses assistive memory devices to recall daily schedule and "to do" lists and record critical information for later use with assistance when requested. Initiates and carries out steps to complete familiar personal, household, work, and leisure tasks independently and unfamiliar personal, household, work, and leisure tasks with assistance when requested. Aware of and acknowledges impairments and disabilities when they interfere with tasks completion and takes appropriate corrective action but requires standby assist to anticipate a problem before it occurs and take action to avoid it. Able to think about consequences of decisions or actions with assistance when requested. Accurately estimates abilities but requires standby assistance to adjust to task demands. Acknowledges others' needs and feelings and responds appropriately with standby assistance. Depression may continue. May be easily irritated. May have low frustration tolerance. Able to self-monitor appropriateness of social interaction with standby assistance.
Level 10 Purposeful and Appropriate Modified Independent	Able to handle multiple tasks simultaneously in all environments but may require periodic breaks. Able to independently procure, create, and maintain own assistive memory devices. Independently initiates and carries out steps to complete familiar and unfamiliar personal, household, community, work, and leisure tasks but may require more than the usual amount of time and/or compensatory strategies to complete them. Anticipates impact of impairments and disabilities on ability to complete daily living tasks and takes action to avoid problems before they occur but may require more than the usual amount of time and/or compensatory strategies. Able to independently think about consequences of decisions or actions but may require more than the usual amount of time and/or compensatory strategies to select the appropriate decision or action. Accurately estimates abilities and independently adjusts to task demands. Able to recognize the needs and feelings of others and automatically respond in appropriate manner. Periodic periods of depression may occur. Irritability and low frustration tolerance when sick, fatigued, and/or under emotional stress. Social interaction behavior is consistently appropriate.

Original scale coauthored by Chris Hagen, PhD, Danese Malkmus, MA, Patricia Durham, MA, Communication Disorder Service, Rancho Los Amigos Medical Center, Downey, CA, 1972. Revised 11/15/74 by Danese Malkmus, MA and Kathryn Stenderup, OTR. Reprinted with permission.

nerve function below the specific cervical lesion will be affected. Spinal cord injuries result in quadriplegia, which means that all four extremities are affected by the injury, or paraplegia, which is loss of function from about waist level down (O'Hare, & Hall, 1997). Quadriplegia results from cervical or upper thoracic spinal injury and paraplegia, from lower thoracic, lumbar, and sacral injury. A SCI is called incomplete when there is some residual "sensory and or motor function in the lowest sacral segments of the cord.... [and is complete] when there is no preservation of function in the lowest sacral segments" (Waters, Sie, Adkins, & Yakura, 1996, p. 13).

The overall incidence rate for SCI in the United States is about 3-5 per 10,000 people (O'Hare, & Hall, 1997), and like TBI, males ages 15-24 are most at risk for incurring a SCI (O'Hare, & Hall, 1997). The most common causes of a SCI stem from automobile and motorcycle accidents, sports, falls, recreational activities, and acts of violence (Eyster, 1993; O'Hare, & Hall, 1997; Waters, Sie, Adkins, & Yakura, 1996).

Working within state and facility guidelines and under the supervision of an OT, the role of the OTA in working with children who have sustained a SCI is to participate in a team oriented care model to recommend and implement adapted techniques and equipment to both maintain and maximize function in all areas of self care, work, and play. The OTA may also play a role in providing family/caregiver education.

Seizure Disorders

A seizure may be likened to an electrical storm in the brain. During a seizure, a child may experience some kind of altered consciousness accompanied by some kind of kinetic or convulsive motor movement, such as an eye blink, staring, shaking, trembling, or jerky type motions (Aytch, Hammond, & White, 2001; Haggerty, 1999). Seizures are the most common neurological disturbance of childhood (Aytch, Hammond, & White, 2001). Although epilepsy, a form of seizure disorder, is attributed to 1 to 2% of the population in the US (Haggerty, 1999), the research literature suggests that as many as 300,000 children under the age of 14 have reoccurring seizures (Shearer, 1999). Most cases of seizure disorder begin in childhood, although they can occur at anytime in life. One of reasons that seizures are more commonly associated with childhood is that the child's brain is immature, and therefore may be more susceptible to seizures (Shearer, 1999).

There are several types of seizures, including the grand mal or generalized seizure that impacts the entire body, absence or petit mal seizures, myoclonic seizures, partial seizures, and partial complex seizures. For many children, the cause of seizure disorder is unknown, yet Atych, Hammond, and White (2001) indicate that seizures may be the result of a birth trauma, head injury, infectious diseases, a degenerative disease, genetic factors, or exposure to teratogens (agents responsible for birth defects).

Children with a known seizure disorder are typically treated with careful medication management. Compliance and adherence to correct medication protocol is essential. Surgical intervention may also be indicated for children with intractable seizures. Seizures may also be treated via diet management, specifically the ketogenic diet. The ketogenic diet is a high fat, low carbohydrate diet that essentially brings on dehydration and starvation, which in turn leads to the production of ketones, a seizure suppressing chemical (Aytch, Hammond, & White, 2001). The diet is initially administered in a hospital setting under the close supervision of a physician, and requires careful, ongoing monitoring to measure its efficacy.

Working within state and facility guidelines and under the supervision of an OT, the role of the OTA in working with children with seizures is to maximize functional capacity in all areas of work, play, and self care.

Summary

This chapter provided a brief overview of several diagnoses commonly associated with childhood that an OTA may encounter when working in pediatrics. It also discussed the role of the OTA in working with children with various diagnoses. An explanation of the *DSM-IV-TR*; one of the most widely reviewed and researched systems to classify and diagnose behavior and symptoms commonly related to disorders was also shared. The interested reader is encouraged to pursue further research into the many diagnoses that he/she may encounter when working with children.

Case Study

One example of the complexities of diagnosing and working with children with mental retardation involves the case of an 11-year-old Latino male. "Noah" presented to a child psychiatric unit following what appeared to be suicidal behavior such as spontaneously running out into traffic and attempting to climb out of windows in his apartment and school. As part of his inpatient treatment, his caregivers were interviewed regarding Noah's history, including pre- and post-natal development, and Noah completed a full psychological evaluation, including intellectual assessment. From the interview with the caregivers it was discovered that while the pregnancy had been normal, the delivery was difficult: Noah was in a breach position during delivery and experienced a brief anoxic period. While his early development appeared normal, by the time Noah was school age he was exhibiting difficulty following instructions and learning age-appropriate behaviors such as dressing himself and reading. By the time he was seen at the child inpatient psychiatric unit at age 11, Noah still had difficulty dressing himself; he would often put his shoes on before putting his pants on, could not tie his own shoes, could not tell time (even with a digital watch), and had little conceptual understanding of the value of money.

Intellectual testing revealed a variety of limitations across a spectrum of cognitive areas. Noah demonstrated well below average attention, impulse control, memory, language, visual motor and reasoning abilities. However, his IQ score was 72, which is considered Borderline intellectual functioning and technically does not fall into the mentally retarded range of intellectual functioning. Attempts to gain Noah and his family services to help them manage his behavior and provide for his high level of care resulted in a conflict between the Department of Mental Retardation (DMR) and the Department of Mental Health (DMH). In Massachusetts, DMR and DMH are mutually exclusive programs; DMR put forth that Noah's behavior was not due to mental retardation but rather emotional disturbance, while DMH put forth that Noah was mentally retarded and not emotionally disturbed. After carefully assessing the family functioning, ruling out language or perceptual problems to explain Noah's behavior, and collecting collateral information from school teachers and previous mental health workers, it was determined that while Noah did not have an IQ that was in the mentally retarded range, the consistency of his low level adaptive behaviors was consistent with him being functionally mentally retarded, and that the focus of his treatment should be on assessing and working with his cognitive limitations. The functional assessment of Noah's behavior was critical in getting him recognized by DMH as mentally retarded and the services that he and his family required to address his needs.

DISCUSSION QUESTIONS RELATED TO CASE STUDY

1. What areas of behavior would you want to make certain to assess to evaluate adaptive behavior?

2. How do you understand the differences between DMH and DMR?

3. What type of collateral information would you want for a case like this?

Application Activities

1. Watch the movie "Mercury Rising" and record behaviors consistent and inconsistent with autism.

2. Read *Driven To Distraction* by Edward Hallowell to gain more information about the nature of ADHD and its impact across the lifespan.

3. Check The APA Monitor website for current articles on many of the disorders discussed (www.apa.org/monitor).

Acknowledgment

I would like to thank Michael Roberts, MS, OTR/L for his assistance with the pediatric cancer section of this chapter.

References

Atych, L. S., Hammond, R., & White, C. (2001). Seizures in infants and young children: An exploratory study of family experiences and needs for information and support. *Journal of Neuroscience Nursing, 33*(5), 278.

Barker, E., Saulino, M., Caristo, A. M. (2002). Spina bifida. *RN, 65*(12), 33-38.

Bennett, F. C. (1999). Diagnosing cerebral palsy: The earlier the better. *Contemporary Pediatrics, 16*(7), 65-73.

Bond, C. (2002). Traumatic brain injury: Help for the family. *RN 65*(11), 60-66.

Bracken, J. M. (1986). *Children with cancer.* New York, Oxford: Oxford University Press.

Brockley, J. A. (1999). History of mental retardation. *History of Psychology, 2*(1), 25–36.

Charman, T., Swettenham, J., Baron-Cohen, S., Cox, A., Baird, G., & Drew, A. (1997). Infants with autism: An investigation of empathy, pretend play, joint attention, and imitation. *Developmental Psychology, 33*(5), 718-789.

Cobham, V. E., Dadds, M. R., & Spence, S. H. (1998). The role of parental anxiety in treatment of childhood anxiety. *Journal of Consulting and Clinical Psychology, 66*(6), 893 – 905.

Davies, M. K., & Hollman, A. (2001). Down syndrome. *Heart, 86*(2), 130.

Doyle, A. E., Biederman, J., Seidman, L. J., Weber, W., & Faraone, S. V. (2000). Diagnostic efficiency of neuropsychological test scores discriminating boys with and without Attention Deficit-Hyperactivity Disorder. *Journal of Consulting and Clinical Psychology, 68*(3), 477–488.

Eley, T. C., Dale, P., Bishop, D., Price, T. S., & Plomin, R. (2001). Longitudinal analysis of the genetic and environmental influences on components of cognitive delay in preschoolers. *Journal of Educational Psychology, 93*(4), 698–707.

Emery, A. H. (2002, 23 Feb). The muscular dystrophies. *The Lancet, 359*(9307), 687-700.

Eyster, E. F. (1993). THINK FIRST: Prevention of head and spinal cord injury. *American Family Physician, 47*(8), 1689-1689.

Ferreri, A. (1995, Sept- Oct.). Cerebral palsy: Equipping children to live full lives. *World Health, 48*(5), 22-23.

Finesilver, C. (2002). Down syndrome: A new age for childhood diseases. *RN, 65*(11), 43-48.

Haggerty, M. (1999). Seizure disorder. *Gale Encyclopedia of Medicine* (1st ed.). p. 2574.

Hoekstra–Weebers, J., Jaspers, J., & Kamps, W. A. (1999) Risk factors for psychological maladjustment of parents of children with cancer. *Journal of the American Academy of Child and Adolescent Psychiatry, 38*(12), 1526.

Honein, M., Paulozzi, L., & Mathews, T. (2001). Impact of folic acid fortification on incidence of neural tube defects. *Nutritional Research Newsletter, 20*(8), 15.

Light, R. Asarnow, R., Satz, P., Zaucha, K., McCleary, C., & Lewis, R. (1998). Mild closed-head injury in children and adolescents behavior problems and academic outcomes. *Journal of Consulting and Clinical Psychology, 66*(6), 1023–1029.

Mattson, S. N., Riley, E. P., Gramling, L., Delis, D. C., & Jones, K. L. (1998). Neuropsychological comparison of alcohol-exposed children with or without physical features of Fetal Alcohol Syndrome. *Neuropsychology, 12*(1), 146–153.

McClure, E. B., Kubiszyn, T., & Kaslow, N. J. (2002). Advances in the diagnosis and treatment of childhood mood disorders. *Professional Psychology: Research and Practice, 33*(2), 125–134.

McMahon, M. A., Noll, R. B., Michaud, L. J., & Johnson, J. C. (2001). Sibling adjustment to pediatric traumatic brain injury: A case controlled pilot study. *The Journal of Head Trauma Rehabilitation, 16*(6), 587-594.

Metules, T. J., & Unkle, D. W. (2000). Spinal cord injury falls into two categories (brief article). *RN, 63*(4), 85.

Miller, L. K. (1999). The savant syndrome: Intellectual impairment and exceptional skill. *Psychological Bulletin, 125*(1), 31–46.

Mosby's Medical, Nursing, & Allied Health Dictionary (5th ed). (1998). St Louis, MO: Mosby.

O'Hare, P., & Hall, K. M. (1997). Preventing spinal cord injuries through safety education programs (Spinal cord injury, Part 3). *American Rehabilitation, 23*(1), 15-18.

Pace, B. (2001). Spina Bifida (JAMA Patient Page). *The Journal of the American Medical Association, 285*(23), 3050.

Palmer, F. B. (2002). First, observe the patient. *Archives of Pediatrics and Adolescent Medicine, 156*(5), 422-423.

Rains, G. D. (2002). *Principles of neuropsychology.* Boston: McGraw-Hill Companies.

Roach, M. A., Barratt, M. S., Miller, J. F., & Leavitt, L. A. (1998). The structure of mother-child play: Young children with Down Syndrome and typically developing children. *Developmental Psychology, 34*(1), 77–87.

Sandler, A. (1997). *Living with spina bifida:A guide for families and professionals.* Chapel Hill, NC and London, UK: University of North Carolina Press.

Scott, M. A., Fletcher, J. M., Brookshire, B. L., Davidson, K. C., Landry, S. H., Bohan, T. C., Kramer, L. A., Brandt, M. E., & Francis, D. J. (1998). Memory functions in children with early hydrocephalus. *Neuropsychology, 12*(4), 578 – 589.

Shearer, A. (1999). Seizures and epilepsy in childhood. *The Exceptional Parent, 29*(8), 64.

Snyder, P. J. & Nussbaum, P. D. (1998). *Clinical neuropsychology.* Washington, D.C.: American Psychological Association.

Wannamaker, C. E. & Glenwick, D. S. (1998). Stress, coping and perceptions of child behavior in parents of preschoolers with cerebral palsy. *Rehabilitation Psychology, 43*(4), 297–312.

Waters, R. L., Sie, I. H., Adkins, R. H., & Yakura, J. S. (1996). Recovery following spinal cord injury. *American Rehabilitation, 22*(4), 13-19.

Wechsler, D. (1944). *The measurement of adult intelligence* (3rd ed.) Baltimore: Williams and Wilkins.

Wechsler, D. (1991). *Wechsler Intelligence Scale for Children Third Edition (WISC-III) Manual.* New York: The Psychological Corporation

Wilson, B. J. (1999). Entry behavior and emotion regulation abilities of developmentally delayed boys. *Developmental Psychology, 35*(1), 214 – 222.

Yirmiya, N., Erel, O., Shaked, M., & Solomonica-Levi, D. (1998). Meta-analyses comparing theory of mind abilities of individuals with autism, individuals with mental retardation, and normally developing individuals. *Psychological Bulletin, 124*(3), 283–307.

Youse, K. M., Le, K. N., Cannazzaro, M. S., & Coelho, C. A. (2002, June 25). Traumatic brain injury: Primer for professionals. *ASHA Leader, 7*(12), 4-7.

POSITIONING IN PEDIATRICS: MAKING THE RIGHT CHOICES

Molly Campbell, MS, OTR/L, ATP

Chapter Objectives

- List at least five issues in pediatrics for which positioning modifications are indicated.
- Explain the benefits of proper positioning.
- Describe at least eight different positioning devices including information about who should use each one, the ideal position prompted by each device, the intended benefit of each piece of equipment, and the precautions that should be taken with each item.
- Access information about resources for purchasing and/or constructing positioning devices.

Introduction

The first question that must be answered before engaging a child with developmental disabilities in feeding, fine motor activities, or therapeutic play is "Is this child positioned correctly?" Unless the child is in a functional position, he or she will not be able to optimally perform the chosen activities. Once you have a child that is properly positioned, it is imperative that meaningful and motivating activity be provided, as positioning alone is boring and frustrating for a child. When providing pediatric treatment, the occupational therapy practitioner must always think about the interplay between the appropriate position and the functional or fun activity.

Another extremely important question to ask is "How much external support should be used to help the child maintain a good position?" It may be that in the context of a therapy session a child with physical disabilities can sit on a bench without any supports for several minutes. Should this child then be expected to sit on a similar bench in the classroom, clinic, or at home? It may be that the child needs to concentrate fairly hard to maintain a good sitting position. Since this might take away from his ability to concentrate on his or her class or seatwork, it might be that he or she should use a more supportive seating system. You never want to over-adapt for a child. It is always important to collaborate closely with the occupational therapist (OT), physical therapist (PT), teacher, family, and other team members to develop a plan for positioning strategies to use in various settings.

The purpose of this chapter is to address positioning options for children. It is important to remember that positioning does not happen in isolation. Physical therapy, occupational therapy, and medical treatments will affect the child's muscle tone, head and trunk control, balance, strength, and endurance. As these abilities change, the child's needs for positioning equipment will also change.

Children who may need positioning interventions include:
- Small children using standard-sized furniture.
- Children with sensory processing problems.
- Children that are very mobile and need clearly defined spaces.
- Children presenting with physical disabilities.

Of these groups of children, it is the final one that warrants the most careful assessment before making positioning recommendations. Children presenting with physical disabilities may have abnormalities in muscle tone, poorly integrated reflexes, musculoskeletal abnormalities, an imbalance between stability and mobility, poor motor control, limited strength, and/or limitations in performance of functional tasks.

MUSCLE TONE

Muscle tone is the state of tension in a resting muscle. Think of the muscle as a rubber band. The normal resting muscle has some tension in it: the rubber band is slightly stretched so that it is ready to pull more tightly when it is called upon to move. A muscle that has increased tone is like an elastic band that is already pulled taut. The joint may constantly be pulled toward the side with the tight muscle, so that movement in the opposite direction may be very difficult for the child. High tone muscle bellies feel very hard. When the OT practitioner quickly stretches a muscle that has high tone, he/she will feel a lot of resistance. A muscle that has low tone is like an elastic band that has little or no tension in it. It is slow to respond when called upon. A child with low tone may tire quickly from activities as basic as sitting or holding up his/her head. A joint surrounded by muscles with low tone may be too mobile. Low tone muscle bellies feel soft and squishy. When the OT practitioner quickly stretches a muscle with low tone, he/she gets very little feeling that the child is pushing back. A child with low muscle tone throughout the body often has poor posture. The youngster's standing posture is characterized by winged scapula (the large flat bones on the back of the child's shoulders seem to protrude in an exaggerated way), a stomach that sticks out, an accentuated curve in the lower back, and locked knees that keep the legs rigidly straight. The child with low tone often has difficulty maintaining weight-bearing positions.

Understanding a child's muscle tone is not always easy. Some children have fluctuating muscle tone, so that they sometimes seem floppy and sometimes seem overly tense. Some children have low tone in the trunk and proximal parts of the body and increased tone in the distal parts. The best way to be clear about a child's tone is to work closely with an experienced OT when treating a child with muscle tone issues.

REFLEXES

Reflexes are automatic movement patterns that occur in response to specific touch or position stimuli. Infants depend on reflexes for survival and early learning. The rooting reflex is an example of a pattern that helps a baby to survive. When the side of the baby's face is touched, he or she automatically turns his/her head in the direction of the touch. This reflexive action is often in response to the touch of the mother's nipple or a bottle's nipple on the child's face, such that the turn enables the child to get milk. Many such patterns are normally present until the child is 6 to 8 months old, when higher level motor skills begin to develop and override the earlier reflexes. However, when motor devel-

opment is atypical, some of these primitive reflexes may continue to be elicited for many years.

The two primitive reflex residuals most often seen in children with atypical development are the tonic neck reflexes and the tonic labyrinthine reflexes.

Symmetrical Tonic Neck Reflex (STNR)

When the head flexes forward, the muscle tone of the flexors in the upper extremities increases and the muscle tone in the extensors of the lower extremities increases. If the head extends backwards (the child looks up), the extensor tone in the upper extremities increases and the muscle tone in the flexors in the lower extremities increases (Figure 11-1).

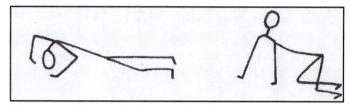

Figure 11-1. Symmetrical tonic neck reflex.

Asymmetrical Tonic Neck Reflex (ATNR)

When the head turns to one side, the tone in the extensors in the limbs on the face side increases and the tone in the flexors increases in the extremities on the back of the head side (Figure 11-2).

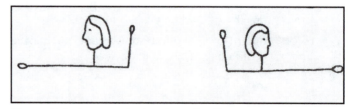

Figure 11-2. Asymmetrical tonic neck reflex.

Tonic Labyrinthine Reflex-Prone

In the prone position (lying on the stomach), flexor tone increases (Figure 11-3).

Tonic Labyrinthine Reflex-Supine

In the supine position (lying on the back), extensor tone increases (please refer to Figure 11-3).

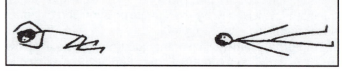

Figure 11-3. Tonic Labyrinthine reflexes.

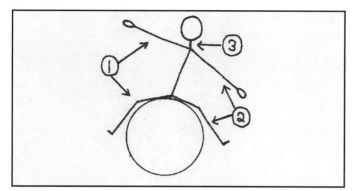

Figure 11-4. Balance and equilibrium responses.

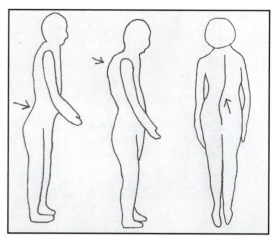

Figure 11-5. Spinal deformities: lordosis, kyphosis, and scoliosis.

Balance and Equilibrium Responses

As previously discussed, most reflexes are present during infancy and become integrated as movement patterns become more complex. Some reflexes, however, emerge somewhat later in the baby's development and remain throughout life. One of these crucial reflexes is the balance and equilibrium response. As the child's body is tipped to the side and his/her center of gravity shifts, the vestibular system is stimulated. The child then demonstrates the following three automatic responses:

1. He or she straightens and abducts his or her arm and leg on the uphill side.

2. He or she straightens the arm and leg on the downhill side and extends these limbs toward the ground as a protective response in case of a fall.

3. He or she rights his or her head so that it is straight up and down in relation to the ground but not in a line with the body (Figure 11-4).

Please also refer to the Major Infant Reflexes Chart and the Developmental Milestones Chart found at the end of this book.

SPINAL ABNORMALITIES

Spinal and pelvic abnormalities need to be considered when choosing positioning options for a child. Common spinal deformities include kyphosis (exaggerated flexion of the upper part of the spinal column), lordosis (exaggerated extension of the lower part of the spinal column), and scoliosis (a lateral asymmetrical curve or twist of the spinal column). These deformities are termed *flexible curvatures* if range of motion is still complete through active movement or passive manipulation. They are *fixed* when full range of motion cannot be attained (Figure 11-5).

A child with a diagnosis like athetoid-type cerebral palsy (CP) presents with uncontrolled, unintentional movement and not enough postural stability. In this case, the positioning devices will need to provide a great deal of stability for the child, especially to the body parts over which the child has the least control. For example, Lucy is a 10-year-old girl whose upper extremities extend and flail without her conscious control. She has better control over her head and lower extremities. When her arms are held, she has enough stability so that she can point to letters on an alphabet board with her left foot. When her arms are released, she loses control of her mobility and can no longer point with her foot. Her seating system includes arm troughs with padded straps so that her forearms can be stabilized.

REFLECTIONS FOR THE OTA

If a positioning device limits a person's mobility, is it a restraint that limits the individual's freedom that could be viewed by some as unethical? This is an important question. When selecting supports that limit movements, the therapy team must always try to choose the least restrictive assistive device components that will meet the child's needs. The team must clearly document that these components are chosen to promote good positioning and optimum control of the body. Many schools and hospitals develop clinical protocols for use of adapted supports so that it is clear that pelvic positioning belts, chest supports, and other straps are therapeutic rather than restrictive.

Meeting the Equipment Needs of Children With Various Disabilities

STARTING SIMPLE

Positioning Device: Footstool

Users: Children whose feet do not reach the floor in the chairs that they have to use (Figure 11-6).

Figure 11-6.
Footstool.

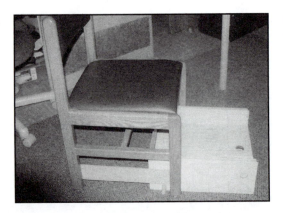

Figure 11-7. Wedge
seat.

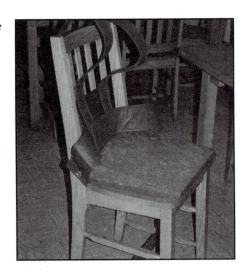

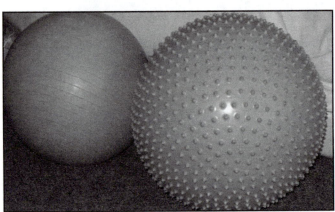

Figure 11-8. Therapy ball.

Set up: The footstool should be high enough so that the soles of the child's feet are completely supported. Ideally, when using a footstool the child should have 90 degrees of flexion at the ankles, at the knees, and at the hips. It should not be so high that the child's knees are raised above the height of the rest of the lap. This latter position may cause increased weight bearing on the ischial tuberosities, the bony prominences in the buttocks.

Benefits: Sitting with firm support under the feet may help children pay better attention to school or sustained work activities. Foot support also prevents heel cord contractures in children with physical disabilities.

Positioning Device: Wedge Seat

Users: Children who have difficulty sitting up straight in their classroom seats may benefit from the use of a wedge seat. Many of these children present with low muscle tone and posterior pelvic tilt (Figure 11-7).

Set up: The wedge is positioned so that the high part is in the back of the child's seat.

Benefits: The wedge facilitates a slight anterior pelvic tilt and improves alignment of the spine. The result is that the child sits up straight in the chair.

Contraindications: If the child's postural control is extremely poor, he/she might slip forward off the wedge and chair.

Other Comments: Inflatable wedges combine positioning modification with some movement input to help keep the child's state of arousal at an optimum level.

Positioning Device: Therapy Ball

Users: Children who squirm and bounce in their regular chairs (Figure 11-8).

Set up: The ball needs to be small enough so that the child's feet can be firmly planted on the floor. Correct sizing should facilitate 90 degrees of flexion at the ankles, knees, and hips. When using the therapy ball as an alternative to a regular chair, the work surface height should be about halfway between the child's waist and chest.

Benefits: Slight bouncing movements while engaged in sustained attentional activities may help students who need some vestibular input in their *sensory diets* stay focused. Automatic balance and equilibrium responses may also be enhanced through use of a therapy ball. In order to maintain his/her balance, the child needs to keep his feet on the floor. Using a therapy ball as an alternative to a regular chair may help with improving attention to task.

Contraindications: The child's posture must be monitored when using the therapy ball as a seat. Some children with low muscle tone may tend to accentuate their lordotic curve in order to stay upright. Unless the child demonstrates good balancing ability, this seating option should not be used without the close supervision of an OT practitioner.

Other Comments: The therapy ball may be used in conjunction with a stand that helps to stabilize the ball.

Figure 11-9. T stool.

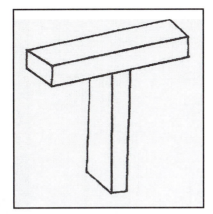

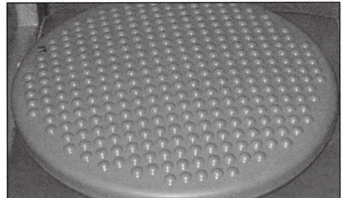

Figure 11-10. Inflatable or pellet-filled seat cover.

Positioning Device: T Stool

Users: A child who is working to refine balance responses might use a T stool. A child who does not typically keep his feet on the floor and has difficulty attending to schoolwork and sustained seatwork tasks might also use the T stool as an alternative to a regular chair (Figure 11-9).

Set up: The height of the stool should facilitate a position of 90 degrees of flexion at the hips, knees and ankles. The child's feet should be firmly planted on the floor.

Benefits: To maintain balance, the child needs to keep his/her feet on the floor. Use of a T stool may facilitate this grounded position.

Contraindications: As with the therapy ball, the child's posture should be monitored to make sure that the unusual seating option is not feeding into any abnormal postural patterns.

Positioning Device: Inflatable or Pellet-Filled Seat Cover

Users: A child without significant physical dysfunction who needs some additional support to maintain stability when seated may use a seat cover filled with a material that conforms firmly to the child's contours. For a child who needs to have a more dynamic seating opportunity, an inflated seat cover or one filled with a very slippery material that allows for more movement may be indicated (Figure 11-10).

Set up: The right seat cover needs to be chosen for the child. Things to consider when recommending a seat cover may include the following: Does the student need more stability or more mobility? The seat cover will raise the seat height a few inches, so that a footstool may be needed to provide foot support.

Benefits: The seat cover may help the child pay better attention in class because stability or mobility needs are being met.

Contraindications: Do not choose the wrong type of seat filling for the child. Carefully consider the child's needs.

Positioning Device: Crescent-Shaped Pillow

Users: Infants or toddlers with delays in gross motor development may be supported with a firmly stuffed crescent-shaped pillow. This cushion replicates the support of the opened legs of an adult sitting with the child on the floor in this "gap". The Boppy® (The Boppy Company, Golden CO) is a brightly colored, washable, commercially available option. Stuffing a pair of pants is a handmade alternative (Figure 11-11).

Set up: The child can be supported in sitting, supine, or side lying using the crescent-shaped pillow.

Benefits: This cushion works best for a child who only requires hip level support, as it is only 5 to 6 inches high. If it is used to assist the child with sitting, it supports the child at the hips, but requires the child to maintain head and upper trunk control.

Contraindications: The crescent-shaped cushion should be used only with close adult supervision in case the child slips out of the intended position.

Positioning Device: Beanbag Chair

Users: Children with multiple disabilities who spend a lot of time in wheelchairs or other very restrictive positioning devices may like the freedom of some down time in a beanbag chair (Figure 11-12).

Set up: Once the child is transferred onto the beanbag, his or her body can be passively moved a little bit to create a supportive trough in which to sit. If extra head support is needed, a second beanbag chair may be propped up behind the first one.

Benefits: This nonrestrictive tactile and proprioceptively rich position may help promote relaxation.

Contraindications: If the child assumes a position that could feed into the development of future deformities, a beanbag should not be used. An OT or PT should be consulted as to the appropriateness of the beanbag chair. If the child is uncomfortable or does not like the position, there is no reason to insist that the child use it.

Figure 11-11.
Crescent-shaped
pillow.

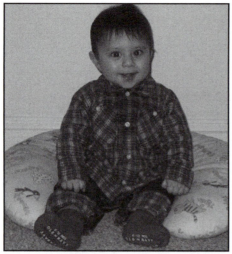

Figure 11-12. Beanbag chair.

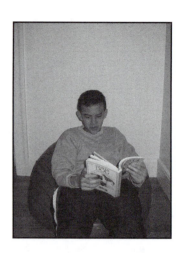

Figure 11-13A. Rifton chair.

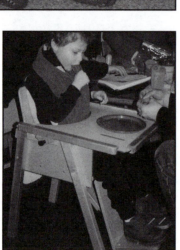

Figure 11-13B. Trip Trap®
chair.

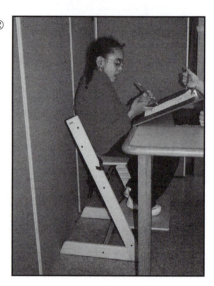

Positioning Device: Chairs That Fit and Provide More Support Than the Standard Child's Chair

Users: Children with mild physical disabilities but fair to good stability in sitting or children with attention deficit disorders may need specialized chairs (Figures 11-13A and 11-13B).

Set up: Cube chairs have side supports that can help the young child who is distractible maintain a sitting position while facing presented activities. Wooden Rifton® chairs (Rifton Equipment, Chester, NY) are toddler-sized and have sides and armrests that encourage good positioning and attention to task. Some versions of these chairs have adjustable angled calf supports, adjustable height footrests, and pelvic positioning belts. (Case-Smith, Allen, & Pratt, 1996). Trip Trap® chairs (Stokke LLC, Kennesaw, NC) were developed in Norway. They have adjustable seat height, seat depth, and footrest heights, and are designed for use in con-

junction with standard height tables. Pummels and pelvic positioning belts can be added to the Trip Trap® chair to provide additional support and stability.

Benefits: These seating options provide extra support and structure for the child presenting with mild physical impairments.

Contraindications: These seats do not provide enough support for a child presenting with more severe physical impairments.

Positioning Device: Floor Sitter

Users: Preschool and early elementary aged children with mild to moderate difficulty staying seated without support and who should be joining peers at floor level for circle time and other activities may benefit from using floor sitters (Figure 11-14).

Set up: Often a floor sitter with a corner chair-shaped back attached to a base on the floor big enough not to tip provides the child with the necessary trunk support for independent sitting.

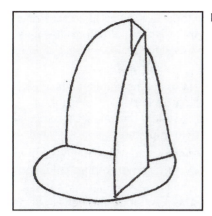

Figure 11-14. Floor sitter.

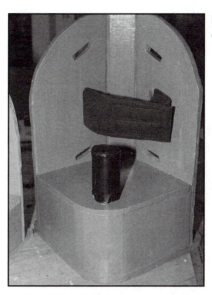

Figure 11-15B. Basic corner chair.

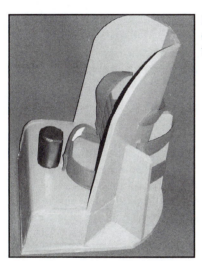

Figure 11-15A. Corner chair with straight seat front.

chair. The corner-shaped back inhibits shoulder retraction and promotes upper extremity midline positioning, placing the child in a good position for visual scanning, attending to objects, breathing, speaking, and eating (Figures 11-15A and 11-15B).

Set up: The child's feet should be flat on the floor with his or her hips and knees flexed to 90 degrees. If head control is inconsistent, the back height of the chair should extend above the head. A child with better head control can sit in a corner chair with the back height even with the superior aspect of the child's shoulders.

Benefits: The corner-shaped back minimizes scapular and shoulder retraction, a pattern of pulling the upper extremities up and back. Scapular and shoulder retraction is a position frequently observed in children who cannot stabilize against gravity. With arms and hands now placed forward, the child is able to use them for exploration, manipulation, and play. In addition, when positioned properly in the corner chair, children with low trunk tone may also demonstrate improved breathing.

Contraindications: Because of the flexed position it encourages, this type of chair is not ideal for children with increased flexor tone. In addition, these chairs are often made with a triangular seat, which may place children in excess hip abduction.

Other Comments: The corner-shaped back can also be used when making a floor seat, giving the seat the benefits of both the corner chair and a floor sitter.

Benefits: Being on the same level as one's peers is very important in building feelings of belonging and increased self-esteem in children.

Contraindications: If the child needs more support than can be provided in a floor sitter, he/she may be better off sitting with an adult. The adult's back and open legs define the sitting space for the child, and the adult's hands can be used to give the child input at the hips and shoulders to prompt better postural control.

Other Comments: Pelvic positioning straps, pummels, and chest supports can be added to basic floor sitters to provide more support.

Positioning Device: Corner Chairs

Users: Children who have adequate head control to maintain an upright position, but have some difficulty with trunk and upper extremity control may benefit from a corner

Figure 11-16. Complex seating system.

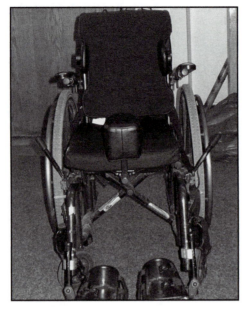

SPECIALIZED SEATING

Positioning Device: Specialized Seats for Children With Multiple Needs

Users: The child with limited head control and trunk stability to maintain a functional position in a corner chair or correctly sized chair with sides will need more external supports in a seat. The child with extremely high or fluctuating muscle tone will also need a more aggressive approach to seating (Figure 11-16).

Set up: Complex positioning systems can be designed for wheelchairs or stationary chairs. PTs or OTs who are experts in seating and positioning must initially evaluate the child's needs and make recommendations about the key features necessary for the seating system. They often will work closely with venders from durable medical equipment companies to make informed choices about specific commercially available equipment.

Some of the key questions addressed in a specialized seating assessment include the following:

- What functional activities is the child expected to perform while seated?

- In what environment will the seating system be used? Is there a lot of room for a large piece of equipment? Do sink or table heights or door widths need to be taken into account?

- Will the seating system need to be transported from one place to another? Will the wheelchair or adapted seat fit in a car or will a special van be needed?

- What are the child's presenting physical abilities and disabilities? What abnormal reflexes are present? What is the child's muscle tone like? Does the child have good head control? Are any postural deformities fixed or are they flexible? How is the child's sitting balance? Can the child shift weight while sitting?

- What features are important to the child and the child's family? This may be the most important question of all. What makes the seating system appealing? Is a special color, decoration or style important?

Some of the important principles for determining a good seating system for a child with complex physical needs include the following:

- Start with the pelvis. The position of the pelvis affects the position of the spine, head, and extremities. The child may present with posterior pelvic tilt, anterior pelvic tilt, pelvic obliquity, or pelvic rotation (various tips and twists of the pelvic girdle). If these differences are not fixed, it is important to provide the seating features necessary to establish the pelvis in a neutral position or position of slight anterior tilt.

- Pay attention to the lower extremities while you are addressing the pelvic position. Ideally, the legs should be positioned in a neutrally abducted position with 90 degrees of flexion at the hips, knees and ankles, with well-supported feet. A child with excessive hamstring tightness may need to be positioned in a less open angle of knee flexion to avoid pulling the pelvis into a posterior tilt, as it will cause the child to slide forward in the chair.

- Look at the trunk. Ideally the child's trunk should be straight up and down along midline and in good alignment. A child with poor balance and postural control may lean to the side. This child will need external supports along the sides of his/her trunk. Some children present with spinal deformities including scoliosis, kyphosis, and lordosis. Seats may need to be contoured to support these differences. A three-point system of control is often recommended to minimize the worsening of a scoliosis. One pad is placed just below the point of the convex curve that is furthest away from midline. Two more pads are placed on the opposite side of the trunk to counteract this force. One is placed at the pelvis and the other is just under the arm.

- Do not forget the head. The child needs to be able to keep the head up and righted to be able to pay attention to activities. The child with poorly integrated primitive reflexes will need to keep the head stabilized to avoid triggering unwanted movements.

- What about the upper extremities? If the child tends to retract the shoulders, some support behind the shoulders may be indicated to promote the ability to engage in fine motor activities at midline. A tray or play table is almost always indicated to go along with a complex seating system. A surface at the right height provides forearm support and a reminder that once well-positioned, the child is ready to do something interesting.

- How can skin integrity be maintained if the child has little volitional movement and is expected to stay in the seating system for long periods of time? If the chair fits the child properly, the potential for skin breakdown is reduced. A seat that tilts in space can shift the pressure from one part of the child's buttocks to another. The choice of cushions for the chair is extremely important. Cushions are often contoured to match the individual's body shape, and can be filled with foam, air, gel, or water. The thickness and density of these materials may vary within the cushion to provide the right combination of support and pressure relief. Good skin hygiene and careful monitoring is always important (Cook & Hussey, 1995; Kreutz, 1999; Trefler, Hobson, Taylor, et al.,1993).

Components of Specialized Seating Systems for Children With Multiple Needs

The following "extras" can be added to most structured seating systems. They are used to place the child in alignment, but should not become too excessive. The child should be comfortable, able to move, and functional while positioned in the device. The components should not restrain the child from being able to complete his/her daily activities. It is important to remember that when creating a specialized seating system, adaptations that are not carefully and individually fitted may do more harm than good.

- *Pummel (medial thigh supports, hip abductor)*: Prevents adduction of the hips and maintains the hips in neutral or a slight amount of abduction. The pummel should be placed at the most distal part of the knee and extend approximately 1/3 the distance of the thigh. *Note:* Pummel should *not* be placed in the groin area to prevent the child from sliding forward in the chair.

- *Lateral Thigh Supports (lateral knee adductor, adduction pads)*: Prevents unwanted or excessive abduction of the hips or can provide a counterpoint for control of hip external rotation.

- *Lateral Pelvic Supports (hip support pads, lateral hip blocks)*: Keep the hip and pelvis in the center of the seat, and help to maintain the pelvis in a vertical position, and minimize the asymmetry of the trunk.

- *Pelvic Belt (hip belt, safety belt)*: Crossing the hip joint and inferior to the anterior superior iliac spines, the pelvic belt controls hip extension and pelvic position. The pelvic belt can be placed at a 45 to 90 degree angle in relation to the seating surface.

- *Posterior Lumbar Support (lumbar roll/bar)*: Provides posterior support for the lumbar spine, and may reduce the amount of pressure in other areas, including the ischial tuberosities. The posterior lumbar support should be placed slightly below the posterior iliac crests.

- *Lateral Supports (lateral trunk pads, trunk control system)*: Provide lateral support to the thoracic spine. Supports placed higher up along the trunk and closer to the body provide more support than those positioned closer to the pelvis and further away.

- *Chest Strap (chest belt, chest panel)*: Provides anterior upper trunk control and controls a kyphotic posture.

- *Headrest (posterior head support)*: Provides posterior support for the head. It is important to allow the head to remain in a neutral position when using a headrest. Care must be taken to avoid pushing the head into too much flexion or extension.

- *Armrest (arm support)*: Support surface for the forearms is imperative to having an appropriate head and neck position. The OT practitioner must be aware of armrests that are too high and may cause scapular elevation and shoulder and neck problems.

- *Anterior Knee Support (knee block)*: Stabilizes the hips and thighs in neutral alignment from the knees. It may also be used to prevent the child from sliding forward in the chair.

Benefits: The complex seating system for the child with multiple needs should have all of the benefits of a "good position" listed earlier in this chapter

Contraindications

This is important! Choosing the right seating system for a child presenting with multiple needs is a very complex process, and only some of the very basic elements have been introduced here. A PT, OT, or assistive technology practitioner with a great deal of experience in assessing and treating children with disabilities and choosing seating systems must take the lead in selecting and obtaining the right equipment for the child. Providing the wrong equipment can do more harm than good. As an OTA, it is important to understand the basics of good positioning for a child presenting with significant physical impairments, but decisions regarding selection of the system are left to the experienced PT, OT, or assistive technology practitioner.

Positioning Device: Seat Insert

Users: Children who want or need to sit in a specific chair but do not fit particularly well in it may need a seat modification or insert. Some children who like to sit cross-legged with their feet tucked in under their thighs, but have difficulty paying attention in such a position, may benefit from an insert.

Set up: To decrease the seat width and/or seat depth to help make a more snug, well-defined sitting space for the child, sometimes all that is needed are some vinyl covered foam cushions that can be strapped to the sides and/or back

Figure 11-17. Vinyl covered foam inserts.

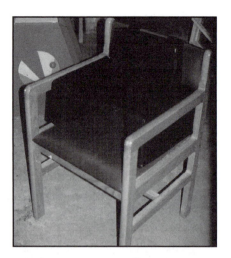

Figure 11-18. Seat insert for dining room chair.

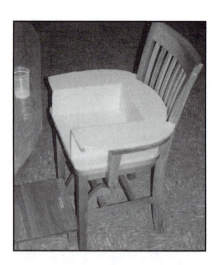

Figure 11-19. Seat insert for rocker.

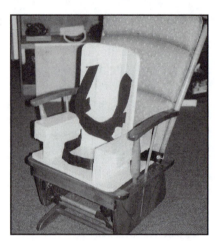

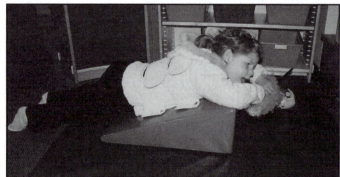

Figure 11-20. Wedge.

of the chair (Figure 11-17). Seat inserts for dining room chairs or rockers are often constructed out of TriWall® (Figures 11-18 and 11-19). These devices may have corner chair style backs, high sides, pelvic positioning belts, or other needed features.

Benefits: The seat insert gives the child a functional sitting position without the expense of purchasing a new chair.

Contraindications: It is important to make sure that the insert is securely attached to the chair. It can be attached with straps to the back or bottom of the seat. Sometimes a generous amount of Velcro® (Velcro USA, Manchester, NH) will do the trick.

Positioning Device: Wedge

Users: Children who need to increase tolerance to the prone position or improve proximal stability or head control may benefit from being positioned on a wedge (Figure 11-20).

Set up: Set up depends on the child and his/her therapeutic objectives. The front edge of the wedge should be the same height as the distance between the child's wrist and his axilla (armpit) if weight bearing on extended arms is the

objective. The height of the front of the wedge should be a bit less that the distance from the child's elbow to the axilla if weight bearing on the forearms is more appropriate for the child. The small end of the wedge should ideally be high enough off the ground so that the child's feet can hang over the edge in a neutral position (to avoid plantar flexion contractures). The positioning wedge needs to be used in conjunction with activities that are fun and meaningful for the child, so that the experience of being on the wedge is a positive one.

Benefits: The child works on head control as he lifts his head to look at toys and people. Weight bearing positions in prone improve strength and proximal stability. This position also helps to stretch muscles in the hips, knees, and shoulders.

Contraindications: If the child is having very little success lifting his/her head, the static wedge may be too advanced for him. Gentle rolling on a ball in a prone position may offer better head support. The child who has difficulty tolerating being in prone should not be required to maintain this position for long periods of time. A graded tolerance program may be effective with such a child.

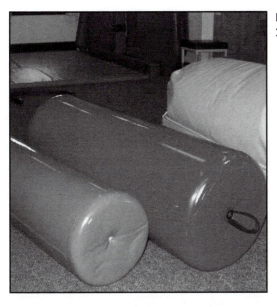

Figure 11-21. Bolster.

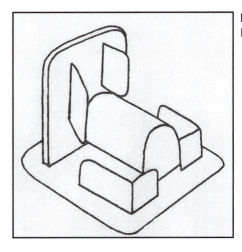

Figure 11-22. Bolster chair.

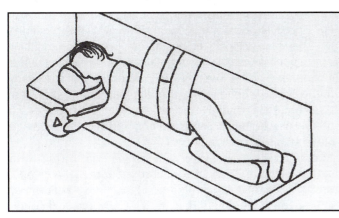

Figure 11-23. Side lyer.

Other Comments: The child that tends to roll may need some side modifications to prevent rolling off the wedge (Warner, 1987).

Positioning Device: Bolster

Users: Children with athetoid or spastic CP who present with lower extremity stiffness that may prevent them from sitting with a wide base of support may be good candidates for bolster use (Figure 11-21).

Set up: The bolster should be small enough so that the child's feet can be planted firmly on the floor. It is also important that the size of the bolster facilitates 90 degrees of hip, knee, and ankle flexion.

Benefits: Straddling a bolster may assist postural control in children who require a wide base of support for stability. It may also be used to decrease hip and knee stiffness, place the child's pelvis in a more neutral position, and approximate normal spinal curves. Bolster chairs maintain hip flexion with abduction and external rotation, a position that promotes movement in sitting and inhibits the deformity influences of W-sitting.

Contraindications: The bolster encourages hip abduction and is therefore not ideal for a child with low tone and excessive hip motion, or a child who overabducts his/her hips in a relaxed position. In addition, children presenting with balance and equilibrium impairments or multiple disabilities may have difficulties remaining seated on top of this chair.

Positioning Device: Bolster Chair

Users: Children presenting with increased muscle tone in their lower extremities may have a tendency to sit with their legs adducted and extended. This increase in extensor tone may overflow into the rest of the body, making purposeful activity difficult (Figure 11-22).

Set up: The bolster chair promotes a position of hip flexion, abduction, and external rotation, as well as knee and ankle flexion.

Benefits: This position breaks up the extensor pattern and may help normalize tone throughout the body. Normalization of tone may help the child gain postural control of the trunk, head, and upper extremities. The bolster chair also provides the child with a wide base of support, which gives the youngster a lot of background stability.

Positioning Device: Side lyer

Users: Children presenting with physical disabilities who cannot move themselves from one position into another may benefit from using a side lyer. This is an especially good position for children whose movements are influenced by the ATNR (Figure 11-23).

Set up: The child is positioned on his side with his back against the back support piece of the side lyer. Thick straps at the hips and chest prevent the child from slipping down into a prone or supine position. To support the head so that it stays in alignment with the trunk, generally the child also needs a pillow or other soft positioning block. To break up high tone, it may also be important to support the child's top leg on a block or pillow in a position of hip flexion and

Figure 11-24. Easy Stand.

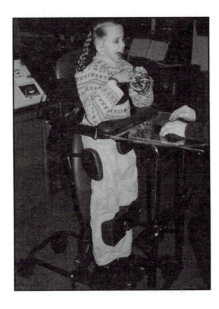

abduction and knee flexion. The side lyer must be used in conjunction with an activity that is motivating for the child. This position will not be well-tolerated if there is nothing fun to do while in it.

Benefits: The head is less likely to turn when it is supported in a neutral position in proper alignment with the spine, a position facilitated by the side lyer. If the head is stable, the ATNR will not be triggered. The child's upper extremities are blocked from retraction in this position, and instead, gravity brings the upper extremities toward midline. In this position the child does not need to reach against gravity so may have greater range of active movement. Children with limited range of motion often have more success reaching for objects at midline when positioned in the side lyer than they do when seated.

Contraindications: The child must be supported and supervised so that proper alignment is achieved and maintained.

Positioning Device: Stander

Users: Children (whether they are ambulatory or not) who are not safe maintaining an unsupported standing position for more than a few minutes may benefit from using a stander (Figure 11-24).

Set up: Choosing the correct standing system for the individual and correctly adjusting the positioning components is a complex process that needs to be carried out by a PT. The trick is to make sure that all areas of the body that need support are properly supported, but also that the parts of the body that the child can control well are not oversupported. There are several types of standers available for use with the pediatric population. A vertical stander is used with children who have good head control and fairly good trunk control but need support and alignment of the lower extremities. A prone stander tips the child slightly forward and provides support along the anterior surface. A child using a prone

stander must have emerging control of the head and trunk. A supine stander tips the child slightly back and provides support along the posterior surface. The supine stander is used for children with less control of the head and trunk, low muscle tone, or limited standing experience. Some standers, such as the Easy Stand® (Altimate Medical, Morton, MN), are designed with a seat to transfer the child to and a transition mechanism to allow the caregiver to easily move the child into a standing position. Some standers have large wheels with rims on the sides so that users can move themselves around freely while in the standing position. Positioning components vary with the type of stander and the child's needs but include pelvic bands, solid pelvic stabilizers, abduction wedges, lateral leg supports, knee blocks, knee pads, fool wells, foot straps, lateral trunk supports, anterior chest supports, and head supports, and trays.

Benefits: While positioned in the stander, tight muscles and joints are passively stretched, which helps to prevent contractures. The child receives the sensory feedback of being positioned with proper joint alignment, which may help improve posture in other positions. Weight bearing increases bone density, and overall increased standing tolerance may help improve strength and endurance needed for ambulation. Further, breathing and digestive processes may improve when a child is on a standing program. Perhaps the most important benefit of using a stander, however, is the uplifting psychological sense that children get when they are able to stand up with their peers.

Contraindications: Never try a stander with a child with multiple physical disabilities without the approval and input from a PT. Bearing weight in a poorly aligned position may increase the likelihood of deformities. Some medical conditions may limit the child's endurance for being upright, so the angle of tilt and the length of time in a stander must be very carefully monitored.

Other Comments: It is imperative that any OT practitioner be properly trained in how to safely transfer the child into the stander. As a rule of thumb, after transferring the child to a stander, the pelvic band should be fastened first so that the child is safely stabilized in standing before the other positioning adjustments are made.

Positioning Device: Dynamic Trunk Splints

Users: Children presenting with a variety of neuromuscular disorders including cerebral palsy, hypotonia, dystonia, and traumatic brain injury may use orthotics to help promote correct biomechanical alignment of the musculoskeletal system (Figure 11-25).

Set up: Both OT and PT practitioners have traditionally employed many strategies to improve trunk stability and posture, including active-assisted activities, handling, adapted chairs, standers, and plastic or rigid braces. A dynamic trunk splint is a new alternative that promotes proper pos-

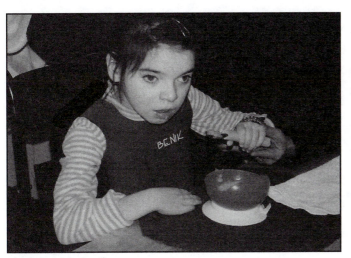

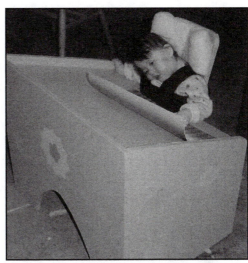

Figure 11-26. Angled play table.

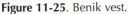

Figure 11-25. Benik vest.

ture. This support, called a thoracic lumbar spinal orthosis or TLSO, is an orthotic that covers the thoracic and lumbar curves of the entire back. Dynamic trunk splints are constructed of multiple layers of lycra or neoprene material (a stretchy, polyester knit fabric) and lined with terrycloth for added comfort. The dynamic trunk splint, worn over clothing, has Velcro® straps to accommodate for variations in clothing thickness as well as the child's growth and comfort. In addition to promoting proper alignment, the garment provides constant pressure to the receptors in muscles and joints. Current examples of dynamic trunk splints include the Benik™ vest (Benik Corp., Silverdale, WA) and TheraTogs™ (TheraTogs, Telluride, CO).

These prefabricated vests are prescribed by a physician and implemented by OTs and PTs, as well as other service providers including OTAs, teachers, and family members. As with any new splint, a wearing schedule is established and closely monitored by the OT or PT practitioner. As the child gains motor control and strength, wearing time of the dynamic trunk splint is decreased to promote independence and skill development.

Benefits: Dynamic trunk splints are more flexible than the traditional rigid plastic splints. They provide sensory cues for proper co-contraction of muscles and help to reeducate the muscles instead of simply correcting biomechanical alignment. Dynamic trunk splints provide stability to the trunk, pelvis, and shoulder girdle, and they may assist in reducing tone in spastic and dystonic muscles.

Research suggests that dynamic trunk splints improve trunk control, posture, and upper extremity function while reducing involuntary movements and self-stimulatory behaviors (Blair et al., 1996; Fertel-Daly, Bedell, & Hinojosa, 2001). Other studies have shown that weighted vests or compression garments increase on-task behavior during fine motor activities (Vandenberg, 2001).

Contraindications: Vest use should be discontinued if decreased respiratory function, increased seizure activity, or excessive extensor tone occur. As some children may be allergic to neoprene, careful monitoring of the dynamic trunk splint is necessary. Additionally, the vest may be uncomfortably sweaty during hot weather, again pointing to the need to carefully monitor its use.

TABLES AND TRAYS

Positioning Device: Tables and Trays

Users: All children need access to work surfaces for school activities and fine motor play. Children with special positioning equipment may not be able to access regular tables or desks, so may need modifications of existing tables or surfaces to go with their other devices (Figure 11-26).

Set up: Tables without support structures right underneath the work surface are best for children in wheelchairs. Sometimes these tables need to be quite high so that the chair can be rolled underneath it, especially if the child's wheelchair tips in space so that the child's knees are raised. Adjustable height tables may work for these children, or blocks of wood (with edges to keep the table legs from slipping off the blocks) can be made to make the table high enough. If the child uses a high joystick to drive his or her chair, it is possible to adapt a table with a cut-out to accommodate the joystick. Some children with limited upper extremity control may benefit from table support that wraps around the sides of the seat so that their elbows and forearms are well supported. A wheelchair tray provides this side surface. If the child is not in a wheelchair, a table or table cover with a rounded cut-out to fit around the child's trunk can either be purchased or fabricated. Floor tables may be used with toddlers who are working on sitting on the carpet.

Figure 11-27.
Volunteer constructing a cardboard chair.

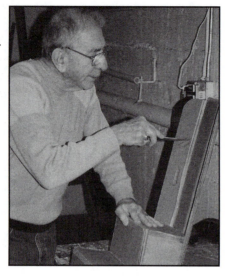

sive, and not too intimidating to work with. Footrests, toddler sized chairs, corner chairs, seat inserts, play tables, and standing boxes can be constructed using this material (Campbell & Truesdell, 2000: Bergen, 1980: Cope & Morrison, 1979: DeBruin, 1988: Blanche & O'Brien, 1984: Horn, Millen, Cavanaugh, & Komisar, 1987: Dilger & Rowe, 1987) (Figure 11-27). Wedges, crescent-shaped pillows, straps, and bolsters can be made using fabric and foam (Table 11-1).

Summary

Evaluating a child who needs positioning equipment is a complex process that should be initiated by qualified OTs and PTs. The OTA's role in pediatric positioning is often to make sure that the child uses the recommended equipment as prescribed. This can, depending on demonstrated competency and state and facility guidelines, include training other staff members in how to correctly and safely use positioning devices. The OTA should always be on the lookout for positioning problems. Is a child sitting with dangling feet? Is another child's wheelchair tray missing? What about the child who leans so far over that his face is practically in his plate at lunch time? All of these issues need to be brought to the attention of the supervising therapists.

REFLECTIONS FOR THE OTA

Many children with visual impairments will see their work better if it is raised up and slanted so that it is closer to their eyes. Book stands for those with visual impairments work best when the slanted part with a lip rests on a box like structure that is set at the right height for the child, while easels are usually used right on a table. Sometimes a nonskid surface is useful under book stands or easels to keep them from sliding.

Benefits: Matching the right table to the child means that he or she can be engaged in functional and meaningful activity while being correctly positioned. Making sure that the table and any stands on the table are at the right height promotes good upper trunk and upper extremity positioning.

REFLECTIONS FOR THE OTA

Small tables with lips around the sides keep toys from falling off and provide a well-defined space for young children.

How Do You Obtain Positioning Equipment?

An Internet search is a good way to begin to get information about the equipment that is available. The website www.abledata.com provides listings of many kinds of assistive technology devices.

Occupational therapy practitioners with a little bit of ingenuity and time can design and construct positioning devices themselves (Warner, 1998). A three-layered corrugated cardboard material (TriWall®) is lightweight, inexpen-

Case Study

Billy is a 2-year-old child with multiple developmental disabilities. He is visually impaired and delayed in cognitive development. Billy presents with low muscle tone, limited trunk control, emerging head control, and evidence of a poorly integrated ATNR reflex. He likes lying on his back but cries whenever he is positioned on his stomach. Billy has a molded plastic-covered Tumble Form® seat (Bergeron Health Care, Dolgeville, NY) that positions him tipped back in space at the floor level. He does not have a play surface to use with this seat. His attention to activities in this tipped back position is fleeting, but the position was chosen for him due to limited head control. Other than his car seat, he does not have any other positioning equipment. During occupational and physical therapy sessions, Billy ring sits on the carpet while the OT/PT practitioner sits behind him and provides input at the pelvis and shoulders. Overall, Billy is showing some nice gains in head and trunk control.

Billy visually attends best to yellow or red items that are at or above eye level. He likes funny sounds. He will keep his hand on a toy for several seconds when it is placed right near his hand, but he does not initiate reaching for objects.

- What positioning options should be tried with Billy?
- What positioning options should be avoided?

Table 11-1

Cardboard Chair and Table Measurements

Name: Contact Person:
Date: Phone Number:

I. __Type of Chair__

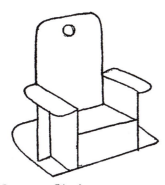

☐ Square Chair

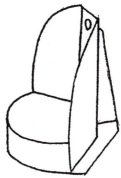

☐ Standard Corner Chair

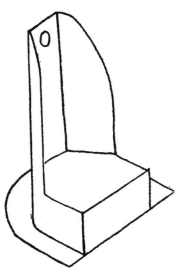

☐ Corner Chair with Straight Front

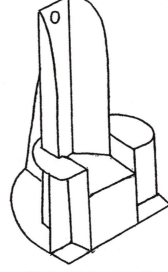

☐ Corner Chair with Straight Front and Arm Rests

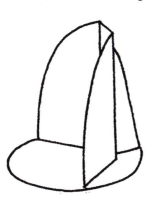

☐ Floor Sitter   ☐ Other: Please Sketch

Table 11-1 (continued)

Cardboard Chair and Table Measurements

II. Positioning Features

A. Seat to Back Angle

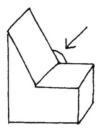

☐ Standard: 90 degrees

☐ Other (measure or draw):

B. Tilt in Space

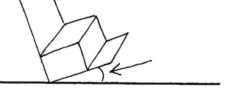

☐ Upright

☐ Tipped back in space
Angle of tilt (measure or draw):

C. Seat Add-Ons

☐ Pelvic positioning belt (seat belt)

☐ Shoulder straps

☐ Chest support straps

☐ Pummel

☐ Head positioning cushions

☐ Lateral supports

☐ Foot straps

☐ Blocks on sides of seat

☐ Other (please describe)

<u>Table 11-1 (continued)</u>

Cardboard Chair and Table Measurements

III. Child Measurements

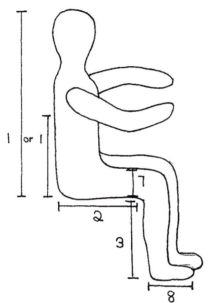 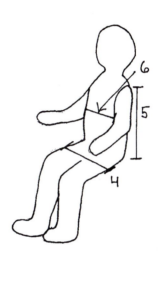

1. **Back Height**
   Child with poor head control:
   Top of head to bottom of buttock

   _____

   Child with good head control:
   Bottom of scapula (shoulder blade) to bottom of buttock

   _____

2. **Seat Depth**
   Base of spine to back of knee

   _____

3. **Seat Height**
   Bottom of foot to popliteal fossa (area behind knee)

   _____

4. **Seat Width**
   Widest distance across hips or lap

   _____

5. **Shoulder Height** (If shoulder straps are needed)
   Bottom of buttock to top of shoulders

   _____

6. **Trunk width** (If chest straps are needed)
   Width across chest

   _____

7. **Lap Height** (If pummel is recommended)
   Height of child's thighs when seated

   _____

8. **Foot Length** (If foot rest is needed)
   Length of feet with shoes on

   _____

Table 11-1 (continued)

Cardboard Chair and Table Measurements

IV. Chair Measurements

The recommendations for chair measurements listed below should provide the child with a good fit immediately. If the chair is made an inch or so bigger in all dimensions then there is room for some growth. Cushions or temporary removable cardboard layers may be needed to get a good initial fit.

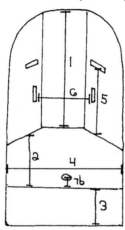 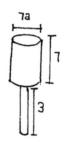

1. **Back Height**
   Same as back height measurement on child
   _____

2. **Seat Depth**
   Subtract 1" from measurement on child
   (Seat depth can be tricky on chairs with corner-shaped backs. The child's bottom does not usually fit all the way to the center of the back. Measure from a few inches out on diagonal side.)
   _____

3. **Seat Height**
   Subtract 1" from measurement on child
   _____

4. **Seat Width**
   Add 2 " to measurement on child
   _____

5. **Shoulder Strap Height**
   Same as measurement on child
   _____

6. **Chest/Trunk Strap Placement**
   Same as measurement on child
   _____

7. **Pummel Height**
   Add 1" to lap height
   _____

7a. **Pummel Diameter**
   (Based on amount of hip abduction required)
   _____

7b. **Pummel Location**
   (Distance in from seat front)
   _____

8. **Foot Rest Depth**
   (Add 2" to foot length)
   _____

Table 11-1 (continued)

Cardboard Chair and Table Measurements

V. Table Measurements

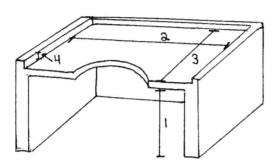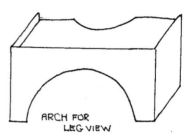

ARCH FOR LEG VIEW

1. **Height** (Allow forearms to rest on table surface with
   90 degrees of elbow flexion.)
   Add 1" to height of pummel or arm rests(whichever is higher)   _____

2. **Width** Based on size of toys. 24" is often used.   _____

3. **Depth** Based on size of toys. Usually 16" to 18".   _____

4. **Lip Height**   _____

Other Features:

Table Surface Shape   (Make paper template if the fit needs
to be exact)

☐ Tummy cut and side angles to fit against the back of the seat

☐ Cut-aways on both sides to allow two children to play at the same time

☐ Long extensions along the sides to give extra support at the elbows

Table Tilt

☐ Flat

☐ Angled surface (_____degrees)

Table Surface

☐ Smooth

☐ With indentations (Describe shapes of desired compartments)

Leg View

☐ Cut arch so the child's foot/leg position can be monitored

• What are some activities that might be set up for him in conjunction with changes in positioning?

Application Activities

1. Complete an Internet search to find out more information about given positioning equipment. Abledata is a resource to start with.

2. Look at a fairly complicated seating system in a wheelchair. Try to name each component and figure out why it might have been chosen.

3. Review adaptive equipment company catalogs to compare similar positioning devices for cost, attractiveness, simplicity, ease of use, and adjustability.

4. Build a simple positioning device for a specific child using low or no cost materials.

5. Design and construct a more complex positioning device for a specific child using low or no cost materials.

Acknowledgments

Several people contributed to this chapter through writing sections, lecturing on positioning at Tufts University, informally discussing the use of positioning devices, or helping with taking photographs of children at Perkins School for the Blind. I would very much like to thank Kim O'Sullivan, Melissa Callaghan, Gary Rabideau, Faith Saftler-Savage, Diane Zuck, and Maryann Girardi for their help with this project.

References

Bergen, A. F. (1980). *TriWall®: Adaptive equipment without tools*. NDT newsletter.

Blair, E., Ballantyne, J., Horsman, S., & Chauvel, P. (1996). A study of a dynamic proximal stability splint in the management of children with cerebral palsy. *Developmental Medicine and Child Neurology, 38(2), 191-193.*

Blanche, E., & O'Brien, M. (1984). Adaptive equipment from boxes. *Teaching exceptional children, 17(1), 23-26.*

Campbell, M., & Truesdell, A. (2000). Creative constructions: Technologies that make adaptive design accessible, affordable, inclusive, and fun. Cambridge, MA: Author.

Case-Smith, J., Allen, A. S., & Pratt, P. N. (1996). *Occupational therapy for children*. St. Louis, MO: Mosby.

Cook, A. M., & Hussey, S. M. (1995). *Assistive technologies: Principles and practice*. St. Louis, MO: Mosby.

Cope, G., & Morrison, P. (1979). *The further adventures of cardboard carpentry*. Arlington, MA: Learning Things, Inc.

DeBruin, J. (1988). *Cardboard carpentry*. Toledo, OH: JED and Associates.

Dilger, N., & Rowe, L. (1987). *Equipment fabrication with TriWall®*. New York: Support Surface, Inc.

Fertel-Daly, D., Bedell, G., & Hinojosa, J. (2001). Effects of a weighted vest on attention to task and self stimulatory behaviors in preschoolers with pervasive developmental disorders. *American Journal of Occupational Therapy, 55*, 629-640.

Finnie, N. (1975). *Handling the young cerebral palsied child at home*. New York: Dutton Sunrise.

Horn, E., Millen, C. E., Cavanaugh, C. L., & Komisar, S. (1987). Chair inserts for preschoolers. *Teaching exceptional children, 20(1), 19-22.*

Kreutz, D. (1999). Characteristics of seating and positioning technologies. In *Fundamentals of assistive technology* (pp. VIII1-VIII30). Arlington, VA: The Rehabilitation Engineering and Assistive Technology Society of North America (RESNA).

Trefler, E., Hobson, D., Johnson Taylor, S., Monahan, L., & Shaw, C. G. (1993). *Seating and mobility for persons with physical disabilities*. Tucson, AZ: Therapy Skill Builders.

Vandenberg, N. (2001). The use of a weighted vest to increase on-task behavior in children with attention difficulties. *American Journal of Occupational Therapy, 55(6),* 621-628.

Warner, D. (1987). *Disabled village children*. Palo Alto, CA: The Hesperian Foundation.

Warner, D. (1998). *Nothing about us without us: Developing innovative technologies for, by, and with disabled persons*. Palo Alto, CA: Health Wrights.

INTRODUCTION TO SENSORY INTEGRATION

Teresa A. May-Benson, MS, OTR/L

Chapter Objectives

- Become familiar with the history of sensory integration.
- Understand the basic premises and neurophysiological basis of sensory integrative theory and its application to occupational performance.
- Describe the components of a comprehensive sensory integrative assessment and identify appropriate evaluations and observations.
- Identify and observe behaviors characteristic of the various sensory integrative dysfunctions.
- Become familiar with the underlying postulates and basic concepts of sensory integration intervention.
- Understand the concepts and application of sensory diets within functional settings.

Life is a sensory experience. During every moment of our life we experience the world through our varied sensory systems. Sensory experiences drive our behavior and contribute to the organization of our thoughts and emotions. (Unknown)

Introduction

Life *is* a sensory experience. Our nervous systems process and use the constant stream of sensory input that assaults every moment of our lives and which impacts our behavior, emotions, arousal level and ability to perform skilled activities. For nearly 40 years occupational therapists (OTs) and

occupational therapy assistants (OTAs) have been concerned with understanding, assessing, and treating problems in sensory processing and motor coordination in children and adults. These problems range from overt disruptions in sensory functioning caused by injury or illness, to more subtle problems in sensory processing and integration in otherwise uninvolved individuals. Today, sensory integration-based occupational therapy reflects one of the most commonly used frames of reference in occupational therapy practice, especially in the area of pediatrics.

Historical Background and Basic Concepts of Sensory Integration Theory

Sensory integration is a term that holds multiple meanings. To many medical and health professionals sensory integration refers to a neurophysiological process that occurs in the central nervous system. To most occupational and physical therapy practitioners, sensory integration refers to a theory linking specialized neurological processes with observable behavior. It also reflects a practice frame of reference to guide occupational therapy assessment and intervention (Miller & Lane, 2000).

Sensory integration theory was developed by occupational therapist, Dr. A. Jean Ayres. Ayres initially observed perceptual, motor coordination, and sensory processing problems in a clinical population of children with learning disabilities. Her primary objective in developing sensory integrative theory was to understand and explain these prob-

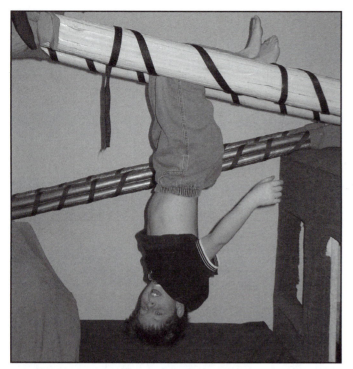

Figure 12-1. Integration of sensory information from movement and one's muscles allows the child to explore the possibilities of his environment and move his body against gravity in joyful play.

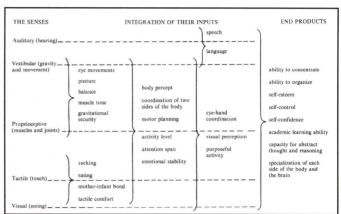

Figure 12-2. The Senses, Integration of Their Inputs, and Their End Products (Ayres, 1982). Reprinted with permission from Western Psychological Services.

lems, and to determine the best interventions to address these difficulties (Spitzer & Roley, 2001).

Ayres (1972) defined sensory integration as "the neurological process that organizes sensation from one's own body and from the environment and makes it possible to use the body effectively within the environment." (p. 11). The normal process of sensory integration reflects a dynamic, self-organizing interaction between the child's abilities and his/her interactions with the environment. This dynamic interactive process is believed to be the natural result of a child's typical sensori-motor development (Turkewitz, 1994). Sensory integration allows the child to engage in and participate in a wide range of meaningful and purposeful occupations of daily life (Parham & Mailloux, 2001; Parham, 2001) (Figure 12-1).

The influence of efficient sensory processing on functional performance in daily life is central to sensory integrative theory. Dysfunction in various aspects of sensory integration may interfere with a child's occupational performance in the areas of play, activities of daily living, and academics, to name a few. For instance, deficits in play behaviors such as participating with others, managing toys, and maneuvering through space have been linked to deficits in sensory integrative functioning in preschool and school-aged children (Schaaf, 1990; Schaaf, Merrill & Kinsella, 1987; Bundy, 1989; Clifford & Bundy, 1989). Difficulties in *praxis* and motor coordination skills have been shown to be related to

functional motor skills in a wide range of children's activities of daily living including dressing, participation in sports, and eating (reviewed by May-Benson, Ingolia & Koomar, 2002). Academic skills such as arithmetic and reading have been shown to be significantly related to sensory integration skills such as praxis and sensory processing of tactile inputs (Parham, 1998). Similarly, sensory integration functions have been shown to influence behavior and emotions (Baranek, Foster, & Berkson, 1997; Kinneally, Oliver, & Wilbarger, 1995), potentially contributing to some individuals making less than optimal occupational choices, such as delinquency (Fanchiang, et al, 1990). Ayres' classic chart in Figure 12-2 demonstrates the relationships between sensory processing and various *functional behaviors*.

Ayres (1972; 1976; 1977; 1987) early studies demonstrated five consistent patterns of sensory integrative dysfunction, which she believed impacted functional performance. These patterns were identified as: 1) difficulties in praxis associated with decreased tactile discrimination, 2) difficulties in sequencing and bilateral coordination associated with decreased vestibular/proprioceptive processing, 3) tactile defensiveness associated with increased activity and distractibility, 4) decreased form and space perception, and 5) decreased auditory–language processing. Mulligan (1998) found a primary problem in generalized sensory integration function with four specific subgroups of deficits including: visual perceptual deficits, bilateral integration and sequencing deficits, deficits in praxis (dyspraxia), and somatosensory deficits. Based largely on Ayres' and Mulligan's work, Bundy and Murray (2002) proposed four major areas of sensory integrative dysfunction:

1. Dysfunction in *sensory modulation* (SMD).

2. Two subtypes of dysfunction in praxis: poor praxis associated with decreased tactile discrimination skills (somatodyspraxia) and bilateral coordination/sequencing deficits.

Table 12-1

Examples of Behaviors of Sensory Integration Dysfunction at Activities and Participation Levels of Occupational Performance

Impairments System/Function	Activities ADLs Occupations Social	Participation Self Maintenance Occupational Roles Social Relationships
SENSORY MODULATION DYSFUNCTION		
Tactile Defensiveness	Avoids wearing certain clothes; avoids haircut and hair washing; nail cutting Avoids finger painting; playing in sand box; walking on grass Hits or pushes others, pulls away from touch; resists cuddles	Unable to wear suit for religious events or special parties. Avoids classroom activities and play activities. Decreased bonding with parents; acting out causes disruption in classroom.
Hypersensitive to Movement	Unable to ride school bus because gets car sick	Avoids school fieldtrips or makes family vacations miserable.
Gravitational Insecurity	Avoids slides, swings and merry-go-rounds on playground	Decreased social interaction with other peers.
Auditory Defensiveness	Attends to humming of florescent lights	Increased distractibility in classroom, decreased attention and classroom participation.
Visual Defensiveness	Sensitive to bright lights; Overloaded by visual stimuli on walls	Increased distractibility or shutdown in the classroom.
Olfactory/Gustatory Defensiveness	Gags and refuses many foods; Avoids eating mixed texture foods	Avoids or tantrums in school cafeteria; unable to eat in restaurants.
DYSFUNCTION IN SENSORY DISCRIMINATION		
Tactile Discrimination Difficulties	Eats with hands; messy eater; unaware of clothing being awry Cannot manipulate pencil or small toys Bumps into things, falls down, trips	Class clown; disrupts classroom; Poor self-esteem; frustration; anxiety about not being able to do tasks.
Movement Discrimination Difficulties	Seeks spinning and swinging Poor balance for bike riding or other gross motor tasks Falls out of seat frequently when leans over	Often in trouble for being overly active. Avoids playing with other children. Often impulsive and gets injured.
Proprioceptive Discrimination Difficulty	Frequently uses hands instead of utensils Drops or breaks things often Uses too much force on pencil and often breaks pencil leads or tears paper; Often seems unnecessarily rough	Poor social acceptance because of sloppy eating habits. Often in trouble for breaking objects and/or spilling things. Frustration from increased time to complete written tasks, tearing school papers. Often in trouble for pushing or shoving others.

3. Dysfunctions in visual perception and visual motor skills.

4. Auditory-language dysfunctions.

These problems in sensory integration are manifested in two major aspects of functioning: behavioral regulation and skilled behavior. Difficulties in functioning in these areas are reflected in a child's behavior at multiple levels. Table 12-1 presents some examples of disruptions in performance in functional life skills in various areas of sensory integrative dysfunction.

The sensory integration theory frame of reference is based on three concepts: 1) that, in the broadest sense, learning and function are dependent on efficient sensory integration, 2) that problems in sensory processing interfere with learning, functional skills, and behavior, and 3) that providing enhanced sensations in the context of a meaningful activity which requires increasingly adaptive responses facilitates learning, skill, and behavior (Bundy and Murray, 2002).

Foundations of Sensory Integration Theory

Sensory integrative theory proposes that foundational mechanisms and functional outputs may be improved through the provision of *enhanced sensory inputs*. These enhanced and intense sensory experiences are provided in a controlled manner in the context of activities and in an environment that is meaningful to the child. Most often this is in the context of play. To encourage and promote the child's ability to demonstrate increasingly more adaptive responses to the environment and task demands, the OTA may, as set forth by state guidelines, demonstrated competency, and under the supervision of an OT, guide and facilitate the selection of therapeutic activities, based on the child's wants and needs. The basic premise of sensory integration therapy is that an increased ability to respond appropriately to environmental demands allows the child to better engage in functional occupations (Figure 12-3).

ASSUMPTIONS OF SENSORY INTEGRATION THEORY

Sensory integration theory is the most researched practice area within the field of occupational therapy (Miller & Kinnealey, 1993; Mulligan, 2002; Parham & Mailloux, 2001). Its underlying assumptions and postulates are firmly based on current neurophysiological research (Mulligan, 2002). Sensory integration theory is comprised of five major underlying assumptions regarding nervous system functioning (Bundy, Lane, & Murray, 2002; Kimball, 1999). The five assumptions are as follows.

Central Nervous System Plasticity

The rationale of sensory integrative intervention is based on the concept of neuroplasticity or the proposed capacity of the nervous system to adapt in response to provision of enhanced sensory inputs (Bundy & Murray, 2002). This process of plasticity occurs as a natural developmental process or as a response to injury or insult to the nervous system (Schaaf, 1994a). Early insults and experiences such as prenatal stress and environmental deprivation may interfere with the development of neural connections. Alternately, enriched early sensory inputs or experiences may facilitate the formation and development of these connections (Jacobs & Schneider, 2001). Sensory integration intervention is believed to encourage neuroplasticity through the child's self-initiated engagement in activities and the provision of an enriched sensory/ motor environment.

Developmental Progressions

Sensory integration is a central nervous system process that occurs as the developing child begins to attach meaning to and gain mastery over the sensory inputs he/she experiences. In the typically developing child these processes emerge effortlessly and without adult intervention, teaching, or guidance to allow the child to master skills and perform daily occupations (Parham & Mailloux, 2001). Please refer to Table 12-2 for examples of specific sensory-motor and adaptive responses. A detailed outline of specific sensory-motor and adaptive responses characteristic of developmental stages from infancy to age seven may be found in Parham and Mailloux (2001) (please refer to References).

Systems Theory and Organization of the Central Nervous System

Sensory integration processes are believed to occur primarily at the brainstem and subcortical levels of the nervous system, however, higher cortical processes are important in the development of praxis and production of adaptive responses. From the onset of her work, Ayres stressed that all levels of brain structures were interactively involved in the sensory integration process. However, she used a simple linear model to illustrate how higher level cortical processes relied upon and were dependent upon adequate functioning and organization of the lower brain centers (Spitzer, 1999) (refer to Figure 12-2). This perspective led many to view sensory integration as a hierarchical process (Kimball 1999). In a hierarchical model neural processes are proposed to develop and function in a pre-determined, linear and specific fashion with lower skills developing before higher ones emerge (e.g. a child must crawl before walking). The process of sensory integration, however, is not a linear neurological process but involves many complex interactions among all levels of central nervous system function. Consequently, behaviors and skills do not emerge in a strictly linear manner, but develop in a more spiral fashion in which a child may simultaneously develop multiple skills at various levels (e.g. a child begins to creep and stand at the same time) (Roley, & Spitzer, 2001). This perspective expands on the hierarchical and spiral models of sensory integration theory and embraces the concept of an open dynamic system to capture the essence of how children are proposed to develop (Spitzer & Roley, 2001).

Adaptive Responses

The primary concept of sensory integrative theory that differentiates it from other models of sensory motor development or sensory stimulation is its emphasis on the promotion of adaptive responses. At its most basic, an adaptive

Table 12-2
Examples of Typical Developmental Sequences Related to Sensory Integration

Developmental Stages	Behaviors
Prenatal Period	• Tactile inputs develop by 12 weeks gestation for hand to mouth exploration. • Vestibular functions appear by 9 weeks gestation to exhibit Moro responses.
Neonatal Period	• Tactile inputs are critical for mother-infant bonding. • Vestibular system is fully functional at birth; movement inputs such as rocking are calming.
2 to 6 Months	• Infant uses tactile system to explore hands and mouth and objects in the environment. • Vestibular system facilitates infant's body movements against gravity; head righting, rolling.
6 to 12 Months	• Tactile system refines with increased precision in fine motor skills. • Vestibular system refines with development of movement against gravity including sitting, crawling, standing, walking. • Motor skills and praxis develop with transfer of objects from hand to hand, hands manipulating objects at midline, self-feeding skills and use of utensils, refinement of object manipulation.
12 to 24 Months	• Integration of vestibular/proprioceptive/visual inputs develops for postural control. • Praxis skills develop with climbing, swinging, exploration of environment.
3 through 7 Years	• Tactile inputs contribute to continuing development of fine motor manipulation skills and body awareness for increased independence in eating, dressing, and play skills. • Vestibular and proprioceptive inputs contribute to development of eye-hand coordination, ball skills, balance skills, bike riding, and so forth.

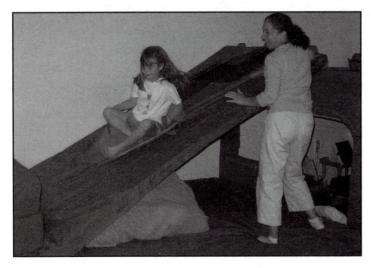

Figure 12-3. In sensory integration intervention, activities provide enhanced movement inputs, challenge postural control, promote adaptive responses and are fun for the child and therapist.

Table 12-3
Levels of Adaptive Response

- Responds to passive stimuli—This is often the *just right challenge* in a low functioning and fragile nervous system, and is where treatment may need to begin. Examples include showing pleasure when vibration is applied or initiating eye contact when pushed on a swing (please refer to Figure 12-4).

- Holding on and staying put—The child is able to maintain a position in a changing environment such as holding onto the ropes of a swing and staying in one position while swinging (please refer to Figure 12-5).

- Alternating contracting and relaxing muscle groups—This is the motor control necessary for pumping a swing and maintaining righting on a changeable surface (please refer to Figure 12-6).

- Initiating an activity but not completing it independently—The child may initiate wanting to climb on a swing, but still needs assistance to accomplish this (please refer to Figure 12-7).

- Moving independently in a somewhat familiar manner—The child initiates and moves independently in an accustomed way, such as walking forwards up a ramp (please refer to Figure 12-8).

- Moving through the environment in an unfamiliar way—Exploration is expanding into more novel ways to move, such as climbing through hanging hoops or swinging on a trapeze and kicking a target (please refer to Figure 12-9).

- Performing complicated activities requiring unfamiliar ways of moving—This level of planning involves multiple sensory adaptations, complicated timing and spatial-temporal adaptation. Examples include setting up and moving through an obstacle or participating in sports activities such as soccer or basketball (please refer to Figure 12-10).

Adapted from the works of A. Jean Ayres c. 1980.

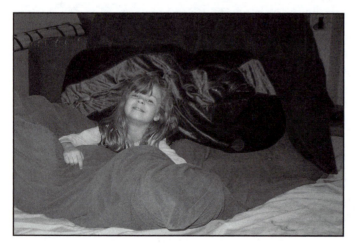

Figure 12-4. The low level of adaptive response may involve responding to passive stimuli and self-regulating arousal level such as often occurs when deep pressure is provided in a "people sandwich".

response is the child's ability to respond actively and appropriately to sensory and environmental demands. Suitable actions for adaptive responses are those that are developmentally appropriate, functional, meaningful, productive, and purposeful (Figure 12-4).

What constitutes an adaptive response for a particular child will vary with the child's level of development, degree of sensory integration, and level of previous skill (Ayres, 1973). Adaptive responses may not be limited to motor responses, but may also include increased organization of postural control, autonomic nervous system processes, affective responses, or spatial-temporal sequencing (Spitzer & Roley, 2001). A child's adaptive responses to environmental demands indicates the ability to "master a challenge and learn something new" (Ayres, 1973, p. 257) in a way that is child-directed, purposeful, and meaningful to the child. Demands that are provided at a "just-right" optimal level of challenge to skill and self-regulation allow the child to grow as an individual (Ayres, 1973). Table 12-3 presents a continuum of adaptive responses that may be observed with children.

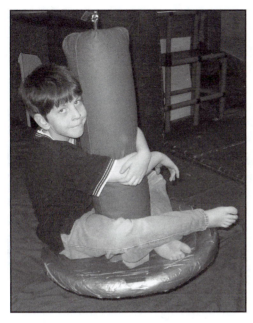

Figure 12-5. The second level of adaptive response involves simply activating postural control to hold on and stay put when environmental demands are made such as holding onto a flexion disc when swinging.

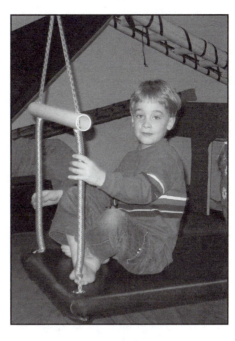

Figure 12-6. Pushing, pumping and propelling one's self while riding on a swing is one example of the third level of adaptive response.

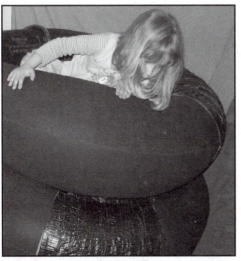

Figure 12-7. Climbing in and out or on and off equipment such as a stack of inner tubes is often initiated but not independently accomplishable early in intervention.

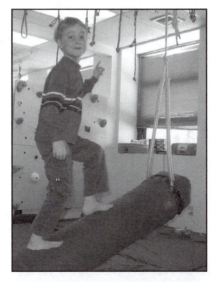

Figure 12-8. Walking up a bolster swing suspended as an incline is a challenging way for a child to move in a novel but familiar way.

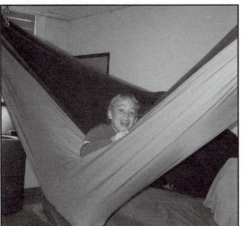

Figure 12-9. Climbing and walking in a suspended hammock made of spandex fabric requires moving through the environment in an unfamiliar and challenging way.

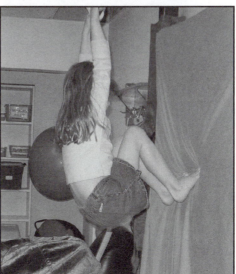

Figure 12-10. Riding on a trolley, lifting one's legs to avoid an obstacle and kicking off the padded wall to return to the starting position is a challenging novel activity requiring timing and complex ways of moving.

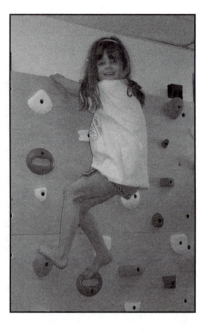

Figure 12-11. A child's inner drive to master a new challenge such as climbing a rock wall is seen in the child's joy in accomplishment.

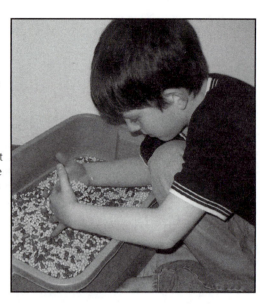

Figure 12-12. Difficulty finding small objects buried in a large bucket of beans is a good indicator of decreased tactile discrimination skills that may impact fine motor functioning.

Inner Drive

A final assumption of sensory integrative theory is that the *inner drive* toward self-actualization is an essential part of the development of sensory integration. Ayres (1973) maintained that humans have an innate drive for self-actualization and development of sensory integration through participation in sensorimotor activities. In the child who is typically developing, this internal drive is seen in the effortless exploration and joy in discovery when confronted with a challenge to achieving a goal (Figure 12-11). However, this internal motivation to seek out, experience, and master challenges is often lacking in the child with sensory integrative dysfunction.

Neurophysiological Processes and Dysfunctions of Sensory Integration Theory

Several neurophysiological processes underlie sensory integrative theory and dysfunctional patterns of behavior and are believed to reflect problems in these specific processes.

SENSORY PROCESSING

Sensory processing refers to the way the central nervous system manages incoming sensory information. The integration and discrimination of sensations, along with sensory reception and modulation are components of sensory processing. These processes are believed to occur throughout the central nervous system, especially at the brainstem and subcortical levels (Miller & Lane, 2000). Efficient sensory

processing is reflected in the child's sensori-motor development and ability to produce adaptive responses. To some extent, all sensory inputs are used in sensory integrative processes, including the "five basic senses" of touch, smell, vision, audition, and taste, and the "hidden senses" of movement and proprioception. A discussion of the tactile, proprioceptive, vestibular, auditory, and visual systems follows. Table 12-4 outlines a summary of the senses, their receptors, major neural pathways, associated brain centers and functions. For more detailed neurological information, please refer to Kandel, Swartz & Jessel, 1991 or Gilman & Newman, 1992.

The tactile system is the largest sensory organ (the skin) in the human body. It consists primarily of a variety of *mechanoreceptors* in the skin, two neural tracts, and sensory receiving areas in the cortex. The tactile system has two primary divisions, the anterolateral system and the dorsal column medial lemniscal system, which work in concert with each other to facilitate self regulation, body awareness, hand skills, praxis and motor performance. The anterolateral system is a diffuse protective system, which responds primarily to sensations of light and unexpected touch, pain, and temperature, and influences autonomic nervous system arousal states. The dorsal column medial lemniscal system is a discriminative system that responds to vibration, deep touch pressure, conscious proprioception, and two-point discrimination, and provides the foundation for hand skills, body awareness and praxis (Kandel, Swartz & Jessel, 1991; Gilman & Newman, 1992). Problems in tactile system processing may be reflected in tactile defensiveness, overresponsivity, or poor discrimination/underresponsivity (Figure 12-12).

The proprioceptive system shares some sensory receptors and neural pathways with the tactile system and functions in

Table 12-4

Sensory Systems, Their Receptors, Neural Tracts, Brain Structures, and Related Functions and Skills

Sensory System	Receptors	Brain Structures	Nervous Tracts	Functions	Skills
Tactile	Mechanoreceptors •Pacini corpuscles •Meissner's corpuscles •Rufini corpuscles •Free nerve endings •Hair cells •Merkel discs	Spinal cord Thalamus Parietal lobes sensory receiving areas 3,2,1	Dorsal Column Medial Lemniscal Anterolateral Spinal Thalamic	•Receptors of deep touch, some proprioception, two-point discrim- ination, vibration •Receptors of light and unexpected touch	•Two point discrimin- nation •Tactile temporal/ spatial awareness •Fine motor skills •Body awareness •Praxis skills
Vestibular	Semi-circular canals Otoliths •Utricle •Saccule	Vestibular Nuclei Midbrain Cerebellum Parietal Lobes	Vestibulospinal tract Vestibulooculo tract Vestibulocerebellar	•Gravity receptors •Angular/ linear accelerometers	•Balance •Muscle tone •Postural control •Bilateral coordination •Projected action sequences
Proprioception	Golgi tendon organs Muscle spindle	Alpha motor neurons Cerebellum	Spinocerebellar tract	Tension and stretch receptors of the muscles and tendons	•Force discrimination •Body awareness of joint position •Force regulation •Postural control and stability •Body awareness
Auditory	Ear •Ear drum •Stapes, hammer, anvil Cochlea	Cochlear nuclei Inferior colliculus Medial geniculate body Temporal lobe	Vestibulocochlear nerve (Cranial Nerve VIII)	Receptors of vibration and sounds Localization of sound	Discrimination of speech Spatial awareness of the environment
Visual	Eye •Lens •Retina	Superior colliculus Lateral geniculate body Occipital lobe	Optic Nerve (Cranial nerve II)	Visual acuity Visual fixation •Saccades •Pursuits •Vergence Visual perception	•Perception of motion, depth, and form •Safety •Directs head, hand and body movement in the environment

concert with both the tactile and vestibular systems to modulate arousal level, facilitate postural control, body awareness, force discrimination, and praxis skills. Proprioception is the body's joint and muscle sense and is sometimes referred to as kinesthesia. Its primary receptors are located in the tendons and muscles of the body and mechanoreceptors of the skin. Problems in proprioceptive processing may be reflected in decreased discrimination, underresponsivity, increased proprioceptive sensitivity, excessive need for proprioceptive inputs for modulation, and *gravitational insecurity* due to poor integration of proprioceptive, visual and vestibular inputs. (Blanche & Schaaf, 2001; Gilman & Newman, 1992) (Figure 12-13).

The vestibular system is the most primal sensory system in the human body. It is developed and working before birth to allow the infant to be secure with gravity. It is located in the inner ear and consists of the semicircular canals and otolith organs. Perception of linear and angular movement information from these receptors forms the foundation for development of balance, muscle tone, posture, and motor coordination of the body in space and time. The vestibular system works in concert with the proprioceptive system to promote body extension and postural control. It also works in conjunction with the visual system and cerebellum to maintain a stable visual field. Problems in vestibular function are reflected in over responsivity to movement, poor

Figure 12-13. The need to fully extend the arms or the inability to use enough force to push back against resistance may reflect decreased proprioceptive processing during heavy work activities such as Barrel War.

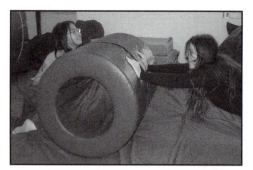

Figure 12-14. Insecurity and poor balance on activities such as the Barrel Roll may reflect decreased vestibular processing.

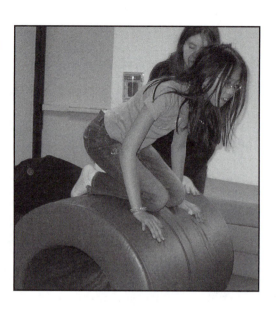

discrimination/ underresponsivity, and gravitational insecurity (Gilman & Newman, 1992; Kandel, Swartz, & Jessel, 1991; Koomar & Bundy, 2002) (Figure 12-14).

The auditory system is important for communication and temporal-spatial awareness of the environment. The auditory system consists of three major components, the outer ear, middle ear, and inner ear or cochlear apparatus (Kandel, Swartz, & Jessel, 1991). The cochlear apparatus of the ear forms a functional and structural unit with the vestibular system for the perception of vibration (Gilman & Newman, 1992) and either system may have an impact on the other. Functionally the auditory system plays an important role in orientation to the environment, regulation of arousal state, emotion, and perception of one's position in the environment (Frick & Hacker, 2002). Deficits in functioning of the auditory system may contribute to poor auditory discrimination, auditory defensiveness, and decreased temporal-spatial awareness, as well as other hearing and communication problems.

Through its role in perception of motion, depth, and form, the visual system influences maintenance of posture, balance, development of visual perception, and spatial awareness (Kandel, Swartz, & Jessel, 1991). The visual system, located in the cerebral cortex consists of the eye and six sets of extra-ocular eye muscles. The visual functions of convergence, accommodation, saccades, pursuits, as well as the vestibuloocular reflex are important to survival, learning, and skill performance. Motion detection, spatiotemporal orientation, the ability to attend, to adapt to a changing environment, and motor coordination are all influenced by functions of the visual system (Moore, 1997). Efficient ability of the eyes to work in concert and in conjunction with vestibular and proprioceptive inputs is vital for spatial orientation and skill performance. Difficulties in visual function may result in poor orientation of the head to environmental stimuli, decreased attention to task, poor eye-hand

coordination, decreased visual perceptual skills, and poor spatial orientation (Henderson, 1992) (please refer to Chapter 16: Visual Perceptual Dysfunction and Low Vision Rehabilitation).

SENSORY MODULATION

The process of adjusting neural information about the intensity, frequency, duration, complexity, and novelty of sensations to allow the nervous system to adapt to new or changing sensory information is called sensory modulation (Miller & Lane, 2000). Behavioral responses associated with sensory modulation are reflected in arousal, attention, emotion, and self-regulation.

Sensory modulation dysfunction (SMD) is identified as one pattern of dysfunction (McIntosh, Miller, Shyu, & Hagerman, 1999; Miller, et al, 1999; Miller & Summers, 2001) and refers to difficulty regulating and organizing the degree, intensity, and nature of responses to sensory input in a graded and adaptive manner. Sensory modulation disorder is thought to disrupt a child's ability to achieve and maintain an optimal range of functioning and interfere with his/her ability to adapt to the sensory and motor challenges of every day life. It may also influence a child's emotional state, attention, and ability to self-regulate (Miller & Summers, 2001).

Sensory modulation problems are proposed to occur when there is a mismatch between what is expected of a child and how the child actually perceives the processing of sensory information. After being registered by the nervous system, sensory inputs are modulated or assessed for relevance, and a positive, negative, or neutral value is placed on them. Inputs assigned a positive value may be sought out and explored, while a negative value will result in defensiveness and withdrawal. A neutral value will typically result in habituation. Deficits in sensory modulation function are generally characterized by a high negative value being

Table 12-5

Examples of Observed Sensory Defensive Behaviors in SMD

Sensory Domains	Sensory Defensive Behaviors	
	EXAGGERATED NEGATIVE RESPONSES	**WITHDRAWAL/AVOIDANCE RESPONSES**
Dysfunction in Tactile Modulation	• Responds aggressively to light or unexpected touch • Upset by bathing, hairwashing, nailcutting • Extremely irritated by waistbands in pants, sock, or certain textures/ types of clothing	• Avoids being in the middle of group activities/ stands at edges of room. • Avoids tactile play or messy substances like finger paint. • Pulls away from physical contact such as hugs, holding hands, caresses.
Dysfunction in Modulation of Vestibular Stimuli	• Becomes sick or nauseous when riding in a car or going on swings or rides • Afraid of climbing jungle gyms or or playground slides • Fearful of having feet leave the ground as in jumping or climbing	• Avoids elevators, escalators, open stairwells. • Avoids movement activities such as bike riding, somersaults.
Dysfunction in Modulation of Visual Stimuli (assumes normal acuity)	• Excessive difficulty with visual scanning of environment • Constantly turning off lights • Becomes upset in rooms with bright florescent lighting	• Avoids eye contact/frequently averts gaze. • Always wears sunglasses. • Covers eyes in bright sunlight. • Covers eyes or turns head to avert gaze in response to visually presented activities.
Dysfunction in Modulating Auditory Stimuli (assumes normal acuity)	• Becomes upset when he or she hears loud sounds like crying, sirens, vacuum cleaners, etc. • Cries or becomes upset with toilet flushing in public restrooms	• Covers ears in noisy environments like classrooms. • Hums, makes noises or grinds teeth frequently.

assigned, resulting in excessive negative responses to sensory inputs that most people do not perceive as being noxious. This type of response is referred to as sensory defensiveness and is manifested in sensory seeking or sensory avoiding behaviors. (Miller, Riesman, McIntosh, & Simon, 2001). Examples of specific behaviors related to sensory modulation dysfunction are found in Table 12-5.

SENSORY DISCRIMINATION

The nervous system distinguishes and organizes the incoming sensory stimuli and determines how those inputs should be used for skill through a process called *sensory discrimination*. Each sensory system has unique qualities that contribute to different functional skill. Tactile inputs provide information on location of touch on the body, and the size, shape, and weight of objects. The vestibular system tells us whether we are right-side up or upside down, whether we are moving or not, and in what direction, and how fast we are moving. Difficulties in sensory discrimination tend to be sensory system specific, although frequently more than one system is disrupted. Problems in sensory discrimination of individual sensory inputs are reflected in deficits in the quality or performance of the various skilled activities associat-

ed with those sensory systems. For instance, deficits in vestibular discrimination are reflected in poor balance skills. Additionally, some problems in performance of functional skills may reflect a deficit in the interaction among several sensory inputs such as poor integration of visual/vestibular/ proprioceptive inputs is seen in poor sports skills like playing baseball. Frequently, a child with sensory discrimination problems appears under responsive to inputs from the impaired sensory system and seeks out excessive quantities of that input such as in the child who spins and twirls constantly to seek vestibular input. Table 12-6 presents some examples of observed behaviors believed to reflect poor sensory discrimination skills in various sensory systems.

Postural skills deficits are believed to result from inadequate sensory discrimination of vestibular and proprioceptive sensory inputs. The development of muscle tone, ability to assume and hold body positions against gravity in prone or flexion, and to utilize equilibrium reactions are important postural mechanisms needed for skilled movement. These postural mechanisms provide the mechanical stability and mobility of the body to allow performance of coordinated and skilled actions. Postural skills difficulties are reflected primarily in the inability to move the body in anti-gravity positions (Figures 12-15 and 12-16), develop mature postur-

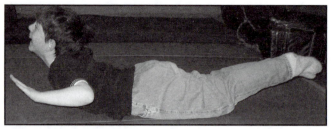

Figure 12-15. The ability to lift the head and move the body against gravity in prone extension is one of the first movement patterns mastered by the infant and is vital for postural control and safety.

Figure 12-16. The ability to achieve supine flexion is important for self-regulation of arousal level and protection.

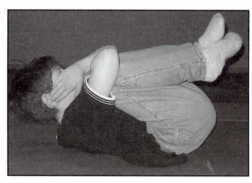

Figure 12-17. Praxis is often seen in a child's ability to climb and maneuver his body in unusual settings such as a ladder suspended on a spandex hammock.

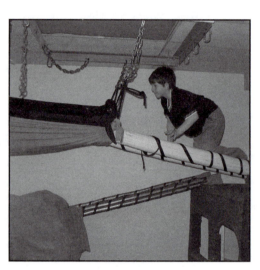

Figure 12-18. Difficulty coordinating flexion of the upper body and extension of the lower body while kicking at a target is characteristic of children with bilateral coordination problems.

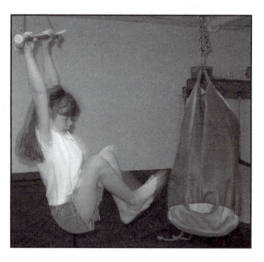

al rotational patterns, or maintain a functional balance of postural stability and mobility. Problems in postural control ultimately impact a child's motor coordination and praxis abilities.

PRAXIS

Praxis is a cognitive process that allows the child to effectively interact with objects and the environment. There are three basic practic processes: *ideation* or conceptualization of the desired act or interaction; *motor planning* of the scheme of the action; and motor execution of the plan itself. Praxis is observed in a child's organization of behavior, motor coordination, sequencing ability, and play (Ayres, 1985; Bundy & Murray, 2002). In the child who is developing typically, these practic processes emerge and are carried out effortlessly to meet everyday motor challenges and to make adaptive responses to changes in the environment (Figure 12-17).

Practice skills allow one to meaningfully interact with and respond adaptively to the demands of the environment, and to engage in the skills, tasks, and occupations of daily life.

Disorders of Praxis

Dysfunctions in praxis may be related to decreased sensory discrimination of tactile, vestibular, or proprioceptive inputs. Problems may occur in any of the component processes of praxis including ideation, motor planning, and execution. Two primary types of practic dysfunctions are discussed below.

Bilateral integration and sequencing problems are associated with poor postural-ocular development and decreased vestibular-proprioceptive processing. This type of motor planning difficulty is believed to be the milder of the two primary practic dysfunctions. It is characterized by poor bilateral coordination skills, difficulties in planning and sequencing actions, and problems with completing projected actions involving timing and spatial skills. Behaviorally, children with bilateral integration and sequencing problems are typically able to complete simple actions but have difficulty sequencing longer actions. They have difficulty coordinating upper and lower parts of the body (such as in pumping a swing), coordinating both sides of the body, developing trunk rotation, and developing skill in tasks that require timing and movement through space (such as in sports and ball skills) (Figure 12-18).

Table 12-6

Examples of Observed Behaviors of Sensory Discrimination Dysfunction

Sensory System	*Observed Behavior*
Dysfunction in Discriminating Tactile Stimuli	• Hands look like "mittens". • Difficulty manipulating small objects out of vision. • Poor awareness of position of clothing on body. • Poor body awareness, frequently bumps into things or trips over uneven surfaces.
Dysfunction in Discriminating Vestibular Stimuli	• Difficulty with balance reactions, especially when moving. • Frequently falls out of seat when leaning over. • Craves movement information, especially spinning or jumping as on beds or sofas. • Rarely, if ever gets dizzy.
Dysfunction in Discriminating Proprioceptive Stimuli	• Uses excessive force when writing with a pencil or using paintbrush. • Appears unintentionally rough or forceful as when giving hugs. • Often "crashes" into other people or furniture. • Frequently leans on or sits too close to others.
Dysfunction in Discriminating Visual Stimuli	• Difficulty with letter reversals. • Difficulty with recognizing, matching, and categorizing color, shape, and size. • Difficulty with or dislikes completing age-appropriate puzzles. • Difficulty with "find the hidden picture" games.

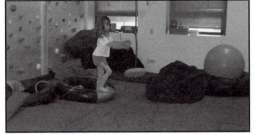

Figure 12-19. The child with somatodyspraxia will have difficulty completing simple obstacle courses such as this one.

Somatodyspraxia is associated with decreased body scheme/awareness and poor tactile discrimination skills. This type of practic difficulty is the more severe of the two. It is characterized by overall difficulties in motor planning (Bundy & Murray, 2002). Behaviorally, children with somatodyspraxia are observed to be clumsy and awkward. They have difficulties with body awareness and often appear disorganized and not well "put together". They tend to have difficulty figuring out how to approach tasks and frequently bump into objects or drop things (Figure 12-19).

Although this area of praxis has not received much attention in the literature, more recently, May-Benson (2001) proposed that difficulties in ideation are more prevalent than previously believed and that problems in this practic process may also be identifiable as another subtype of practic dysfunction. Children with ideational problems have difficulties knowing how to use objects or initiating ideas for interactions with objects or their environment. While these children often are able to complete actions when given an idea by another person, they tend to have a very limited repertoire of motor actions and interact with objects in the same way regardless of the nature of the object. In children, these limitations may be reflected in poor independent play skills.

Assessment and Identification of Sensory Integrative Dysfunction

Identification of sensory integrative dysfunction is dependent upon a combination of careful observation and formal assessment data. The role of the OTA in sensory integrative assessment depends upon the licensure laws of the state in which they practice, as well as demonstrated service competency. Good observation skills and an ability to understand assessment data are important for any OTA working with children with sensory integrative dysfunction. An initial comprehensive assessment of sensory integrative functioning completed by an OT, serves three purposes:

1. To identify the impact of sensory processing and praxis problems on a child's function.

2. To identify specific sensory integrative problems and determine the need for intervention.

3. To provide information to assist with treatment planning (Spitzer & Roley, 2001).

Table 12-7

Examples of Sensory History Information

Developmental History

1. Did the mother have any unusual stresses, illnesses or complications during pregnancy?
2. Was the child born full term? Was assisted delivery necessary?
3. Did the child have jaundice?
4. Was the child colicky?
5. Did the child have any feeding problems? Sleeping problems?
6. Were developmental milestones of rolling, crawling, sitting, and walking achieved within average limits?

Sensory History

Does the child...

VISUAL
1. become easily distracted by visual stimulation?
2. blink at bright lights or seem irritated by them?
3. avoid or have difficulty with eye contact?

AUDITORY
1. become distracted by background noises such as refrigerators, fluorescent lights?
2. seem overly sensitive to sounds?
3. seem fearful of loud noises such as toilets flushing or vacuum cleaners?

MOVEMENT
1. hesitate or avoid climbing on equipment such as jungle gyms?
2. hesitate or have difficulty going down stairs?
3. dislike elevators or escalators?
4. jump a lot on beds or other surfaces?
5. like to spin self around?
6. become carsick easily?

TACTILE
1. become irritated by tags in the back of shirts?
2. strongly dislike haircutting or shampooing?
3. complains if socks aren't on correctly?
4. avoid getting hands into paste, finger paints, or messy things?

PROPRIOCEPTION
1. frequently grasp objects very tightly?
2. feel heavier when lifted than anticipated?
3. slump while sitting?
4. have difficulty with handling eating utensils?

SENSORY INTEGRATIVE ASSESSMENT PROCESS

By definition, a sensory integrative assessment is a comprehensive and individually specific process of gathering information about the child's strengths and needs as well as family goals. A sensory history is administered to gather information about the child's sensori-motor development, play preferences, school performance and ability to perform daily routines from the parent and/or teacher's perspective. Other relevant information gathering involves interviews with parents, teachers, and other team members, as well as identifying the presenting problems. After this information is gathered, and if indicated, formal evaluation commences (Dunn, 1988). Table 12-7 presents an example of sensory history information.

FORMAL ASSESSMENT OF SENSORY INTEGRATION

Sensory integration assessment may take the form of a formal, objective, standardized assessment; a more informal, subjective clinical assessment process; or some combination of both procedures. Formal standardized assessments may be norm-referenced, in which the child's performance is compared to the performance of other peers. One example of a norm-referenced sensory integrative-based assessment is the Sensory Integration and Praxis Test (SIPT) (Ayres, 1989). The purpose of the SIPT is to provide diagnostic and descriptive information related to sensory integrative and praxis functions in children aged 4 to 8. The SIPT consists of seventeen tests, which assess the areas of tactile, vestibular, and proprioceptive sensory processing; form and space per-

Table 12-8

Sensory Integration and Praxis Tests With Related Functions Assessed

SIPT Tests	*Functions Assessed*
VISUO-PERCEPTUAL TESTS	
Space Visualization	Motor-free visual perception; mental rotation
Figure-Ground Perception	Motor-free visual figure-ground perception
SOMATOSENSORY TESTS	
Manual Form Perception	Recognition of forms held in hands; spatial visualization
Kinesthesia	Somatic perception of arm position and movement of joints
Finger Identification	Tactile perception of individual fingers
Graphesthesia	Tactile perception of simple designs; praxis; spatial visualization
Localization of Tactile Stimuli	Identification of place on arm or hand touched
PRAXIS TESTS	
Praxis on Verbal Command	Translation of verbal direction into action
Postural Praxis	Planning and executing bodily movements
Oral Praxis	Imitating tongue/lip/jaw movements
Sequencing Praxis	Sequencing movements, bilateral integration
Bilateral Motor Coordination	Functional integration of the two sides of the body
VISUO-MOTOR/CONSTRUCTION	
Design Copying	Visuopraxis; two-dimensional construction
Constructional Praxis	Three-dimensional visual space management
Motor Accuracy	Eye-hand coordination; somato praxis
VESTIBULAR/PROPRIOCEPTIVE TESTS	
Standing and Walking Balance	CNS processing of muscle, joint, gravity input
Postrotary Nystagmus	CNS processing of vestibular input

Adapted from Sensory Integration and Praxis Tests Report, WPS, 1989. Reprinted with permission.

ception; visuomotor coordination; practic ability; and bilateral integration and sequencing. Table 12-8 presents a summary of the SIPT tests and the functions they assess. Occupational therapists must complete a rigorous certification process to administer and interpret this assessment.

As the SIPT (Ayres, 1989) is normed primarily for school aged children, preschool children between 2.8 and 5.10 years may also be evaluated for sensory integrative concerns using the Miller Assessment of Preschoolers (Miller, 1988) or screened for problems using the First Step (Miller, 1993).

Alternatively, the assessment may consist of criterion- referenced tests in which the child's performance is compared to established criteria. An example of a sensory integrative-based criterion-referenced assessment is the DeGangi-Berk Test of Sensory Integration (Berk & DeGangi, 1983) (please refer to Chapter 8: An Overview of Developmental Assessments). Other assessments frequently used by pediatric occupational and physical therapists may provide observational information on sensory processing and praxis skills at various levels of occupational performance. Table 12-9 provides a list of some of these assessments.

CLINICAL ASSESSMENT OF SENSORY INTEGRATION

Clinical assessment of sensory integration may consist of formal clinical observations initiated by the OT practitioner (Ayres, 1973; Ayres, 1980, Dunn, 1981; Windsor, Roley, & Szklut, 2001); or informal skilled observations made in a naturalistic setting such as the SI room, classroom, home, and/or playground. Formal clinical observations provide qualitative information on aspects of sensory integrative functioning that are not easily quantifiable for standardized assessment and primarily serve to assess aspects of postural control, oculo-motor control, coordination and sensory processing. This type of assessment is administered by the OT practitioner in a formal manner but is scored using qualitative and subjective criteria. Please refer to Table 12-10 for examples of the most commonly used clinical observations. Informal skilled observations may be most desirable for children who are not able to participate in standardized or formal assessment, and are an important part of ongoing monitoring of progress during intervention. This type of assessment consists of a list of observable behaviors that are

Table 12-9

Examples of Standardized/Formal Assessments That Provide Information on Sensory Integrative Functioning at Various Levels

Assessment	*Functions Related to Sensory Integration*
SCHOOL AGE ASSESSMENTS	
Participation Level:	
Coping Inventory (Zeitlen, 1986)	Ability to handle environmental and internal stressors.
School Function Assessment (Coster, Deeney, Haltiwanger, & Haley, 1998)	Ability to complete functional tasks, navigate environment, participate across settings
Touch Inventory for Elementary School Aged Children (Royeen & Fortune, 1990)	Child's self-perception of sensitivity to functional tasks and interpersonal experiences.
Activities Level:	
Assessment of Motor and Process Skills (AMPS) - School Version (Fisher, A. G., Bryze, K., & Atchison, B. T. , 2000)	Motor and cognitive processing skills required to complete a desired activity of daily living or functional task.
Bruininks Oseretsky Test of Motor Proficiency (Bruininks, 1978)	Gross and fine motor skills including balance, bilateral coordination, and manipulation skills.
Movement ABC (Henderson & Sudgen, (1991)	Gross and fine motor skills including balance, manipulation skills, and ball skills.
Impairment Level:	
Clinical Observations of Motor and Postural Skills -2 (Wilson, Pollack, Kaplan, & Law, 2000)	Foundational postural skills and soft neurological signs.
Sensorimotor Performance Analysis (SPA) (Richter & Montgomery, 1989)	Foundational postural skills, fine and gross motor coordination skills.
Sensory Integration and Praxis Tests (Ayres, 1989)	Tactile, visual perceptual, proprioceptive and movement sensory processing as well as praxis skills.
Sensory Profile (Dunn, 1994)	Parent/teacher report of behaviors associated primarily with sensory modulation problems.
Quick Neurological Screening-II (Mutti, Sterling, Martin & Spalding, 1998)	Soft neurological signs.
PRESCHOOL AGED ASSESSMENTS	
Participation Level:	
Early Coping Inventory (Zeitlin, Williamson, & Szczepanski, 1988)	Infant's constitutional responsivity to the environment and self-regulation, coping competencies and coping patterns.
Pediatric Evaluation of Disability Inventory (PEDI) (Haley, Coster, Ludlow, Haltiwanger, & Andrellos, 1992)	Child's capability and performance of functional activities in self-care, mobility, and social function.
Activities Level:	
Peabody Developmental Motor Scales-2 (Folio & Fewell, 2000)	Fine and gross motor skills.
Impairment Level:	
Miller Assessment for Preschoolers (Miller, 1982)	Tactile, proprioceptive and movement sensory processing, praxis, postural, fine motor and perceptual skills.
DeGangi-Berk Test of Sensory Integration (Berk & DeGangi, 1983)	Postural, bilateral coordination and reflex integration.
FirstStep (Miller, 1993)	Screening for gross motor, fine motor skills.

Table 12-10

Most Common Clinical Observations of Sensory Integrative Functioning

Clinical Observations	Description
Muscle Tone	The resting state of the muscle fibers. Evaluated by extending the arm, wrist and fingers and looking for hyperextensibility of the joints and softness of the muscle bellies.
Proximal Stability	The ability to stabilize and cocontract muscles around the shoulder and hip joints as well as the trunk so precise movement may occur at more distal joints. Evaluated by having the child stabilize shoulders, neck, arms and trunk as the therapist attempts to move the child.
Prone Extension	The ability to lift or extend the head, neck and trunk against gravity while on one's stomach. Evaluated with the prone extension posture.
Supine Flexion	The ability to flex or curl one's head, neck, trunk and extremities into a ball while on one's back. Evaluated with the supine flexion posture.
Equilibrium/Righting Reactions	The ability to maintain and regain one's upright position when one's balance is challenged. Assessed by having the child sit on a large therapy ball, which the therapist tips from side to side.
Gravitational Insecurity	The irrational fear of movement of the head out of an upright position or having the feet leave the ground. Evaluated by having the child lie supine on a large therapy ball and tipping the ball backward unexpectedly.
Projected Action Sequences	The ability to complete various activities requiring timing and movement through space. Assessed with throwing and catching ball skills, hopscotch, etc.
RAMP Movements	The ability to complete slow controlled bilateral movements of the upper extremities reflecting proprioceptive processing. Assessed by having the child slowly extend both arms at shoulder level and then flex to touch the shoulders.
Diadochokinesis	The ability to complete rapid alternating forearm movements from supination to pronation reflective of motor planning and proprioceptive processing. Assessed by counting the number and quality of forearm rotations within 10 seconds.
Stride Jumps/Jumping Jacks	The ability to coordinate bilateral limb movements to complete ipsilateral and contralateral stride jumps as well as jumping jacks.

believed to reflect a child's processing of various sensory inputs (please refer to the Sensory Modulation/ Discrimination Evaluation in Roley, Blanche, Schaaf, 2002). Such observations, made in a naturalistic setting, may provide information on a child's sensory processing skills and reflects the child's functional performance. While the OTA may or may not be able to conduct portions of the formal evaluation, they may be a vital contributor to observing and understanding the child's functional performance.

Sensory Integrative Intervention

Sensory integrative intervention is an art and a science. As a science it involves an understanding of the neurological foundations of sensory integration theory and its application to behavior. As an art, it involves a skillful interplay between the child and the therapist. Sensory integration intervention is unique from other sensory motor therapies in its interplay of the use of specialized equipment, therapist-child interactions, and eliciting of adaptive responses. By definition it is the use of activities that are meaningful to the child, provide sensory input, invite planning and produce an adaptive response. Most often these activities involve the use of suspended equipment. This section will present an overview of the basic principles of occupational therapy intervention using sensory integration. More detailed information on interventions for specific dysfunctional areas is available in resources such as Bundy, Lane and Murray (2002); Kimball (1999); Parham and Mailloux (2001); and Roley, Blanche, and Schaaf (2001).

PRINCIPLES OF INTERVENTION

Sensory integrative-based intervention is based on six basic principles.

Goal Setting

Sensory integrative intervention begins with testing and determining the goals of treatment. These are determined by

Figure 12-20. The therapist provides support and encouragement as needed to facilitate the child's confidence and ability to accomplish difficult tasks.

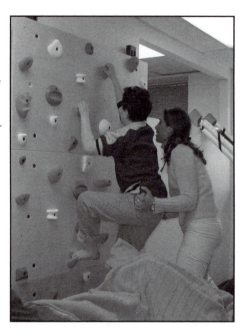

Figure 12-21. When an activity provides the right amount of sensory input and appropriate level of challenge the child has fun and wants to repeat the activity.

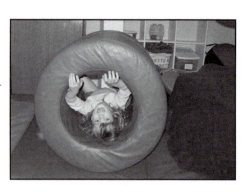

identification of specific aspects of sensory integrative dysfunction that are impacting the occupational performance areas valued by the child and family/caregivers (Spitzer & Roley, 2001). Most often intervention will begin by addressing modulation problems such as tactile and auditory defensiveness followed by addressing sensory discrimination difficulties. Development of postural control and stability and body scheme are built upon foundations of sensory discrimination, which are followed by improving praxis skills (Lane, 2002).

Child-Directed Therapy and the Therapeutic Relationship

Occupational therapy practitioners must learn to be a partner with the child in the intervention process. The OT practitioner's role is to facilitate the child's actions, set up and modify the environment and task, and guide interactions. The therapeutic relationship allows the child to feel safe to explore and take risks (Bundy & Koomar, 2002) (Figure 12-20).

Inner Drive and the Just-Right Challenge

Sensory integration treatment taps into a child's inner drive or *intrinsic motivation* to interact with the environment and make use of it. Children are attracted to activities that organize sensory inputs and offer an achievable challenge (Ayres, 1973). The OT practitioner scaffolds the child's performance to provide a challenge that stretches the child's skills just beyond his/her current abilities. When there is a match between the child's abilities and the demands of the task, the just-right challenge is achieved. The child feels masterful and enters into a state of *flow*, or total involvement with the activity (Bundy & Koomar, 2002).

Safe Environments

Sensory integrative intervention provides the child with the opportunity to take risks in an emotionally and physically safe environment. The practitioner stays close enough to the child to be an active participant in the therapeutic process and to prevent injury, but far enough away to allow the child to be self-directed and experience challenges in a safe environment. A physically safe environment provides adequate space, appropriately installed and maintained suspension system for hanging equipment, floor padding, and well constructed equipment (Koomar & Bundy, 2002).

Fun

Ayres (1973) stated, "the ultimate goal of sensory integrative treatment is a being which wants to, can, and will direct himself [sic] meaningfully and with satisfaction in response to the environmental demands" (p. 257). At its best, sensory integrative treatment is fun and looks like play (Figure 12-21). The OT practitioner facilitates fun, enjoyment, and exploration through creative, imaginative play, and playful competition. For instance the child may be empowered when the therapist takes a less powerful role or "loses", allowing the child to be the successful partner in play (Bundy & Koomar, 2002).

Artful Vigilance

In sensory integrative intervention, the OT practitioner practices *artful vigilance* or the ability to constantly balance the child's need for structure and freedom to explore, initiate, and choose activities. The practitioner's role is to be a non-invasive guide, to constantly anticipate needs, evaluate performance, support actions, adapt the environment and provide challenges at a just right level (Ayres, 1973; Bundy & Murray, 2002).

Intervention Principles for Specific Aspects of Dysfunction

Sensory input is provided in a controlled manner based on a child's ability to intake sensory information in terms of

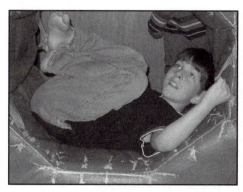

Figure 12-22. Children love small enclosed "womb" spaces that promote flexion, have low light, and allow close face-to-face interaction with the therapist. Such spaces promote self-organization and calming.

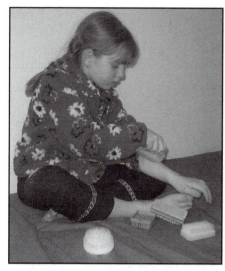

Figure 12-23. Use of a variety of different textured brushes to provide deep touch inputs can facilitate tactile discrimination and body awareness skills and facilitate decreased tactile defensiveness.

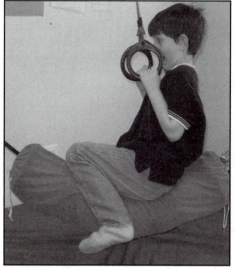

Figure 12-24. Children who are sensitive to movement may do best with activities that provide linear vertical movement that they can control such as is provided by the whale swing and which is combined with heavy work proprioceptive inputs such as pulling on the rings.

the frequency, duration, rhythm or intensity of the inputs. Controlled sensory inputs and a structured therapeutic environment also facilitate self-regulation in terms of the child's ability to attain and maintain a flexible window of *homeostasis*.

SENSORY MODULATION DYSFUNCTION

Sensory modulation problems are most often seen behaviorally as distractibility, defensiveness, or oversensitivity to various sensory inputs resulting in a state of over arousal, and sometimes shut down. Inputs that are too intense, too frequent, too long in duration, or dysrhythmic will increase a child's arousal level and promote disorganized behavior. Inputs that are low intensity, low frequency, and rhythmic will tend to decrease arousal level and promote organized behaviors (Koomar & Bundy, 2002).

The goal of sensory integration intervention is to facilitate the child's ability to attain and maintain a central nervous system state of functional and flexible homeostasis. This is accomplished through reduction of environmental stimuli, provision of calming and organizing womb spaces (small,

enclosed, low light environments) and provision of organizing sensory inputs that are slow, repetitive, rhythmical, and are presented at the body's midline to promote whole body flexion (Richter & Oetter, 1990; Oetter, Richter, & Frick, 1993) (Figure 12-22). Most children find proprioceptive and deep touch pressure organizing, but slow linear movement and oral inputs may be organizing as well.

Sensory Defensiveness

Sensory defensiveness is characterized by flight, fright, and fight responses to individual or multiple sensory inputs such as loud sounds, bright lights, or light and unexpected touch. Most often intervention to decrease sensory defensiveness is aimed at decreasing the response to noxious environmental stimuli by providing deep touch pressure and proprioceptive inputs to reduce defensiveness. Deep pressure tactile activities, such as brushing the arms or legs are often effective (Figure 12-23), although proprioceptive activities that provide active resistance such as holding onto a tire swing for a "rough ride" are typically most organizing (Wilbarger & Wilbarger, 1991). Inputs are most effective when self-administered by the child in a quiet, enclosed space.

Intolerance to Movement

Intolerance to movement is characterized by an over sensitivity to movement inputs (such as car sickness) and is manifested by *vertigo*, nausea, and autonomic nervous system responses such as dilated eyes, sweating, and pallor. The goal of intervention is to facilitate the child's tolerance of common movement experiences such as riding in a car. Treatment involves provision of linear movement (horizontal and vertical) as tolerated, and resistive proprioceptive activities (Kimball, 1999; Koomar & Bundy, 2002) (Figure 12-24).

Figure 12-25. Children who are gravitationally insecure do well with swings that are well supported, such as adding a tire to a platform swing, and which they can control.

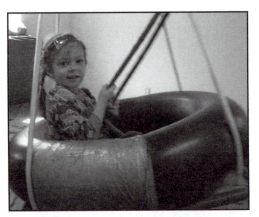

Figure 12-26. As the child with gravitational insecurity feels more comfortable with movement she may initiate and explore equipment in different ways including moving the body in prone.

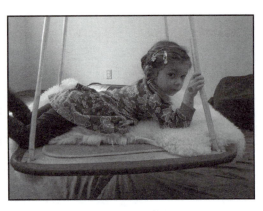

Figure 12-27. Going prone over a therapy ball or engaging in other activities which invert the head may be initially very frightening for the gravitationally insecure child and the ability to so may only emerge later in treatment.

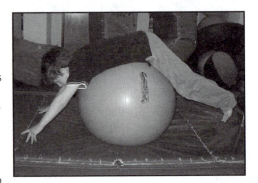

Figure 12-28. Finding jingle balls in a pit of bubble balls provides deep touch pressure and is a good activity to promote tactile discrimination skills.

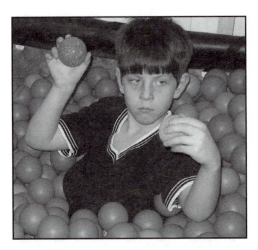

Gravitational Insecurity

Gravitational insecurity is characterized by extreme fear reactions to movement, such as having the head tipped backwards, having the feet off the ground, or of heights. This insecurity in movement is most often due to a sensory modulation problem, but may be due to a poor ability to integrate several sensory inputs such as vestibular, proprioceptive, and/or visual information. In either case, intervention first and foremost involves respecting the child's fears and not forcing or imposing movement on the child. The earliest activities should be those that incorporate swings that have a firm base of support and are low to the ground, such as a platform or glider swing (Figures 12-25 and 12-26) Slow linear movements combined with resistive or heavy work proprioceptive inputs are also initially provided. Later, as tolerance increases, the child may work in prone positions on and off swings with the head moved out of an upright position (Figures 12-25 through 12-27) (Kimball, 1999; Koomar & Bundy, 2002).

SENSORY DISCRIMINATION DYSFUNCTION

Sensory discrimination problems are most often seen through deficits in skills associated with difficulties in pro-

cessing specific sensory inputs (such as poor tactile discrimination is reflected in decreased body awareness). Treatment of skill-related problems is directed at providing enhanced sensory inputs to facilitate sensory processing of the impaired sensory systems. Development of specific skills are further facilitated through the provision of practic activities that provide a challenge to those skills. For instance, body awareness is facilitated by crawling through tunnels (Ayres, 1973; Ayres, 1979; Kimball, 1999; Koomar & Bundy, 2002).

Tactile Discrimination

Tactile discrimination problems are related to difficulties in body awareness, body scheme, hand function, fine motor skills, and praxis skills. Treatment of tactile discrimination problems involves provision of whole body deep touch pressure inputs (such as being made into a person sandwich by "squashing" the child under large pillows), textures (such as finding objects in a bucket of beans or rice), spatial information on size and shape of objects (matching objects by touch), and temporal information in the form of vibration (using a hand held vibrator to remove shaving cream from the arms and legs) (Ayres, 1973; Ayres, 1979; Kimball, 1999; Koomar & Bundy, 2002) (Figure 12-28).

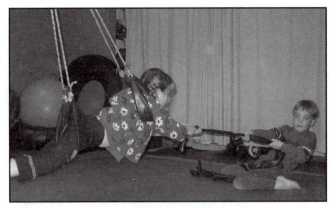

Figure 12-29. Using stretchy ropes made of bicycle inner tubes and having children pull and propel each other on swings is a good way to incorporate proprioception and heavy work into an activity.

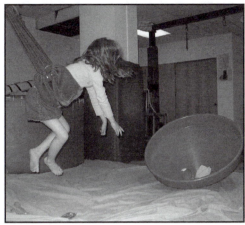

Figure 12-30. Single point suspension swings such as the frog provide intense rotary movement inputs that are easily controlled by the child and are amenable to adaptation by the therapist for increased skill.

Proprioceptive Discrimination

Proprioceptive discrimination problems are related to difficulties in body awareness, poor gradation and smooth control of movements, decreased force discrimination, and postural problems such as decreased postural stability. Intervention for proprioceptive discrimination problems involves use of activities that provide resistance to muscles through heavy work against gravity or cocontraction of muscles around joints. Resistive activities include any activities, which involve holding, pushing, pulling, carrying, jumping, and crashing. Favorite proprioceptive activities often include jumping on a mini-trampoline or inner tube, carrying heavy beanbags or weighted balls, and pulling on stretchy ropes when swinging (Figure 12-29). Use of bungee cord on suspended equipment provides increased proprioceptive input. Joint traction or compression also provides some proprioception (Ayres, 1973; Ayres, 1979; Blanche & Schaaf, 2001; Kimball, 1999; Koomar & Bundy, 2002).

Vestibular Discrimination

Vestibular discrimination problems are typically reflected in a under responsiveness to movement and are characterized by decreased balance, decreased righting and equilibrium responses, low muscle tone, poor postural control, and decreased bilateral coordination. Intervention for decreased vestibular discrimination involves provision of enhanced vestibular inputs, especially rotary or angular movement, which are best provided by single-point suspension swings such as a net swing, square platform swing, or frog swing (Figure 12-30). Intensity of movement sensations may be increased through varying the type of movement provided (including rotary versus linear) and the speed of the movement (fast versus slow). Activities should involve frequent starting and stopping to vary the speed of inputs and are best provided in all planes and directions of movement (Ayres, 1973; Ayres, 1979; Kimball, 1999; Koomar & Bundy, 2002).

DEFICITS IN POSTURAL CONTROL

Postural control problems may be seen as low muscle tone, poor postural stability, decreased equilibrium reactions, and difficulty assuming and holding body positions against gravity in flexion and extension. In general, postural responses depend on efficient discrimination of vestibular and proprioceptive inputs. Intervention for improving postural responses begins with the provision of enhanced vestibular and proprioceptive sensations embedded within the context of activities that challenge the postural mechanism being addressed, such as bouncing on a therapy ball while throwing and catching beanbags to promote balance reactions and eye hand coordination.

Postural extension is addressed by having the child engage in activities done in prone positions working against gravity and that provide linear movement, including swinging on a glider swing in prone to promote whole body extension. Postural flexion responds to resistive activities done against gravity, especially those that require the neck to be flexed and the whole body to be wrapped around the therapeutic equipment, like going for a rough ride on a bolster swing (Figure 12-31).

Postural stability and muscle tone are facilitated as these anti-gravity responses are developed. Equilibrium reactions and postural mobility are facilitated by angular vestibular inputs provided through activities with an unstable surface and which have opportunities for reaching and weight shifting off the body's base of support, such as reaching down to pick up bean bags off the floor while riding on a glider swing (Ayres, 1973; Ayres, 1979; Kimball, 1999; Koomar & Bundy, 2002) (Figure 12-32).

Figure 12-31. Holding on under a bolster swing with all extremities and having the therapist vigorously shake the bolster for a "rough ride" provides intense proprioceptive inputs and facilitates whole body flexion.

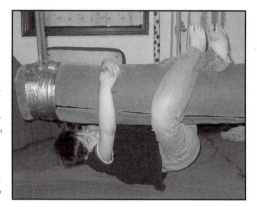

Figure 12-32. Fishing off a moving glider swing using a magnetic fishing rod promotes trunk rotation and equilibrium reactions.

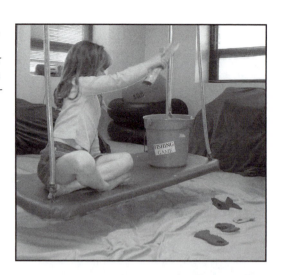

DYSFUNCTIONS IN PRAXIS

Praxis problems are widely variable and may be characterized by difficulties in creating ideas for actions in the environment, problems varying activities, sequencing tasks, coordinating both sides of the body, planning actions, problem solving, or organizing actions.

Ideation Problems

Ideation problems are characterized by difficulties in generating ideas for actions in the environment or interactions with objects. Children with ideational problems may have difficulties recognizing what actions their bodies are capable of, or what they can do with objects in the context of their environments. Intervention for ideational problems tends to be cognitively oriented in that the OT practitioner assists the child with labeling actions, recognizing object properties, relating previous experiences with current activities, and questioning or providing cues to facilitate the child's ability to generate new ideas (Ayres, 1985, Koomar & Bundy, 2002; May-Benson, 2001).

Motor Planning Problems

Problems in motor planning are characterized by difficulties with body awareness, planning and sequencing difficulties, and problems producing feedback dependent actions. Intervention for motor planning problems initially involves provision of tactile and/or proprioceptive inputs to facilitate development of body awareness. Activities are graded from simple activities requiring a low level of adaptive response that the child can do well (such as crawling through a barrel or pumping a swing), to more complex and challenging activities requiring sequencing and timing (such as swinging on a trapeze and kicking a suspended ball). Altering the task demands so as allow the child to master the activity without frustration or anxiety is vital in achieving the just-right challenge. Facilitating the child's ability to recognize feedback from his body and actions in the environment is also an

Figure 12-33. Landing on a stack of inner tubes after riding on a trolley requires motor planning and postural control.

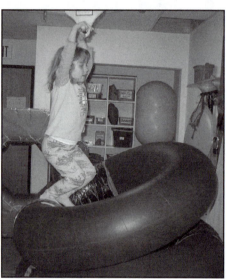

important part of intervention (Ayres, 1973; Ayres, 1979; Ayres, 1985; Kimball, 1999; Koomar & Bundy, 2002) (Figure 12-33).

Bilateral Coordination Problems

Bilateral coordination problems are characterized by difficulties using both sides of the body together effectively, crossing the midline, coordinating upper and lower extremities, and also with trunk rotation. Intervention for bilateral coordination problems involves provision of vestibular and proprioceptive sensations in the context of activities that require bilateral upper and/or lower body coordination responses, like pulling on ropes to propel a swing. Activities are best introduced along continuums of simple to complex, feedback to feedforward dependent tasks, and symmetrical movements to alternating movements (Ayres, 1973; Ayres, 1979; Ayres, 1985; Kimball, 1999; Koomar & Bundy, 2002) (Figure 12-34).

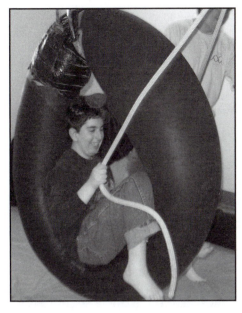

Figure 12-34. Pulling on ropes to propel oneself in a tire swing facilitates upper extremity bilateral coordination as well as whole body flexion.

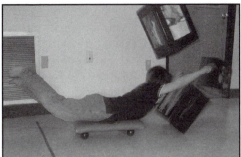

Figure 12-35. Projected action sequences involve timing and movement through space. Riding on a scooter to knock over blocks is a medium-level projected action activity that also provides strong vestibular input and promotes whole body extension.

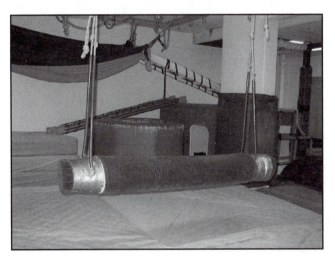

Figure 12-36. A sensory integrative clinic will be an inviting, safe environment with adequate floor padding, multiple suspension points for hanging equipment, opportunities for climbing and planning, a variety of suspended equipment and womb spaces for calming and organization.

Projected Action Sequence Problems

Problems in projected action sequences are characterized by difficulties effectively completing activities that involve anticipation of future events in the environment and the ability to adjust actions to meet those conditions. Problems with projected action sequences are seen primarily in activities that have strong temporal and spatial qualities, such as moving across a soccer field to be in the right place to kick a moving ball. Intervention involves provision of vestibular and proprioceptive inputs and opportunities to engage in graded activities that have increasing spatial and temporal (timing) demands. The relative contribution of feedback and feedforward demands contributes to the difficulty of the activity, with feedback tasks being easiest (like standing still and throwing a beanbag into a target) and feedforward tasks generally being more difficult (such as swinging on a trapeze and landing in a stack of inner tube tires). The extent and speed of the child's movements and the target's movements also contribute to the task complexity. Easier tasks are those in which both the child and target are stationary and harder activities are those in which both the child and the target are moving quickly. A spatial task may be graded by increasing or decreasing the extent and speed of the child's movement, for example, sitting on a square platform swing and swinging slowly or running across the room to jump over a hurdle into a pile of pillows. Temporal demands may be graded by changing the rate at which the target moves or by having the child move rapidly (Koomar & Bundy, 2002) (Figure 12-35).

Considerations in Provision of Services

Classic sensory integrative-based occupational therapy services emphasize remediation of problems and require the availability of a clinic space well-equipped with specialized equipment, adequate suspension system, as well as the opportunity for a child to engage in a one to one therapeutic relationship with the OT practitioner (Figure 12-36). Intervention may be in a clinic setting or in a specialized room within the school setting. For children with mild problems or nearing the end of services, small groups of two to four may work well for developing social interaction skills as well as sensory and motor performance. The OTA, depending on state guidelines, with demonstrated competency and under the supervision of an OT, may provide direct sensory integrative-based intervention services, may use sensory-integrative techniques within the context of a sensory-motor program or group, or may provide consultation and supervision of sensory diet and accommodation programs. In a school setting, the goal of sensory integrative based services is to enable the child to function in the school environment, while in a private clinic or hospital, setting goals may emphasize improvement in the child's ability to function at home. (Koomar, 1990; Koomar, 1997; Tryon, 1997). Similarly, the goals of intervention may be to use sensory integrative principles to develop accommodation and sensory diet programs to promote functioning in a naturalistic setting.

Developing Sensory Diet and Accommodation Programs

While not classic sensory integration intervention, development of a sensory diet program involves application of sensory integrative intervention principles and necessitates the understanding of sensory integration theory, specifically an understanding of the impact of intensity, frequency, and duration of sensory inputs on arousal and skill. In contrast to the classic, clinic-oriented, remediation-based sensory integrative intervention program, sensory diets are individualized strategies and activities that the child uses to make temporary changes in his/her ability to maintain/achieve a functional level of arousal, such as use of a squeezy ball or chewing gum for self-regulation (Wilbarger & Wilbarger, 1991, Wilbarger & Wilbarger, 2002).

To address sensory modulation problems, the sensory diet program is designed to help the child be alert and adaptable in order to function to the best of his/her ability in his/her environment (Wilbarger & Wilbarger, 1991, Wilbarger & Wilbarger, 2002). Sensory diet programs may also be implemented to address sensory discrimination problems through the provision of intense sensory inputs at salient times to prepare the body for skill, like bouncing on a therapy ball to increase muscle tone and postural stability prior to doing a writing, table-top task. The OTA, depending on state and school district guidelines, as well as demonstrated level of competency, and working under the supervision of an OT, may be able to develop and monitor sensory diet and accommodation programs for children to use in the classroom, and possibly, home environments.

Because sensory diet programs are not remedial in nature and tend to be situation specific, they should always be part of a total therapeutic program. Sensory diet programs are rarely effective when used exclusively in place of direct intervention. They are primarily maintenance and accommodation programs and do not typically result in long-lasting changes in sensory processing. Instead, they may be

thought of as an effective adjunct to individual treatment to facilitate carryover of therapeutic interventions within the home and school environment. Sensory diets may also be a logical "next" step in a child's treatment program as the need for direct services decreases and strategies for life-long self-regulation need to be developed.

A total sensory diet program will typically involve both accommodations and sensory diet strategies. Accommodations, as developed by an OT, are personalized strategies that assist in temporarily overcoming a deficit. What works for one child may not work for another. Specific accommodations may be environmental modifications (including decreasing lights or carpeting floors to decrease noise), changes in interactional styles (such as always approaching the child from the front or using a firm touch when interacting), or involve changes or the use of specialized materials or equipment (like using pencil grips or inflatable seat cushions). Each child's sensory diet program will be unique and individualized to their own set of sensory needs and behaviors. A good sensory diet involves the "just right" combinations of input to maintain a functional level of arousal. There are four components to a sensory diet program:

1. Regularly scheduled activities and routines (sensory meals).

2. Environmental accommodations and supports.

3. Sensory snacks used on an as-needed basis.

4. Supportive leisure activities.

Selected activities must provide appropriate intensity and duration of sensory inputs. Sensory diets are variable and depend on close observation of how different inputs impact behavior, interaction, learning, play, and communication. They may change from day to day and there is no set "recipe" that works all the time. Constant awareness of the environment, the immediate situation, and the cumulative effect of daily events are needed to monitor and change activities, or make additional accommodations (Wilbarger & Wilbarger, 1991).

When preparing a sensory diet, the OT must figure out the necessary timing, duration, and intensity of inputs. Generally, one to four regularly scheduled activities are selected and carried out at specific times during the day, such as jump on trampoline for 10 minutes before school. Routines for particularly difficult times during the day are developed (like using a heavy towel to provide deep pressure after bathing) and a "hideout" or escape for each environment should be identified to allow opportunities for reorganization (including providing a "cubby corner" or small clubhouse in a corner of the classroom). A menu of sensory snacks to be used throughout the day on an "as needed" basis should be provided to maintain the child's level of alertness or help with particularly difficult or unexpected situations, such as small items like squeezy balls, paperclips to bend, and/or gum to chew. Finally, teacher, parents and

---

Table 12-11
Example of a Sensory Diet Program

Child's Name: Sarah   Age: 7 years   Intended Setting for Sensory Diet: Home and School

Part 1: Accommodations

Home:
- A large monthly calendar was obtained to list all family appointments, events, and changes in schedules to ease Sarah's transitions.
- A heavy bed quilt and room darkening shades for Sarah's bedroom helped to facilitate her sleep.
- A hand-held showerhead was installed in the bathtub to make hairwashing easier.

School:
- Sarah's seat was moved near the teacher but at the edge of the classroom where there was little traffic.
- She was given an inflatable cushion for her seat.
- Sarah entered the school 5 minutes before the rest of her class to hang up her coat and get settled in the classroom before her classmates arrived, allowing her to avoid the crowds and unsettling tactile inputs at the lockers.

Part 2: Regular Sensory Meals

Sarah had two time periods during the day that were particularly difficult for her.
- Bathing in the morning: Sarah was encouraged to shower in the morning using a loofa sponge to provide deep touch pressure to organize her along with deep touch pressure provided by a heavy, thick towel.
- After lunch regrouping: After lunch, Sarah bounced on a large therapy ball placed in a quiet corner of her classroom for 5 minutes while the class had a quiet time.

Part 3: Sensory Snacks

Sarah was provided with a small box of "fidgets" to use at will throughout her day, which included:
- A squeezy ball
- Therapy putty
- Large paperclips to bend
- Straws to chew on
- A waterbottle with a spout top to drink out of.

Part 4: Supportive Leisure Activities

- Weekly swimming and karate classes at the local YMCA.
- Daily bicycle riding when the weather permitted.

---

caregivers should be instructed in the best ways to interact with the child, ways to modify the environment to support the child's arousal level, and facilitate their recognition of the child's signs of inappropriate arousal (Wilbarger & Wilbarger, 1991) (please refer to Table 12-11 for a detailed example of a sensory diet).

Summary

In conclusion, an understanding of sensory integrative theory, assessment and intervention is an important part of pediatric occupational therapy practice. Based on state guidelines, demonstrated competency, and under the supervision of an OT, the OTA may assist with clinical and naturalistic observation of the child, may carry out the treatment plan, and may play a role in implementing and monitoring sensory diets and accommodation programs.

Case Study

Name: Sarah
Age: 7 years 8 months
Grade: One
Medical/Developmental History: Sarah was born prematurely by emergency C-section at 25 weeks gestation at 1 ¼ lbs, and was hospitalized for three months. Early developmental milestones were grossly within normal limits. She is left hand dominant. She has a diagnosed learning disability, attention deficit disorder, and language processing problems. She was not on any medications at the time of evaluation.

Referral Information: Sarah's parents were concerned about her high state of arousal and oversensitivity as evidenced by extreme emotionality and frequent meltdowns. They were afraid that Sarah's limited social interactions and acceptance by peers were affected by her poor hygiene and sloppy dress. They also expressed concern about Sarah's lack of independence in dressing, self care, and hygiene. They believed that her problems with fine motor skills and handwriting impacted her ability to complete her school-work. They wanted home life to be easier and less stressful for all family members. In addition they wanted Sarah to experience overall better self-esteem, and feel less frustrated and more successful in school.

Assessment Results: Based on referral difficulties in social participation and functional performance at home and school, Sarah was evaluated using the Sensory Integration and Praxis Tests, parent-completed developmental/ sensory history, and informal clinical observations. Assessment results indicated that Sarah was very tactile defensive and had definite sensitivities to touch, visual, and auditory sensory inputs. She often sought proprioceptive input as a means of self organization. Sarah also demonstrated decreased tactile, proprioceptive, and vestibular discrimination skills, which contributed to problems in postural control and praxis. In the area of praxis she demonstrated good ideation skills, but had difficulties with motor planning, sequencing skills, and bilateral coordination.

Intervention Plan: Sarah's occupational therapy program involved one-hour, once weekly, direct, individual sensory integrative based occupational therapy services in a private clinic setting; individual occupational therapy services for fine motor and handwriting skills development in the school system setting, and monthly consultation to the parents and school system therapist and teachers provided by the clinic occupational therapist. A sensory diet program was implemented and is outlined in Table 12-12.

Discharge from Sensory Integration Intervention Services: Sarah was discharged from direct, individual sensory-integrative based occupational therapy services after two years. Her parents noted that she was emotionally less volatile and there were fewer meltdowns at home. She was able to take showers regularly and although she stated it still felt "yucky" when the water ran down her face, Sarah washed her hair without complaint. She was able to wear loose cotton pants with elastic waists and pullover cotton shirts instead of stretch pants, t-shirts and sweat suits. Her parents reported that her self-esteem was much improved

and she rarely got frustrated when she could not learn a new task "the first time." Transitions and schedule changes were easier, but Sarah was most successful when given advance warning of changes and had a written schedule to follow. Overall, Sarah and her parents believed that her therapy services had accomplished their goals.

DISCUSSION QUESTIONS

1. How might the OTA implement and monitor Sarah's sensory diet?
2. If you were Sarah's parents, how might you explain sensory integration based treatment to a friend or relative?

Application Activities

1. Examine and analyze your own sensory preferences. Think about the activities and sensations you like, crave or dislike, then answer the following questions.
2. What morning routines and activities do you use to wake up and get going in the morning?
3. What sensory inputs do these activities provide you?
4. Are there activities or experiences you avoid because they are unpleasant or overwhelming for you?
5. What activities do you use to calm yourself down when you are stressed or upset?
6. What sensory inputs do these activities provide you or remove from your environment to allow you to be calm?
7. Are there activities that you regularly engage in because they meet a sensory need that you enjoy or crave?
8. What sensory inputs do these activities provide? Do they calm you, get you going, or make you feel more organized and able to function?

Table 12-12

Case Study Supplement—Sensory Diet

Case Study Examples of Functional Limitations, Evaluation Results, and Treatment Strategies for Sensory Integrative Dysfunctions.

Identified Sensory Integration Dysfunctions	Limitations in Social Participation at Home and School	Limitations in Activities at School	Limitations in Activities at Home	Evaluation and Clinical Observation Results	Treatment Activities and Strategies
Sensory Modulation Problems	At school, Sarah was generally very quiet and shy around others with few friends. At home, Sarah was emotional; frequent temper tantrums and fights with her younger brother.	Sarah was very distracted at school and had difficulty attending in class.	Sarah had difficulty sleeping alone, falling asleep, and sleeping through the night. Sarah often sought proprioceptive input as a means of self-organization through jumping on beds and chewing on her clothing and other objects.	Sarah was noted to be very distracted and overly active during testing.	Decreasing the lights in the clinic Using deep pressure under large pillows Allowing opportunities to regroup following over-stimulating activities in a small quiet space such as a "cave" under some pillows or a small clubhouse
Tactile defensiveness	Sarah had difficulties standing in line at school and often got into trouble for pushing or yelling at others.	Sarah refused to do messy art projects.	Sarah was very particular about her clothing, and was sensitive to certain clothing textures, tags in shirts, and socks. She generally wore stretch pants and t-shirts that made her look unkempt. Sarah strongly resisted hair cutting and hair brushing.	Sarah was observed to pull away from light and unexpected touch during the tactile tests of the SIPT.	A deep pressure program was implemented along with a sensory diet.
Auditory defensive	Sarah became upset in gym class due to her frustration and over-sensitivity to sounds in the gym.	Sarah could not tolerate the toilet flushing in the school bathroom.	Sarah could not tolerate her mother vacuuming the house in her presence.	Sarah was distracted by noise in the hallway outside the testing room.	Headphones and accommodations were put in place to reduce intolerable noise.

Table 12-12 (continued)

Case Study Supplement—Sensory Diet

Identified Sensory Integration Dysfunctions	Limitations in Social Participation at Home and School	Limitations in Activities at School	Limitations in Activities at Home	Evaluation and Clinical Observation Results	Treatment Activities and Strategies
Sensory Discrimination Problems					
Tactile Discrimination	Other children often did not want Sarah to play with them on the playground because she was clumsy and often dropped the ball in play.	Sarah had difficulties with fine motor skills such as handwriting, cutting, drawing, and pasting.	Sarah was a messy eater, had difficulties handling utensils, often knocked over glasses, and spilled or broke things.	Sarah scored below average on all four tactile discrimination tests of the SIPT.	Provision of opportunities for tactile inputs within the natural context of her environment, such as covering the swings with textured materials. Crawling through a path of large pillows covered in velour material. Finding small plastic animals in a large bucket of dried beans or rice. Writing and drawing on a paper hung on the wall with colored foam soap. Pretending to paint herself using a large 2-inch soft bristle paintbrush.
Proprioceptive Discrimination	Sarah was often un-intentionally rough with other students.	Sarah pushed very hard on her pencil and often broke pencil leads or tore paper when erasing mistakes.	Sarah often "waited until the last minute" to indicate the need to use the bathroom.	Scored below average on the Kinesthesia test of the SIPT.	Heavy work activities such as holding onto the bolster swing for a rough ride. Pushing heavy medicine balls across a mountain of large pillows.
Vestibular Discrimination	Sarah played alone on the playground, preferring to swing instead of playing running games with peers.	Sarah often fell out of her seat in class and preferred to stand to work at her desk.	Sarah had poor balance, which made it hard to learn how to ride a bicycle.	Scored below average on the Standing and Walking Balance and Post Rotary Nystagmus tests of the SIPT	Swinging on a variety of swings such as the bolster, square platform swing, or frog swing.
Postural Control Difficulties	Sarah fatigued quickly and could not keep up with her mother when shopping at the mall or supermarket.	Due to decreased strength, Sarah was afraid of climbing on slides and jungle gyms and descending stairs.	Sarah often stood at the table instead of sitting, sat on the edge of her seat, and frequently fell out of her chair.	Decreased muscle tone with decreased shoulder and trunk stability and strength. Easily fatigued. Difficulty assuming and holding body positions against gravity in prone or in flexion positions.	Carrying a large pillow on her back like a turtle while crawling across the clinic to increase shoulder strength. Holding onto a flexion disc or inner tube tire swing while being given a rough ride. Propelling herself around cones on the floor while prone on a scooter board to deliver mail from one end of the room to another.

Table 12-12 (continued)

Case Study Supplement—Sensory Diet

Identified Sensory Integration Dysfunctions	Limitations in Social Participation at Home and School	Limitations in Activities at School	Limitations in Activities at Home	Evaluation and Clinical Observation Results	Treatment Activities and Strategies
Praxis Problems	On the playground, Sarah was often reluctant and hesitant to engage with others. At home, Sarah had difficulty with changes in routines, had difficulty handling new situations, and required a lot of structure from others.	Sarah often got lost navigating around her school. She had difficulty following the teacher's directions to complete tasks.	Sarah had difficulties dressing herself, managing fasteners, and tying her shoes. Sarah was slow to learn to ride a bicycle. Sarah had problems organizing herself to clean up her room or complete household chores.	Sarah scored below average on all praxis tests of the SIPT.	Provision of activities that progressed through the adaptive response levels. Finding jingle balls in a ball pit of plastic bubble balls, holding onto the flexion disc while riding, or holding onto a bolster swing on her stomach with arms and legs and dropping off into a pile of pillows. Ride a "frog" sling swing on her stomach and knock down foam bowling pins with her feet. 2 to 3 step obstacle courses incorporating individual activities that were accomplishable by her, then progressing to 5 to 6 steps over time. More complex activities involving swinging on swing and targeting games were incorporated as skills developed.

References

Ayres, A. J. (1972). Types of sensory integrative dysfunction among disabled learners. *American Journal of Occupational Therapy, 26*, 13-18.

Ayres, A. J. (1972). *Southern California sensory integration tests manual.* Los Angeles: Western Psychological Services.

Ayres, A. (1973). *Sensory integration and learning disorders.* Los Angeles: Western Psychological Services.

Ayres, A. J. (1975). *Southern California postrotary nystagmus test.* Los Angeles: Western Psychological Services.

Ayres, A. J. (1976). *The effect of sensory integrative therapy on learning disabled children: The final report of a research project.* Los Angeles: University of Southern California.

Ayres, A.J. (1977). Cluster analyses of measures of sensory integration. *American Journal of Occupational Therapy, 31*, 362-366.

Ayres, A. J. (1979). *Sensory integration and the child.* Los Angeles: Western Psychological Services.

Ayres, A.J. (1980). *The adaptive response.* (videotape). Sensory Integration International.

Ayres, A.J. (1985). *Developmental dyspraxia and adult-onset apraxia.* Torrance, CA: Sensory Integration International.

Ayres, A.J. (1989). *Sensory integration and praxis tests manual.* Los Angeles: Western Psychological Services.

Baranek, G., Foster, L., & Berkson, G. (1997). Tactile defensiveness and stereotyped behaviors. *American Journal of Occupational Therapy, 51*, 91-95.

Berk, R. & DeGangi, G. (1983). *DeGangi-Berk test of sensory integration.* Los Angeles: Western Psychological Services.

Blanche, E. & Schaaf, R. (2001). Proprioception: A cornerstone of sensory integrative intervention. In S. Roley, E. Blanche, and R. Schaaf (Eds.). *Understanding the nature of sensory integration with diverse populations.* Tucson, AZ: Therapy Skill Builders.

Bruininks, R. (1978). *Bruininks-Oseretesky test of motor proficiency manual.* Circle Pines, MN: American Guidance Services.

Bundy, A. (1989). A comparison of the play skills of normal boys and boys with sensory integrative dysfunction. *Occupational Therapy Journal of Research, 9*, 84–100.

Bundy, A., & Koomar, J. (2002). Orchestrating intervention: The art of practice. In A. Bundy, S. Lane, & E. Murray (Eds.), *Sensory integration: Theory and practice* (2nd ed.). Philadelphia: F. A. Davis.

Bundy, A., Lane, S., & Murray, E. (2001). *Sensory integration: Theory and practice* (2nd ed). Philadelphia: F. A. Davis.

Bundy, A. & Murray, E. (2001). Sensory integration: A. Jean Ayres' theory revisited. In A. Bundy, S. Lane, & E. Murray (Eds.), *Sensory integration: Theory and practice* (2nd ed). Philadelphia: F. A. Davis.

Clifford, J. & Bundy, A. (1989). Play preference and play performance in normal boys and boys with sensory integrative dysfunction. *Occupational Therapy Journal of Research, 9*, 202-217.

Coster, W. J., Deeney, T., Haltiwanger, J., & Haley, S. (1998). *School function assessment.* San Antonio, TX: The Psychological Corporation/Therapy Skill Builders.

Dunn, W. (1988). Assessment of sensory integrative dysfunction: An educator's perspective. *Sensory Integration Special Interest Section Newsletter, 11*(4), 3-4.

Dunn, W. (1981). *A guide to testing clinical observations.* Rockville, MD: American Occupational Therapy Association.

Dunn, W. (1999). *Sensory profile user's manual.* San Antonio: Psychological Corporation.

Fanchiang, S., Snyder, C., Zobel-Lachiusa, J. (1990). Sensory integrative processing in delinquent-prone and non-delinquent-prone adolescents. *American Journal of Occupational Therapy, 44*, 630-639.

Fisher, A. G., Bryze, K., & Atchison, B. T. (2000). Naturalistic assessment of functional performance in school settings: Reliability and validity of the School AMPS scales. *Journal of Outcome Measurement 4*, 504-522.

Folio, M. R. & Fewell, R. (2000). *Peabody Developmental Motor Scales -2.* Austin, TX: Pro-Ed.

Frick, S. & Hacker, C. (2001). *Listening with the whole body.* Madison, WI: Vital Links.

Gilman, S. & Newman, S. (1992). *Manter and Gatz's essentials of clinical neuroanatomy and neurophysiology* (9th ed). Philadelphia: F. A. Davis.

Haley, S. M., Coster, W. J., Ludlow, L. H., Haltiwanger, J. T., & Andrellos, P. J. (1992). *Pediatric evaluation of disability inventory: Development, standardization, and administration manual,* Version 1.0. Boston, MA: New England Medical Center.

Henderson, A. (1992a). A functional typology of spatial abilities and disabilities. Part I. *Sensory Integration Quarterly, 20*(3), 1–6.

Henderson, A. (1992b). A functional typology of spatial abilities and disabilities. Part II. *Sensory Integration Quarterly, 20*(4), 1-5.

Henderson, S. & Sugden, D. (1992). *Movement assessment battery for children manual.* New York: Psychological Corporation.

Jacobs, E. & Schneider, M. (2001). Neuroplasticity and the environment: Implications for sensory integration. In S. Roley, E. Blanche, and R. Schaaf (Eds.). *Understanding the nature of sensory integration with diverse populations.* Tucson, AZ: Therapy Skill Builders.

Kandel, E., Swartz, J, & Jessel, T. (1991). Principles of neural science (3rd ed). Norwalk, CT: Appleton & Lange.

Kimball, J. (1999). Sensory integration frame of reference. In P. Kramer and J. Hinojosa (Eds.). *Frames of reference for pediatric occupational therapy* (2nd ed). Philadelphia: Lippincott, Williams & Wilkins.

Kinnealey, M., Oliver, B., & Wilbarger, P. (1995). A phenomenological study of sensory defensiveness in adults. *American Journal of Occupational Therapy, 49*, 444-451.

Koomar, J. (1990). Sensory integration treatment in the public schools. In S. Merrill, Ed. *Environment: Implications for occupational therapy.* Rockville, MD: American Occupational Therapy Association.

Koomar, J. (1997). Statement of services. *Sensory Integration Special Interest Section Quarterly, 20*(4), 3.

Koomar, J. & Bundy, A. (2002). Creating direct intervention from theory. In A. Bundy, S. Lane, & E. Murray (Eds.). *Sensory integration: Theory and practice* (2nd ed). Philadelphia: F. A. Davis.

Lane, S. (2001). Sensory modulation. In A. Bundy, S. Lane, & E. Murray (Eds.). *Sensory integration: Theory and practice* (2nd ed). Philadelphia: F. A. Davis.

May-Benson, T. (2001). A theoretical model of ideation in praxis. In S. Roley, E. Blanche, and R. Schaaf (Eds.). *Understanding the nature of sensory integration with diverse populations.* Tucson, AZ: Therapy Skill Builders.

May-Benson, T., Ingolia, P., & Koomar, J. (2001). Daily living skills and developmental coordination disorder. In S. Cermak & D. Larking (Eds.), *Developmental coordination disorder.* Albany, NY: Delmar.

McIntosh, D., Miller, L., Shyu, V., & Dunn, W. (1999). Development and validation of the Short Sensory Profile. In W. Dunn (Ed.), *The sensory profile: Examiner's manual.* San Antonio, TX: Psychological Corporation.

Miller, L. (1988). *Miller assessment of preschoolers.* San Antonio, TX: Psychological Corporation.

Miller, L. (1993). *First STEP.* San Antonio, TX: Psychological Corporation.

Miller, L. & Kinnealey, M. (1993). Researching the effectiveness of sensory integration. *Sensory Integration Quarterly, 21*(2), 1-5.

Miller, L., & Lane, S. (2000). Toward a concensus in terminology in sensory integration theory and practice: Part 1: Taxonomy of neurophysiological processes. *Sensory Integration Special Interest Section Quarterly, 23*:1.

Miller, L. & McIntosh, D. (1998). The diagnosis, treatment and etiology of sensory modulation disorder. *Sensory Integration Special Interest Section Quarterly, 21*: 1.

Miller, L., McIntosh, D., McGrath, J., Shyu, V., Lampe, M., Taylor, A., Tassone, F., Neitzel, K., Stackhouse, T., & Hagerman, R. (1999). Electrodermal responses to sensory stimuli in individuals with Fragile X syndrome: A preliminary report. *American Journal of Medical Genetics, 83*(4), 268-279.s

Miller, L. & Summers, C. (2001). Clinical applications in sensory modulation dysfunction: Assessment and intervention considerations. In S. Roley, E. Blanche, and R. Schaaf (Eds.). *Understanding the nature of sensory integration with diverse populations.* Tucson, AZ: Therapy Skill Builders.

Moore, J. (1997). Course notes from Moore, J. & Baker Nobles, L. *Evaluation and treatment of the child with visual impairment.* VisAbilities rehab Services and Boston University-Sargent College, Boston, MA. September 27 – 28, 1997.

Mutti, M., Sterling, H., Martin, N., & Spalding, N. (1998). *Quick neurological screening test* (QNST-II). East Aurora, NY: Slosson Educational Publications, Inc.

Mulligan, S. (1998). Patterns of sensory integrative dysfunction: A confirmatory factor analyses. *American Journal of Occupational Therapy, 52,* 819-828.

Mulligan, S. (2002). Advances in sensory integration research. In A. Bundy, S. Lane, & E. Murray (Eds.). *Sensory integration: Theory and practice* (2nd ed). Philadelphia: F. A. Davis.

Neill, L.P. (1999). Thinking about Jean Ayres. *Sensory Integration Quarterly, Spring/Summer, 1,* 10-11.

Oetter, P., Richter, E. & Frick, S. (1995). *MORE: Integrating the mouth with sensory and postural functions* (2nd ed.). Hugo, MN: PDP Press.

Parham, D. (1998). The relationship of sensory integrative development to achievement in elementary students: Four year longitudinal patterns. *Occupational Therapy Journal of Research, 18*(3), 105-127.

Parham, D. (2002). Sensory integration and occupation. In A. Bundy, S. Lane, & E. Murray (Eds.). *Sensory integration: Theory and practice* (2nd ed). Philadelphia: F. A. Davis.

Parham, L. & Mailloux, Z. (2001). Sensory Integration. In J. Case-Smith, A. Allen, & P. N. Pratt. (Eds.). *Occupational therapy for children* (4th ed.). St. Louis: Mosby.

Richter, E. & Montgomery, P. (1989). *Sensorimotor performance analysis.* Hugo, MN: PDP Press.

Richter, E. & Oetter, P. (1990). Environmental matrices for sensory integrative treatment. In S. Merrill (Ed.), *Environment: Implications for occupational therapy practice.* Rockville, MD: American Occupational Therapy Association.

Roley, S., Blanche, E., & Schaaf, R. (2001). *Understanding the nature of sensory integration with diverse populations.* Tucson, AZ: Therapy Skill Builders.

Royeen, C. & Fortune, J. (1990). TIE: Touch Inventory for School Aged Children. *American Journal of Occupational Therapy, 44,* 165-170.

Schaaf, R. (1990). Play behavior and occupational therapy. *American Journal of Occupational Therapy, 44,* 68-75.

Schaaf, R. (1994). Neuroplasticity and sensory integration: Part 1. *Sensory Integration Quarterly, 22*(1), 1–5.

Schaaf, R., Merrill, S. & Kinsella, N. (1987). Sensory integration and play behavior: A case study of the effectiveness of occupational therapy using sensory integrative techniques. *Occupational Therapy in Health Care, 4*(2), 61-75.

Spitzer, S. (1999). Dynamic systems theory: Relevance to the theory of sensory integration and the study of occupation. *Sensory Integration Special Interest Section Quarterly, 22*(2), 1-4.

Spitzer, S. & Roley, S. (2001). Sensory integration revisited: A philosophy of practice. In S. Roley, E. Blanche, & R. Schaaf (Eds.), *Understanding the nature of sensory integration with diverse populations.* Tucson, AZ: Therapy Skill Builders.

Tryon, P. (1997). Communication and collaboration with parents and between school- and clinic-based therapists. *Sensory Integration Special Interest Section Quarterly, 20*(4), 1 – 2.

Turkewitz, G. (1994). Sources of order for intersensory functioning. In D. J. Lewkowicz & R. Lickliter (Eds.), *The development of intersensory perception: Comparative perspectives* (pp. 3-17). Hillsdale, NJ: Lawrence Erlbaum and Associates, Publishers.

Wilbarger, P. (1995). The sensory diet: Activity programs based on sensory processing theory. *Sensory Integration Special Interest Section Newsletter, 18*: 2.

Wilbarger, P. & Wilbarger, J. (1991). *Sensory defensiveness in children aged 2–12: An intervention guide for parents and other caregivers.* Denver, CO: Avanti Educational Programs.

Wilbarger, J. & Wilbarger, P. (2002). The Wilbarger approach to treating sensory defensiveness. In A. Bundy, S. Lane, & E. Murray (Eds.). *Sensory integration: Theory and practice* (2nd ed). Philadelphia: F. A. Davis.

Williams, M. & Shellenberger, S. (1994). The alert program for self-regulation. *Sensory Integration Special Interest Section Newsletter, 17*:3.

Wilson, B., Pollock, N., Kaplan, B., Law, M., & Faris, P. (2000). *Clinical observations of motor and postural skills–2.* Framingham, MA: Therapro.

Windsor, M., Roley, S., & Szklut, S. (2001). Assessment of sensory integration and praxis. In S. Roley, E. Blanche, & R. Schaaf (Eds.), *Understanding the nature of sensory integration with diverse populations.* Tucson, AZ: Therapy Skill Builders.

Zeitlin, S. (1986). *Coping Inventory.* Bensenville, IL: Scholastic Testing Service.

Zeitlin, S., Williamson, G., & Szczepanski, M. (1988). *Early coping inventory.* Bensenville, IL: Scholastic Testing Service.

13

ORAL MOTOR SKILLS AND FEEDING

Jean Lyons Martens, MS, OTR/L

Chapter Objectives

- Gain an understanding of the development of oral motor control and oral motor reflexes.
- Understand and identify problems of feeding and self-feeding in infants and children.
- Recognize the role of the OT and OTA in developing and implementing an oral motor program.
- Understand the role of the OT and OTA in developing and implementing a feeding program.

Introduction

The purpose of this chapter is to provide a general overview of normal oral motor development and feeding skills, signs of feeding problems, and an overview of assessment and treatment strategies associated with oral motor and feeding skills. Emphasis is on infancy and the preschool years, as they are the early years for learning to feed and self feed. Information about oral motor and feeding skills associated with medically fragile and medically complicated child are not included in this chapter as working with these children require specialized training that extends beyond the scope of a general pediatric occupational therapy assistant text.

The foundations for treatment and treatment strategies found within this chapter are compiled from this author's treatment experiences over the years. Similar techniques and theories can also be found within the literature and even through Internet sources. The reader is referred to *Pre-*

Feeding Skills, by Suzanne Morris and Marsha Klein, and *Feeding and Swallowing Disorders in Infancy*, by Lynn Wolf and Robin Glass for more detailed information on the foundational skills and specific treatment techniques found within this chapter.

The Feeding Team

The team members involved in planning and implementing a feeding program depends on the treatment setting and the needs of the child. Children with feeding issues often present with a combination of physiological and behavioral components associated with feeding difficulties (Burklow, Phelps, Schultz, McConnell, & Rudolph, 1998). To meet the multiple medical and feeding needs of the child, an integrated interdisciplinary feeding team approach is often necessary (Miller, Burklow, Santoro, Kirby, Mason, & Rudolph, 2001; Vergara, 1993).

Typically, feeding team members include the pediatrician, nutritionist/dietician, speech and language pathologists, occupational therapy (OT) practitioners, child behaviorist, developmental psychologist, dentist, nurse, social worker, teachers, childcare providers, and of course, the parents/caregivers. Generally the child's *pediatrician* coordinates and determines which team members are necessary. All team members must communicate with the pediatrician and obtain medical authorization before implementing new feeding treatment strategies (Clark, 1993). For instance, an OT practitioner working with a child on a restricted diet or tube feedings needs to consult with the pediatrician before making any changes to an oral/feeding program. The pediatrician also prescribes and monitors medications to assist in efficient feeding, to prevent reflux, to increase appetite, or to aid in digestion.

A *nutritionist* or *dietitian* is included on the team when caloric intake and expenditure need to be monitored. Based on the child's age, size, and activity level, the dietitian provides the team with information regarding ideal caloric intakes. For instance, increasing caloric intake may include adding butter, oil, and cream to foods. The dietitian also helps determine schedules of meals and types and quantities of formulas to be used for each child (Miller, Burklow, Santoro, Kirby, Mason, & Rudolph, 2001).

A *nurse* may monitor medical complications and help with the implementation of treatment techniques (Glass & Wolf, 1992).

Occupational therapy practitioners and/or speech and language pathologists assess and develop treatment plans to improve a child's oral motor skills. Occupational therapy practitioners have knowledge and competency in reflex activity, oral motor skills, and sensory processing skills as they relate to oral motor and feeding skills (Morris, & Klein, 2000). Speech and language pathologists often have knowledge and competency in feeding and swallow evaluations, and assess oral structures, swallow dysfunction, and look for signs of aspiration. It is important to understand that aspiration cannot be seen without a videofluoroscopic study. Speech and language pathologists may also have advanced competency with videofluoroscopic swallowing studies (Miller, Burklow, Santoro, Kirby, Mason, & Rudolph, 2001; Glass & Wolf, 1999). A child identified as having aspiration issues may require oral dietary changes and possibly suction during meal times to prevent pneumonia damage to the lungs (Morris & Klein, 2000). The OT practitioner and/or speech and language practitioner assess and implement adapted feeding equipment, proper food texture and consistency, and proper feeding positions. When a child's posture and tone interfere with proper positioning, an occupational or *physical therapy* consultation may also be indicated to determine optimal seating positions or devise adapted seating devices (Wolf & Glass, 1992).

Mealtime is not a pleasurable experience for a child with oral hypersensitivity or weak oral musculature. Children with these problems often develop avoidance behaviors around feeding time, which, in turn, interferes with food intake. A *child behaviorist or a developmental psychologist* works with the team to develop a behavioral plan that diminishes avoidance behaviors without decreasing the amount of food intake.

The *social worker* helps the family/caregivers sort out the overwhelming circumstances and feelings around having a child with multiple medical and feeding issues (Satter, 1992; Glass & Wolf, 1992).

A *dentist* monitors oral care and oral health. Children with oral motor and feeding issues often have medical complications such as seizures, anatomical anomalies, or oral hypersensitivity. These complications may require modified daily oral hygiene programs such as fluoride supplements or use of adaptive toothbrushes. Some children with feeding issues also require daily doses of medications. Many of the medications given to young children contain sugars not normally included in their regular diet. This requires even more vigilant oral care and tooth brushing to prevent dental decay. Some children with oral motor and feeding issues refuse to brush or have their teeth brushed. To ensure good oral health and prevention of cavities, these children will also require extra dental monitoring. It is important to keep in mind that cavities are very painful and are an additional barrier to developing efficient oral motor and feeding skills (Kenny, & Judd, 1988).

Those members of the feeding team carrying out the oral and feeding programs on a daily basis include *school teachers, babysitters, childcare providers* and most importantly, the *parents/caregivers*. These team members must understand how to follow through with mealtime goals and objectives, and perhaps most importantly, to be provided with an efficient and workable communication system through which to discuss changes with the rest of the team. Parents/caregivers are responsible for carrying out the feeding program when other professionals are not present. This is for most mealtimes. Because of this responsibility, when developing a feeding plan, it is essential for the parents to be involved in setting feeding goals and objectives that realistically reflect the families' needs at mealtimes.

When working towards achieving feeding goals, overlap in service provision between the feeding team members often occurs. A team effort on the behalf of the child requires the team members to have a "clearly defined professional role and related goals" (Miller, Burklow, Santoro, Kirby, Mason, & Rudolph, 2001, p. 214) to stay within the scope of their professional expertise, and to balance this expertise in order to provide "best practice" services.

Feeding times are social times and times of connection for young children. It "is one of the first social contacts between parent and child" (Chamberlin, Henry, Roberts, Sapsford, & Courtney, 1991, p. 907). It may be a very positive emotional time for the parent/caregiver and child. There is nothing as gratifying as feeding a willing baby or young child. Seeing a baby's look of comfort and engaging in social interaction with a young child when feeding is rewarding. However, it can be a very distressing time when oral and feeding issues exist. If a child is not getting enough to eat he/she may be in distress. If parents/caregivers are unable to meet the basic nutritional needs of the child, they may feel incompetent in their role. Because of the key role that parents/caregivers play in feeding their child, providing proper ongoing, and understandable team based education and support is critical (Figure 13-1).

Development of Oral Motor and Feeding Skills

REFLEX DEVELOPMENT

An infant develops the reflex base needed for survival while still in utero (Morris & Klein, 2000). At birth physiological flexion dominates. This is a reflex that flexes the limbs and spine (including the neck) towards the center of the body. When a limb is extended away from the body, it recoils back towards the center. In prone, the infant turns its head just enough to clear space to breathe. In supine, the pull of gravity rotates the limbs and spine into a little more extension. (Alexander, Boehme, & Cupps, 1993; Conner, Williamson, & Siepp, 1983; Morris, & Klein, 2000).

Active motor control occurs *cephalocaudally*, or in a head to toe direction. A child initially gains control of extension high in the neck, and then gains control of neck flexion concurrently with development of extension further down the neck/spine. This pattern continues down through the spine, into the hips, and finally, to the legs and feet. Voluntary control is first gained in the head/neck, and then in the shoulder girdle, before the trunk, hips, and legs. As a child gains control of voluntary motor functions, there is less reliance on reflex activity. With practice, repetition, and success in acquiring motor skills, the reflex influence diminishes and eventually disappears (Alexander, Boehme, & Cupps, 1993; Conner, Williamson, & Siepp, 1978; Morris, & Klein, 2000).

A similar pattern occurs with oral motor development. An infant is born with several reflexes dominating motor control in the oral area. Many of these reflexes develop while the infant is in utero (refer to Table 13-1 and Major Infant Reflex Chart). At birth, these reflexes are well developed, thus allowing the full-term infant to suck and feed minutes after birth. For instance, following stimulation to the cheek or side of mouth, infants automatically orient their head and mouth towards the nipple. This *rooting* reflex allows the infant to find the nipple and begin feeding before eyesight and motor control are well developed (Morris & Klein, 2000).

Glass and Wolf (1999) describe three intricately connected processes that lay the foundation for infant feeding. They consist of <u>sucking</u>, swallowing, and breathing. These processes are related both functionally and anatomically. Some of the anatomical structures involved in feeding (sucking and swallowing) and breathing overlap, as they are in close proximity to each other. This proximity calls for precise coordination of the anatomical structures to ensure proper feeding and breathing (Alexander, Boehme, & Cupps, 1993; Glass & Wolf, 1992).

Sucking is elicited through rhythmic coordination of the

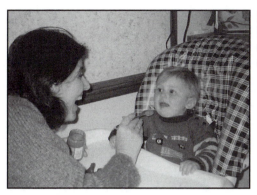

Figure 13-1. Feeding a child can be a joyous experience.

tongue, lips, cheeks, and jaw (Alexander, Boehme, & Cupps, 1993; Wolf & Glass, 1992). Typically developing infants crave sucking, and automatically suck when a nipple or other stimulus is placed in the mouth. This sucking reflex ensures nutritional intake and state regulation or calming when a nipple is presented to the mouth (Wolf & Glass, 1992).

An infant uses an up and down motion of the tongue and jaw to suck. Sucking uses positive and negative grades of pressure to bring liquid into the mouth. Positive pressure occurs when the nipple is compressed and the liquid is expelled. Negative pressure is like a vacuum, suction occurs when the oral cavity is sealed. The tongue, pressed to the top of the mouth and around the lower surface of the nipple, expels the liquid (positive pressure). A downward motion of the tongue slightly enlarges the space pushing the liquid from the front of the mouth to the back (negative pressure). There is little loss of liquid to the sides of the mouth as the tongue is cupped and the suck pads fill up the sides of the oral cavity. Suck pads are embedded within the cheeks of full term infants. Suck pads give structural stability within the mouth, support tongue movements, and help provide a strong lip seal for suction around the nipple. This provides a simple reflexive and very efficient pattern for liquid intake (Glass & Wolf, 1999; Morris & Klein, 2000; Wolf & Glass, 1992).

Swallowing consists of three separate phases: the oral, pharyngeal, and esophageal phases (Lundy-Ekman, 1998; Wolf & Glass, 1992). Food moves from the mouth through the pharynx to the esophagus and stomach. The pharynx is the cavity behind the nose and mouth. Its muscles are involved in swallowing and the esophagus is the tube that connects the pharynx to the stomach (Wolf & Glass, 1992).

Breathing provides the oxygen requirements necessary for survival. To prevent aspiration, breathing must be well coordinated with the suck and swallow processes (Glass & Wolf, 1999). Specifically, air and food pass through the oral cavity to the pharynx before splitting off to the lungs and stomach respectively. Air passes through the trachea to the lungs and food through the esophagus to the stomach. The larynx is a structure at the opening of the trachea that keeps

Table 13-1
Oral Motor Reflexes

Movement	Develops	Diminishes
Swallow	13-14 weeks gestation	2-5 months
Suck	15-16 weeks gestation	4-6 months
Gag Reflex	18 weeks gestation	6-7 months
Rooting Reflex	present at birth	4-5 months
Bite Reflex	present at birth	3-5 months

Compiled from Ianniruberto & Tajani, 1981; Morris & Klein, 2000; Mueller, 1972; Oetter, Richter, & Frick, 1995.

food from entering the lungs during a swallow (Glass & Wolf, 1999; Morris & Klein, 2000).

A reflexive coordination of sucking, swallowing, and breathing provides a smooth, efficient, and undisturbed rhythm for eating. The infant sucks, swallows, and breathes through several repetitions, rests, then begins the pattern again. The infant's mouth stays engaged around the nipple through the entire pattern. This coordinated suck, swallow and breath rhythm is not possible for adults or even young children. Anatomical changes in the epiglottis and soft palate begin at around 4 to 12 months. At this time the infant is no longer able to swallow and breathe in the same coordinated manner (Glass & Wolf, 1999; Morris & Klein, 2000; Wolf & Glass, 1992). As the child grows, the structures grow further apart and rely upon more coordinated muscle activity (Morris & Klein, 2000).

The *suck and swallow reflex* relies on physiological flexion of the spine and neck. Without physiological flexion, the suck pads will not provide structural stability in the oral cavity for a strong seal for suction, the lips will not seal, and the tongue will flatten (a cupped position is ideal for sucking and swallowing). This causes more loss of liquid out of the mouth and to the sides inside the mouth. Ideally, infants should be fed while cradled in the caregivers arms so the neck is flexed, thus maximizing reflexive control and ultimately, efficient feeding (Alexander, Boehme, & Cupps, 1993; Morris & Klein, 2000).

REFLECTIONS FOR THE OTA

Experiential:

1. Tip your head back into hyperextension, keeping your mouth relaxed. Notice how your lips automatically open up.

2. Swallow a sip of liquid with your head/neck in flexion, then in neutral, and then in extension. Notice the increase of space in your mouth and the increase in tongue activity as you move out of neck/head flexion.

ORAL MOTOR PROTECTIVE REFLEXES

At birth, the full term infant has two protective oral motor reflexes, the *gag reflex* and the cough reflex. The gag reflex is a safety mechanism that prevents solids from being swallowed. It is very sensitive in the middle and back thirds of the mouth (Morris & Klein, 2000). If the nipple or other solid object enters past the first third of the mouth, the baby will gag and may even vomit. The purpose of the cough reflex is to protect the airway. If something goes down the trachea, the cough reflex is elicited to expel the substance. A cough is necessary for safe feeding, but does not always mean that feeding is safe (Wolf & Glass, 1992). Often, children with oral motor and feeding issues have a cough reflex, but it is not strong enough or sensitive enough to expel all substances. These children may be aspirating food without any visible signs of aspiration (Morris & Klein, 2000).

ORAL MOTOR REFLEX INTEGRATION

By 4 to 6 months, an infant's head and neck control has increased and he/she may now maintain a supported sitting position with less external head support (Conner, Williamson, & Siepp, 1978). Additionally, in relation to head, neck, and spine control, the infant is developing more voluntary and refined oral motor control. A combination of random and controlled movements from the shoulder girdle, arms, and hands are more prevalent as physiological flexion is being replaced by voluntary control of flexion and extension. The *grasp reflex*, which allows the child to grasp toys with his/her hands is replaced by a voluntary grasp pattern. The infant is now able to grasp a toy and bring it to his/her mouth (Alexander, Boehme, & Cupps, 1993). As infants grow, they learn to discriminate between edible and nonedible items, though mouthing toys may persist into the first year. Mouthing of toys stimulates voluntary and random tongue and lip movement. In turn, with exposure to hands and toys in the mouth, the gag reflex becomes less sensitive and moves to the back third of the mouth (Figure 13-2). New nonreflexive bound tongue and lip movements derived from mouthing transfers to more voluntary tongue and lip movements at feeding times. Additionally, introduction of non-*pureed* foods that require biting and chewing action to process food further diminishes the gag reflex (Alexander, Boehme, & Cupps, 1993; Connor, Williamson, & Siepp, 1978: Morris & Klein, 2000; Vergara, 1993).

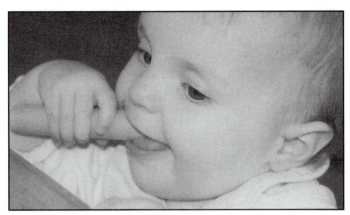

Figure 13-2. Babies will mouth any object they can bring to their mouths.

VOLUNTARY ORAL MOTOR CONTROL

Chewing

Chewing develops in a sequential manner and begins with an automatic or reflexive up and down motion elicited through touch to the gums or biting surfaces. This is called a phasic bite-release (Alexander, Boehme, & Cupps, 1993; Morris & Klein, 2000). With experience, this *munching* pattern turns into voluntary bite or chewing motions (Gisel, 1991). Once all chewing patterns have emerged, the motions used depend on the food being eaten. There are also three directions associated with chewing; vertical, diagonal, and rotary or grinding. Vertical chewing emerges at around 6 months with the first introduction of soft foods. Vertical chewing consists of up and down motions of the jaw. Diagonal chewing emerges at around 9 to 15 months and consists of up and down and up and diagonal jaw movements with associated side to side tongue movements. The tongue is moving food from one side to the other. Rotary chewing develops at around 24 months, and consists of rotary or circular jaw movements. Vertical and diagonal chewing motions are used for soft foods and *rotary chewing* and grinding for meats (Morris & Klein, 2000; Oetter, Richter, & Frick, 1995). Solid foods take the longest time to chew, followed by viscous, and lastly, pureed foods (Gisel, 1991).

Tongue Movements

Tongue movements support sucking, swallowing, and chewing, as well as provide structural support for the oral mechanisms. An infant's tongue fills the oral cavity, moving up and down with the jaw. Cupping of the tongue helps direct the liquid to the posterior portion of the mouth (Alexander, Boehme, & Cupps, 1993). At around 3 to 5 months the up and down motions of the tongue become more voluntary and are coupled with a back and forth motion to bring foods in to the mouth. It is normal to see some tongue thrusting or protrusion out of the mouth with new and different textures. While chewing, lateral tongue movements bring food from one side of the mouth to the other to break the food down before swallowing. Diagonal tongue movements develop at around 9 months to support diagonal chewing (Alexander, Boehme, & Cupps, 1993; Morris, & Klein, 2000).

There is a balance between emerging voluntary motor control and diminishing reflex activity to allow for efficient feeding. As children grow, voluntary oral motor control improves so that oral motor reflexes are used only for protection. By age 2 children's oral motor skills are more refined as they learn to eat an increasingly varied diet with improved utensil skill (Alexander, Boehme, & Cupps, 1993; Morris & Klein, 2000; Oetter, Richter, & Frick, 1995). Table 13-2 summarizes the developmental progression of feeding skills.

Signs of Feeding Problems

Feeding or eating is an activity of daily living, a performance area we participate in several times a day. It is necessary for survival. Successful feeding entails a sequence of turn taking interactions between the infant and his/her parents/caregivers (Stevenson, Roach, VanHoeve & Leavitt, 1990). It is through this interaction that the feeding relationship grows (Satter, 1992). For instance, the infant indicates wanting to be fed and the parent or caregiver responds. To ensure a smooth feeding process, a parent or caregiver must be responsive to the infant and interpret his/her cues, while the infant must learn to signal hunger and fullness (DeGangi, 2000). When an infant/child has difficulties with feeding it may become a time of considerable anxiety for a parent or caregiver instead of a time for relationship building, fun, and social communication (DeGangi, 2000).

Cross culturally, different social expectations and norms exist around feeding. This translates to differences in mealtime routines and differences in when and how foods are introduced (DeGangi, 2000). For instance, some families find it acceptable to introduce solids after the first year, in others, parents are not concerned about the amount of time it takes to feed a child, and yet others prefer to feed versus encourage self-feeding until the child can do so without spilling. What may seem like a problem to the OT practitioner may not be a problem for the family and as such it is important to keep in mind that "both parents and therapists have different understandings about what characteristics contribute to a child's success" (Humphry, & Thigpen-Beck, 1998, p. 841). As OT practitioners we must weigh the families' values and expectations with our own and come to a common understanding before a child is diagnosed as having a feeding problem.

What follows are descriptions of specific feeding problems, typical feeding patterns, performances, and behaviors. Wolf and Glass (1992) suggest there is a feeding problem

Table 13-2

Development of Feeding Skills

1 Month:
Poor head control
Poor lip closure, liquids run out of the corners of the mouth
Bite and gag reflex present.
Oversensitive gag reflex in the back two-thirds of the mouth
Suckle swallow pattern to bring liquids in (using a back and forward motion of the tongue)
Rooting reflex present
Suck pads present
Need neck flexion and chin tuck for efficient suck/swallow

3 Months:
Beginning of head control
Can bring hand to mouth with increased purpose
Pre-language sounds, first sounds are with exhalation and observed when baby moves
Increased up and down tongue movements to swallow
Hands and toys placed in the mouth may cause gagging

4 Months:
Increased head control as neck musculature develops
Increasingly brings hands and toys to mouth
Holds bottle with two hands and brings it to mouth with two hands (strong midline orientation)
More active lip movement, better lip closure
Can eat with head in neutral, decreased need for chin tuck
Suckling decreases and tongue movements increase
More cupping and flattening of the tongue emerge as suck pads begin to diminish
Introduction of strained foods, may gag at first

5 Months:
Increased mouthing and oral exploration
Gag reflex moves back to last 1/3 of the mouth
Increased hand to mouth activity
Teething may begin, increased mouthing/biting and drooling
Munching appears with introduction of soft solids

6 Months:
Good lip control
Voluntary sucking, tongue moves in and out with foods
As tongue goes in and out, infant may push some food back out
Beginning lateral tongue movements
Voluntary chewing movements
Gag decreases with feeding as more texture is tolerated
Supported sitting for spoon feeding begins
Food is scraped off the spoon and on to the gums
First interest in drinking from a cup, no lid

7 Months:
Upper lip comes down to take food off the spoon
Lower lip moves out to support bottle or cup

8 Months:
Beginning of diagonal chewing (coincides with trunk rotation and mid-line crossing)
Finger feeding begins
Holds and bangs spoon
Biting and chewing on toys increases as teething increases
Beginning of babbling; sounds no longer related only to body movements
No loss of liquid around nipple as lip control continues to develop

10 Months:
Bites through soft foods
Lip closure over a spoon good

12 Months:
Good *tongue lateralization*
Good jaw movements and control
Lip control for cup drinking emerging, may see biting on cup for stability
Removes food from a spoon with lips
Using teeth to chew
Sits to drink liquids
Can take sips out of a cup no lid

15-18 Months:
Scoops and brings food to mouth with spoon
Some spilling of foods off spoon
Beginning to drink from a cup with no lid, some spilling

Table 13-2 (continued)

Development of Feeding Skills

24 Months:	Automatic rotary chewing Good lip control around a cup, no spilling with no lid Holds a cup with one hand Holds eating utensil palm up when self-feeding Likes to play with food
36 Months:	Feeds self with minimal assistance and minimal spilling Pours from a pitcher Uses a fork to stab food Chews with mouth closed

Compiled from Alexander, Boehme, & Cupps, 1993; Case-Smith, 2001; Glass & Wolf, 1992; and Morris & Klein, 2000.

---

when the typical expected performance for a particular infant is not met. These descriptions are presented to guide an occupational therapy assistant (OTA) working under the supervision of an occupational therapist (OT) to determine which behaviors may be more associated with normal development and therefore not a feeding issue, and which are interfering with the child's ability to feed.

ORAL MOTOR CONTROL

Oral motor control is influenced in part by muscle tone, reflex development, anatomical structures and anomalies, and a child's sensory processing abilities. Diagnoses often influenced by oral motor control issues include: cerebral palsy, prematurity, facial anomalies such as cleft palate or Pierre-Robbin syndrome, low tone as seen in Down syndrome, or a child with sensory integration dysfunction.

When the team assesses oral motor/feeding problems, oral motor reflexes should be examined first as they provide a sense of the function of the oral structures (Mueller, 1972). Treatment will be explored in more detail in the Oral Stimulation Section.

Components of Oral Motor Control

1. Suck: The infant may have problems with lip seal for suction, a weak suck, arrhythmic suck, or incoordination with the suck, swallow, breathe pattern (Morris & Klein, 2000; Vergara, 1992). Nutritive suck should be looked at separately from *non-nutritive suck*, as the rhythm for each suck is quite different (Wolff, 1968).

2. Swallow: The swallow may be weak or inefficient causing aspiration (Morris & Klein, 2000; Vergara, 1993).

3. Bite Reflex: May be over or under reactive. An overactive (hyper active) bite reflex results in a forceful biting down on the spoon/food without a timely release. With an under reactive (hypo reactive) bite reflex the child does not perceive the food on the gums, and

does not begin a bite or to chew (Morris & Klein, 2000; Case-Smith, 2001).

4. Jaw Control: Difficulties with jaw control influence cheek, lip, and tongue movements. There may be poor jaw closure, *jaw thrust* and/or tonic jaw closure (Morris and Klein 2000). Decreased *jaw stability* as seen in hypotonia will affect chewing and cup drinking (Case-Smith, 1989). Hypertonia may result in hyperactive reflexes interfering with jaw excursions (Case-Smith 1989). In addition, the upper and lower teeth may not meet to allow for a good bite/chew, resulting in misalignment of the lips for removing food from the utensil (Morris & Klein, 2000; Vergara, 1992).

5. Tongue control: The tongue may thrust, retract, or not lateralize. A *tongue thrust* occurs when the tongue extends out past the lips when food is presented. This may be a forceful movement (Case-Smith, 2001). Tongue thrust is normal with the presentation of new foods. It becomes a problem when the thrust persists after a few months of consistent food presentation, when the thrust does not allow the presentation of food or a utensil into the mouth, and/or when the child is not able to meet nutritional needs. *Tongue retraction* is the retraction of the tongue into the posterior portion of the oral cavity. Retraction does not allow for movement of the food or for a safe swallow. Tongue lateralization refers to the horizontal motions of the tongue. (Morris & Klein, 2000; Vergara, 1993). These motions are required to break up the food through tongue movements and/or biting and munching. A child with uncoordinated tongue and jaw movements is at risk for aspiration (Case-Smith, 1989).

6. Lip control allows for a strong lip seal around the nipple. Poor lip seal will not produce the suction needed to expel liquid from the nipple. In an older child, poor lip control effects the ability to remove food from a spoon and to control liquid from a cup. Different lip

Figure 13-3. Note the lip, chin, and cheek muscles used for successful cup drinking.

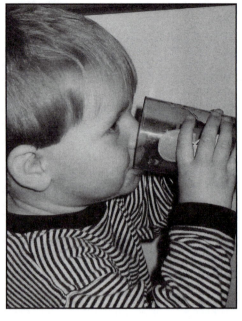

control patterns are needed to drink from a straw, a cup with a lid, or a cup with no lid. Lip seal with suction is used with a straw and a cup with a lid, and *lip pursing* is needed for an open cup (Morris & Klein, 2000; Vergara, 1993) (Figure 13-3).

POOR FEEDING ENDURANCE

Typically, a newborn is fed every three hours. Toddlers eat three meals and two or three snacks a day, and a school aged child eats three meals and one or two snacks a day. If it takes more than 30 to 40 minutes to complete a feed/meal or snack, there may be a feeding problem. When much of the child's day is spent feeding/eating there is less time for other activities. Because most of the typically developing infant's awake time is spent eating, if *all* the time is spent eating, there is no time left for socialization and exploration. Poor endurance is a primary reason for a feeding or meal to take longer than 30 minutes to consume.

Causes of Poor Feeding Endurance

1. *Weak oral motor musculature causing a slow sucking rhythm or a disorganized suck.* The child does not have the strength or endurance to suck, use efficient tongue movements, and/or bite patterns for an entire meal. Due to decreased proprioceptive response the reflexive oral mechanisms are more difficult to elicit (Case-Smith, 1989). This may continue into the toddler years.

2. *Medical issues such as those seen in prematurity.* Premature infants need a great deal of sleep and a high concentration of calories to sustain themselves. These infants need to consume enough calories to grow and strengthen, but often have poor coordination of oral reflexes and fatigue before they can consume enough

(Measel, & Anderson, 1979). These children often fall asleep before the meal is finished. The parent/caregiver must then use techniques to try to keep the child awake, take breaks during a feed, or offer more, smaller feeds through the day.

Cassie was born with very low tone and sensory hypersensitivity. Feeding endurance was decreased from birth. Mom stopped breast feeding after a few months because of the amount of effort, energy, and time it took for Cassie to eat. Mom switched to a bottle with a larger hole in the nipple. When Cassie transitioned to table foods, she fatigued before finishing a meal. Cassie lived with her extended family. The solution for this family was to have Cassie eat small meals several times a day with different family members. She ate breakfast with her father before work, then with her grandfather when he got up. Lunch was at school, and she ate two dinners, one with an uncle and one with her parents. In this family, providing several small meals fit in with the preexisting schedule.

REFUSAL OF FOOD

Toddlers are notorious for being picky eaters. The amount they eat from one day to the next varies, as do the types of foods they eat. To allay concerns, pediatricians often advise parents/caregivers to look at what the child has eaten over the course of a week versus over the course of one day. It is also typical for a child to need numerous neutral exposures to a new food before they will try and enjoy it (Birch 1984). It is important to react to a child's food refusals in a very matter of fact manner to avoid unnecessary conflict and to promote greater willingness to try new and varied foods (Roberts & Heyman, 2000).

Results of the Mennella & Beauchamp (1993) study on taste in infants found that taste and smell are well developed in infants; so that even with repeated neutral exposures, infants and children will reject some flavors and foods.

Introduction of new and/or different textures are some of the more common reasons for food refusal. Determining the reason or reasons for the refusals must be thoroughly assessed prior to choosing the appropriate treatment approach. Treatment approaches must balance the child's acceptance of foods and nutritional needs with the therapeutic goal to tolerate more texture and taste. There is a risk of increased food refusal if the expectations around taste and texture are more than the child can handle. Nutrition should not be compromised to increase texture and consistency of foods (Case-Smith 1989). These issues must be carefully considered with the parent/caregiver before a feeding program is developed.

Reasons for Refusal of New and Different Textured Foods

1. *Uncoordinated or weak oral motor control.* The child may not have the oral mechanisms to safely chew and swallow textures (Morris and Klein, 2000). Food refusal becomes a way of staying safe and not choking on foods that cannot be chewed and swallowed safely and efficiently.

2. *Hypersensitivity to taste or texture.* A child with oral hypersensitivity may also have increased muscle tone and abnormal oral motor control seen as, tongue thrust, bite reflex, and *lip retraction* (not allowing lip seal or lip pursing) following tactile input during feeding (Case-Smith, 1989; Morris & Klein, 2000). A child with hypersensitivities may gag on a new or heightened taste or texture. A child experiencing oral hypersensitivity will demonstrate feeding issues (Mueller, 1972). As hypersensitivity may be systemic, treatment must be holistic in nature (please refer to Chapter 12: Introduction to Sensory Integration).

3. *Hyposensitivity to taste or texture.* A child with hyposensitivity may not have the precise oral motor control needed to tolerate increased food texture. Less efficient patterns of moving the food around in the mouth, including chewing and swallowing secondary to decreased muscle tone and generalized weakness are noted in children with oral motor hyposensitivity. This makes introducing increased food texture consistency a choking hazard. Children with hyposensitivity are at risk nutritionally because they take longer to eat, may avoid textures they cannot chew properly, and may display less interest in eating (Case-Smith, 1989; Morris & Klein, 2000).

4. *Limited repertoire.* Children with autism spectrum disorders often eat a limited repertoire of foods. Morris and Klein (2000) described these children as "limiting sensory input" (p. 673) in an effort to control the amount of sensory information they are receiving orally. The foods these children typically eat are often bland and white; pasta, bread, cheese, yogurt, chips, french fries, and some cereals. Desensitizing the oral area (Table 13-3) before a meal may diminish the tactile over responsiveness so the child with autism will try a new food (Quill, 1995).

BEHAVIOR PROBLEMS RELATED TO FEEDING

Many typically developing children exhibit behaviors around mealtimes that interfere with eating. Toddlers play with their food and do not remain at the table as long as adults. Mealtimes may occur when the child is not ready, and he/she refuses to come to the table. Parent/caregivers may not give the child a favored cup or spoon, or the child may not want the food being offered. These same behaviors are seen in children with feeding issues but may be magnified due to decreased communication skills, diminished oral motor skills, or sensory processing issues.

Many emotional issues arise when dealing with a child with feeding difficulties (Harris, 1986). A parent/caregiver may feel pressure to persuade the child to eat for nutritional purposes, and in extreme cases to prevent him/her from having a *feeding tube*. Children with feeding difficulties may have little interest in eating. They may not connect hunger with eating, be able to give cues around how much they want, what, and when to eat. In other words these children do not have the ability to adequately communicate needs and desires about feeding. Mealtimes turn from a fun interactive playtime between parents/caregivers and the child, to an intensive period of focused or even forced food intake.

Resistive Behaviors Around Feeding Are Often Seen in Children With These Issues

1. *Communication*: Children with communication issues are not always able to make their needs known. Developing a communication board with pictures of food choices, or having the child look at the desired food item offers some control in food selection.

2. *Cue reading*: Due to decreased motor abilities, delayed language skills and/or decreased body awareness, some children have a diminished ability to give verbal and/or nonverbal cues. Frequently, when verbal cues are not understood, nonverbal cues are given. These situations may arise when an infant has not yet developed language, or when an older child has speech and language delays. Examples of nonverbal cues include closing the mouth or turning the head to indicate "all done," opening the mouth for more, or looking at the cup for a drink (Roberts, & Heyman, 2000). When nonverbal cues are not responded to appropriately, a child may exaggerate them in order to be understood, or may get upset and reject feeding (DeGangi, 2000). Children may also resort to vomiting or gagging as a way to communicate, as it elicits a strong, quick reaction from the parent or caregiver. A parent or caregiv-

Table 13-3

Treatment of Oral Motor Skills

Treatment of oral motor skills often occurs away from the feeding or mealtime experience. This allows the child time to tolerate oral motor stimulation while learning new oral motor movements without the expectation to eat a meal. The child's new oral motor skills can be integrated into feeding and the mealtime at a pace that is comfortable for the child.

General Area of Concern	Specific Area of Concern	Treatment Strategies
Outside the Mouth	Positioning	• Placing a mirror in front of the child with the parent/caregiver sitting behind the child allows the child to see and model activities. • A younger child may sit in the OT practitioner's or parent/caregiver's lap; this position allows molding of the child into a more flexed position with the child's arms in towards midline. This sets up a comfortable position for oral activities (Figure 13-4).
	Sensory Play	• When working in the mouth with a child with hypersensitivity: use deep pressure, constant rhythm.· • When working in the mouth with a child with hyposensitivity: use lighter touch, and irregular intermittent patterns (Ayres, 1979; Case-Smith, 1989). • Any play around the mouth and face with safe toys should be encouraged, at least through the first year. Keeping child's hands in midline facilitates spontaneous toy to mouth play. • Encourage parents/caregivers to kiss, blow raspberries, play around the child's face (e.g., sing "Head Shoulders Knees and Toes," touching the child's body parts with exaggeration at the mouth sequence of the song). • Play with differently textured toys on the face and around the mouth. • Scented toys increase oral motor awareness and promote sucking and swallowing. • When wiping the mouth, use quick firm dabs of the cloth instead of a full swipe. • Let the child have as much control with oral motor stimulation as possible in treatment. Active muscle movement will lay the pathways for automatic feeding control. *Cautionary note*: The lips and tongue are among the most sensitive areas of the body (Farber, 1982). Sensory input may result in whole body reactions, which must be carefully monitored.
	Strengthening Oral Mechanisms: Mouth and Lip Closure	• Use deep pressure on the upper lip. • Rub the bottom lip up and the upper lip down. • Place two fingers at midline under the nose and quickly abduct them to the sides of the upper lip. • Rubbing circles with fingertips around the lips will promote suck and lip closure.
	Strengthening Oral Mechanisms: Jaw Control	• Making sure your thumb is out of the child's line of vision, gently placing two fingers under the chin and two fingers on the chin provides jaw stability for lip and tongue movement (Figure 13-5).
	Strengthening Oral Mechanisms: Suck and Swallow	• Rub from under the chin down the neck, but do not rub too hard. • To close lips for a suck, place ice or popsicles on the lips. • With the nipple in child's mouth, put your fingers on one cheek and thumb on the other cheek to promote a suck pattern.

Table 13-3 (continued)

Treatment of Oral Motor Skills

General Area of Concern	Specific Area of Concern	Treatment Strategies
	Strengthening Oral Mechanisms: Active Lip Movements	• Pucker lips to kiss; a mirror may help. • Simply blow or use a straw to blow. Blow cotton balls across a tabletop. • Blow bubbles using a long wand. • Blow on horns and whistles. • Bottle nipples and cup lids come in a variety of sizes, shapes, and varying degrees of flexibility. Changing the seal surface may improve lip seal and suction for successful bottle and cup drinking.
Inside the Mouth		• Respect the child's emotional state relative to play inside the mouth. • To promote participation, play games with songs and turn taking. • Allow the child to hold any of the toys/utensils going into the mouth. This provides the child more control as well as a sense of safety. • Ayres (1979) outlines how tactile input initiated by the child is often more tolerable than input initiated by someone else. • The child will be more comfortable with the mother versus a stranger. If the child is not familiar with or comfortable with the OT practitioner, instructing the parent/caregiver on proper techniques is indicated. • Placing a mirror in front of the child with the parent/caregiver sitting behind the child allows the child to see and model the activities. • Sitting in front of the child while bringing something to their mouth may be too much for some children to process. • A younger child may sit on the OT practitioner or parent/caregivers lap. This position allows molding of the child into a more flexed position with the child's arms in towards midline (Figure 13-4).
	Sensory Stimulation	• For a child with hypersensitivity, use deep pressure, constant rhythm. • For a child with hyposensitivity, use lighter touch, and irregular intermittent patterns (Ayres, 1979; Case-Smith, 1989). • Use an index finger wrapped in a washcloth to rub gums, walk back on the tongue, and /or stretch the lips and cheeks. • To increase sensory awareness of the mouth and/or to decrease stuffing of food, brush teeth before a meal. This increases tactile awareness of the mouth and allows for more efficient oral motor control. Do not use toothpaste, as you do not want to add taste. • Dip toothbrush or toys in juice or food for a child to taste, with no expectation to eat a meal. This provides a way to try new tastes away from mealtimes. • Invite the child to play with a spoon with and without food on it. Often the child will put the spoon in his/her mouth and explore with it when he/she has complete control. • To amplify taste, increase the spice level on foods. Many children with feeding issues need spicier foods to register the tastes, such as pickles, lemons, and mustard. • Try toys and food of varying temperatures. Freeze pops and popsicles may be used to facilitate oral awareness and swallowing. Plastic and metal toys have different temperatures. • Encourage teething and mouthing with different textured toys. Each provides different tactile stimulation resulting in different oral motor responses. • Soft, chewy rubber animals with protruding arms and legs promote chewing and increase tactile stimulation in the mouth.

Table 13-3 (continued)

Treatment of Oral Motor Skills

General Area of Concern	Specific Area of Concern	Treatment Strategies
		• Sucking and chewing on toys and food may be very organizing for a child with sensory needs (Oetter, Richter, & Frick, 1995). As the body is interconnected, working on tolerance of sensory input to the hands, feet, and face while working to increase tolerance in the mouth may be necessary (Ayres, 1979).
	Strengthening Oral Mechanisms: Suck *Many of these children have been* *on tube feeds, resulting in oral* *hypersensitivity.*	• To increase strength, gently pull on the nipple of a bottle when the infant is sucking. • Non-nutritive sucking – use of a pacifier, a different nipple, or the tip of your little finger. • Non-nutritive sucking can also be used to strengthen sucking muscles and increase endurance. Non-nutritive suck supports nutritive sucking in strengthening and in decreasing tactile aversion. • Help establish a sucking rhythm with a feed. Gently pulling finger or pacifier in and out of the mouth gets the rhythm going. Remember, nutritive sucking and non-nutritive sucking rhythms are different (Wolff 1968). • Sucking pudding or a thickened shake through a straw. • Drinking from a water bottle.
	Strengthening Oral Mechanisms: Chewing	• Chewing, sucking, and mouthing toys in play. • For a child who has teeth, place crunchy food on the molars and assist with chewing if necessary. Long thin pieces of crackers work well. • Eating scrambled eggs and fish may stimulate munching movements in the jaw. • Long thin grilled cheese strips, microwaved carrots strips, and roll-up fruit snacks can be placed on the gums or molars to stimulate munching. Chewing dried fruit and raisins or fruit snacks also helps facilitate munching.
	Strengthening Oral Mechanisms: Tongue Movements	• Lick items such as popsicles or lollipops. • Place a pretzel rod, strip of cheese, or licorice strip in the mouth. Encourage the child to search for it and move it with his/her tongue. Make certain the child can chew the item if a piece breaks off. • Promote tongue lateralization by placing a piece of food on the teeth or between the gums and teeth, and encourage the child to search for the food with his/her tongue. • If tongue retraction is strong, firmly walk back on the tongue using a toothbrush, small spoon, or fingers. Try this before a meal and a few times during the meal. • For tongue thrusting, place bowl of a spoon on center of tongue in the first third of the mouth and push gently down with a rocking motion from front of tongue towards the back. The lips will come down around the spoon as the tongue rounds around the bowl of the spoon. • Place a raisin or piece of cereal on the upper lip to promote tongue movement out of the mouth. Dipping the food in peanut butter will help it stick to the lip. • Place a piece of food such as a piece of cracker or pretzel on the child's lips that he/she needs to bring into the mouth using only the lips. • Have the child use his/her tongue to find your finger. Move your finger around to different places on the outside of the cheeks for the child to find.

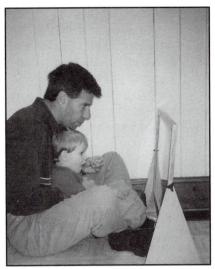

Figure 13-4. Sitting in front of a mirror allows for eye contact while providing needed support for oral motor play.

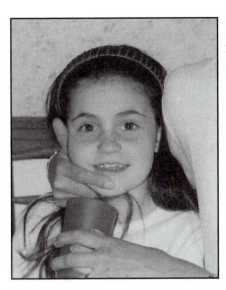

Figure 13-5. Providing jaw stability allows the child to have more lip control.

er who is skillful in reading the child's signals tends to be more successful with the feeding process (DeGangi, 2000).

3. *Transitions*: Transitions in feeding and mealtime routines are difficult for some children. It may be a large transition such as from a bottle to a cup or from formula to solids, or a more subtle one as in transitioning from one type of spoon to another (plastic to metal) or from formula to milk. These transitional difficulties are often due to comfort level. The child has figured out how to be successful with the current method of food intake and it is meeting his/her needs. A child with sensory processing difficulties will often detect a slight change in taste or texture. A child with motor planning difficulties may not know the new motor plan for a different type of cup, and the child with poor motor control will have to come up with a new way to use the different spoon. Avoiding negative feeding behaviors requires flexibility and ingenuity of the part of the feeding team to support the child, as well as parents/caregivers.

REPEATED GAGGING AND HICCUPPING

Young children frequently hiccup at mealtimes. It is cause for concern in an older child and also when it regularly occurs at mealtimes. Hiccuping is a signal that too much air is being swallowed while eating. As the air temporarily fills the stomach, hiccuping may result in reduced food intake and even may cause vomiting.

Until about 8 to 10 months of age, it is normal for infants to spit up some food and liquid. This usually diminishes as solid foods replace liquids as the main source of nutrition. Gagging is not usually a concern with the introduction of new textures, strong tastes, and nonpreferred tastes. When children gag because they cannot chew foods into small enough pieces, have an overactive gag reflex, or are gagging

as a mode of nonverbal communication, it is a cause for concern (Morris & Klein, 2000).

VOMITING AFTER OR DURING A FEEDING

If a child vomits soon after a meal or during a feeding, a medical check up is warranted to rule out physical anomalies and obstructions. Gastroesophageal Reflux (GER) is a common cause of vomiting. Gastroesophageal Reflux is the backward flow of stomach contents to the esophagus and pharynx. Some amount of GER is common in all infants after a feeding. If a child is not gaining weight, esophageal irritation is present, and/or there is aspiration, intervention is required (Morris and Klein, 2000). As there is a correlation between GER and respiratory illness, keeping the child in an upright position for up to one hour after a feed and when sleeping is recommended (Wolf & Glass, 1992). Elevating the head of the crib mattress or having the child nap in a car seat achieves this upright position. For many children with GER, medication may also be required (Morris & Klein, 2000; Wolf & Glass, 1992).

A child with oral hypersensitivity may vomit or gag during and/ or soon after a mealtime, as the sensory experience is too intense for them. The vomiting or gagging may be the only way a child can communicate to the caregiver (Morris & Klein, 2000). It may mean "I am over full," "I do not like that food," "I am too anxious to eat," or simply, "look and talk to me." Behaviorally, a child may get a kind of reaction from the caregiver through vomiting that they cannot get through more subtle forms of nonverbal communication.

CHILD ON A FEEDING TUBE

Nonoral feedings are implemented when a child is unable to take an oral feed or when oral feeds do not meet nutritional and growth requirements. Premature infants may not have the oral reflexes to allow for safe oral feedings, as they develop between 33 to 36 weeks of gestation (Wolff,

1968). These infants often have feeding tubes inserted at birth, which remain until they can learn to feed on their own. Children with neurological conditions who are unable to coordinate oral reflexes or oral musculature for a safe swallow, those with respiratory or cardiac issues who may not have the energy to suck and swallow, and children with oral hypersensitivities that may be so severe that the child cannot tolerate oral feeding may also require tube feeding (Morris & Klein, 2000; Wolf & Glass, 1992).

A nasal-gastric tube or NG-tube is used as a temporary or short-term method for increasing nutritional intake. It goes through the nose and down to the stomach. In addition to the discomfort from the tape required to hold it in place on the face, this tube may be very uncomfortable in the nasal cavity. A gastric-tube (G-tube) or jejunum-tube (J-tube) is used for longer or permanent tube placements. Gastric and Jejunum-tubes require minor surgery for insertion into the gastric system. A G-tube enters the stomach while a J-tube enters the large intestines, bypassing the stomach. Both G- and J-tubes are used for children with GER. A button at the end of the tube may be opened for a feed and closed when it is done (Morris & Klein, 2000; Wolf & Glass, 1992).

Morris and Klein (2000) describe how many children who have been on feeding tubes in the past or are transitioning off feeding tubes have had negative experiences with oral feedings and in the general oral area itself. When hypersensitivity in the oral area interferes with reflexes or makes feedings sensorily overwhelming, the child may be wary of anything approaching the oral area. Children born with medical issues may have had many aversive procedures in and around their mouth, and come to view the mouth as a place of negative, not pleasurable input (Wolf & Glass, 1992). For instance, when a NG-tube is used, it is taped to the nasal area and requires routine changing of the tube. The liquid and tube going down the back of the throat is described as uncomfortable and may cause irritation. Additionally, children with tonal and/or reflexive issues may have a history of choking. Choking on food is a very frightening experience that even very young children may remember (Morris & Klein, 2000).

Morris and Klein (2000) discuss potential issues in children with feeding tubes (or are status post feeding tube fed) when they are referred for feeding assessments. In these situations, the feeding problem has already been identified. For a child still on the tube, the goal is to transition from the tube to oral feedings. For a child off the tube, the feeding problem is often related to early sensory experiences, diminished oral motor control, and/or aversive behaviors around feeding.

Children transitioning from feeding tubes to oral feeding may not feel hungry. The tube feeds are often done at night with a pump, not three times a day like "meals." Without hunger, a child lacks the natural motivation to eat. As the child begins to transition from the tube, timing tube feeds with oral feed times may set the pattern for more typical feeding behaviors. In fact, premature infants that sucked during tube feedings transitioned to bottles sooner than those who did not (Measel & Anderson, 1979). For some children, the pump can be stopped earlier in the night to allow the sensation of hunger upon awakening. Pediatrician orders *must* be obtained to make the changes in tube feeds and/or transition from a tube to oral feeds.

ASPIRATION

Signs of aspiration include gagging and/or choking during or just after drinking and eating, wet mouth, difficulty managing saliva, wet sounding voice, and frequent respiratory infections (Geyer & McGowan, 1995; Wolf & Glass, 1992). As previously discussed, aspiration cannot always be identified through clinical assessment. If there is a question of aspiration, a *videofluoroscopic swallow study* is indicated, as it will provide a more definitive etiology and information for treatment solutions (Zerilli, Stefans, & DiPietro, 1990).

DECREASED ARTICULATION

Clear precise articulation of words requires well coordinated, sequenced, and timed movements of the tongue and lips. Proper breath support allows for modulation of volume and pitch and for appropriate length of word utterances. The lips and tongue bring the food in, the tongue moves the food around the mouth, and then to the back for a swallow. The oral movement patterns for feeding parallel the oral patterns for sound production (Morris & Klein, 2000).

Supervision

Entry-level competencies for both OTs and OTAs are clearly defined by the American Occupational Therapy Association (AOTA, 2000) (please refer to Appendices following this chapter). Working with children with oral motor and feeding issues may require additional training beyond entry-level competency. For example, specialized training is required to work with the child who is medically fragile or dependent upon technology. All OT practitioners must determine their individual level of competence and seek out additional training as appropriate (AOTA, 1993). The level of supervision provided to the OTA regarding feeding issues are further determined according to individual level of expertise, the level of service required by each child, as well as state and facility guidelines.

Through supervision, the OT and OTA work together to develop and implement effective treatment programs. Several models of supervision with reference to oral motor and feeding issues are listed below:

a) Observation of the OTA working on a feeding plan by the OT. The OT gives input on and modifies the treatment plan while the OTA that the child is most comfortable with carries out the program.

b) Each OT practitioner works with the child on the feeding plan at least one time a week so each have first hand knowledge of the current status of the child.

c) Videotaping treatment sessions and sharing the videotapes with the OT practitioners and the parent/caregiver. Will need parent/caregiver permission before videotaping.

Developing a viable supervision model with regard to oral motor and feeding issues requires "professional accountability and effective channels of communication between the OTR and OTA..." (Clark, 1993, p. 54) This ensures development and implementation of safe, appropriate, and coordinated therapy services.

Assessment of Oral Motor Feeding Skills

An infant feeding assessment should focus on sucking, as that is primarily how an infant feeds (Wolf and Glass 1992). The assessment of an older child needs to combine the control and sensory awareness of oral motor structures with the ability to coordinate self-feeding skills. It is important to concentrate on self-feeding skills in the older child, as that may be more important to the child than their oral motor abilities. For example, a 5 year old may be more concerned with being able to set up and open all the contents of their lunch and use utensils in the cafeteria rather than being able to chew meat.

REFLECTIONS FOR THE OTA

Always adhere to sound universal precautions such as wearing gloves when working in and around a child's mouth.

Any assessment of feeding and oral motor control must contain the following.

- A *medical history*, including past medical procedures, allergies, and medical complications

- A *parent/caregiver interview*, to obtain information on feeding history. The feeding history is often a checklist or form for the parent/caregiver to complete. The history should contain questions about problem areas, strategies that have been tried, child preferences and dislikes in food tastes and textures, information on how food is prepared and presented, specialized equipment, and average consumption of liquids and solids.

- *Observation* of the parent/caregiver feeding the infant/child in a naturalistic setting is very important. Positioning of child/infant, food textures, food presen-

tation, and time of the day should be as typical for the child as possible. If the child is in school, it may be helpful to see the child eat with the teachers as well as with the parent/caregiver. Feeding behaviors may differ depending on the context.

- *Oral motor control and reflex development, formal assessments* and *normal oral motor milestones* may be used to determine neuromotor functioning and its influence on feeding behavior. One example, the Oral-Motor/Feeding Rating Scale (Jelm, 1990) is used for ages 1 though adulthood. It is a rating scale for oral-motor/feeding patterns and related areas of feeding function.

- *Sensory motor processing. The Sensory Profile* (Dunn, 1999) and the *Infant/Toddler Sensory Profile* (Dunn, 2002) look at oral motor sensitivities in children aged 3 to 10 years and birth to 36 months, respectively. These Likert scale checklists can be completed by a parent/caregiver.

A parent/caregiver may be reluctant to admit or talk about their child/infant's feeding problem. Often the first contact with the parent/caregiver involves completing the feeding questionnaire and an observation of the parent/caregiver feeding the child. This can be a very emotional experience for the parent/caregiver. Wolf and Glass (1992) describe how a mother's confidence in her mothering skills are intimately linked to infant feeding. It is with sensitivity to these very personal and emotional experiences that the OT practitioner proceeds with the assessment process (please refer to Table 13-3).

Getting Ready for Feeding

POSITIONING

A child should be positioned as upright as tolerated to elicit the most efficient suck and swallow patterns. Emphasis should be on chin tuck, neck elongation, and a symmetrical trunk position (Case-Smith 1989). A more upright position allows for ease of arm movements to assist in self-feeding, and promotes eye gaze with both the parent/caregiver and the food.

For optimal self feeding, a child needs slight head flexion, hip flexion, and the hands positioned towards midline or the mouth. The child should feel comfortable enough to move around, but also safe and secure. An older child should be seated with feet firmly on the ground (or on a footrest), hips flexed to 90 degrees, with table or tray height about 1 or 2 inches above the elbows. If the child needs additional support, a chair with sides and arm rests as well as a tray may be used. When head control is limited, a slightly reclined position may be achieved by tilting the chair back. Most commercially available high chairs have variable tilt options (please refer to Chapter 11: Positioning in Pediatrics: Making the Right Choices).

A high chair can be adapted for smaller children by rolling up large bath towels and sliding them into the sides of the chair. This offers lateral support without taking away active trunk control or restricting arm movements (Figure 13-6).

Proper positioning depends on the infant or child's postural tone (Walker & Gorga, 1992). Maintaining postural alignment is essential for respiration, oral-pharyngeal control, and overall motor function (Geyer & McGowan, 1995). There is an artful balance in finding a position that allows for support without restricting too much trunk, head, and arm movement.

STATE REGULATION

The child should be awake, alert, and calm before a feeding or oral motor session. As has been discussed, children with feeding issues often have self-regulation difficulties, difficulty giving and reading signals around feeding, may be fearful of choking and new textures, or have to work extra hard to successfully coordinate oral musculature. If a child is agitated and distressed before and during a meal, he/she may be unable to successfully do the hard work associated with feeding. Keep in mind that because it is hard for children with feeding issues to eat, they may refuse to open their mouths. It may be very tempting to feed a child while he/she is crying, as the mouth is open. Think about the mouth position needed to actively remove food from a spoon. The lips are pursed and protracted and the tongue is forward and cupped. During a cry, the lips are retracted and the tongue retracted and arched. The food may get into the mouth, but it will not be brought to the back of the mouth and swallowed with the planned, controlled, and voluntary movements that need to be practiced for success in achieving the next level in feeding/self-feeding. Further, a child is at high risk for choking when fed while crying.

Experiential:
Put your head back and retract lips.
Imagine food, or nipple from a bottle coming at you.
Try to swallow.

Things to Keep in Mind When Feeding

- Babies often cough during a feed. Coughing clears the airway passage and strengthens the muscles involved in swallowing.
- Make certain respiration is okay. If you hear signs of distress you may need to stop feeding. Premature infants' respiration may increase due to the extra ener-

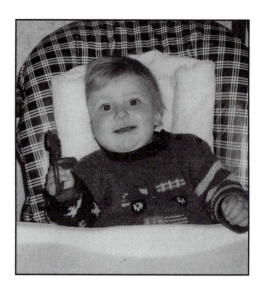

Figure 13-6. A rolled up towel can provide a child the lateral support needed when sitting in a highchair.

gy expenditure needed to feed (Wolf & Glass, 1992). It may be more important for the child to expend less energy (burn less calories) during this particular feed. A child with sensory processing issues may become so distraught with new tastes and textures during a meal that respiration increases. The fear may be so intense that new learning does not occur.

- A child needs to be hungry before a meal. Children with feeding issues may not be eating three meals at regular intervals, so they are not hungry at typical meal times. Children who are tube fed and children that do not take in much at each meal may not experience hunger. For a child on tube feeds, a tube meal might need to be delayed or skipped. This must be monitored and supported by the primary caregiver and the pediatrician.
- Timing tube feedings with oral stimulation may help the child connect eating and hunger with oral motor activity (Satter, 1992).
- Follow the infant and young child's signals (Satter 1992). These signals and cues are early attempts at communication. A child who can communicate what and when they want something will be more receptive to trying new and more difficult foods and textures. Often, a child's facial expressions during a meal will communicate his/her wants and needs.

PREPARATION OF FOOD FOR MEAL TIME

Tongue movements increase with the introduction of soft solid foods such as rice cereal. These foods are typically introduced between 4 and 6 months (Knight & Lumley 1985). Thicker and heavier foods are easier to control in the mouth than thinner and lighter foods. They also give more solid sensory information as to location in the mouth. Thicker and heavier foods require less motor control to consume than thinner foods. Mashed potatoes, oatmeal, nectar juices, and yogurt are examples of thicker foods. These foods stay together as they move to the back of the mouth to be swallowed and are less likely to run off the tongue to the sides of the mouth or under the tongue. Cooler and room temperature foods are thicker and easier to control in the mouth than heated foods. Very thick foods require more energy to eat; moving peanut butter to the back of the mouth to swallow or sucking a thickened liquid out of a cup requires a great deal of energy.

A child who fatigues easily should be monitored when being fed thickened food. Avoid foods that have both a solid and liquid consistency. Vegetable soup, cereal with milk, and jello with fruit all contain a solid and a liquid. A food with both a solid and liquid component requires the highest level of oral motor control as the child must separate the solid from the liquid, swallow the liquid, and then chew the solid.

Children with increased muscle tone may be over-responsive to some food tastes, textures, or consistencies. The additional taste and/or texture may stimulate already overresponsive oral reflexes or exaggerate unwanted oral motor mechanisms. Children with decreased muscle tone may benefit from introducing increased taste experiences to stimulate delayed or underreactive reflexes.

MEAL TIME

It is important for the child to be as actively involved as possible during the mealtime. It is through the child's active and self-initiated movements that they learn new and more efficient motor control and sensory processing. It is also helpful to think about the feeding environment before food is presented to the child. What is the noise level and distraction level in the room? Can the child eat with a group of children present or TV on, does the child need soothing music, and should the child have only one bite of food on the plate at a time (Morris & Klein 2000)? The purpose of altering the environment is to provide a safe organizing place where the child can concentrate on eating (Case-Smith, 1989).

Respect family/caregiver mealtime values. Every family has unique mealtime expectations, rules and routines. Some families/caregivers prefer to introduce solid foods earlier than others, while some prefer to feed the children separately from the adults, or to continue bottle-feeding longer (DeGangi, 2000). The family/caregivers already have to balance their child's feeding difficulties with their own expectations, as well as follow the pediatrician and nutritionists' tations, as well as follow the pediatrician and nutritionists'

recommendations. One of the roles of the OT practitioner is to help the family successfully put it all together.

Table 13-4 presents suggestions for providing opportunity for an optimal mealtime experience.

Oral Motor/Feeding Therapy Groups

A therapy group may be a more effective way to treat some children with refusal to eat feeding issues. In a group situation, children will experience multiple exposures to different foods just by sitting with peers at lunch or snack. The food each child brings from home provides an interesting assortment of textures, smells, and tastes. In a group situation there is no external pressure to try new foods as they belong to another child. In fact, Roberts and Heyman (2000) discuss the importance of avoiding persuasion in developing a more healthy diet. A group situation may provide a safe neutral setting to try new things.

Therapy groups that center around food, but not eating the food is another way to provide exposure without pressure. Art projects that use food, cooking foods, reading books about food, and pretend food games all provide exposure with the emphasis on the activity, and not the food. Placing a snack made up of the foods presented in the activity close to the child may tempt him/her to eat it while working on the activity.

Many children need to work on oral motor exercises, but find them repetitive and not fun. Taking turns and doing the exercises in a group provides more of a game-like atmosphere that may increase participation and lead to faster goal attainment.

Table 13-4

Components of an Optimal Mealtime

- Present the food to the child at eye level. If the food is too high, the child will have to extend the neck, presented too low, the child will not see it. *Remember, if your neck is extended it is very difficult to swallow.*

- A child needs to see the food coming towards them to anticipate and prepare the mouth for food.

Experiential:
Have someone prepare to give you a drink from a cup, and notice how you purse your lips and cup your tongue *before* the cup reaches your lips.

- If a child does not seem fully prepared by the time the spoon or cup reaches the lips, or he/she is visually impaired, touching the food to the lips first provides a physical cue to ready the mouth themselves. Wait a few seconds and tap again, but do not put food into the mouth if the child is not actively prepared. As it is typical for a child to refuse the first bite of food, leaving a small taste on the lips often encourages exploration.

- Wait a few seconds for the child to close his/her mouth around the food/spoon/cup. It may take longer for a child with feeding difficulties to process the input for action. Provide jaw control techniques if the mouth does not close or if there is not a tight seal around the food/cup/utensil.

- Make sure the cup or nipple rests on the lips and not the teeth. If the cup or nipple rests on the teeth, it could stimulate the bite reflex.

- If the top lip does not come down to take the food off the spoon, gently press the spoon down on the front third of the tongue and wait a few seconds for the lip to come down.

- Do not put too much food on the spoon. The child should be able to safely manage the full amount of food on the spoon.

- To reinforce voluntary control with the verbal request, combine verbal cues with facilitation techniques. An example of this is to say, "Close your lips" while gently pressing the spoon down on the front third of the tongue.

- Let the child touch and play with the food, and bring it to the mouth even if you are doing the nutritive feeding. This is especially important for children on feeding tubes. These techniques help foster a sense of mealtime rituals.

- Limit the special equipment needed for feeding. Special equipment is often essential for safe feeding, more independence in self-feeding, and increased ease during a mealtime. These issues must balance with the cost of special equipment, the availability of the equipment, and the parent/caregiver stress around having special equipment. The parent/caregiver may view the equipment as one more thing that visually separates their child from typically developing children, or as one more thing to remember at mealtime.

In a group situation, several students and teachers may eat together under the guidance of an OT practitioner. Students and teachers will have the opportunity to learn the techniques to be implemented on the days when the OT practitioner is not present.

Summary

This chapter provided an overview of oral motor and feeding issues. It is not intended to be a comprehensive source, but a resource for the OTA practitioner to use in conjunction with the supervising OT in implementing oral motor and feeding treatment plans.

Case Study

Sara is 3 1/2 years old and was born with oxygen deprivation due to a difficult birth. Sara does not have the ability to sit on her own, communicate verbally or with a board, or feed herself. She is dependent in all areas of self-care. She was referred for additional home-based occupational therapy when she turned 3 to address feeding issues. The mother showed the OT practitioner how she fed Sara. Sara was positioned in a custom fitted highchair with footrests and a tray for arm support. Back and side head supports were also used. The chair was slightly reclined about 15 degrees to allow for more head control. During mealtimes, Sara moved her head from side to side while her mother attempted, whenever possible, to get a spoonful of food in her mouth. Sara would accept some mouthfuls, but more frequently closed her mouth or pushed the food back out with her tongue. Her mother said she frequently held Sara's head still with one hand while prying her mouth open with her other hand to get a spoonful of food into her mouth. This made Sara cry. The consistency of Sara's food was soft ground, meaning that there were some lumps in it. It was apparent that Sara had no control over when food was presented to her. Therapy sessions began with finding a way for Sara to tell her parents when she was ready for the next bite. Foods were placed in the center of the tray at mouth level for Sara to first see and smell. As she moved her head from side to side Sara began to brush her lips and tongue against the spoon to taste the foods being presented at the center of the tray. Sara had found a way to control when, what, and how much she put in her mouth. In just a few weeks' time, the closing her mouth and pushing the food out behaviors dramatically decreased. Once Sara was able to give signals that could be read by caregivers regarding when she wanted to eat, she began to make food choices. Two different foods were presented at eye level, and Sara would look at the one she wanted. After 2 months of therapy, Sara began to accept more texture in her food. Now that the feeding experience was more pleasant and she had some control, Sara felt safe and was calm enough to attempt more chewing.

DISCUSSION QUESTIONS

1. Think about and discuss how Sara's mother felt about mealtimes with Sara before and after occupational therapy intervention.

2. How could the communication system at mealtime be expanded to other functional activities?

3. What activities would you include in a chewing program for Sara?

Application Activities

1. Have the students break up into pairs to feed each other. One student acts as the practitioner and one as the child. After each trial stop and have the practitioner/child discuss the experience from their perspective.

   Have applesauce, spoons, juice, cups, graham crackers, pretzel rods, and gloves available for:

   a. drinking from a cup, no talking

   b. drinking from a cup eyes closed

   c. drinking from a cup with verbal cues to help the child prepare for the cup coming

   d. give jaw stability with cup drinking (see Figure 13-5 for example)

   e. feed from a spoon, no talking

   f. feed from a spoon, scrape food off of teeth

   g. feed from a spoon, wait for lips to come down to take food off

   h. gently depress the first third of tongue and "feel" mouth closure

   i. chew crackers, count how many times tongue moves the food

   j. chew crackers, count how many directions the tongue goes to move the food

   k. place pretzel rod on teeth gums to "facilitate" bite

   l. move the pretzel around inside and outside the mouth, wait for the tongue to find it before moving to the next location

2. Practice oral stimulation techniques discussed in this chapter on a partner.

   a. jaw stability

   b. lip closure

   c. lip movements

   d. swallow

   e. tongue movements

References

Alexander, R., Boehme, R., & Cupps, B. 1993. *Normal development of functional motor skills.* Tucson: Therapy Skill Builders.

Ayres, A. J. (1979). *Sensory integration and the child.* Los Angeles: CA: Western Psychological Services.

American Occupational Therapy Association (2000). Specialized knowledge and skills in eating and feeding for occupational therapy practice. *American Journal of Occupational Therapy, 54*(6), 629-640.

Birch, L.L., Marlin, D. W., & Rotter, J. (1984). Eating as the "means" activity in a contingency: Effects on a young child's food preference. *Child Development, 55*(2), 431-439.

Burklow, K. A., Phelps, A. N., Schultz, J., R., McConnell K., & Rudolph, C. (1998). Classifying complex pediatric feeding disorders. *Journal of Pediatric Gastroenterology and Nutrition, 27*, 143-147.

Case-Smith, J. (2001). *Occupational therapy for children.* St Louis, MO: Mosby.

Case-Smith, J. (1989). Intervention strategies for promoting feeding skills in infants with sensory deficits. *Physical and Occupational Therapy in Pediatrics*, 129-141.

Chamberlin, J., Henry, M., Roberts, J., Sapsford, A., & Courtney, S. 1991. An infant and toddler feeding group program. *American Journal of Occupational Therapy, 45*(10), 907-911.

Clark, G. F. (1993). *Oral-motor and feeding issues.* The American Occupational Therapy Association Self Study Series.

Conner, F. P., Williamson, G. G., & Siepp, J. M. (1983). *Program guide for infants and toddlers with neuromotor and other developmental disabilities.* New York: Teachers College Press.

DeGangi, G. (2000). *Pediatric disorders of regulation in affect and behavior.* London: Academic Press.

Dunn, W. (1999). The sensory profile. San Antonio, TX: The Psychological Corporation.

Dunn, W. (2000). The infant/toddler sensory profile. San Antonio, TX: The Psychological Corporation.

Farber, S. (1982). *Neurorehabilitation: A multisensory approach.* Philadelphia, PA: W. B. Saunders.

Geyer, L. A., & McGowan, J. S. (1995). Positioning infants and children for videofluoroscopic swallowing function studies. *Infants and Young Children, 8*(2) 58-64.

Gisel. E. (1991). Effect of food texture on the development of chewing of children between six months and two years of age. *Developmental Medicine and Child Neurology, 33,* 69-79.

Glass, R. P., & Wolf, L. S. (1999). Feeding management of infants with cleft lip and palate and micrognathia. *Infants and Young Children, 12*(1) 70-81.

Harris, M. (1986). Oral management of the high risk neonate. *Physical and Occupational Therapy in Pediatrics, 6,* 217-254.

Humphry, R., & Thigpen-Beck, B. (1998). Parenting values and attitudes: Views of therapists and parents. *American Journal of Occupational Therapy, 52,* 835-843.

Ianniruberto, A., & Tajani, E. (1981). Ultrasonographic study of fetal movements. *Seminars in Perinatology, 5,* 175-181

Jelm, J. (1990). *Oral motor/feeding rating scale.* Tucson, AZ: Therapy Skill Builders.

Kenny, D., & Judd, P. (1988). Oral care for developmentally disabled children: The primary dentition stage. *Infants and Young Children, 1*(2) 11-19.

Knight, K., & Lumley, J. (1985). *The baby cookbook.* New York: Quill.

Lundy-Ekman, L. (1998). *Neuroscience fundamentals for rehabilitation.* Philadelphia, PA: W. B. Saunders.

Measel, C. P., Anderson, G. C. (1979). Non-nutritive sucking during tube feeding: Effect on clinical course in premature infants. *JOGN, 8*(5):265-272.

Mennella, J. A., & Beauchamp, G. (1993). Early flavor experiences: When do they start? *Zero to Three, 14*(2) 1-7.

Miller, C. K., Burklow K. A., Santoro, K., Kirby, E., Mason, D., & Rudolph, C. D. (2001). An interdisciplinary team approach to the management of pediatric feeding and swallowing disorders. *Children's Health Care, 30*(3) 201-218.

Morris, S. E., & Klein M. D. (2000). *Pre-feeding skills.* Tucson, AZ: Therapy Skill Builders.

Mueller, H. (1972). Facilitating feeding and prespeech. In P. H. Pearson and C. E. Williams (Eds.), *Physical therapy services in the developmental disabilities.* Springfield: Charles C. Thomas.

Oetter, P., Richter, E. W., & Frick, S. M. (1995). *M.O.R.E. Integrating the mouth with sensory and postural functions* (2nd Ed.). Hugo MN: PDP Press.

Quill, K. A. (1995). *Teaching children with autism: Strategies to enhance communication and socialization.* New York: Delmar Publishers Inc.

Roberts, S. B. & Heyman, M. B. (2000). How to feed babies and toddlers in the 21st century. *Zero to Three, 21*(1)24-28.

Satter, E. 1992. The feeding relationship. *Zero to Three, 12*(5) 3-9.

Stevenson, M. B., Roach, M. A., Ver Hoeve, J. N., & Leavitt, L. A. (1990). Rhythms in the dialogue of infant feeding: Preterm and term infants. *Infant Behavior and Development, 13,* 51-70.

Vergara, E. 1993. *Foundations for practice in the neonatal intensive care unit and early intervention* Volume 2. Rockville MD: AOTA.

Walker, L., & Gorga, D. 1992. Clinical considerations in feeding the medically ill, hospitalized infant. *Occupational Therapy Practice, 3*(2) 35-50.

Wolf, L. S., & Glass, R. P. (1992). *Feeding and swallowing disorders in infancy: Assessment and management.* Tucson, AZ: Therapy Skill Builders.

Wolff, P. H. 1968. The serial organization of sucking in the young infant. *Pediatrics, 42,* 943-955.

Zerilli, K. S., Stefans, V. A., & DiPietro, M. A. (1990). Protocol for the use of videofluoroscopy in pediatric swallowing dysfunction. *American Journal of Occupational Therapy, 44*(5), 441-446.

Appendix 13-1

Entry Level Knowledge and Skills Assessment—Context

Occupational Therapists and Occupational Therapy Assistants will have entry level knowledge and skills to:	OT	OTA
	Based on the establishment of competency and under the supervision of an OT	
Cultural components that affect feeding: utensils, food types, meanings/symbolism of food, mealtime practices and rituals, dietary restrictions	X	X
Attitudes and values of client, family or caregivers, and friends toward feeding and mealtime	X	X
Settings where feeding/eating take place	X	X
Social opportunities during mealtime that support or interfere with social interaction	X	X
Aspects of the client's developmental status/life phase that support or interfere with eating/feeding	X	
Effect of medical condition/disability status on feeding performance	X	
Factors in the environment that support or interfere with feeding/eating (available: foods, seating, time, feeders, etc.)	X	

X = able to perform the task.

Reprinted with permission from the American Occupational Therapy Association. Specialized knowledge and skills in eating and feeding for occupational therapy practice (2000). *American Journal of Occupational Therapy, 54*(6), 629-640.

Appendix 13-2

Entry Level Knowledge and Skills Assessment—Pre-Oral Phase

	OT	OTA
Occupational Therapists and Occupational Therapy Assistants will have entry level knowledge and skills to:	**Based on the establishment of competency and under the supervision of an OT**	
The role of appetite and hunger sensation.	X	X
Tactile and proprioceptive qualities of food and equipment in both the hands and mouth.	X	X
Ability to see/locate food/drink/utensils.	X	X
Ability to appreciate smell—pleasant, noxious.	X	X
Need for use of auditory cues (verbal cues, utensils hitting plate).	X	X
Ability to achieve a position of proximal postural control that allows upper extremity and oral function for eating.	X	X
Nature of communication during feeding/mealtime.	X	X
Feeding experience as satisfactory to self.	X	X
Ability to bring food to mouth as supported or prevented by factors such as figure ground, depth perception, spatial relations, and motor planning.	X	
Neuromotor components that support or interfere with adequate positioning.	X	
Upper extremity function and hand manipulation adequate for self-feeding.	X	
The influence of motor activity involved in bringing food to mouth.	X	
Ability to orient mouth to receive food (timing, positioning of structures).	X	
Initiation of eating as supported/prevented by level of alertness/arousal, orientation to task, recognition, and memory.	X	
Persistence with feeding is supported/prevented by level of arousal, attention span, initiation of activity, memory, and sequencing.	X	
Carryover of skill to future feeding tasks is supported/prevented by level of memory, learning, and generalization.	X	
Factors that influence the willingness or unwillingness to eat (self-image, self-esteem, caregiver, family, feeder interaction, eating history, dying).	X	

X = able to perform the task.

Appendix 13-3

Entry Level Knowledge and Skills Assessment—Oral Phase

Occupational Therapists and Occupational Therapy Assistants will have entry level knowledge and skills to:	OT	OTA
	Based on the establishment of competency and under the supervision of an OT	
Behaviors or reports that indicate pain or discomfort in the oral area.	X	X
Behaviors that interfere with the oral phase (spitting foods, pocketing foods, refusing to swallow).	X	X
Level of awareness/sensation in the oral motor area.	X	
Level of reception and perception of tactile (texture), temperature, proprioception, and gustatory qualities of food and utensils.	X	
Factors supporting/interfering with secretion management.	X	
Respiratory control factors that permit safe and efficient bolus manipulation (mouth breathers, Adult Respiration Distress Syndrome, bronchopulmonary dysplasia).	X	
Structural or neuromotor factors (reflexes, range of motion, muscle tone, strength, endurance) that support or interfere with oral motor function.	X	
Level of coordinated movements (praxis) of oral structures (cheeks, lips, jaw, tongue, palate, teeth) with or without foods.	X	
Oral structures' ability to work together to contain, form, and propel the bolus.	X	
Bolus manipulation supported/compromised by memory, attention span, orientation, and problem solving.	X	
Speed of the oral phase adequate to support sufficient oral intake.	X	

X = able to perform the task.

Reprinted with permission from the American Occupational Therapy Association. Specialized knowledge and skills in eating and feeding for occupational therapy practice (2000). *American Journal of Occupational Therapy, 54*(6), 629-640.

Appendix 13-4

Entry Level Knowledge and Skills Assessment—Pharyngeal Phase

Occupational Therapists and Occupational Therapy Assistants will have entry level knowledge and skills to:	OT	OTA
	Based on the establishment of competency and under the supervision of an OT	
Behaviors or reports that indicate pain or discomfort localized to the pharyngeal area.	X	
Presence of signs and symptoms of aspiration.	X	

X = able to perform the task.

Reprinted with permission from the American Occupational Therapy Association. Specialized knowledge and skills in eating and feeding for occupational therapy practice (2000). *American Journal of Occupational Therapy, 54*(6), 629-640.

Appendix 13-5

Entry Level Knowledge and Skills Assessment—Esophageal Phase

	OT	OTA
Occupational Therapists and Occupational Therapy Assistants will have entry level knowledge and skills to:	**Based on the establishment of competency and under the supervision of an OT**	
Behaviors or reports that indicate pain or discomfort in the esophageal area.	X	
Inappropriate return of food from the stomach into the esophagus, pharynx, or oral cavity.	X	

X = able to perform the task.

Reprinted with permission from the American Occupational Therapy Association. Specialized knowledge and skills in eating and feeding for occupational therapy practice (2000). *American Journal of Occupational Therapy, 54*(6), 629-640.

Appendix 13-6

Entry Level Knowledge and Skills Assessment—Instrumentation

	OT	OTA
Occupational Therapists and Occupational Therapy Assistants will have entry level knowledge and skills to:	**Based on the establishment of competency and under the supervision of an OT**	
Understand formal instrumentation used by therapists or other professionals to evaluate the oral, pharyngeal, and esophageal phase of the swallow, including, but not limited to, videofluoroscopy, ultrasonography, fiberoptic endoscopy, scintigraphy, and manometry.	X	

X = able to perform the task.

Reprinted with permission from the American Occupational Therapy Association. Specialized knowledge and skills in eating and feeding for occupational therapy practice (2000). *American Journal of Occupational Therapy, 54*(6), 629-640.

Appendix 13-7

Entry Level Knowledge and Skills Intervention—Pharyngeal Phase

	OT	OTA
Occupational Therapists and Occupational Therapy Assistants will have entry level knowledge and skills to:	**Based on the establishment of competency and under the supervision of an OT**	
Facilitate head and neck positioning for swallowing (e.g., chin tuck).	X	
Facilitate compensatory swallow techniques (e.g., double swallow).	X	

X = able to perform the task.

Reprinted with permission from the American Occupational Therapy Association. Specialized knowledge and skills in eating and feeding for occupational therapy practice (2000). *American Journal of Occupational Therapy, 54*(6), 629-640.

Appendix 13-8

Entry Level Knowledge and Skills Intervention—Esophageal Phase

	OT	OTA
Occupational Therapists and Occupational Therapy Assistants will have entry level knowledge and skills to:		**Based on the establishment of competency and under the supervision of an OT**
Modify position before, during, and after feeding task.	X	

X = able to perform the task.

Reprinted with permission from the American Occupational Therapy Association. Specialized knowledge and skills in eating and feeding for occupational therapy practice (2000). *American Journal of Occupational Therapy, 54*(6), 629-640.

14

Childhood Occupations

Jan Hollenbeck, MS, OTR/L

Chapter Objectives

- Describe the importance of occupation to occupational therapy and identify the primary occupations of childhood.

- Define play and play development through the work of major theorists, including the contribution of occupational therapy.

- Describe the impact of various disabilities on play development.

- Describe intervention strategies to enhance play skills, playfulness, and the development of other performance skills and client factors through the use of play.

Introduction: The Nature of Occupations

Occupation is the very essence of occupational therapy. Occupation frames our profession and defines who we, as occupational therapists (OTs) and occupational therapy assistants (OTAs), are. The *Occupational Therapy Practice Framework* (2002) describes the domain and process of occupational therapy. The domain of practice is what is unique to occupational therapy and is what sets us apart from other professions. Occupational performance is the domain of concern for the occupational therapy profession (Kramer & Hinojosa, 1993). That is, engagement in occupation in order to support participation in context is the focus and targeted end objective of occupational therapy intervention. (AOTA, 2002). This is derived from the belief that

engagement in meaningful activities promotes health and well-being (Roley, 2002).

The *Occupational Therapy Practice Framework* defines occupation as "activities...of everyday life, named, organized, and given value and meaning by individuals and a culture. Occupation is everything people do to occupy themselves, including looking after themselves...enjoying life...and contributing to the social and economic fabric of their communities...." (AOTA, 2002; Law, et al, 1997, p. 32) The *Occupational Therapy Practice Framework* (2002) identifies the following areas of occupation: activities of daily living (ADL), instrumental activities of daily living (IADL), education, work, play, leisure, and social participation (Table 14-1).

Childhood Occupations

The occupations of children are not unique to childhood; however, occupational areas are influenced by several factors including the child's age, stage of development, sociocultural background, and environment. The extent to which an occupational area is relevant to a particular child depends on these factors (Llorens, 1991; Kramer & Hinojosa, 1993). The Areas of Occupation most typically relevant for children include ADL, education, play, and social participation. That is not to say, however, that these are the only occupations in which children engage. As indicated above, the relevancy and importance of each area of occupation must be considered with regard to each child. For example, while it is clear that not all IADL are relevant to all children there are some aspects that may be relevant to a particular child. Caring for pets, assisting with the care

Table 14-1
Areas of Occupation

Various kinds of life activities in which people engage, including ADL, IADL, education, work, play, leisure, and social participation.

Activities of Daily Living (ADL)

Activities that are oriented toward taking care of one's own body (adapted from Rogers & Holm, 1994, pp. 181-202), also called basic activities of daily living (BADL) or personal activities of daily living (PADL).

- Bathing, showering—Obtaining and using supplies; soaping, rinsing, and drying body parts; maintaining bathing position; and transferring to and from bathing positions.
- Bowel and bladder management—Includes complete intentional control of bowel movements and urinary bladder and, if necessary, use of equipment or agents for bladder control (Uniform Data System for Medical Rehabilitation [UDSMR], 1996, pp. III-20, III-24).
- Dressing—Selecting clothing and accessories appropriate to time of day, weather, and occasion; obtaining clothing from storage area; dressing and undressing in a sequential fashion; fastening and adjusting clothing and shoes; and applying and removing personal devices, prostheses, or orthoses.
- Eating—"The ability to keep and manipulate food/fluid in the mouth and swallow it" (O'Sullivan, 1995, p. 191; AOTA, 2000, p. 629).
- Feeding—"The process of [setting up, arranging, and] bringing food [fluids] from the plate or cup to the mouth" (O'Sullivan, 1995, p. 191; AOTA, 2000, p. 629).
- Functional mobility—Moving from one position or place to another (during performance of everyday activities), such as in-bed mobility, wheelchair mobility, transfers (wheelchair, bed, car, tub/shower, toilet, chair, floor). Performing functional ambulation and transporting objects.
- Personal device care—Using, cleaning, and maintaining personal care items, such as hearing aids, contact lenses, glasses, orthotics, prosthetics, adaptive equipment, and contraceptive and sexual devices.
- Personal hygiene and grooming—Obtaining and using supplies; removing body hair (use of razors, tweezers, lotions, etc.); applying and removing cosmetics; washing, drying, combing, styling, brushing, and trimming hair; caring for nails (hands and feet); caring for skin, ears, eyes, and nose; applying deodorant; cleaning mouth; brushing and flossing teeth; or removing, cleaning, and reinserting dental orthotics and prosthetics.
- Sexual activity—Engagement in activities that result in sexual satisfaction.
- Sleep/rest—A period of inactivity in which one may or may not suspend consciousness.
- Toilet Hygiene—Obtaining and using supplies; clothing management; maintaining toileting position; transferring to and from toileting position; cleaning body; and caring for menstrual and continence needs (including catheters, colostomies, and suppository management).

Instrumental Activities of Daily Living (IADL)

Activities that are oriented toward interacting with the environment and that are often complex - generally optional in nature (i.e. may be delegated to another) (adapted from Rogers & Holm, 1994, pp. 181-202).

- Care of others (including selecting and supervising caregivers)—Arranging, supervising, or providing the care for others.
- Care of pets—Arranging, supervising, or providing the care for pets and service to animals.
- Child rearing—Providing the care and supervision to support the developmental needs of a child.
- Communication device use—Using equipment of systems such as writing equipment, telephones, typewriters, computers, communication boards, call lights, emergency systems, Braille writers, telecommunication devices for the deaf, and augmentative communication systems to send and receive information.
- Community mobility—Moving self in the community and using public or private transportation, such as driving, or accessing buses, taxicabs, or other public transportation systems.
- Financial management—Using fiscal resources, including alternate methods of financial transaction and planning and using finances with long-term and short-term goals.
- Health management and maintenance—Developing, managing, and maintaining routines for health and wellness promotion, such as physical fitness, nutrition, decreasing health risk behaviors, and medication routines.
- Home establishment and management—Obtaining and maintaining personal and household possessions and environment (e.g., home, yard, garden, appliances, vehicles), including maintaining and repairing personal possessions (clothing and household items) and knowing how to seek help or whom to contact.
- Meal preparation and cleanup—Planning, preparing, serving well-balanced, nutritional meals and cleaning up food and utensils after meals.
- Safety procedures and emergency responses—Knowing and performing preventive procedures to maintain a safe environment as well as recognizing sudden, unexpected hazardous situations, and initiating emergency action to reduce the threat to health and safety.
- Shopping—Preparing shopping lists (grocery and other); selecting and purchasing items; selecting method of payment; and completing money transactions.

Table 14-1 (continued)

Areas of Occupation

Education

Includes activities needed for being a student and participating in a learning environment.

- Formal educational participation—Including the categories of academic (e.g., math, reading, working on a degree), nonacademic (e.g., recess, lunchroom, hallway), extracurricular (e.g., sports, band, cheerleading, dances), and vocational (prevocational and vocational) participation.
- Exploration of informal personal educational needs or interests (beyond formal education)—Identifying topics and methods for obtaining topic-related information or skills.
- Informal personal education participation—Participating in classes, programs, and activities that provide instruction/training in identified areas of interest.

Work

Includes activities needed for engaging in remunerative employment or volunteer activities (Mosey, 1996, p. 341).

- Employment interests and pursuits—Identifying and selecting work opportunities based on personal assets, limitations, likes, and dislikes relative to work (adapted from Mosey, 1996, p. 342).
- Employment seeking and acquisition—Identifying job opportunities, completing and submitting appropriate application materials, preparing for interviews, participation in interviews and following up afterward, discussing job benefits, and finalizing negotiations.
- Job performance—Including work habits, for example, attendance, punctuality, appropriate relationships with coworkers and supervisors, completion of assigned work, and compliance with the norms of the work setting (adapted from Mosey, 1996, p. 342).
- Retirement preparation and adjustment—Determining aptitudes, developing interests and skills, and selecting appropriate avocational pursuits.
- Volunteer exploration—Determining community causes, organizations, or opportunities for unpaid "work" in relationship to personal skills, interests, location, and time available.
- Volunteer participation—Performing unpaid "work" activities for the benefit of identified selected causes, organizations, or facilities.

Play

"Any spontaneous or organized activity that provides enjoyment, entertainment, amusement, or diversion" (Parham & Fazio, 1997, p. 252).

- Play exploration—Identifying appropriate play activities, which can include exploration play, practice play, pretend play, games with rules, constructive play, and symbolic play (adapted from Bergen, 1988, pp. 64-65).
- Play participation—Participating in play; maintaining a balance of play with other areas of occupation; and obtaining, using, and maintaining, toys, equipment, and supplies appropriately.

Leisure

"A nonobligatory activity that is intrinsically motivated and engaged in during discretionary time, that is, time not committed to obligatory occupations such as work, self care, or sleep" (Parham & Fazio, 1997, p. 250).

- Leisure exploration—Identifying interests, skills, opportunities, and appropriate leisure activities.
- Leisure participation—Planning and participating in appropriate leisure activities; maintaining a balance of leisure activities with other areas of occupation; and obtaining, using, and maintaining equipment and supplies as appropriate.

Social Participation

Activities associated with organized patterns of behavior that are characteristic and expected of an individual or an individual interacting with others within a given social system (adapted from Mosey, 1996, p. 340).

- Community—Activities that result in successful interaction at the community level (i.e., neighborhood, organizations, work, school).
- Family—"[Activities that result in] successful interaction in specific required and/or desired familial roles" (Mosey, 1996, p. 340).
- Peer, friend—Activities at different levels of intimacy, including engaging in desired sexual activity.

of younger siblings, use of the telephone and computer, managing an allowance, cleaning one's own room, and knowing basic emergency procedures are all examples of IADL that may be relevant to childhood.

ACTIVITIES OF DAILY LIVING & INSTRUMENTAL ACTIVITIES OF DAILY LIVING

Activities of daily living (ADL) refer to the activities involved in caring for oneself. These self-care activities include bathing, bowel and bladder management (control of bowel and bladder functions), dressing, eating (managing food in the mouth and swallowing), feeding (getting food from the cup and plate/bowl to the mouth), functional mobility, personal device care (using and caring for items such as glasses, hearing aids, orthotics or adaptive equipment necessary for the performance of ADL), personal hygiene and grooming (i.e., hair care, nail care, brushing teeth, etc.), sexual activity, sleep/rest, and toilet hygiene (managing materials needed for toileting such as clothing and toilet paper, transferring on/off toilet, cleaning self after toileting, etc.) (AOTA, 2002).

Instrumental activities of daily living (IADL) include care of others, care of pets, child rearing, communication device use, community mobility, financial management, health management and maintenance, home establishment and management, meal preparation and clean up, safety procedures and emergency responses, and shopping (AOTA, 2002). A more detailed discussion of the OT and the OTAs role with ADL and IADL may be found in Chapter 15: Self-Care.

EDUCATION

Educational activities include both formal and informal education. Children typically do not encounter formal education until age 5 or 6 when they enter elementary school. However, child development center, nursery, or preschool, instructional classes such as dance, karate, or arts and crafts, as well as religious education may all be considered educational activities (AOTA, 2002).

WORK

Activities demands for paid or volunteer work experiences fall into the occupational area of work. Consideration of the cultural context of the child must be given when determining the relevancy of work. In the United States, young children typically do not participate in paid work activities. As children get older, they may begin to take on paid responsibilities such as paper routes, mowing lawns, or shoveling snow (Kramer & Hinojosa, 1993). Children may also be involved in volunteer work activities such as fund raising, participating in a community clean-up day, or making and donating gifts or food for charity.

PLAY

The *Occupational Therapy Practice Framework* (2002) defines play as "any spontaneous or organized activity that provides enjoyment, entertainment, amusement, or diversion" (Parham & Fazio, 1997, p. 252). The occupational area of play includes two subcategories: play exploration and play participation. Play exploration involves identifying appropriate play activities, which may include exploration play, practice play, pretend play, games with rules, constructive play, and symbolic play (adapted from Bergen, 1988). Play participation includes participating in play; maintaining a balance of play with other areas of occupation; and obtaining, using, and maintaining toys, equipment, and supplies appropriately (AOTA, 2002). Play is a primary occupation of childhood and will be addressed at length in this chapter.

LEISURE

Leisure is defined as "a nonobligatory activity that is intrinsically motivated and engaged in during discretionary time, that is, time not committed to obligatory occupations such as work, self-care, or sleep" (AOTA, 2002; Parham & Fazio, 1997, p. 250). This occupational area consists of leisure exploration and leisure participation. Leisure exploration includes identifying interests, skills, opportunities, and appropriate leisure activities. Leisure participation includes planning and participation in appropriate leisure activities; maintaining a balance of leisure activities with other areas of occupation; and obtaining, using, and maintaining equipment and supplies as appropriate (AOTA, 2002).

The play and leisure areas of occupation are not mutually exclusive in that using the description of each as put forth in the AOTA's *Occupational Therapy Practice Framework* (2002), some play activities might also be considered leisure activities, and the reverse is also true. The distinction between play and leisure still needs more clarification (personal notes from conference lecture, Mary Jane Youngstrom, MS, OTR, FAOTA, 2002).

SOCIAL PARTICIPATION

Social participation includes activities associated with organized patterns of behavior that are characteristic and expected of an individual or an individual interacting with others within a given social system (AOTA, 2002). Social participation includes activities that result in successful interaction with family and friends, and also within the larger community.

The term *occupation* is at the very core of the occupational therapy profession. Occupations are the meaningful activities in which individuals engage that are a part of every day life. Occupations have value to the individual as well as to the culture of that individual. Occupations are broader

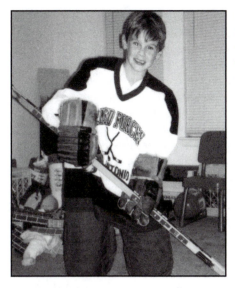

Figure 14-1. Dressing skills are reinforced through pretend play with Dad's hockey gear.

than activities. Engaging in occupation is more than simply participating, performing, or doing. Engagement recognizes the importance of personal choice and personal meaning as well as the psychological/emotional and physical aspects of performance. Occupation is individually based, what is work for one person may be play to another. The primary occupations of childhood include ADL, education, play, and social participation.

The contribution of occupational therapy is to link activities and participation through engagement in occupations. The overarching goal of pediatric occupational therapy is engagement of the child in occupation to support participation in context. Context supports and mediates engagement in occupations. Context, in this case, refers to more than simply the physical environment of the child. The OT and OTA considers and addresses the cultural, physical, social, personal (age, gender, educational and socioeconomic status), spiritual, temporal, and even virtual contexts (AOTA, 2002) of the individual child in order to achieve active engagement in occupation within the child's real life situation.

Play History

BACKGROUND

Play contributes to a child's development in many ways. Play is believed to have a role in the development of cognitive and language skills, and promotes problem solving, social interaction, creativity and self-expression. In play, children expand their understanding of themselves and others, their knowledge of the physical world, and their ability to communicate with peers and adults (Fernie, 1988). Play facilitates the development of physical abilities and sensory integration and provides children with a sense of mastery

over their bodies and their environment. Play is imitation of adult life and prepares children for adult roles (Mack. Lindquist, & Parham, 1982; Anderson, 1997). Through play, children learn societal roles, norms, and values (Reiber, et al., 1998).

Despite the importance of play and its critical role in development, play is a difficult concept to define. In fact, there is no universally accepted definition of play (Parham & Primeau, 1997). Many different academic disciplines including developmental psychology, anthropology, sociology, evolutionary biology, and, more recently, occupational therapy, have studied play. Play theorists have attempted to define play, categorize aspects of play, and outline developmental sequences of play. The relevance of play to occupational therapy is discussed below.

RELEVANCE TO OCCUPATIONAL THERAPY

Play is a primary occupation of childhood and as such, holds an important place in the field of occupational therapy. Play serves many functions for the OT and OTA. Play, as occupation is an end goal of intervention. Play is also a medium for intervention, and play, in the form of *playfulness* is a style or attitude important in both intervention and in life.

Of primary importance to occupational therapy is the focus on play as occupation. If play is considered the primary occupation of children, then the development of play skills becomes, in itself, an important goal for intervention (Missiuna & Pollock, 1991). When intervention is aimed at increasing a child's ability to engage in the occupation of playing, the outcome of therapy is that the child is better able to engage in play in naturally occurring contexts. For example, intervention may be aimed at getting a child to engage with and explore a toy, encouraging a child to begin to explore the multiple ways in which a toy or object may be "played with", determining alternate methods of participating in play activities with peers, adapting games and toys for access, or increasing the complexity or length of a child's play experience.

OTs and OTAs regularly use play as a medium for intervention to motivate and engage a child so that he/she may achieve goals in other areas. For example, a child may develop eye-hand coordination while playing a game of jacks, improve balance reactions while playing on a platform swing pretending to be fishing in a pond on a windy day, or improve independence in dressing skills by donning and doffing dress-up clothes while playing 'house' with a peer (Figure 14-1).

Play is also a style, an approach to daily life events in the form of playfulness (Bundy, 1993; 2002). Bundy (1993) states that playfulness is intimately related to play both as occupation and as a medium for intervention and "without playfulness, all activities become work" (p. 217). Activities can be more or less playful depending on several factors or criteria, which will be discussed later in this chapter.

PLAY THEORIES/THEORISTS

The study of play has led to many and varied attempts to describe, define, and classify play. Through studying and theorizing, play researchers and scholars are better able to observe, analyze, and understand play. Some of these theorists (i.e., Piaget, Vygotsky, and Parten) describe play in terms of a developmental sequence of skill acquisition or types of play activities. Others (i.e., Rubin, Neumann, and Lieberman) have attempted to define play by identifying criteria or characteristics present in play. And finally, Csikszentmihalyi attempts to answer the question of motivation, or why we play. When providing intervention with children, occupational therapists draw upon many different models and theories. Some of the prominent play theories as well as those with relevance to occupational therapy are introduced below.

DEVELOPMENTAL SEQUENCES

Perhaps the most familiar developmental theorist is Jean Piaget, a developmental psychologist who described play in terms of a developmental sequence of skill acquisition. Piaget (1962) believed that play was important for a child's intellectual development and later cognitive functioning. In fact "Piaget's interests focused on the active involvement of the child as an individual working with objects and making sense of the world through that activity" (Rogoff, 1990, p. 34). Piaget viewed the development of intellect as involving two processes: assimilation and accommodation. Assimilation occurs when individuals fit information from outside of themselves into schemes representing what they already know. In the process of accommodation, individuals modify these schemes when they do not fit adequately with their developing knowledge. Piaget described a developmental sequence consisting of three types of play reflective of children's acquisition of cognitive skills: 1) practice play (also described as sensorimotor play) characterized by exploration of sensations and movements (Parham & Primeau, 1997); 2) symbolic play in which children engage in games that involve imagination, make believe, or pretend play and; 3) games with rules typically characterized by games that contain socially constructed rules involving the cooperative play of at least two individuals (Piaget, 1962; Bundy, 1991; Miller, 1993). Piaget's work provides a framework for much of the current research on play development (Bergen, 1988).

Lev Vygotsky also developed a theory of cognitive development based, in part, on play. Vygotsky theorized that children develop cognitive capacities through social interaction that eventually becomes internalized. He described what he termed the zone of proximal development (ZPD) as the "distance between the actual developmental level as deter-

mined by independent problem solving and the level of potential development as determined through problem solving under adult guidance or in collaboration with more capable peers" (Vygotsky, 1978, p. 86; Miller, 1993). Specifically, children develop and learn through the help of a more capable other. Vygotsky did not propose a specific set of developmental stages, though did suggest some possible themes for developmental stages. These themes included affliction (infancy), play (early childhood), learning (middle childhood), peer activity (adolescence), work (adulthood), and theorizing (old age). Different from Piaget, in Vygotsky's theory, an active-child-in-cultural-context is what develops (Miller, 1993). In essence, Vygotsky's theory is based on the belief that a child's intellectual development cannot be understood without reference to the social milieu in which the child is embedded (Rogoff, 1990).

The theories of Piaget, Vygotsky, and other developmental psychologists most often focused on cognitive development, with play being somewhat incidental or peripheral (Cohen, 1993). Differentially, Parten developed a theory and sequence specific to play. Parten's (1932) Social Play Hierarchy identifies the following six levels of sequentially more sophisticated social play:

1. Unoccupied Play—random activity.

2. Solitary Play—the child plays independently even if there are other children near by (typical of 2-year-olds).

3. Onlooker Play—the child watches others but does not participate.

4. Parallel Play—the child plays independently beside or near other children; is aware of other children present but plays separately.

5. Associative-group play (common among 3- and especially 4-year-olds)—engagement of a group of children focusing on a common activity with sharing, lending, taking turns, and attending to the activities of one's peers, but without a common goal.

6. Cooperative-group play—a high level of play that represents the child's social and cognitive maturity; play and/or activity that is organized cooperatively and involves a division of labor in order to achieve a common goal. (Bergen, 1988; Greene, 1997; Tobias & Goldkopf, 1995).

ELEMENTS AND CHARACTERISTICS OF PLAY

Several sets of play criteria identifying characteristics of play are found in research literature. There is a great deal of overlap in these sets of play criteria. The contributions of developmental researchers Rubin, Neumann, and Lieberman led to the identification of play as described below.

Based on a review of literature, Rubin et al. (1983), identified six traits or characteristics that distinguish play from nonplay:

1. Intrinsic motivation.
2. Attention to the means rather than the end.
3. Activity is dominated by the child rather than the object or stimulus. For instance, what can I do with this object, rather than what does this object do?
4. Nonliteral, simulative behavior.
5. Freedom from externally imposed rules.
6. Active engagement.

Lieberman (1965) developed a set of five criteria for what she considered to be playfulness: physical spontaneity; social spontaneity; cognitive spontaneity; manifest joy; and a sense of humor.

In *The Elements of Play*, Neumann (1971) analyzed the literature on play and further simplified play characteristics, proposing that play transactions have three criteria. The three criteria are:

1. Internal control vs. external control—to the extent that control is internal, the activity is play, to the extent that control is external, the activity is nonplay.
2. Internal reality vs. external reality—the ability of the player to *suspend reality*, to act "as if", to pretend, to make believe.
3. Internal vs. external motivation—to the extent that an activity is internally motivated, it is play, to the extent that it is externally motivated it is nonplay. One may judge an activity and determine whether or not it is play by assessing the activity for these three criteria. The degree to which each of these three elements is present determines where the activity falls on a play - nonplay continuum.

MOTIVATION FOR PLAY: WHY DO WE PLAY?

Csikszentmihalyi attempts to answer the question of motivation or, "why do we play?" with his theory of flow. Csikszentmihalyi (1990) uses the term *flow* to describe an individual's state of being fully engaged in an enjoyable activity. Flow is defined as "...the state in which people are so involved in an activity that nothing else seems to matter; the experience is so enjoyable that people will do it even at great cost, for the sheer sake of doing it" (Csikszentmihalyi, 1990, p. 4). Csikszentmihalyi goes on to say that in order to experience flow, one must have the ability to focus attention and to concentrate without distraction. Flow is marked by the following eight criteria, one or more which must be present in order to achieve flow:

1. The activity provides optimal challenge.
2. Attention is completely absorbed.

3. The activity has clear goals.
4. The activity provides clear and consistent feedback.
5. The activity completely absorbs the individual.
6. The individual feels completely in control of the activity.
7. All feelings of self-consciousness disappear.
8. The individual is unaware of or loses track of time passing while engaged in the activity (Csikszentmihalyi, 1990).

The concept of optimal or "just right" challenge is important and one that is useful to the OT practitioner. If the activity is too easy, one may become bored with it; if the activity is too difficult, it may produce anxiety. (Ayres, 1972; Bundy, 2002; Csikszentmihalyi, 1990; Rieber, 1996).

Arousal-seeking theory, as proposed by Berlyne (1960) and Shultz (1979) also attempts to explain why we play. This theory proposes that all individuals have an optimal level of arousal that they seek to maintain. Too much stimulation causes discomfort and too little stimulation causes the individual to shut down. Play is one method of mediating the amount of stimulation in the quest for an optimal level of arousal (Bergen, 1988).

Contributions of Occupational Therapy to Play Research and Theory

Researchers of many disciplines relate the importance of play to children's emotional, social, physical/motor, gender/sex role, language, moral development, and cognitive development (Bergen, 1988). However, as discussed, distinguishing play from nonplay is not an easy task. Theories, definitions, and characteristics of play do not encompass all that OT practitioners consider to be play. These theorists also do not necessarily define play in terms that are necessarily useful for occupational therapy. Further, some of the problems with the definitions or characteristics in the play literature from other disciplines as described earlier in this chapter, preclude the use of play as medium and as an end for intervention. For example, when play is used as an intervention medium, someone other than the child (i.e. the OT practitioner) exerts some degree of control over the transaction. This may cause the child to feel externally controlled, thus impacting intrinsic motivation, two of the key characteristics of play behavior (Bundy, 2002).

Today, contributions to the body of play theory and research within the field of occupational therapy are growing. Occupational therapy practitioners are studying play in order to better define, operationalize, and develop tools to assess play. Assessments of a child's play and of his or her abilities as seen through play provide the OT practitioner with tools to analyze play and to plan treatment (Knox, 1997). Systematic applications of play principles in practice are also being developed in the profession (Parham & Primeau, 1997). Currently, considering play as an occupation, as well as recognition of the concept and importance of playfulness are gaining greater acceptance in the field of occupational therapy.

Mary Reilly was one of the first occupational therapists to take an in depth look at children's play (Pierce, 1997). In *Play as Exploratory Learning*, instead, Reilly (1974) proposed that play has an organizing effect on behavior and children learn rules of people, objects, and movement during play.

Reilly proposed three hierarchical stages of play development, exploratory, competency, and achievement. Exploratory behavior is play behavior seen in early childhood and stems from an interest in the environment, is engaged in for its own sake (intrinsically motivated) and has a focus on sensory experiences. Exploratory behavior is dependent upon a safe environment, which allows doing something for its own sake, and in turn generates hope and trust. Competency behavior, based on White's theory of competence motivation suggests that people receive satisfaction from developing competency (Bergen, 1988). Competency behavior is characterized by a drive to deal with the environment, to actively influence it, and to be influenced by it. The prevailing attitude is, "I want to do it alone" in which the child displays concentration and persistence when engaged in the activity. This "wanting to do it alone" attitude fosters the development of self-confidence and self-reliance. Achievement behavior is the third phase of play development that incorporates the learning of the first two phases. Achievement behavior focuses on performance and outcomes such as success or failure and winning or losing and involves a more competitive element than do the first two stages. Achievement behavior is more extrinsically motivated and also involves a higher level of excitement, danger, and risk taking, as the child develops the ability to strategize leading toward greater control and mastery over his or her environment. The hope, trust, self-confidence, and self-reliance developed during the first two phases of development are transformed into a state of courage (Reilly, 1974).

Linda Florey (1971) described play as a learning process occurring throughout every child's day. Therefore, based on Florey's theory, OT practitioners address play both in the treatment session and in the contexts in which play naturally occurs. Florey also identified potentially adverse effects of a child's disability on play in that the environment and state of the child may inhibit or nurture play (Parham & Primeau, 1997; Tobias & Goldkopf, 1995). Florey classified human and nonhuman objects and described play as action on human and nonhuman objects that change over time and with development. Human objects include parents, peers, siblings, and the child's body. Nonhuman objects are divided into three subcategories. Type 1 objects include creative and unstructured media that can change shape and form

when directly manipulated by the child (i.e., clay, sand, paint) Type 2 objects can be changed when combined with other objects (i.e., beads + string = necklace). Type 3 objects maintain their original form (i.e., bicycles, dolls, balls) (Morrison, et al, 1996; Tobias & Goldkopf, 1995).

According to Nancy Takata, play and development are intertwined. Development, and thus play, follows an orderly and predictable sequence and increases in complexity over time. Takata (1974), based on a review of the literature, proposed an age-based classification of play, Takata's Play Taxonomy, so as to better observe and analyze play. The following play epochs were proposed to describe play behavior: Sensorimotor (0 to 2 years), Symbolic and Simple Constructive (2 to 4 years), Dramatic and Complex Constructive and Pre-Game (4 to 7 years), Games (7 to 12 years), and Recreational (12 to 16 years) (Takata, 1974; Tobias & Goldkopf, 1995). Takata (1974) developed a play assessment, the Play History, based on these play epochs. This tool was developed to diagnose and treat play dysfunction in children and through interview and observation to evaluate the play development of children. The Play History assesses a child's play history and play competence over time and is divided into three sections: general information, previous play experiences, and actual play examination (Morrison, et al, 1996; Parham & Primeau, 1997; Tobias & Goldkopf, 1995).

The Preschool Play Scale (PPS), originally named the Play Scale, was developed by Susan Knox (1974) and later revised by Bledsoe and Shepherd (1982). The PPS analyzes four dimensions of play in yearly increments: space management, material management, imitation, and participation (Knox, 1997; Tobias & Goldkopf, 1995). The PPS has been used as a research tool to demonstrate differences in the play behavior of different populations and to assess pre- and post-intervention status (Knox, 1997). Clinically, the PPS is used for assessment and to guide the developmental nature of play (Knox, 1997). The PPS is an observational assessment designed to describe development of play behavior in children from birth to 6 years of age.

Anita Bundy's contributions to the study of play provide OT practitioners with a useful model for identifying the degree to which an activity is play. Bundy (1991; 1993; 1997; 2002) expanded upon the play–nonplay continuum first developed by Neumann (1971). Bundy believes a child's ability to play should be of primary concern to the OT and OTA. There is growing attention within the OT profession on play as a primary occupation of children. To this end, Bundy (1997) proposes the following working definition of play.

"Play is a transaction between an individual and the environment that is:
- Relatively intrinsically controlled
- Relatively internally controlled
- Free of some of the constraints of objective reality" (Bundy, 2002, p. 229).

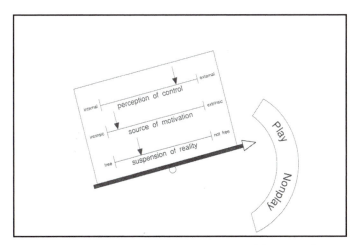

Figure 14-2. Play-nonplay continuum. Reprinted from Bundy, A., Lane, S., & Murray, E.A. (2002). *Sensory integration: Theory and practice* (2nd ed.). Philadelphia: F. A. Davis Co. Used with permission.

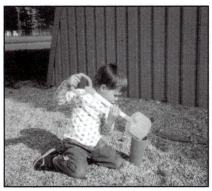

Figure 14-3. A child engaged in exploratory play: dumping and filling.

Depending on the degree that each of these criteria is present, a play transaction will fall somewhere on a continuum of behaviors that are more or less playful (Figure 14-2). This play-nonplay continuum is a useful tool that may help the OT practitioner determine the degree to which an activity is play vs. nonplay. By observing and manipulating the child's perception of control, source of motivation, and ability to suspend reality, the OT practitioner may be able to shift an activity along the play-nonplay continuum facilitating the child's ability to engage in the occupation of play. Bundy also recognized a need for assessment tools to evaluate children's ability to play and developed The Test of Playfulness (ToP). The Test of Playfulness (ToP) is a play observation consisting of 68 items designed to examine these same three elements in play transactions: intrinsic motivation, *internal control*, and freedom to suspend reality.

Typical Development of Play

While, as previously stated, there is no single accepted sequence of play development, it is generally acknowledged that play skills follow a general sequence of development. Toys and play activities vary according to the age and stage of development of the child. It is necessary for the OT and OTA to have an understanding of play development in order to generate effective goals and intervention plans.

As described earlier in this chapter, play includes both exploration and participation. Based on the work of multiple researchers and theorists, Bergen (1988) provides an overview of the stages of play development, participation, and exploration from infancy through middle childhood. This overview is shared below.

A. Exploratory and Sensorimotor-Practice Play begins in infancy and involves repetitive motor movements such as dumping and filling containers with objects, push-pull toys, examining objects and determining their characteristics, via mouthing, looking, touching or repetitive actions (Figure 14-3). This is the primary mode of play in infancy and the early toddler years in which children experiment with bodily sensation, motor movements, objects, and people (Fernie, 1988). Children engage in more exploration when exposed to novel or more complex toys and more sensorimotor play when exposed to toys that are less complex and more familiar. Exploratory and sensorimotor- practice play is needed throughout life whenever mastery of new mental or physical skills are required, such as for effective performance of games and sports.

B. Pretend play, also called symbolic play or dramatic play, begins by around 2 years of age when toddlers begin to represent their world symbolically. In this stage, children take on roles and transform objects in dramatic and make-believe play (Fernie, 1988). Pretend play continues to be a primary form of play during preschool and kindergarten years (4-5 years) and continues, though less so, into the elementary years. In pretend play, the child uses an object as if it were something else, such as pretending a block is a truck or pretending to be someone else such as being the mommy and feeding the baby doll (Figure 14-4).

C. Constructive play combines physical repetitive activity with symbolic representation of objects and ideas and becomes predominant in the third year of life continuing on into elementary and middle school years in the form of more complex and abstract play. Constructive play involves transforming objects into a new configuration. Building with blocks, arts and craft projects, molding with clay, assembling models, and making a beaded necklace are examples of constructive play (Figure 14-5).

D. Games with rules are games played with accepted rules that are either pre-established or made up and agreed upon by those involved. Children become involved in games with rules by around age five with games such as hide-and-seek, tag, and hopscotch.

Figure 14-4.
Pretend play:
Spacemen.

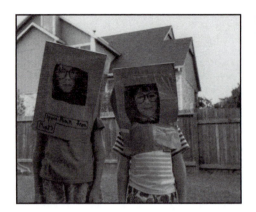

Figure 14-5.
Constructive
play.

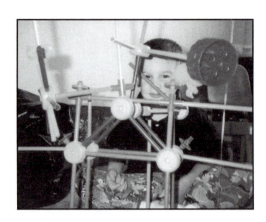

Games with rules increase in quantity and complexity during early elementary years and peak in middle elementary years. Young children follow rules of games not so much to win, but so that everyone is able to enjoy the game. In later years, games with rules develop into more formal games such as board games and sports that include competition and agreed upon criteria as to how to determine a winner (Table 14-2).

Effects of Disability On Play

It is difficult to accurately describe the impact of a disability on the development of children's play, play skills, and playfulness, particularly since there is no universally accepted definition of play. In addition, there is limited research on the play of children with special needs and much of the research that is available has been identified to have methodological flaws (Block & King, 1987). Compared to the literature available relative to the development of cognitive, language, social emotional, and motor skills, there is surprisingly little research that describes the play development of typically developing children. Thus, it is not surprising that so little is known about the play of children with disabilities (Hellendoorn, et al, 1994; Knox & Mailloux, 1997). Hellendoorn, et al, (1994) speculates that this may be because historically, play has not been considered to be as important for these children as are, for instance, cognitive and language development. Another factor limiting research is that children who have special needs are often quite unique in the degree and functional impact of their disability, even among those with the same diagnosis (Hellendoorn, et al., 1994; Knox & Mailloux, 1997). Because play generally parallels other areas of development, some general statements can be made as to the impact of disability on play development. Knox & Mailloux (1997) emphasize the need to use caution in generalizing descriptions and problems with play across or within disabilities. In practice, each child must be considered individually. The information contained in this section is based on available research and general knowledge of the impact of disabilities on children. However, given the lack of methodologically sound research and the highly individual needs of children with disabilities, it is important to use caution when generalizing this information for use in planning and providing intervention for children with disabilities.

The presence of a disability may influence a child's ability to play in many ways. Limited and abnormal movement patterns, reduced cognitive and communication abilities and sensory impairments may impact a child's play development, limit their ability to engage in play, and reduce playfulness. Children with special needs often have an impaired ability to explore, interact with, and master their environment, therefore distorting normal childhood experiences (Knox & Mailloux, 1997). This impaired ability to explore, interact with, and master the environment, in addition to other limiting factors, may contribute to feelings of inadequacy, loss of control, and learned helplessness. The impact of a child's disability may result in a limited play repertoire and repetitive and stereotyped play behaviors. Behavioral difficulties may also arise due to a child's cognitive, communication, and motoric impairments.

Factors related to the care of a child with special needs may result in fewer opportunities for social interaction and play time. The time needed to perform tasks related to the day-to-day care, medical management, and scheduling demands of the various therapy services required for a child with special needs reduces time available for play. The dynamics between a child with special needs and the caregiver may be different than those of a caregiver and a typically developing child, and as such, development of typical play routines may be affected (Okimoto, et al., 2000). For instance, caregivers' perceived limitations of the child with special needs might result in lowered expectations of the child, which in turn may contribute to limited play experiences.

Table 14-2

Stages of Play Development by Age

Infant/Toddler Play: Birth to 2 years

- Exploratory/sensorimotor play is primary.
- Beginnings of symbolic play.
- Emergence of reciprocal social games.

Preschool/Kindergarten Play: 3 to 5 years

- Exploratory/sensorimotor play is seen though less time is spent in this type of play than in infancy and toddlerhood.
- Constructive play is the most common type of play seen in 3- to 5-year-olds.
- Pretend/symbolic/dramatic play is at its peak in children 4 to 5 years old.
- Games with rules are emerging at this stage/age.

Elementary Play: 7 to 12 years

- Games with rules primary type of play during middle childhood.
- Constructive and symbolic play are also seen.

Adolescence/Adulthood Play

- Games with rules, symbolic play, and constructive play continue through adolescence and into adulthood.

Reflections for the OTA

Okimoto, et al (2000) found that children with cerebral palsy and developmental delay face more challenges than do their typically developing peers, not only due to their physical limitations, but also to their limitations as perceived by their caregivers and playmates.

Cultural and societal beliefs may also impact play for children with disabilities and limit the child's options for play. Family and societal beliefs and views about disability, the role of the child, the size of the support network, the value of play and types of play activities, and the attitude toward professionals are examples of factors that may vary among cultures and warrant consideration by the OT practitioner.

PERFORMANCE SKILLS AND CLIENT FACTORS

Limitations in performance skills and client factors (AOTA, 2002) may influence a child's ability to play in many ways. Performance skills are features of what one does related to observable actions when engaged, in this case, in play activities. Performance skills include motor skills, process skills, and communication/interaction skills. Motor skills involve moving and interacting with tasks, objects, and the environment. Process skills are those used in managing and modifying actions during the performance of daily life tasks. Communication/interaction skills involve conveying intentions and needs and coordinating social behavior to act

together with people. Client factors are those factors that reside within the client (child) that may affect occupational (play) performance. Client factors consist of body functions (including the psychological functions of body systems) and body structures (anatomical parts of the body such as organs, limbs, and their components) (AOTA, 2002).

The Impact of Limitations in Motor Skills, Neuromusculoskeletal and Movement-Related Functions on Play

Limitations in motor skills, neuromusculoskeletal status, and movement are typically present in children with diagnoses such as cerebral palsy, juvenile rheumatoid arthritis, and spina bifida (please refer to Chapter 10: Diagnoses Commonly Associated With Childhood). These children experience limited or abnormal movement patterns resulting in limited ability to access, explore, and physically interact with toys, and others. Children with multiple handicaps may also be extremely limited in the ability to play and interact with the environment in an active way (Nakken et al., 1994). Further, difficulties with fine motor control and coordination often result in limited ability to manipulate toys. Children with physical impairments often experience reduced endurance and may also have to put forth substantially greater effort than that of their typically developing peers in order to act upon their environment. These children, therefore, are likely to fatigue more quickly than their typically developing peers, which impacts the amount of time they are able to sustain participation in play activities. External and environmental factors may further inhibit the play experiences of the child with a physical disability.

Splinting and bracing, for example, required for some children with physical limitations, may impact a child's ability to participate in play experiences by further reducing the ability to assume typical play positions or to effectively manipulate toys.

The Impact of Limitations in Process Skills, and Affective, Cognitive and Perceptual Mental Functions on Play

Mental retardation, attention deficit/hyperactivity disorder (ADHD), nonverbal learning disabilities, depression, and other psychiatric disorders are some of the diagnoses that may affect a child's processing skills, cognitive, and play function (please refer to Chapter 22: Pediatric Psychosocial Therapy). In children with mental retardation, early play development appears to follow approximately the same sequence as that of normally developing children, but at a much slower rate (Nakkan et al, 1994). Children with mental retardation have cognitive delays that may influence their ability to initiate, sequence, and persist at play activities. This means that the same types of play and play abilities can be seen at the same developmental age, but with a wide variation of chronological ages (Nakkan et al, 1994). A child with mental retardation will progress through the stages of play development following the same sequence as his/her typically developing peers, but may remain in each stage for a longer period, moving ahead to the next stage at a later chronological age. Depending on the degree of disability, the child with mental retardation may never reach the later stages of play development. Nakkan (1994) speculates that the impact of mental retardation on play is due at least as much to lack of specific stimulation, opportunities, and training, as it is due to innate disability.

The child with attention deficit/hyperactivity disorder often has difficulty sustaining attention and participation in play activities. Difficulty organizing tasks is also seen with these children. Impulsivity and a tendency to act without thinking (lack of self-control) may result in poor safety awareness, particularly during large motor play activities. Impulsivity may also cause the child with ADHD difficulty with the social aspects of play due to problems with turn taking, sharing materials (may grab without asking), disruptive behaviors, and a tendency to interrupt others. Decreased attention may also result in decreased task persistence and impact regarding the development of play skills.

A child with a nonverbal learning disability may lack both the eye-hand as well as gross and fine motor coordination necessary for engaging in play activities requiring coordination and confidence. These children may have a tendency to withdraw as they grow older as games and play activities rely more heavily on coordinated actions and become more competitive.

Depression is marked by decreased activity and an inability to experience pleasure and may substantially limit a child's participation in play experiences. Social withdrawal and irritability may also interfere with a child's social play. Motor retardation, reduced energy and diminished interest, symptoms of depression, may also result in difficulty initiating play activities as well as persisting with play activities through to completion (DSM IV, 1994).

The Impact of Limitations in Communication/interaction Skills, Sensory Functions and Pain on Play

Autism/Pervasive developmental disorders (PDD), blind/visually impaired, deaf/hearing impaired, sensory integrative dysfunction, medical conditions and chronic pain are examples of diagnoses that may cause limitations in interaction skills and/or sensory function and result in reduced participation in play experiences (please refer to Chapter 10: Diagnoses Commonly Associated With Childhood, Chapter 12: Introduction to Sensory Integration, and Chapter 22: Pediatric Psychosocial Therapy).

Autism/PDD is characterized by impairment in several areas of development that impact play including social interaction, language as used in social communication, and symbolic/imaginative play. Children with Autism/PDD may also demonstrate stereotyped behaviors, interests, and activities, which may significantly limit a child's interest in, awareness of and participation in typical play activities (DSM IV, 1994).

The typical play characteristics of children who are blind or visually impaired include reduced hand use for exploration, gross motor/mobility delays related to a lack of visual stimulation, avoidance of gross motor activities due to fear and reduced balance, and a tendency to be passive and withdraw from their environment (Reed, 1991). These children may also experience difficulty with constructive play, delays in developing complex play routines with others, and decreased imitative and role-play due to reliance on audition (Knox & Mailloux, 1997). Children who are deaf or hearing-impaired may show increased time spent in non-interactive construction play, decreased symbolic play, decreased organization of play, decreased social play, and increased solitary play (Knox & Mailloux, 1997).

Children with sensory integration dysfunction may also experience problems with play. Overall, children with decreased motor planning/praxis experience a lack of coordination and difficulty with multi-step tasks, which may, in turn, result in decreased self-esteem. A child with dyspraxia may present with uneven performance/abilities from day to day, and perform only in adult-mediated activities where play is broken down into manageable steps. This child's play may also be limited to simple and familiar games due to his or her difficulty with motor planning (Ayres, 1979). The child with gravitational insecurity is restricted in play by fear and anxiety in response to movement and having the feet leave the ground (Ayres, 1979) resulting in an avoidance of gross motor play, roughhousing, and playground activities. The child with tactile defensiveness may avoid certain types of play (sand, water, paint, and other "messy" substances) and may avoid playing with other children because he/she does not like other children touching him or her (Ayres, 1979) (please refer to Chapter 12: Introduction to Sensory Integration).

A child with chronic pain may avoid play activities to reduce the likelihood of causing pain and therefore display a tendency to withdraw from social play situations. Pain may also cause reduced energy and concentration, further limiting a child's participation and persistence in play activities (Reed, 1991; Knox & Mailloux, 1997).

The child with medical issues may experience pain, discomfort, weakness, and reduced endurance for physical activity, thus limiting participation in play activities. These children may have decreased time and opportunity for social play and experience estrangement from their peer group due to frequent hospitalizations, treatments, or physical restrictions. Children with medical issues may also show a delay in development of social and play skills resulting from decreased opportunity for social experiences (Knox & Mailloux, 1997).

These descriptions, while far from complete, provide examples of the many and varied ways in which a disability may impact the play participation and play development of a child. The OTA is again cautioned against making generalizations regarding the impact of disability on play, and reminded of the importance of considering each child's play skills and abilities individually.

EFFECTS OF THE ENVIRONMENT/CONTEXT ON PLAY

Environmental factors may also influence children's play skills and play development. The impact of environmental factors may be seen in the play characteristics of children who have experienced neglect. These characteristics may include self-stimulation, immature play skills, limited play repertoire, increased or decreased fantasy, and reduced imitation (Knox & Mailloux, 1997). Further, the effects of extended hospitalization on children's play behavior may include decreased attention span, decreased endurance and movement, and decreased initiative, curiosity and creativity; reduced playfulness, decreased affect, and increased anxiety (Knox & Mailloux, 1997; Kielhofner et al., 1983). Extended hospital stays may also reduce the opportunities for social play experiences. For a child with a disability, the play environment may impose both physical and social restrictions that may be as limiting as the disability itself (Blanche, 1997). Physical limitations of the environment may include decreased accessibility to appropriate toys, play environments, or social groups.

Children who have physical disabilities often spend more time in structured activities and have fewer opportunities to make decisions about what to do, where to go and how to do something. In fact, Blanche (1997) points out that these factors can seriously impede a child's freedom to explore their environment and engage in play. Children with disabilities are restricted not only by the inherent limitations of the diagnosis, but also by sociocultural constraints imposed by others and the environment. Social barriers occur as a result of other's values and beliefs. For example, it is not uncommon for individuals who lack experience in interacting with children with disabilities to assume that these children cannot participate in typical play experiences. Such a belief may inadvertently limit a child's opportunities for play. Blanche (1997) stresses the important role the OT practitioner has in being aware of an adult's responsibility in either facilitating or inhibiting a child's play.

Play Assessment

Many factors influence a child's play development and ability to play. A disability in the form of a developmental lag may result in immature play skills. There may also be a mismatch between what the child wants to do and what he/she is actually capable of performing (Morrison et al, 1991), such that playfulness may be diminished. In order to maximize a child's ability to function to the best of their ability, play assessment, and intervention must then consider all of these factors. Assessment of a child's play must consider the impact of the disability on the child, the child's play development, opportunities for and participation in play experiences, play preferences, and the degree of playfulness displayed by the child. The child's developmental level, chronological age, interests and motivation—including activity demands of those interests, client factors, performance skills and context(s) (social, cultural, physical, temporal, etc.)—are also important factors to assess. To maximize a child's capacity to function to the best of their ability, play assessment, and intervention must then consider all of these factors.

Examples of play assessments were provided earlier in this chapter and included Takata's (1974) Play History; The Preschool Play Scale (Knox, 1974; Bledsoe & Shepherd, 1982); and Bundy's (1997) Test of Playfulness (ToP). Assessment of play may include a combination of standardized assessments, play observation, caregiver interview, child interview, and specific evaluation of client factors and performance skills.

Intervention

UNIQUE PERSPECTIVE THAT OT BRINGS TO THE FACILITATION OF PLAY SKILLS

Engagement in the occupation of play is the unique focus and expected outcome of pediatric occupational therapy. Ultimately, the meaningfulness of the activity to the child makes the activity occupation-based. This focus on occupationally based activity is at the very core of occupational therapy. Play stands apart from other childhood occupations in that it is something children do because they want to, not because they have to. That play must be child-directed and intrinsically motivated in order to "qualify" as play makes occupational therapy - with its focus on engagement in meaningful occupations - uniquely suited to address play deficits in children.

The OT practitioner views the child's strengths, weaknesses, and areas of need in relation to their ability to participate in the occupation of play. The OT practitioner also considers the context and the demands of the activity as well as the child's performance skills, performance patterns, and client factors and how these factors interact with each other to influence occupational performance (play). Further, context is always considered, as the OTA does not look at the child or the child's skills in isolation. The goal of occupational therapy is to enhance a child's ability to function within the naturally occurring context. Interventions are designed to foster engagement in the occupation of play to support participation in life, not only in the treatment room or clinic, but also in the child's home, at school, on the playground, and in the neighborhood. Occupational therapy utilizes a holistic approach through intervention that engages the child with consideration of both the subjective (emotional or psychological) and the objective (physically observable) aspects of performance.

DOMAIN OF OT/PRACTICE IN PLAY INTERVENTION

The domain of occupational therapy frames intervention. The overarching statement: engagement in occupational to support participation in context or contexts describes the domain in its broadest sense (AOTA, 2002). The other areas included in the domain (Table 14-3) identify the various aspects that OTs and OTAs attend to in intervention, so are important to present here. Performance skills and performance patterns describe the observed performance the child carries out when engaging in occupations, in this case, play. Context, activity demands, and client factors are areas that influence performance skills and patterns (AOTA, 2002).

SELECTING APPROPRIATE INTERVENTION

The *Occupational Therapy Practice Framework* (2002) delineates five types of intervention: to promote/create, establish/restore, maintain, modify, and prevent. Examples of each intervention type relevant to children can be found in Table 14-4.

When working with children, the focus of intervention is most typically to restore and modify. It is important to consider, however, that OT practitioners are uniquely qualified to address the broader needs of children, groups of children, and society as related to children through other intervention approaches as described in Table 14-4.

USE OF PLAY IN INTERVENTION

Play as an Intervention Outcome/Goal/Occupation/End

Consider that "if play is considered the primary [occupation] of children, then, the development of play skills becomes, in itself, an important goal for intervention" (Missiuna & Pollock, 1991, p. 882). When play is the desired outcome of intervention, the occupational therapist must address the individual child's skills and the dimensions of that child's environment as they combine to enable participation in the occupation of play in the naturally occurring context (Pierce 1997). The acquisition of typical developmental patterns of play is both an important goal and a powerful means through which to reach other goals (Pierce, 1997).

When a child demonstrates a deficit with play, intervention focuses on improving play skills (Morrison et al., 1997). Intervention begins where the child is, such as getting the child to engage with and begin to explore a toy or other object in the environment or to gradually increase the complexity or length of the play experience. For instance, for a child who is developmentally immature, intervention focuses on facilitating play development. Intervention is designed to move the child toward a specific developmental stage of play. Increasing the child's ability to engage in constructional play or pretend play, or increasing social interactions to move the child beyond solitary play activities to play with peers are examples of intervention for children who are developmentally immature (Figure 14-6).

When a sensory or motor deficit is present, intervention may focus on broadening the range of play activities in which a child engages by addressing the specific sensory or motor deficit, such as increasing tolerance of tactile-based play activities. When disability and environmental constraints combine to limit a child's opportunity to engage in play, the OT practitioner seeks to expand the child's ability to interact with his or her environment through play. The

---

Table 14-3

Domain of Practice

Performance in Areas of Occupation include the life activities in which people engage, including ADL, IADL, education, work, play, leisure, and social participation.

Performance Skills are observable elements of action (e.g. bends, chooses, gazes). Performance skills fall into three categories: motor skills (e.g. posture, coordination, strength); process skills (e.g., knowledge, initiates/sequences, organizes, attends); and communication/interaction skills (e.g., nonverbal communication, articulates, asks, collaborates). The effective execution of performance skills depends on client factors, activity demands, and context.

Performance Patterns are habits, routines, and roles. Performance patterns develop over time and are influenced by context.

Client Factors can influence performance and include body functions (e.g. attention, memory, perception, seeing, hearing, joint mobility, strength, respiration, etc.) and body structures (e.g., structures related to the nervous system, the eyes, the ears, cardiovascular system, etc.).

Activity Demands are the aspects of an activity that are inherent in or generic to that activity, the steps, skills, objects needed to perform an activity.

Context (cultural, physical, social, personal, spiritual, temporal, and virtual) refers to a variety of interrelated conditions within and surrounding the person that influence performance.

Adapted from the Occupational therapy practice framework: Domain and process (2002). *American Journal of Occupational Therapy, 56*, 611. Adapted with permission from the American Occupational Therapy Association, Inc.

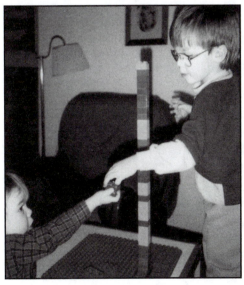

Figure 14-6. Children playing together to construct a block tower.

the underlying deficiencies, such as balance; fine motor skills; exposure to other types of play that the child could be successful at; or modifying the desired play activity, materials or environment to allow participation (including allowing the child to jump with both feet when playing hopscotch; slowing the response speed required of the video game, mounting the control on a stable surface, or changing controls to a joy stick) (Parham & Primeau, 1997).

Play as Medium/Means

While some children with disabilities need to be taught to "play", others may be taught other skills through the use of play as a treatment modality. An OT practitioner frequently and routinely uses play activities in intervention to achieve objectives and promote skill development. Play may be used as a therapeutic modality to facilitate specific areas of development such as gross motor, fine motor, social, self-help, cognitive, and communication skills. Play may also be a powerful motivator, enhancing the child's enthusiasm and effort to participate in activities they might otherwise resist. When children are engaged in play activities, the consequences are somehow diminished, as it is a release from real life and thus allows for playfulness. Play may also be used as a reinforcer in intervention.

Facilitating Playfulness

In addition to facilitating a child's play skills and developing other skill areas thorough play, OTAs must also address the child's playfulness and motivation to engage in play. Playfulness is a quality of a child's play that involves flexibility and spontaneity rather than simply the child's skill in performing specific play activities (Morrison et al, 1997;

focus of intervention may be decreasing isolation and stimulating play through providing a safe, accessible, and appropriate environment, and opportunities for engagement in play for its own sake.

Another approach to play as occupation intervention is to look at the mismatch between a child's play preferences and play skills (Clifford & Bundy, 1989). A child who wants to play hopscotch at recess with his or her peers but lacks the balance to hop, or a child who wants to play a video game with his or her siblings but lacks the fine motor skills to do so, illustrate a mismatch between desire and skill. Intervention for this type of play deficit may include treating

Table 14-4

Occupational Therapy Intervention Approaches

Intervention Approach	Focus of Intervention	Examples
1. Create, promote (health promotion)— • Does not assume a disability is present • Focuses on enriching the context or activities in order to enhance the performance of everyone who encounters the particular context or activity • Universal design is an example of this.	Performance Skills Performance Patterns Context(s) Activity Demands Client Factors	Creating a workshop series to educate early childhood teachers on how to facilitate the development of hand skills through play activities. Creating a parent newsletter designed to teach parents about typical child development and how to facilitate their child's development through play. Enhance the home play environment of a child by providing developmentally appropriate toys and activities. Provide a preschool classroom with a variety of materials, equipment and activities to increase exposure to developmentally appropriate play activities while facilitating cognitive, social, and motor skill development. Create a variety of equipment at a public playground to promote diverse sensory play experiences. Promote increased strength and endurance of elementary school aged children by increasing the time spent on playground equipment.
2. Establish, restore (remediation)— • Designed to change client variables • Involves establishing a skill or ability that has not yet developed or restoring a skill or ability that has been impaired	Performance Skills Performance Patterns Client Factors	Improve fine motor manipulation skills to allow for participation in arts and craft type activities. Improve gross motor skills and coordination to allow participation in a desired organized sport with peers. Improve ability to tolerate touch input to improve social play with peers. Reduce distractibility by establishing a daily routine of sensory movement activities in order to allow for participation in play with others. Restore mobility needed for play activities.
3. Maintain— • Designed to provide the supports to allow preservation of performance capabilities that have been regained	Performance Skills Performance Patterns Context(s) Activity Demands Client Factors	Maintain ability to keep play area free of clutter by providing pictures designating where each item belongs. Maintaining safe and independent access for a child with a vision impairment by providing increased lighting and high contrast play materials. Maintain independent grasp for a child with progressive condition by providing drawing and coloring implements with modified grips. Teach a caregiver range of motion exercises designed to allow a child with increased muscle tone to continue to be able to achieve a seated position on the floor for play with peers.
4. Modify (compensation, adaptation)— • Directed at "finding ways to revise the current context of activity demands to support performance in the natural setting… [includes] compensatory techniques, including enhancing some features to provide cues, or reducing other features to reduce distractibility" (Dunn et al., 1998, p.533).	Performance Patterns Context(s) Activity Demands	Modify playground equipment to allow a child who is non-ambulatory to access equipment. Modify computer mouse and chair to allow child to participate in computer games with his peers. Modify daily routine to provide consistency and predictability to support child's performance. Modify daily routine to minimize fatigue to support the child's participation in after school play with sibling or peer. Modify game pieces by building up size so that a child with limited grasp can grasp and move them to play the game. Carpet a playroom floor to minimize auditory distraction for a child with a hearing impairment
5. Prevent (disability prevention)— • Designed to address individuals with or without a disability who are at risk for occupational performance problems • To prevent barriers to performance from occurring. • Interventions may be directed at client, context, or activity variables.	Performance Skills Performance Patterns Context(s) Activity Demands Client Factors	Prevent social isolation by enrolling in an after-school recreation program. Prevent poor posture when sitting to play board games with peers by providing a chair with proper support and positionings. Prevent fatigue and injury when playing on outdoor climbing structures by providing instruction in appropriate techniques for safety and energy conservation.

Occupational therapy practice framework: Domain and process (2002), *American Journal of Occupational Therapy, 56,* 627. Adapted with permission from the American Occupational Therapy Association, Inc.

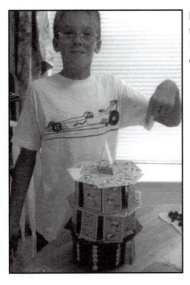

Figure 14-7. A sense of mastery or "look what I did" is an indicator of the "just right challenge".

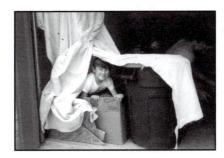

Figure 14-8. Freedom to suspend reality.

Parham & Primeau, 1997). Knox (1996) examined playfulness in preschoolers and identified actions and behaviors that appeared to characterize playful children: curiosity, imagination, joy, physical activity, and social and verbal flexibility. The less playful children seemed to lack the spontaneity and flexibility of the playful children and were characterized by negative affect/verbalizations, withdrawal or refusal to participate, lack of control over a situation, preference for adults and younger children, and emotional immaturity (Knox, 1996). Strategies for increasing playfulness include setting up a (safe) environment, facilitating a sense of control, building trust, providing the child with "just right challenge", and integrating a playful attitude into other aspects of intervention (Figure 14-7).

STRATEGIES FOR INTERVENTION

To be considered play, an activity must be intrinsically motivating, internally controlled, and free from objective reality (Figure 14-8). When OT practitioners use play in intervention, these three elements may be distorted. It is important for the OTA to be aware of these three elements and support them as closely as possible when attempting to set up play experiences in intervention (Musselwhite, 1986)

The OTAs Role in Play

Preparation is one of the most powerful strategies the OTA uses to facilitate play. Preparation involves organizing the physical setting, space and materials so that it is conducive to productive play (Bergen, 1988). The OTA must set up the environment to facilitate play with appropriate materials, toys and equipment, and consider environmental factors such as lighting, visual clutter, ambient noise, and how they can be modified to maximize the play experience. The OTA must also give thought as to how the elements of intrinsic motivation, internal control, and suspension of reality will be facilitated during the play intervention. Play activities

should be selected to offer the "just right challenge": not too easy and not too hard, so that they are challenging yet attainable for the child.

During intervention the OTAs role may be:

1. To get and sustain the child's attention.
   - Be animated.
   - Add or remove items from play area based on the child's abilities and needs.
2. To teach specific skills, to instruct.
   - Have a short planning/discussion period with the child prior to playing to help the child identify what he/she may do during the session (Bergen, 1988).
   - Discuss the purposes, uses, and limitations of the materials.
   - Model or demonstrate specific skills.
3. To observe—to watch or give play-by-play commentary of the play action.
4. To participate in (and model play) initiate, respond, and encourage the child to take his or her turn. Play intervention may require a suggestion, a supportive comment, or the addition of accessories to encourage the child to engage in a play activity (Bergen, 1988).
   - Guide play by participating; interact, ask the child what he or she needs, suggest materials, or model/demonstrate, suggest new roles in pretend play.

There is a fine line between too much guidance or structure and not enough. The key is to intervene in such a way as to enhance the development of play without sacrificing its essence (Bergen, 1988).

STRATEGIES TO FACILITATE PLAY SKILLS

Bergen (1988) identified several strategies designed to assist the teacher in intervening in order to make play educationally productive. These strategies are outlined below and are highly applicable for the OT practitioner in facilitating play skills with children.

- Instruction: teach a fact or concept that will move play along.
- Praise: to show approval and encourage repetition of a particular play behavior.

- Maintenance: strategies to help cope with problems arising from crowded space, insufficient materials or equipment, or disagreements.
- Conversation: to engage in a dialogue about a child's interests and activities.
- Demonstration: to show child the way to do something.
- Redirection: to suggest alternate activities.
- Participation: join the play activity.

Combinations of the above strategies are often used by the OTA to enhance the productivity of children's play.

THE "JUST RIGHT CHALLENGE"

When using play in treatment, the OT practitioner:

1. Constructs an environment to facilitate play and make the child feel safe in order to encourage exploration of the environment, objects, and materials.
2. Facilitates the child's sense of control over the play situation by following the child's lead and entering into play only when invited, giving the child the message that they are in control; also helps to establish trust.
3. Once trust is established, the OT practitioner may then build on the child's strengths and begin to expand on the child's repertoire of playful behaviors by providing the "just right challenge" (Ayres, 1979). The "just right challenge" is achieved by setting up the play experience so that the child's skills are at a level to meet the challenge. If the play activity is too hard, the child may become anxious or give up. If the play activity is too easy, the child may become bored. The challenge of the play activity must be just right so that the child is stretching just beyond their current functioning to develop and expand skills. The child must be able to practice the "just right challenge" safely and without consequences. (Morrison, et al., 1991).

Determining when and how much an OT practitioner should intervene in a child's play behavior is highly situational. The type, timing, and amount of intervention provided depend on the goal of intervention, the child's particular abilities and need areas (such as performance skills, performance patterns, and/or client factors), the demands of the activity, and the context(s) in which the play event is occurring. Caution must be exercised to avoid providing too much intervention by exerting too much external control and extrinsic motivation, as this can inhibit play by tipping the scales toward nonplay. However, the absence of inter-

vention may keep a child from achieving their full play potential, so the therapist must strive for balance. The challenge for OT practitioners is to intervene in order to optimize the development of play skills and play behavior without sacrificing its essence (Bergen, 1988).

ESTABLISHING A POSITIVE THERAPEUTIC ENVIRONMENT

Cronin (1996) identifies three methods for establishing a positive therapeutic environment:

1. Use of positive feedback and reinforcement: this should be directed at specific behaviors, such as "I liked the way you caught that ball with both hands" or "nice job coloring inside the lines", rather than general comments such as "good job" or "good girl". Specific verbal praise and positive feedback may increase the desired behavior and make the child aware of specific expectations.
2. Repeat or paraphrase the child's speech: this lets the child know that you are listening and also shows respect for the child and his or her ideas.
3. The OTA's affect should clearly demonstrate enjoyment in spending time with the child. Interacting with laughter, playfulness and ease and help the child to feel valued, and also increases the child's positive feelings about the therapy experience.

SELECTING DEVELOPMENTALLY APPROPRIATE PLAY

In order to establish developmentally appropriate play patterns, OT practitioners must have an understanding of normal development. However, facilitating normal patterns of play sequences in therapy is difficult due to the lack of research describing these patterns (Pierce, 1997). Child development is usually orderly, predictable, and sequential, though children develop at different rates. Consideration must be given to the naturally occurring differences in rates of development when determining what is "normal" or "typical". The same is true for play development. Intervention should incorporate activities that support the appropriate developmental stage. Establishing developmentally appropriate play is accomplished through practitioner-facilitated play progressions. If the child is not playing, then the goal will be for the child to briefly engage by showing interest in objects. If the child is not motivated, a playful spirit can be incorporated into the activity to make it more enjoyable, placing the emphasis on having fun with the activity (Pierce,

1997). Goals for establishing developmentally appropriate play may address the frequency and amount of the child's play time and the types and complexity of the child's play content. The OTA selects activities, toys, and games that are appropriate for the child's developmental age and abilities. It is also important to consider the child's interests when selecting play activities for intervention.

MANAGING DISCIPLINE ISSUES AT HOME AND IN THE CLINIC

Children with disabilities may present with inappropriate behaviors. These behaviors may occur for a number of reasons including attention-seeking, to communicate something, sensory-seeking, and also to avoid something. Children may have problems controlling impulses, focusing attention, or, due to the fact that they have a disability, may not have been held to the typical societal standards of manners and appropriate social interactions. Inappropriate behaviors may limit the child's ability to focus on and show progress towards his or her therapy goals.

Additional considerations when working with children exhibiting interfering behaviors:

1. Consider the level of structure a particular child is able to handle when determining play interventions.

2. Establish clear rules, guidelines and expectations early on in therapy rather than waiting until there is a problem. Often these rules and guidelines may be related to safety and common courtesy. Review them periodically and as often as necessary.

3. It is important to set limits with children. Children need to know what is expected of them and also where the line is drawn.

4. The intervention for a disruptive or inappropriate behavior will depend on the reason for the particular behavior.

   • If the child is attempting to communicate something (e.g., head banging in a nonverbal child may signify an ear infection, throwing materials may signify that a task is too difficult) the OTA may acknowledge what the child is trying to communicate and determine a more appropriate method of communicating that need.

   • If the child is rocking his or her body with some intensity, they may be seeking vestibular sensory input and the behavior may be reduced or eliminated by providing the child with regular opportunities for vestibular input.

   • Attention-seeking and task avoiding behaviors are often best dealt with by ignoring the behavior and neutrally redirecting the child back to the task at hand. Obviously, this can only be done if the behaviors are not posing a safety risk for the child or others. It is critical that this ignoring and redirection be done with neutral affect so that the child is not being reinforced by the OTAs response (anger, frustration).

5. Alternate preferred with less preferred activities during intervention.

6. Engage child in favorite/preferred play activities.

7. Reward the child with a preferred activity for the completion of a less preferred activity.

8. It is important for the OTA to be in control of the therapy session. If a child stops part way through an activity or throws the materials on the floor and is allowed to end the task in this manner, the child will learn that he or she is in control. In a situation like this, it is very important that the child follow through with the task to completion, even if this entails shortening, simplifying, or increasing the amount of assistance necessary to complete the task.

9. Consistency is a critical factor of any behavior plan. If a child has a specific plan for dealing with problem behaviors in another setting (such as home, school), then typically, the same strategies should be used during therapy. Behavioral strategies must be consistently used if they are to be effective.

ADAPTING PLAY EXPERIENCES

Depending on the needs of the child with a disability, there are several ways in which a play experience may be adapted. A child's ability to access a play situation may be achieved through adapting the environment, positioning, or materials. For example, for the child with motor problems, an OTA may adapt position (of body and play surface) and tools, materials, and equipment used for an activity. The environment may be adapted to enhance exploration and sensorimotor experiences, such as altering the positioning of the child in order to enhance independent exploration, manipulation, and participation. For example, a child may be positioned on the floor, with positioning devices/support, seated at table, or moving in and out of positions. Positioning and stabilization of play materials may facilitate access and the child's ability to manipulate the play materials. Adapting play materials may facilitate grasp and manipulation. A game or sport may need to be adapted so that a child is able to join peers in play. A playground may also be adapted for access.

Activity Demands: Selecting and Adapting Toys and Games

Webster's Dictionary (1979) defines a toy as "something for a child to play with" (p. 874). DuBois (1997) describes toys as the media of play. OT practitioners use toys/play-things to support developmental stages, to restore or support human function, to motivate, and to affect the quality of interaction with the environment (DuBois, 1997). When selecting toys for play, consideration must be given to the developmental level, skills, and interests of the child. It is sometimes necessary for the OT practitioner to adapt toys and games, particularly for the child with significant physical limitations.

Games and play activities provide a wealth of opportunities for the development of skills and in addressing the needs of children with disabilities. Games and play activities may also provide opportunities to work on needed skills in a fun and motivating way. Personal and social skills such as patience, honesty, task persistence (seeing the game through to the end), turn taking, and cooperation, frustration tolerance, the ability to deal with success and failure in a socially acceptable manner, following and giving directions, asking and answering questions, negotiating, communication, pragmatic skills, social interaction, auditory attention and discrimination, visual discrimination, visual attention, academic and cognitive skills, can all be easily incorporated into games (Satterfield & Shockley, 2002). In order to take advantage of all of these qualities inherent in the many available games and play activities, these games may need to be adapted so that children with disabilities can participate and thus benefit from all they potentially have to offer.

Tips for Individualizing Games, Toys, and Activities

1. Increase (or decrease) the game/toy/activity's level of difficulty.
   - Alter the size of materials (use larger or smaller beanbags for target games depending on the ability level of the child).
   - Minimize steps of the task (simplify a craft activity so that it involves fewer steps).
2. Vary levels of support to make the activity more or less difficult.
   - Provide additional support in positioning the child to facilitate ease of participation in play activity (provide a chair with arms and footrest to provide a stable base of support in order for the child to more easily and effectively use his or her hands/arms for a table top activity).
   - Increase difficulty by adding demands or challenges to the play activity (have the child standing on a balance board while playing catch with a ball).
   - Simplify the process or change the game, rules, sequence, etc.
3. Vary materials used for the activity without changing the activity. This allows the use of alternate and developmentally appropriate materials.

- Use of a balloon or beach ball instead of a volleyball.
4. Alternate ways in which activities are performed, thus changing the purpose of the activity.
   - Placing a game board or activity on a *vertical surface* can facilitate development of hand skills.
   - Placing a game board or activity on a vertical or slanted surface can reduce head control demands on a child with low muscle tone and poor head control.
   - Allow the child to go right up to a target so that he or she can place (rather than throw) a ball into it.
5. Adapt games to allow the child greater ability to actively participate.
   - Enlarge game pieces/use large objects for game pieces.
   - Make a giant game board with sidewalk chalk and have the children be the game pieces and move themselves around the board in wheelchairs or not (Satterfield & Shockley, 2002).
   - Fabricate a switch-operated spinner.
   - Eliminate time constraints or shorten a game to work on task persistence.
   - Increase contrast and provide tactile cues for the child with visual impairment or attentional difficulties.
   - If the game cannot be adapted to include a physically involved child, let him/her have a different role, such as being the spinner for Twister® (Hasbro, East Longmeadow, MA) or controlling the music via a switch in musical chairs.

When selecting games and play activities to use in treatment, the OTA uses activity analysis to determine the activity demands or generic components of the game or activity. The OTA has the ability to choose a game or activity based on the individual child's abilities, interests, needs, and goals. Consideration should be given to games appropriate to the child's age and/or developmental level. Ask, will the child be playing the game with typical peers, you, the OTA, or other children with disabilities similar or different from the child's? Setting the game environment up for success is important while providing the "just right challenge".

Consideration of Context or Contexts – Adapting/Modifying Environments

The interventions discussed thus far have focused primarily on the individual child (performance skills and client factors) and the demands of the activity. Performance patterns and context(s) also need to be considered. Rubin, et al (1983) identified some of the environmental components that are commonly used by researchers to elicit play. These traits are thought to increase the likelihood that play will occur and include:

1. An array of familiar and engaging objects and/or peers.

2. An awareness on the part of the child that he/she is free to choose whatever he/she wishes.

3. Minimally intrusive or directive adult behavior.

4. A friendly, comfortable, and safe atmosphere.

5. Scheduling to reduce the likelihood of bodily stress (hunger, fatigue, illness, etc.) (Rubin, et al., 1983; Bundy, 1991).

Bundy (1991) goes on to succinctly summarize these environmental components in the following statement: "...when a child is in a safe environment, surrounded by interesting toys and nondirective adults, the chances increase that the child will be intrinsically motivated and free of external rules. This, the chance for play to occur is maximized" (p. 233).

When preparing the environment for therapy, Morrison et al. (1991) proposed that the therapist do the following.

1. Set up the treatment environment to facilitate play and to make the child feel safe to engage in exploration of the environment.

2. Facilitate practice of play skills in the treatment environment while eliminating the consequences of failure.

3. Modify aspects of the environment which, through observation, are determined to facilitate or constrain the child's play.

4. Generalize effective characteristics of the treatment environment to other, naturally occurring environments in the child's world.

Blanche (1997) identifies several considerations for setting up and encouraging play outside of the treatment setting. These include:

Play Materials
- Type of toys
- Variety of toys (constructive, dramatic)
- Need for adaptive toys

Play Space
- Consideration of Distractions
- Seating and positioning
- Adapted playgrounds

Play Time
- Individual play at home
- Play with others at home
- Play dates
- Play in the community with others

Playmates
- Typically developing children (siblings, neighbors, classmates)
- Children with similar disabilities

OT practitioners must always keep in mind that it is the child's ability to engage in occupational performance, beyond the clinical setting, that they are targeting for change (Pierce, 1997).

FAMILY INVOLVEMENT—WORKING WITH FAMILIES

Play may be a powerful means of enhancing normalization and helping the child develop within the family, the classroom, and the community. Burton White (1979), the Director of the Harvard Preschool Project spoke to the importance of family variables on children's development and concluded that the informal education, which parents provide, makes more of an impact on a child's overall development than does the formal education system. (McConkey, 1994). The role of the therapist in working with the families of children with disabilities should not be underestimated. Children with disabilities may take longer to respond, make less obvious responses, and initiate play activities less frequently. Parents and others involved with a child's care need to be more directive when interacting with children with disabilities. Without careful planning, the end result may be experiences that are externally controlled and motivated that are not, in fact, play. It is therefore important for the OTA to explore the families' attitudes about their child's play.

McConkey (1994) outlined 4 advantages to a family-oriented approach to play development relevant for the OT practitioner concerned with play.

1. Using games which parents and other family members are familiar with reduces the need for training. Also, the inadequacy some parents feel when instructed to carryover home "therapy" programs are reduced. For interventions that are familiar, families may be more likely to continue to use them (McConkey, 1994; Baker, 1989).

2. A family-centered approach reinforces or extends existing family routines rather than requiring changes in routine and procedures that may be disruptive to the family (McConkey, 1994; McConachie, 1986).

3. The activities are drawn from the local culture, assuring the ecological validity of the intervention and possibly even strengthening the cultural identity of the child (McConkey, 1994; Ivic, 1986).

Play-based interventions may offer a better opportunity for successful integration into the family and the life of the local community, particularly for the child with a marked disability (McConkey, 1994; Richardson & Ritchie, 1989).

Hinojosa & Kramer (1997) note that the nature of play within a family is strongly influenced by the family's collective values. A family that values reading and knowledge seeking may tend toward more sedentary play activities whereas the play demands of a family who value sports and fitness will stress more physically active play activity. Because play is so dependent on the individual family unit, it may not be possible to impose play on a family because, if not relevant to the family, these imposed activities may not, in fact, be play at all (Hinojosa & Kramer, 1997). The OTA must then, determine the types of activities that the family of a child with a disability does consider to be play, and then establish strategies to allow the child to participate. Providing the child with increased opportunities for occupation (play) designed to facilitate everyday opportunities for newly learned and emerging skills in the home environment may have a positive influence on the child's participation and performance (Kellegrew, 1998). The OTA works with the family in order to ensure that play objects are available, which facilitate the type of play toward which the family and therapist wish the child to move (Hinojosa & Kramer, 1997). Okimoto, et al (2000) found that when the shared goal of parents and therapists was to enable children to express their inherent playfulness, intervention to improve parent-child interactions could be more effective than intervention directed at improving the child's developmental skills. Promoting play by optimizing the naturally occurring interactions, which all children may experience within their families and communities, is an important goal of occupational therapy.

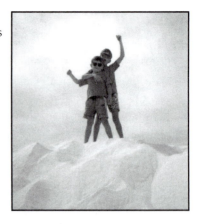

Figure 14-9. For these children, reaching the top of this giant sand dune was an intrinsically motivated and internally controlled play activity.

incorporate play activities into the family routine. The contributions of occupational therapy practitioners may have a profound impact on the play development, play experiences, skill development, and playfulness of a child with a disability.

Summary

Play has been studied by scholars of many disciplines, yet there remains less available research on play than in other areas of child development. Key theories and definitions of play have been presented, including those from within the field of OT. Play is one of the primary occupations of childhood and is thus an important aspect of intervention. Intervention addresses play in three ways: play as occupation/development of play skills; play as a means to motivate the child in order to address other areas of deficit; and play in the form of playfulness. Play is a transaction between the child and the environment, which is intrinsically motivated, internally controlled and free from objective reality (Figure 14-9).

Occupational therapy addresses the play development of a child with a disability through varied means including the selection of and adaptation of appropriate play activities, designing play environments to promote access, participation and skill development, and working with families to

Case Study

Zachary is a 7-year-old boy who has right hemiplegia. He receives occupational therapy services through an outpatient clinic as well as in his school setting. Zachary has difficulty with balance. He has difficulty negotiating around obstacles in school, home and other environments and frequently trips. Due to reduced postural control, Zachary struggles to maintain a sitting position on the floor or in a chair for more than 10 minutes at a time, which makes it difficult for him to participate in many school and play activities. Right upper extremity use is limited due to increased muscle tone, reduced active range of motion and poor motor control. This impacts Zachary's ability to perform tasks requiring bilateral hand use such as manipulation of clothing fasteners, food items, classroom tools (scissors, ruler, computer), and play materials as well as participating in typical playground activities such as ball play, swings, and climbing structures. Treatment goals focus on increasing Zachary's ability to participate in typical play activities with his peers, improving independence in ADLs in both school and home environments and increasing participation in school-related fine motor activities. Intervention strategies (see Table 14-4) include remediation of balance, postural control and use of right upper extremity; maintenance of range of motion of right upper extremity; and modification of the environment, activities or objects to minimize the impact of right hemiplegia and facilitate successful participation in occupational areas.

Zachary has been receiving multiple therapies for most of his life and both the outpatient clinic OT practitioner and the school-based OT practitioner have been experiencing difficulty motivating him. Zachary has recently begun to refuse to participate in treatment activities. The OT practitioners collaborated in order to determine what strategies each had found successful in motivating and engaging Zachary in therapy sessions. They identified that the following activities and strategies had been effective in engaging Zachary in therapy sessions. They were then able to expand upon use of similar activities, thus increasing Zachary's motivation and participation in therapy sessions, and ultimately his progress toward goals.

- Zachary was typically not interested in working on bilateral hand skills but when these same skills were made into a game where Zachary shook (using both hands) and rolled dice to determine which activity he would participate in, he was able to do so.

- Zachary was strongly motivated to develop the computer skills needed so that he would be able to play computer games with his older brother. He displayed difficulty negotiating the mouse and keyboard and had resisted previous attempts to work on these skills. By incorporating use of computer games into the therapy session, Zachary was motivated to participate and thus able to improve his computer skills for both games and school-related use.

- Zachary required assistance to open various types of containers and refused to attempt these tasks on his own. Stickers motivated Zachary. Instead of simply rewarding Zachary for attempting to open containers by presenting him with a sticker, stickers were incorporated into a game. Stickers were placed various "treasure" containers, which were then hidden around the room. Zachary had to find the "treasure" (this involved negotiating over, through, and around various obstacles challenging his balance and postural control), open the containers (a functional skill and goal), and place the stickers into his sticker book (a bilateral and extremely motivating task). If Zachary was able to find all of the treasure, he was permitted to have a peer join him for his next session (another big motivator for Zachary).

QUESTIONS

1. Discuss how play is used as a motivator, to develop play skills, and as a means to address skill acquisition in other areas.

2. Describe three strategies that the OT practitioner used to facilitate Zachary's participation in therapy.

3. Describe two more ways that the OT practitioner might be able to promote a more playful experience.

4. One of Zachary's goals is to participate in typical play activities with his peers. What might the OT practitioner do to facilitate play and play opportunities to address this goal outside of therapy sessions?

5. Give an example of a toy or play activity that might be difficult for Zachary to play with or participate in. Describe how and why you would modify or adapt the toy or play activity for Zachary.

Application Activities

1. Consider and describe how limitations in each of these areas—movement, sensory processing, cognition, and the environment—may impact on the development of play skills. How might you, as the treating OTA, address each of these types of limitations?

2. Describe how play might be used as a motivator; to develop play skills; and as a means to address skill acquisition in other areas for each of the three children described below:

   a. A 3-year-old boy with spastic quadraplegia (cerebral palsy)

   b. A 7-year-old girl with autism/PDD

   c. A 9-year-old boy with ADHD

3. Visit a toy store. List 3 to 5 toys or games appropriate for each of the three children described above. Select one toy or game for each of these three children that would require modification and describe how and why the toy/game could be modified.

4. Describe ways in which the environment can facilitate or inhibit play.

5. Describe the role of the family in developing play skills in the child.

6. Observe children playing. Describe and categorize the children's play activities using Bergen's stages of play development (exploratory and sensorimotor practice play, pretend play, constructive play, and games with rules).

7. Identify three activities, toys, or games that are examples of each stage of play development (exploratory and sensorimotor practice play, pretend play, constructive play, and games with rules).

8. Observe children in a treatment session, classroom or other adult-mediated setting. Using Bundy's model of playfulness, identify and describe an activity that you feel was play and an activity you feel was not play and why.

References

American Occupational Therapy Association (2002). Occupational therapy practice framework: Domain and process. *American Journal of Occupational Therapy, 56,* 609-639.

Ayres, A. J. (1979). *Sensory integration and the child.* Los Angeles: Western Psychological Services.

Baker, B. (1989). *Parent training and developmental disabilities.* Washington: American Association on Mental Retardation.

Bergen, D. (1988). *Play as a medium for learning and development.* Portsmouth, NH: Heinemann.

Berlyn, D. E. (1960). *Conflict, arousal and curiosity.* New York: McGraw-Hill.

Blanche, E. I. (1997). Doing with – not doing to: Play and the child with cerebral palsy. In Parham, L. D. & Fazio, L. S. (Eds.). *Play in occupational therapy for children* (pp. 202-218). St. Louis, MO: Mosby.

Block, J. H., & King, N. R. (1987). *School play: A source book.* New York: Teachers College Press.

Bundy, A. C. (1991). Play theory and sensory integration. In Fisher, A. G., Murray, E. A., & Bundy, A. C. (Eds.), *Sensory integration theory and practice* (pp. 46-68). Philadelphia: F. A. Davis Company.

Bundy, A. C. (1993). Assessment of play and leisure: Delineation of the problem. *The American Journal of Occupational Therapy, 47*(3), 217-222.

Bundy, A. C. (1997). Play and playfulness: what to look for. In Parham, L. D. & Fazio, L. S. (Eds.), *Play in occupational therapy for children* (pp. 52-66). St. Louis: Mosby.

Bundy, A. C. (2002). Play theory and sensory integration. In Bundy, A. C., Lane, S. J., & Murray, E. A. (Eds.). *Sensory integration theory and practice* (2nd ed.). (pp. 228-241). Philadelphia: F. A. Davis Company.

Clifford, J. M. & Bundy, A. C. (1989). Play preference and performance in normal boys and boys with sensory integrative dysfunction. *Occupational Therapy Journal of Research, 9*, 202-217.

Cronin, A. F. (1996). Psychosocial and emotional domains of behavior. In Case-Smith, J., Allen, A. S. & Pratt, P. N. (Eds.), *Occupational therapy for children* (3rd ed.). (pp. 387-429). St. Louis, MO: Mosby.

Cohen, D. (1993). *The development of play* (2nd ed.). London: Routledge.

Csikszentmihalyi, M. (1990). *Flow: The psychology of optimal experience.* New York: Harper & Row.

Diagnostic and Statistical Manual of Mental Disorders (4th ed.). (1994). Washington D. C.: American Psychiatric Association.

DuBois, S. A. (1997). Playthings: Toy use, accessibility, and adaptation. In B. E. Chandler (Ed.), *The essence of play: A child's occupation,* p. 107-130, American Occupational Therapy Association.

Dunn, W., McClain, L. H., Brown, C., & Youngstrom, M. J. (1998). The ecology of human performance. In M. E. Neistadt & E. B. Crepeau (Eds.), *Willard & Spackman's Occupational Therapy* (9th ed., pp. 525-535). Philadelphia: Lippincott Williams & Wilkins.

Fernie, D. (1988). *The nature of children's play.* Urbana, IL: ERIC Clearinghouse on Elementary and Early Childhood Education.

Florey, L. (1971). An approach to play and development. *American Journal of Occupational Therapy, 25*(6), 275-280.

Greene, S. (1997). Playmates: Social interaction in early and middle childhood. In B. E. Chandler (Ed.), *The essence of play: A child's occupation,* p. 131-157, American Occupational Therapy Association.

Hellendoorn, J., van der Kooij, R., & Sutton-Smith, B. (1994). Play and intervention. In A. D. Pelligrini (Ed.), *Children's play in society.* Albany, NY: State University of New York Press.

Hinojosa, J., & Kramer, P. (1997). Integrating children with disabilities into family play. In Parham, L. D. & Fazio, L. S. (Eds.), *Play in occupational therapy for children* (pp. 159-170). St. Louis, MO: Mosby.

Ivic, I. (1986). The play activities of children in different cultures: The universal aspects and the cultural peculiarities. In I. Ivic, & A. Marjanovic, (Eds.), *Traditional games and children of today.* Belgrade: OMEP (World Organization for Early Childhood Education).

Kielhofner, G. (1983). Comparison of play behavior in non hospitalized and hospitalized children. *The American Journal of Occupational Therapy, 37*, 305-312.

Knox, S. (1974). A play scale. In M. Reilly (Ed.), *Play as exploratory learning* (pp. 247-266). Beverly Hills: Sage Publications.

Knox, S. (1996). Play and playfulness in preschool children. In R. Zemke & F. Clark (Eds.), *Occupational science: The evolving discipline.* Philadelphia: F. A. Davis.

Knox, S. (1997). Development and current use of the Knox preschool play scale. In Parham, L. D. & Fazio, L. S. (Eds.), *Play in occupational ther-*

apy for children (pp. 35-51). St. Louis, MO: Mosby.

Knox S., & Mailloux, Z. (1997). Play as treatment and treatment through play. In B. E. Chandler (Ed.), *The essence of play: A child's occupation* (pp. 175-204). American Occupational Therapy Association.

Kramer, P. & Hinojosa, J. (1993). *Frames of reference for pediatric occupational therapy.* Baltimore: Williams & Wilkins.

Law, M., Polatajko, H., Baptiste, W., & Townsend, E. (1997). Core concepts of occupational therapy. In E. Townsend (Ed.), *Enabling occupation: An occupational therapy perspective* (pp. 29-56). Ottawa, ON: Canadian Association of Occupational Therapists.

Levitt, S. (1975). A study of the cross-motor skills of cerebral palsied children in an adventure playground for handicapped children. *Child Care, Health, and Development, 1,* p. 29.

Lieberman, J. N. (1965). Playfulness and divergent thinking: An investigation of their relationship at the kindergarten level. *Journal of Genetic Psychology, 107*(2), 219-224.

Llorens, L. A. (1991). Performance tasks and roles throughout the life span. In C. Christiansen & C. Baum (Eds.), *Occupational therapy: Overcoming human performance deficits.* (pp. 45-66). Thorofare, NJ: SLACK Incorporated.

Mack, W., Lindquist, J. E., & Parham, L. D. (1982). A synthesis of occupational behavior and sensory integrative concepts in theory and practice, Part 1. Theoretical Foundations. *American Journal of Occupational Therapy, 36,* 365-374.

McConachie, H. (1986). *Parents and young mentally handicapped children: A review of research issues.* London: Croom Helm.

McConkey, R. (1994). Interventions for children with developmental handicaps. In Hellendoorn, J., van der Kooij, R., & Sutton-Smith, B. Eds. Play and intervention. In A. D. Pelligrini (Ed.), *Children's play in society.* Albany, NY: State University of New York Press.

Miller, P. H. (1993). *Theories of developmental psychology,* 3rd ed. New York: W. H. Freeman and Company.

Missiuna, C. & Pollock, N. (1991). Play deprivation in children with physical disabilities: The role of the occupational therapist in preventing secondary disability. *The American Journal of Occupational Therapy, 45*(10), 882-888.

Morrison, C. D., Bundy, A. C., & Fisher, A. G. (1991). The contribution of motor skills and playfulness to the play performance of preschoolers. *The American Journal of Occupational Therapy, 45*(8), 687-694.

Morrison, C. D., Metzger, P., & Pratt, P. N. (1996). Play. In Case-Smith, J., Allen, A. S. & Pratt, P. N. (Eds.), *Occupational therapy for children* (3rd ed.). (pp. 504-523). St. Louis, MO: Mosby.

Musselwhite, C. R., (1986). *Adaptive play for special needs children: Strategies to enhance communication and learning.* San Diego: College-Hill Press.

Nakken, H., Vlaskamp, C., & van Wijck, R. (1994). Play within an intervention for multiply handicapped children. In Hellendoorn, J., van der Kooij, R., & Sutton-Smith, B. Eds. (1994). Play and intervention. In A. D. Pelligrini (Ed.), *Children's play in society.* Albany, NY: State University of New York Press.

Neumann, E. (1971). *The elements of play.* New York: MSS Information.

Okimoto, A. M., Bundy, A., & Hanzlik, J. (2000). Playfulness in children with and without disability: Measurement and intervention. *The American Journal of Occupational Therapy, 54*(1), 73-82.

Parham, L. D. & Fazio, L. S. (Eds.). (1997). *Play in occupational therapy for children.* St. Louis, MO: Mosby.

Parham, L. D. & Primeau, L. (1997). Play and occupational therapy. In Parham, L. D. & Fazio, L. S. (Eds.), *Play in occupational therapy for children* (pp. 2-21). St. Louis, MO: Mosby.

Parten, M. (1932). Social play among school children. *Journal of Abnormal Psychology, 28,* 136-147.

Piaget, J. (1962). *Play, dreams and imitation in childhood.* New York: W. W. Norton & Co.

Pierce, D. (1997). The power of object play for infants and toddlers at risk for developmental delays. In Parham, L. D. & Fazio, L. S. (Eds.), *Play in occupational therapy for children* (pp. 86-111). St. Louis, MO: Mosby.

Reed, K. L. (1991). Quick reference to occupational therapy. In R. R. Zukas (series ed.), *Aspen series in occupational therapy*. Gaithersburg, MD: Aspen Publishers, Inc.

Reilly, M. Ed. (1974). *Play as exploratory learning*. Beverly Hills: Sage Publications.

Richardson, A., & Ritchie, J. (1989). *Developing friendships: Enabling people with learning difficulties to make and maintain friendships*. London: Policy Studies Institute.

Rieber, L. P. (1996). Seriously considering play: Designing interactive learning environments based on the blending of microworlds, simulations, and games. *Educational Technology Research & Development, 44*(2), 43-58.

Rogoff, B. (1990). *Apprenticeship in thinking: Cognitive development in social context*. New York: Oxford University Press.

Roley, S. S. (2002). *Application of sensory integration using the occupational therapy practice framework*. Sensory Integration Special Interest Section Quarterly, 25(4), 1-3. American Occupational Therapy Association.

Rubin, K. H., Fein, G. G., & Vandenberg, B. (1983). Play. In P. H. Mussen (series ed.) Handbook of child psychology (vol. 4) E. M. Hetherington (vol. ed.) *Socialization, personality and social development* (p. 693-774). (4th ed.) New York: John Wiley.

Satterfield, P. & Shockley, C. (2002). Games: Engaging environments for developing skills. *Closing the Gap: Computer Technology in Special Education and Rehabilitation, 21*(3), p. 1.

Shultz, T. R. (1979). Play as arousal. In B. Sutton-Smith (Ed.), *Play and learning* (pp. 7-22). New York: Gardner Press.

Takata, N. (1974). Play as a prescription. In M. Reilly (Ed.), *Play as exploratory learning* (pp. 209-246). Beverly Hills: Sage Publications.

Tobias, M. V., & Goldkopf, I. M. (1995). Toys and games: Their role in hand development. In Henderson, A., & Pehoski, C. (Eds.), *Hand function in the child: Foundations for remediation*, (pp. 223-254). St. Louis, MO: Mosby.

Vygotsky, L. S. (1978). *Mind in society: The development of higher psychological processes*. Cambridge, MA: Harvard University Press.

Webster's New Collegiate Dictionary (1979). Springfield, Massachusetts: G. & C. Merriam Company.

White, B. (1979). *The first three years of life*. London: W. H. Allen.

15

SELF-CARE

Christina Monaco, COTA/L
Jennifer Kaldenberg, MSA, OTR/L, CLVT
Amy Wagenfeld, PhD, OTR/L

Chapter Objectives

- Compare and contrast activities of daily living and instrumental activities of daily living as they apply to children.

- Recognize that cultural and ethnic differences influence the way in which activities of daily living and instrumental activities of daily living are introduced to children.

- Understand and recognize the various categories (and sub groups) of activities of daily living and instrumental activities of daily living and how they apply to children.

Introduction

For all children, self-care is important in order to maintain a healthy lifestyle. Serious health risks such as bacterial infections, painful skin breakdown, and even loss of life may result if a child is not properly cared for. Children with special needs are at risk for inadequate every day care simply because a parent/caregiver may not know how to correctly care for the child. An Occupational Therapy Assistant (OTA) working under the supervision of an Occupational Therapist (OT) plays an important role in teaching a child with special needs and his/her parent/caregiver adaptive ways to facilitate and maximize involvement with self-care tasks. For example, facilitating independence with dressing or grooming may make life easier for the parent/ caregiver, thus allowing more time and energy to be spent on other areas of care.

Basic self-care tasks or Activities of Daily Living (ADLs) are an integral part of everyday life. A child may engage in the everyday tasks of bathing, toilet hygiene, personal hygiene and grooming, dressing, eating and feeding, as well as functional mobility (AOTA, 2002). Activities of daily living may also be referred to as personal activities of daily living (PADL) or basic activities of daily living (BADL) (AOTA, 2002). More elaborate self-care tasks are called Instrumental Activities of Daily Living (IADLs) (AOTA, 2002). These activities, or self-care tasks, are used to measure independent living capabilities at home, school, or at work. IADLs involve being able to use communication devices, move about the local community, manage finances, manage and maintain health, keep up with household chores, prepare and clean up after a meal, and follow safety procedures and emergency responses (AOTA, 2002). Unlike ADLs, and depending on a child's level of function, as well as his/her cultural background, IADLs are often volitional tasks a child may perform (AOTA, 2002). In some cases, a parent or caregiver may be responsible for IADLs, such as preparing a meal or managing money (AOTA, 2002).

This chapter discusses specific ADLs and IADLs that a child participates in at home or at school, as well as compensatory techniques and adaptations that may be made for a child with special needs to become successful with self-care skills. Exploration of family/caregiver influence on the development and progression of these skills is also discussed in this chapter. The discussion begins with ADLs.

Family Influence on ADL Skills

When treating a child with special needs, it is important to consider the parent's/caregiver's expectations for their child which may, in part, be greatly influenced by culture, values, and/or beliefs. These cultures, values, and beliefs provide meaning to a specific task, so that what one may find meaningful may not be for another. It is important for all practitioners to be mindful of these effects. Before beginning treatment sessions, interviewing parents/caregivers about their views and values on ADLs and IADLs may help identify those ADL or IADL tasks or goals most important for treatment. A parent's cultural background may also determine other factors relative to self-care and IADL skills. These factors include, but are not limited to the type of clothes a child wears, how or what a child eats, as well as how other health care needs are met. Further, a parent's socioeconomic status may characterize how ADLs or IADLs are carried out (Shepard, 2001). If a family/caregiver's financial resources are limited, considerations as to available funds for self-care items may, in turn, be limited.

Sharing personal information about values, beliefs, and socioeconomic status may make a parent/caregiver feel uncomfortable or uneasy. As an OTA working with children, it is important to take adequate time to explain and make sure the parent/caregiver understands that this information will be extremely helpful in planning and carrying out their child's treatment.

Activities of Daily Living

DRESSING

Dressing is an important part of a child's daily living skills. According to Orelove and Sobsey (1996), a typically developing child begins to engage in helping with dressing at about 12 months of age. The first dressing task a child engages in is holding out his/her arm for a sleeve or his/her foot for a sock or shoe. By age 4, most typically developing children are able to dress and undress, given minimal assistance. It is not until a child is 5 years of age that he/she may be completely independent in dressing.

However, for a child with a disability, these milestones may be delayed or unachievable. Depending on the child's level of functioning, the monumental task of clothing selection and then donning the outfit may be formidable. One of the roles that the OTA, working under the supervision of an OT facilitates is to actively participate in recommending and implementing adapted equipment/clothing as well as specialized techniques to maximize a child's dressing skills.

When teaching a child with disabilities to dress, it is important to consider the child's strengths and limitations. It is important to work with the OT to gain an understanding of the child's active and passive range of motion throughout upper and lower extremities, to assess whether he/she has adequate coordination and endurance, and to determine if he/she has any visual, perceptual, cognitive, or other sensory impairments. When recommending clothing, the OTA, working under the supervision of an OT, may recommend the child wear looser fitting clothing, soft stretchy materials, or wear clothes with Velcro® fasteners (Velcro USA, Manchester, NH) (Jones & Machover, 2000).

Reflections for the OTA

Undressing is usually the precursor to dressing, since undressing is generally considered to be an easier task (Shepherd, Procter, & Coley, 1996).

When teaching dressing skills, it may be useful to break the entire dressing sequence down into steps, gradually working through each step until the child is as independent as possible with dressing. Steps may be added or removed as necessary. Pictures may also be helpful to illustrate the steps of dressing. An excellent way to teach the steps of dressing is through the use of backward chaining, (the OT practitioner teaches the child all of the steps and then has the child do the last step independently, then the last two, the last three, etc., until the child is independent with the task), and forward chaining, (the OT practitioner has the child perform the first step independently and then, working with the practitioner, completes the rest of the steps, then the first two, three, etc.) (Pedretti & Wade, 1998; Shepard, 2001). Adaptive devices and adaptive strategies that may assist with dressing are discussed below.

Donning and Doffing: Underpants, Pants, Shorts, Skirts (Pull Up Garments)

With all dressing tasks, the key to success is matching the specific devices and strategies to the strengths and weaknesses of the individual. When teaching skills necessary for pull up garments keep in mind comfort, function, and the child's and parent/caregiver's wishes.

Suggested Adaptive Devices
- Elastic waistbands, loose fitting clothing
- Trouser pulls, trouser loops
- Dressing sticks, reachers
- Velcro® closures
- Zipper pulls

Suggested Adaptive Strategies
- Rolling side to side from supine
- Depending on trunk control, sitting in a chair with or without back support
- Sit to stand to sit

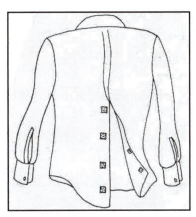

Figure 15-1. Velcro® fastened shirt.

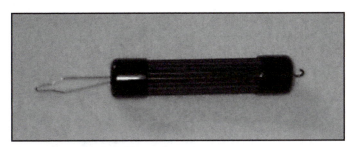

Figure 15-2. Zipper pull.

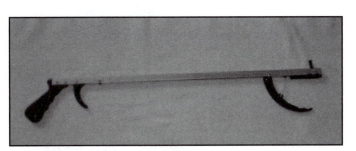

Figure 15-3. Reacher.

- Use of grab bars or sturdy furniture to stabilize self
- Dress involved side or weaker side first and undress uninvolved or stronger side first (Figures 15-1 through 15-3).

Reflections for the OTA

When working on dressing skills with a child with hypertonicity, it is important to remember appropriate positioning to reduce tone. Keeping hips and knees flexed, or positioning the child in sidelying may reduce tone.

Illustrative Case Study

Ryan is a 7-year-old who suffered a spinal cord injury at T-8. He has control of his arms and hands, but poor trunk control. The OTA is working on lower extremity dressing while Ryan is lying supine in bed. The OTA has Ryan roll (using side rails) from side to side to pull up his pants, and has adapted the pants by adding trouser pulls, a helpful assistive device for pulling up pants. These pulls are made of large loops, which may be clipped to the waistband that the child grasps in order to pull up his pants. A trouser pull may also be used to help with donning underpants, skirts, or shorts. Dressing sticks and reachers are also useful tools for children with limited range of motion in their lower extremities and/or poor trunk control.

Another practical technique for donning pants or other lower extremity garments is a sit to stand to sit method. This method requires the child to sit in a chair while he/she dons one leg of a pair of pants, shorts, or underpants at a time. Once this step is done, the child may then shift from side to side using his/her arm for support, until he/she is able to pull the garment past his/her knees. At this time the child may stand to finish pulling up his/her pants and then may sit back down to button or zip pants, shorts, or skirts, if necessary (Jones & Machover, 2000) (Figure 15-4).

Shirts, Sweaters, Capes, Jackets (Pullover Garments)

As with pull up garments, matching the specific devices and strategies to the individual strengths and weaknesses of the child is important for success in donning pull over garments.

Suggested Adaptive Devices
- Large openings for head and neck.
- One size larger to allow for ease of dressing.
- Comfortable, stretchy, loose fit garments.

Suggested Adaptive Strategies
- Lay garments face down on a flat surface, put one arm in an arm hole at a time, push hands and wrist through arm holes, then flip over the head.
- Dress involved or weaker side first, undress uninvolved or stronger side first.
- Pull garment over the head and then push arms through arm holes.

Illustrative Case Study

Kelly is a 6-year-old who suffered a stroke in utero. Kelly has right hemiparesis and fair sitting balance. One adapted technique the OTA is teaching Kelly for donning a shirt or sweater is to lay the garment face down on a flat surface such as a table. Kelly then takes

Figure 15-4A. Sit to stand to sit method sequence.

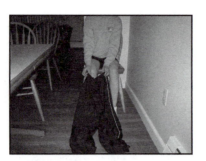

Figure 15-4B.

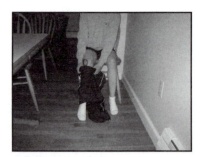

Figure 15-4C.

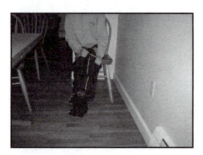

Figure 15-4D.

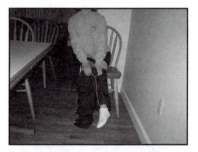

Figure 15-4E.

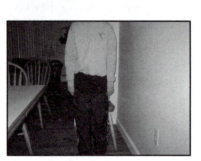

Figure 15-4F.

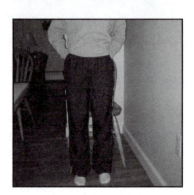

one arm (her right arm) and pushes it through the garment with help from the left arm until the arm is through the sleeve. Kelly then repeats the procedure with her left arm. Next, using her left arm (uninvolved side), Kelly pulls the garment over her head. This is called the flip over method. Due to Kelly's limited sitting balance, the OTA recommends that she complete these tasks while seated, and to provide increased support, that the chair should have a back rest.

Another technique is to have the child do the reverse of the above-mentioned method. The child first pulls his/her head through the garment and then pushes the arms through the sleeves. This technique may be used most effectively with children who have good trunk control as well as adequate bilateral upper extremity active range of motion. Both of these methods may also be used with jackets or capes (Shepherd, Procter, & Coley, 1996).

Button Down Shirt or Jacket

In treatment planning and implementation, working to find the "just right fit" when choosing methods and media includes the articles of clothing used during treatment sessions. Remember success is important. Button down shirts, or jackets generally would not be the first item to teach a child to don, however, this may be preferred by the child and/or his/her parent/caregiver, and as such, must be respected and appropriately attended to.

Suggested Adaptive Devices
- Loose fitting, comfortable materials
- Button hook
- Velcro® closures
- Short sleeves are easier than long sleeves

Figure 15-5A. Flip over method sequence.

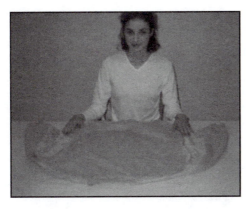

Figure 15-5B.

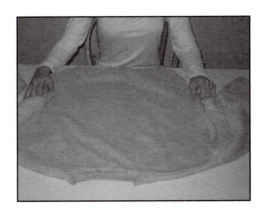

Figure 15-5C.

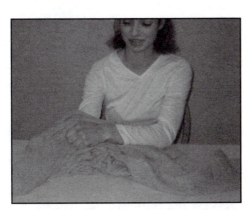

Figure 15-5D.

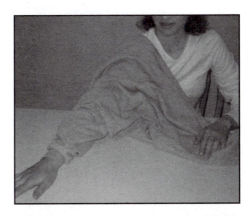

Figure 15-5E.

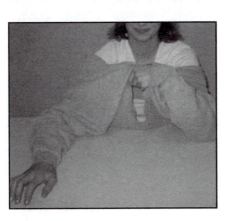

Figure 15-5F.

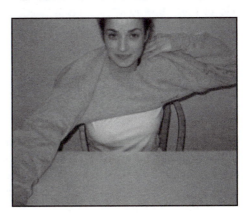

Suggested Adaptive Strategies

- Place involved or weaker arm in sleeve of shirt making sure the sleeve is placed as far up on the arm as possible, bring shirt around the back and dress the uninvolved or stronger side
- Place both arms in sleeves and flip over the head; this technique may be used most effectively with children who have good trunk control as well as adequate bilateral upper extremity active range of motion (Figure 15-5A-F).

The hardest part of donning a button down shirt may be buttoning itself. For a child with insufficient fine motor skills, hemiparesis, or even visual deficits (see fasteners section for ideas), buttoning may be a major challenge. However, using adapted equipment and adapted techniques may prove to be beneficial.

Illustrative Case Study

John is a 10-year-old with limited grasp. The OTA introduces John to a buttonhook (Figure 15-6). Due to his limited grasp, the OTA chose a buttonhook with a built up handle. The OTA instructs John to use one hand to grasp the buttonhook, and place it through the buttonhole. John is then instructed to loop the buttonhook over the button and pull it through the buttonhole (Pedretti & Umphred, 1998).

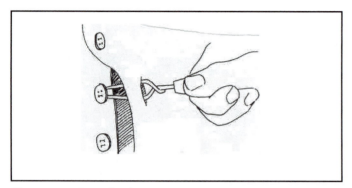

Figure 15-6. Buttonhook.

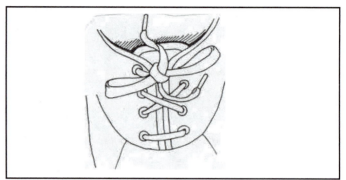

Figure 15-7. Elastic shoelaces.

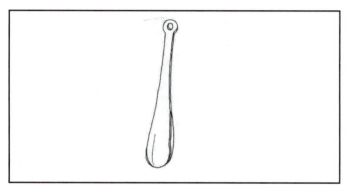

Figure 15-8. Shoe horn.

Shoes

When it comes to recommending and selecting footwear, begin with safety, which means recommending properly fitted, good supportive shoes with nonskid soles. Children who wear orthotics or prosthetics may require increased assistance with choosing appropriate footwear that will accommodate the brace. Adaptations that can be made to sneakers or dress shoes, which encourage independence in donning and fastening shoes, include the following:

Suggested Adaptive Devices
- Elastic shoe laces
- Contrasting colored shoe laces
- Velcro® closures
- Slip on shoes
- Long handled shoe horn

Suggested Adaptive Strategies
- Sit to don shoes
- Use a foot stool

Illustrative Case Study

Katie is a 7 year old with cerebral palsy, who experiences difficulty and frustration when trying to manage regular shoelaces. The OT and OTA discuss Katie's functional limitations and frustrations with the family who then ask about potential adaptations that Katie might use as an alternative to tying shoe laces. The OTA replaces Katie's shoelaces with elastic shoelaces (Figure 15-7). Elastic shoelaces do two things for Katie. They remain tied and they temporarily expand the width of the shoes to allow for easier slip on. The OTA also recommends a long handled shoehorn (Figure 15-8), which allows Katie to easily slide her foot into her shoe.

For safety reasons, when putting the shoe or sneaker on, it is important for a child to be sitting. To further assist in the process and for easier access to the shoe or sneaker, have a child rest his/her foot on a stool when donning the shoe or sneaker. Encouraging a child to flex his/her legs and point his/her toes downward when donning the shoe or sneaker may also make the process simpler (Shepherd, 2001).

There are many ways for the OTA to teach a child with physical, cognitive, and perceptual challenges to tie his/her shoes. For instance, try teaching the child or work together to create a rhyme or song to help remember the steps of shoe tying. Replace white laces with bright colored or alternating colored laces to increase the visual contrast between the shoe and the laces or each of the laces. It may also be fun to work on shoe tying skills by using fun shaped lace-up cards. Lace up cards may be purchased or may be fabricated out of simple pieces of 12" x 12" (approximately) sturdy cardboard and yarn, string, or actual shoelaces. Learning to tie shoelaces may be a frustrating task for any child. In order to maintain their interest in learning to tie, be sure to offer praise for each step that is done correctly (Jones & Machover, 2000) (Table 15-1).

Table 15-1

Shoe Tying Methods

Method 1

- Begin by holding one lace in each hand.
- Make an X with the laces.
- Put the lace held by the dominant hand under the X, and grasp it again with the dominant hand
- With the non dominant hand, grasp the other lace and pull tightly with both hands
- With the dominant hand make a loop
- Pinch the loop with the thumb and index finger and hold it against the shoe
- With the non dominant hand wrap the other lace around the loop.
- Push the loop through the hole using the thumb of the non dominant hand
- Grab the loop with your non dominant hand while still holding on to the other loop with your dominant hand and then pull tightly

Method 2 (Rabbit Ear Method)

- Start the same way as Method 1
- Make an X, then with the dominant hand, place the lace held by the dominant hand under the X and grab it again with the dominant hand. Pull tight.
- Make 2 loops.
- Cross one loop over the other and hold at the middle with thumb and index finger of the nondominant hand.
- With dominant hand bring loop under through the hole.
- Grab loops and pull tight (Egan, 1992; Borel, 1994).

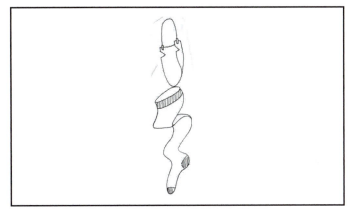

Figure 15-9. Stocking aide.

Socks

Like all lower extremity garments, learning to don socks requires a combination of balance and motor skills, as well as the ingenuity of the OT practitioner to make this a successful self-care task.

Suggested Adaptive Devices

- Loose fitting, tube sock rather than anklet
- Soft, stretchy material
- Sock aid
- As a motivator, consider fun, colorful socks (if they meet the above criteria)

Suggested Adaptive Strategies

- Sit to don socks

Illustrative Case Study

Christopher is a 9-year-old boy with Spina Bifida. One of his goals is to be able independently don his socks. The OTA recommends a stocking aide (Figure 15-9) to help with this task. The stocking aide keeps the sock open as Christopher first slides his foot into the opened sock and then uses the straps connected to the stocking aide to pull the sock up above his ankles. Having Christopher seated in a chair, with a back support, if possible, is the best way to put on his socks because it reduces the risk of loss of balance and of falling (Jones & Machover, 2000).

Fasteners

Successful manipulation of fasteners such as zippers, snaps, buttons, and Velcro® closures involves making use of sensory, cognitive, and perceptive skills. Not only does it involve these skills, fastening may also be facilitated through the use of various adaptive devices. Learning to fasten clothing takes time and patience, and may first be taught through use of a dressing board (Table 15-2).

Suggested Adaptive Devices

- Large, textured, contrasting colored buttons
- Button hook
- Zipper pulls
- Rings or loops

Suggested Adaptive Strategies

- Sit or lay down to complete fasteners, if applicable

Table 15-2

Making a Dressing Board

Materials Needed:

Picture frame
Buttons
Snaps
Zippers
Laces
Sewing machine
Staple gun or hammer and upholstery
Nails
Fabric (sturdy)

Attach several layers of fabric to each side of the frame by stapling, or nailing. Attach at middle either by buttons, snaps, a zipper, etc.

- Use adaptive devices based on specific needs. For instance, children with visual impairments may require high contrast or increased sensory input such as textured fasteners
- Practice with dressing boards

Finding and recommending clothing and adaptive equipment for a child may take some perseverance. Proper instruction and implementation to the child and his/her family/caregivers will take time, patience, and creativity on the part of the OTA. There are many Internet web sites and catalogues that distribute adapted clothing and equipment and may serve as important references for the OT practitioner.

PERSONAL HYGIENE AND GROOMING

Engaging in personal hygiene and grooming is an important developmental task necessary for maintaining a healthy lifestyle. The most common hygiene and grooming tasks for children and adolescents include hair care (washing, drying, combing, and styling hair), oral hygiene (brushing and flossing teeth), skin care (washing hands and face, applying lotion to the body), blowing the nose, eye care (cleaning glasses or contact lens care), applying cosmetics, applying deodorant, shaving, as well as nail care for the hands and feet (AOTA, 2002). Successful engagement in personal hygiene and grooming often affords a child a sense of personal accomplishment and pride.

Hair Care

Hair care may not be as simple as it seems. A child with sensory defensiveness may find this to be a painful task. Techniques that may assist in making hair care easier on the parent/caregiver, as well as the child, may include applying deep pressure to the head before shampooing, which is

calming and organizing (*Note*: this technique should be taught to the parents/caregivers by an experienced OT who has extensive background in sensory integration based therapy) (please refer to Chapter 12: Introduction to Sensory Integration).

To help with washing hair, recommend use of a hand held showerhead to control pressure and spray and keep water out of the child's eyes. Additionally, suggest that parent/caregiver count to 10 while holding a washcloth over the child's eyes when rinsing hair. This will prepare the child for the water and let him or her know when rinsing will be done. When combing the child's hair, using even strokes, going from scalp to hair end is organizing and calming (Jones & Machover, 2000). If drying hair is a challenge for the child, consider recommending use of a dryer set on a low setting, or if weather and health permit, allowing the hair to air dry. It is important to remember that providing the child with an explanation of what is happening and what the next step is going to be allows him/her to prepare for each successive step in a hair care protocol.

Ideas for Adapted Equipment and Techniques

- While combing hair, have the child use a table to rest both arms on to act as extra support (Shepherd, Procter, & Coley, 1996).
- Place a mirror at the appropriate height so that the child can see what he/she is doing (Shepherd, Procter, & Coley, 1996).
- Recommend large handled combs/brushes for better over all grasp (Shepherd, Procter, & Coley, 1996).
- For children with limited range of motion use a goose-neck mount for longer handled hairbrushes and hairdryers. (Shepherd, Procter, & Coley, 1996).

Oral Hygiene

Brushing and flossing teeth is a vital self-care task that is necessary for overall good health and hygiene. Failure to maintain proper oral hygiene may result in unpleasant breath, cavities, gum disease, loss of teeth, pain, or may even interfere with eating. Choosing the right toothbrush for a child may be difficult. There are a number of commercially available toothbrushes ranging from manual to electric, soft to hard, and short head to full head size. Electric spin brushes may be better suited for a child who has difficulty bringing the toothbrush to his/her mouth and/or moving it around. When first introducing oral care, the OT practitioner may consider the Nuk® brush (Gerber Products Co., Fremont, MI), as its bristles are pliable and gentle on the gums and teeth. It is important to note that children should be supervised during oral care until they can demonstrate independence with the task. Children must be supervised to assure that they do not use an excess amount of toothpaste (too much fluoride is not healthy), do not accidentally damage the gums or palate with the brush, and that brushing is done thoroughly and carefully (Jones, & Machover, 2000).

Ideas for Adapted Equipment and Techniques

- Use a small, soft, bristled toothbrush instead of a larger sized toothbrush. A small toothbrush is easier to maneuver in the child's mouth (Shepherd, Procter, & Coley, 1996).
- Recommend toothbrushes that have built up handles for better grasp (Shepherd, Procter, & Coley, 1996).
- Tube squeezers are available to help with pushing toothpaste out of the tube (Shepherd, Procter, & Coley, 1996).

Skin Care and Applying Lotion

Proper skin care is extremely important when working with a child with special needs and his/her parents/caregivers and thus begins with proper hand washing. For all children, hand washing is an important self-care task. It is important for all individuals working with children to educate them on not only the importance of hand washing, but to incorporate it into their daily routines. Children must understand that the most important times to wash the hands are after sneezing or coughing, after toileting, before meals, and after play. How and when to apply lotion should also be taught to children who live in cold or dry climates (Jones, & Machover, 2000).

There are many ways to make hand washing fun for children, from using certain types of soap or dispensers to singing songs. A note of caution: Be sure that you are aware of any allergies or sensitivities before using any skin care products. Children who wear splints or other orthotic devices should also be taught, if possible, to care for their devices and incorporate this care into a hand washing routine.

Due to the potential for limited ability to change positions or the use of orthotic equipment (braces, hand splints, etc.), children with disabilities are at a greater risk of developing skin breakdown. Sores, blisters, or uncomfortable red areas may result if a child is not repositioned frequently or if orthotics have come into contact with bare skin for extended periods of time. Teaching the parent/caregiver as well as the child ways to prevent skin damage, such as discussing how often the child should be repositioned, proper ways to put equipment on, and even how often skin should be checked may, depending upon demonstrated competency and state and facility guidelines, be done by the OTA. For instance (when deemed suitable), mirrors may be easily adapted to allow the child to independently check for skin issues.

Nose Blowing

For a child with special needs, nose blowing may be extremely challenging. This task is difficult for even the OT practitioner to demonstrate since nose blowing is only heard and not seen. As suggested by Jones and Machover, (2000) there are a variety of methods that may be useful in teaching a child to blow his/her nose:

- Use a dampened or soft tissue to blow or wipe with if a child is hypersensitive.
- For a child with poor sensation in the facial region, cue the child to use a mirror to see if he/she needs to blow and if his/her nostrils are clear.
- Place the child's hand under the OT practitioner's nose as he/she is blowing to have the child feel the air flow that comes during nose blowing.
- Demonstrate how the tissue is supposed to move as air is blown into it.
- Sprinkle a powdery like substance on dark paper and have the child visually track the powder as it is blown by the nostrils (p. 242-243).

Eye Care

For children who wear glasses for functional vision, it is important to learn to care for them. Glasses are expensive and depending on the child's family financial status, broken glasses may not be easily or quickly replaced. An OTA may help the child work out the best ways to clean his/her glasses on a daily basis as well as find safe places to store them.

Children may not enjoy wearing glasses. They may slip off his/her nose, may leave uncomfortable red marks, or the child may simply not like how he/she looks when wearing them. An OTA may need to remind the child how much better he/she sees when wearing them as well as make any necessary modifications such as adding nose grips (from a commercially available eyeglass kit) or eye glass straps to keep the glasses on the child's face.

Other eye care tasks may include contact lens care and application of eye drops. Contact lens application may be a difficult task to teach and may need to be left to the optometric professional, however the care and management of the contact lenses is important to encourage. Teaching proper hygiene, care, and management of the contact lenses is important. As children may also experience eye irritation or dry eyes, it may be recommended by their optometrist or ophthalmologist to use eye drops. The OT practitioner can assist by teaching the child how to manage the dropper, adapt the dropper, or provide adaptive devices for the child or his/her parent/caregiver. Children with low vision may also use specific devices to assist with visual tasks and may need to be educated in proper care and storage. These devices are discussed in Chapter 16: Visual Perceptual Dysfunction and Low Vision Rehabilitation.

Applying Cosmetics

Applying makeup may be challenging for an adolescent girl who may have an unsteady hand, poor arm strength, grasp, or even cognitive deficits. The OTA may need to work with the adolescent on adapting handles of brushes or other makeup applicators to ensure a better grasp. To help with sequencing and the application process, providing pictures of the steps and how to apply each cosmetic may be a useful therapy tool. Given the wide variety of makeup products available, it may also be necessary to work with the adolescent on selecting age appropriate and medically appropriate (allergies, skin type, etc) cosmetic choices.

Applying Deodorant

Applying deodorant is also an important part of personal hygiene and should be recommended when appropriate. Adolescents should be reminded to apply deodorant to their underarms at least once a day, preferably after donning undergarments. Depending on the child's strength in his/her hand and wrist, range of motion in his/her upper extremities, and coordination, either a roll-on antiperspirant or aerosol may be recommended.

Ideas for Adapted Equipment and Techniques
- If a child is able to use an aerosol can, there are spray adapters with long handle triggers available to help with spraying.
- Lever handles may also be used with aerosol can deodorants (Shepherd, Procter, & Coley, 1996).
- Using equipment or furniture to hold UE in position, teach positioning of the UE to allow for application.

Shaving

Shaving is a typical personal hygiene task of adolescence. When working on shaving, adhering to strict safety precautions is extremely important. Electric razors are often recommended for adolescents with special needs as they are considered to be safer than straight edge razors, they require less precision, and the blades are covered (Shepard, Procter, Coley, 1996).

Reflections for the OTA

Be aware of and take the necessary precautions when working with adolescents on shaving who may have any type of circulatory issue or communicable disease.

Ideas for Adapted Equipment and Techniques
- Razors can be modified with built up or extended handles for easier access.
- Electric razors and disposable razors do not require new blades therefore making these razors a safer choice than a standard straight edge razor (Shepherd, Procter, & Coley, 1996).

Nail Care

Nail care is an important grooming task. Uncut and ragged nails may cause accidental self injury or injury to others. Long nails can trap dirt and germs, which may transmit disease. Providing finger and toe nail care for a child with a disability may be a difficult task. For instance, a child with sensory defensiveness may not enjoy having his/her nails trimmed or filed, let alone having his/her hands touched.

Ideas for Adapted Equipment and Techniques
- For single hand use, attach both nail file and clippers to a height appropriate table (Shepherd, Procter, & Coley, 1996).
- Attach an adapted nail clipper to a board fitted with suction cups to allow for single handed use (Jones, & Machover, 2000).
- Recommend using a larger sized emery board for better handling while filing nails (Jones, & Machover, 2000).

Reflections for the OTA

Remember that unsupervised nail clipping and filing may be unsafe for children to do.

Contractures and Nail Care
- When a child's hand is contracted, the muscles or joints are not easily moved or may not move at all. Fabrication of a hand splint may help to decrease or prevent a contracture, therefore making nail care easier. Additionally, an OT practitioner may implement a range of motion treatment to increase range in the child's fingers. As the child's parent/caregiver may be responsible for cutting their child's fingernails, this treatment program should be taught to them in order for it to be implemented as part of the child's daily routine.

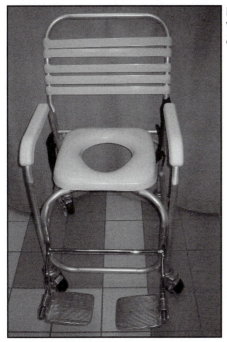

Figure 15-10. Wheeled shower chair.

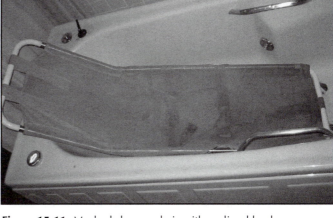

Figure 15-11. Meshed shower chair with reclined back.

BATHING AND SHOWERING

For any child who loves the water, bath time is usually considered to be an extension of playtime. However, for a child with special needs, bathing/showering may easily become a daunting chore that neither participant nor helper may want to be a part of. Bathing/showering is necessary and, in an ideal world, should be an enjoyable time for both child and caregiver. Bathing has other benefits besides cleanliness and hygiene. Warm water may help relax the tight muscles of a child with hypertonia. Soft bath toys may also aid in a child's exploration of tactile materials. An OTA, working under the supervision of an OT, works with the child with special needs and caregivers in determining which adaptations and safety measures are needed in order to make bathing/showering a positive experience for all involved parties.

Positioning

Proper positioning of the child is needed during the bathing process. Improper positioning not only makes bathing troublesome and awkward, but may also cause serious harm to the child. The OTA should educate the parent/s/caregiver/s on proper body mechanics, as improper lifting may result in injury.

There is a variety of adapted seating equipment available. Before making a decision about which equipment is best for the child, it is important to consider tone, sitting balance, endurance, trunk and head control, arm and leg movements, as well as overall safety awareness (Shepard, Procter, & Coley, 1996). For instance, a child who does not have suf-

ficient trunk control would not be ideally suited for a bath bench. A reclined tub chair with safety straps would be a better choice for this child. Another adapted seating option available is called a wheeled shower chair (Figure 15-10). This chair is useful for larger or heavier children since the chair can be easily rolled and maneuvered into and out of a walk-in shower stall. Mesh chairs (Figure 15-11) are also available with reclined or straight backs to accommodate a child with low tone. However, for smaller or lighter children who can be easily lifted in and out of the tub, bath chairs that fit securely inside a tub are available. One such example is a corner chair with a suction cup base that provides proper positioning and an adjustable handrail for extra security. For a small child who has more active movement, yet requires additional stability when seated in the tub, a wraparound bath support might be recommended. This adapted seat has a wide base and cushioned back support with safety belt. The child is free to move his/her arms and legs without fear of falling when seated in a wraparound bath support. Bath benches may also be recommended as part of a bathroom modification. Bath benches make transfers to and from a wheel chair more manageable. Adapted seating for bathing is always changing, such that the OTA is strongly urged to stay abreast of current trends in adapted bathing options.

Safety Adaptations

There are many modifications that may be made to a bathroom in order to make it more readily accessible. Removing thresholds may create a barrier free room. A roll-in shower stall instead of a bathtub may be useful for larger sized children, as a parent/caregiver may easily maneuver a wheeled shower chair in and out of the stall. Other modifications include adaptive equipment such as using a hand held showerhead as well as soap and shampoo dispensers

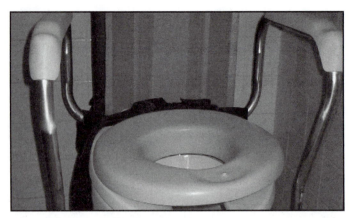

Figure 15-12. Raised toilet seat with armrests.

(Jones, & Machover, 2000). Additional bathroom modification information will be discussed in other ADL areas included in this chapter.

The bathroom contains many hidden dangers. All daily activities that take place in the bathroom should be done with safety in mind. The following are recommendations that should be provided to all parents/caregivers. To prevent burns, water heaters should be set at 110 degrees or below. Make sure all razor blades and cleaning supplies are kept out of a child's reach. Nonskid mats should be placed inside and outside of the tub or shower area to prevent falls. Also, parents/caregivers should consider having grab bars professionally installed in the shower/tub area to provide extra support and safety. To make transfers safer and easier, the OTA must educate parents/caregivers on proper body mechanics when lifting and transferring, such as emphasizing bending the knees and keeping the back straight when lifting and transferring. When lifting a heavier child, the OTA may recommend, as an alternative to standard transfer methods, that parents/caregivers make use of a hydraulic lift (Shepard, Proctor, & Coley, 1996).

TOILET HYGIENE/BOWEL AND BLADDER MANAGEMENT

Achieving independence with toileting is a major developmental milestone for any child. However, this self-care task is not necessarily an easy one to master. Like all self-care tasks that a child with special needs participates in, toilet training may be frustrating for both child and parent/caregiver. Toilet training requires the parent/caregiver to have time, patience, and the ability to feel comfortable assisting the child with special needs to master this skill. Not all children with special needs become independent with the toileting process. Many children will require instruction in adapted techniques as well as adapted equipment to assist in achieving the highest level of functioning with regard to toileting.

Developmental Progression of Toileting

Before introducing a toileting program, it is important for not only the OT practitioners, but for the entire team to determine whether physiologically the child is ready for the program. According to Shepard (2001),

At birth a newborn voids reflexively and involuntarily. Changes in position, handling by others, and other stimuli can trigger maturation. As the child matures, the spinal tract is myelinated to a level for bowel and bladder control at the lumbar and sacral areas and the child learns to control sphincter reflexes for the volitional holding of urine and feces. Children are often physiologically ready for toileting if they have a pattern of urine and feces elimination (Shepard, 2001, p. 508).

As with other areas of development, a typically developing child proceeds through an orderly series of steps to achieve control of his/her bowels. Table 15-3 presents an overview of the development of bowel and bladder control.

Adapted Equipment

There is a variety of adapted equipment available to help with the toileting process. For instance, raised toilet seats and toilet safety frames (Figure 15-12) may help a child who has poor sitting balance remain stable while on the toilet. There are also commercially available toilet supports with contoured backs and safety straps that provide additional safety for toileting. Toilet supports may also be fitted with armrests and footrests. Toilet supports are designed to fit any toilet and enable the child to remain secure while on the toilet.

For children who have difficulty getting to the bathroom during the night, a bedside commode may be an option. Bedside commodes are adjustable in height and since they are portable, may be placed anywhere. Another option for toileting includes the use of urinals. Urinals are available for both males and females. They may best be suited for children who have the ability to control their bladder but are unable to ambulate, or are primarily wheelchair or bed bound. Additional adapted equipment for toileting will be discussed in the hygiene portion of this section. Also refer to bathing section for additional ideas on how to make the bathroom barrier free.

Illustrative Case Study

Tim is a 7-year-old boy with spastic quadriplegia. Tim's parents would like him to be involved in the toileting process. Tim has poor sitting balance and requires minimal assistance to maintain an upright position once seated. Tim is petite and his feet do not touch the floor when seated on a standard sized toilet. When looking for adaptive equipment for Tim what does the OT/OTA need to consider?

Table 15-3
Toileting Milestones

Age	Milestone
1 year	Child may show emotional distress when soiled.
2 years	May begin to initiate interest in potty training
30 months	Child is able to let his/her parent/caregiver know if he/she needs to use the toilet. Can determine if he she needs to urinate or have a bowel movement. Requires parent/caregiver assistance with managing clothing and wiping.
3 years	Will often toilet on own.
4 years	Has few accidents.
4 ½ years	Child is able to toilet independently and pull up and adjust clothing.
5 years	Washes hands after toileting.

Adapted From: Kurtz, L. (1996). Developmental Milestones. In L. Kurtz, P. Dowrick, S. Levy, M. Batshaw. In Handbook of Developmental Disabilities Resources for Interdisciplinary Care. (pp. 30-52) Gaithersburg, MD: Aspen Publication.

Parks, S. (1997). Inside HELP Hawaii Early Learning Profile Administration and Reference Manual. Palo Alto, CA: VORT Corporation.

Potty training study offers answers (4/22/03). www.ynhh.org/healthlink/pediatrics Retrieved May 23, 2003.

Toileting Programs

Toileting programs are useful in helping a child become familiar with the process and procedures associated with bowel and bladder management. Toileting programs may be implemented at home or in a school setting, and are typically developed by the entire team of professionals working with the child. The OT practitioner's role in developing a toileting program may be to recommend, teach, and monitor the child and involved adults in the correct use of adapted equipment, to advise about positioning, and to help with developing a schedule. When a child is at home, either the parent or caregiver may carry out the toileting program, and when at school, the child's teacher or aide may be responsible for the child's toileting program. Ongoing communication between OT practitioners, teachers, and parent/caregivers is critical for ensuring success with a child's toileting program.

When developing a toileting program, it is helpful to break down the entire toileting process into steps, gradually working through each step until the child is as independent as possible with toileting. Steps may be added or removed as necessary. A toileting program may include specific information regarding the time of day the child is to use the toilet, the place in which the child will be toileted, how the child is to be positioned when on the toilet, all necessary equipment that will be needed, and any specific instructions or guidelines that would be helpful during the toileting process. Guidelines may include listing any precautions that

may need to be taken when carrying out the program, or any reward system that is to be used to motivate the child. Another important component of a toileting program is a comment section in which progress or challenges may be documented. This program then serves as a communication tool for all parties involved in working with the child on the toileting program. A sample toileting program is shown in Table 15-4.

Toileting Hygiene

There is more involved with toilet hygiene than one may realize. Before starting the toilet hygiene process, there are basic skills that a child may need in order to be successful and include, "...visual and/or tactile recognition of cleanliness, adequate sitting balance, trunk rotation, shoulder extension and rotation (for reaching), and sufficient strength and proprioceptive discrimination to apply pressure for wiping"(Jones, & Machover, 2000 p. 244). Limitations with any of these skills as they apply to toileting will call upon the ingenuity of the OT practitioner to introduce and implement adapted strategies, techniques, and equipment in order to maximize function. The OTA, working under the supervision of an OT, plays an important role in facilitating this process.

Toilet hygiene involves being able to gather and make use of toileting supplies, manage clothing and fasteners, to maneuver on and off the toilet or commode, maintain the safest possible position while on the toilet or commode, cleaning one's body, and even caring for menstrual and con-

Table 15-4

Daily Toileting Program

Name:
Age:
Brief Summary of Status:

Date:
Equipment Needs (be specific):

Positioning Instructions:
(Include Photo of Child Properly Positioned Here)

Precautions:

Where Is Child To Be Toileted:
Classroom _____   Nurses Clinic _____
Hall Bathroom _____   Home _____

Toileting Schedule:
Time   Successful? Y = Yes/ N=No, Bowel Movement Y = Yes/ N=No, Urinated Y = Yes/ N=No

8:00 AM	10:30 PM
8:30	11:00
9:00	11:30
9:30	12 Midnight
10:00	12:30
10:30	1:00
11:00	1:30
11:30	2:00
12 Noon	2:30
12:30	3:00
1:00	3:30
1:30	4:00
2:00	4:30
2:30	5:00
3:00	5:30
3:30	6:00
4:00	6:30
4:30	7:00
5:00	7:30
5:30	
6:00	
6:30	
7:00	
7:30	
8:00	
8:30	
9:00	
9:30	
10:00	

Did Child:
Pull Down Lower Extremity Garments   Level of assistance
Wipe self   Level of assistance
Pull Up Lower Extremity Garments   Level of assistance
Wash/Dry Hands   Level of assistance

Reward System (please list):

Comments:

tinence needs (AOTA, 2002). Toileting supplies may include tissue paper, wet wipes, briefs/incontinence pads (if used for added protection), or any other objects that a child requires when toileting. Managing clothing while toileting may be difficult, especially if a child has limited or restricted range of motion and/or balance. It may be best to have the child seated on the toilet first, and then, with assistance (as needed), doff and don lower extremity garments. Having the child use a dressing stick or reacher (see dressing section) to help with lower extremity clothing management during toileting are alternatives for the OT practitioner to consider.

As previously discussed, there are many adapted devices that may help a child maintain his/her position while on the toilet. For example, a toilet armrest frame with footrests or safety straps may help keep a child from losing his/her balance.

Reflections for the OTA

While a child is voiding or having a bowel movement, privacy should be respected and assistance given only when necessary.

With a female adolescent, and depending on her level of functioning, teaching about menstrual care may be part of the treatment program. It is important to explain the use of the sanitary pad, to demonstrate how and when to change the pad, and how to properly dispose of the items.

Toilet hygiene is important to maintain a healthy lifestyle. For instance, it is important for children to understand that hand washing after toileting is important for good health. Understanding may not be enough; children must also practice and carry out good hand washing after toileting. In addition, infections and rashes may occur if the peri area is not properly cleaned. Supervision and assistance should be provided in all aspects of toileting until the child is able to demonstrate independence in these tasks.

Illustrative Case Study

Tim is a 7-year-old boy who is aware when he needs to void but has not been an active participant in the toileting and hygiene process. Tim has limited upper extremity ROM due to increased tone. Tim is quite conscious of hygiene and enjoys washing his hands. Tim's parents have had limited education in toileting and hygiene. What would be an age-appropriate goal for Tim? What can the OT/OTA do to maximize Tim's independence with hygiene tasks?

EATING AND FEEDING

Proper nourishment is essential for maintaining a healthy lifestyle. For a child with oral motor impairments this simple and otherwise often enjoyable ADL becomes a complex challenge for the child as well as for his/her parent/caregiver. An OTA, working under the supervision of an OT, may play a key role in developing adapted techniques, adapted equipment, and the best position for the child during meals.

Oral motor skills, methods, and equipment will be discussed in detail in Chapter 13: Oral Motor Skills and Feeding.

FUNCTIONAL MOBILITY

Functional mobility is a term used to describe transferring or moving from one position to another, and includes ambulation and wheelchair transfers as well as wheelchair mobility. Functional mobility describes daily activities involving transfers to and from bed, to and from the shower, as well as to and from the toilet (AOTA, 2002). Specific transfer techniques are designed or chosen to meet each child's specific strengths and needs, and vary significantly, based on the child's ability to assist.

Transfers

The transfer status of each child varies. Depending on the child's size, weight, and functional abilities, a one-person, two person, or hydraulic lift may be necessary to ensure a safe transfer. An OTA may be asked to instruct the child and his/her parent/caregiver in the best methods of transferring or assisting in the transfer. As part of this instructional process, it is also important to educate the child and his/her parents/caregivers on ways to prevent injuries when lifting and transferring through teaching and demonstrating proper body mechanics and safety procedures.

Adler, Tipton-Burton and Lehman (1998) suggest eight basic principles of body mechanics to consider when lifting and transferring children:

1. Move as close as possible to the child or move the child close to you.

2. Face the child head on.

3. Keep knees bent, making sure to use your legs and not your back.

4. Keep your back straight.

5. Maintain a wide base of support.

6. Do not raise your heels; keep them down.

7. If you feel that you are unable to lift the child by yourself, ask for help.

8. Avoid twisting your body when lifting.

Before beginning a transfer, make sure the child is aware of what is about to happen, and that there is a clear path to the wheelchair, tub, bed, etc. If transferring to a wheelchair, the parent/caregiver must make sure it is locked, and be aware of any limitations or medical precautions the child may have that might interfere with the transfer.

When working with a child with a disability and his/her parent/caregiver, it is always important to stress safety issues. The child and parent/caregiver may become accidentally injured if a transfer is done incorrectly or a wheelchair is left unlocked.

Ideas That May Help to Prevent Accidents

- Remember to apply the brakes on the child's wheelchair during transfers.

- Make sure all pathways are clear of clutter, loose rugs, or wires to prevent falls during transfers, ambulation, or allow the child to complete wheelchair mobility.

- For a child who is capable of maneuvering a manual or power wheelchair, make sure he/she is able to maneuver it in tight spaces while watching out for others walking by.

- Make sure the child's feet are resting on the footrests of the wheelchair and that his/her arms are resting on the armrest of the wheelchair, and not dangling off the sides of the chair.

- For children using walkers or wheelchairs, make sure they are able to safely maneuver on different textured floors such as carpet, wood flooring, and tile.

- Clearly indicate thresholds and stair risers by marking them with bright paint or marking tape (Jones, & Machover, 2000).

Activities of Daily Living Summary

Engaging in ADLs is an important part of a child's life. In order to support a best practice (Dunn, 2000) model of treatment when working with children and their families/caregivers on self-care skills, the OTA must be well educated, respectful, and compassionate in his/her implementation skills. Please refer to Developmental Milestones Chart in the back of the book.

Instrumental Activities of Daily Living

As children grow and develop, so too do their occupational roles. Like ADLs, children may also actively participate in Instrumental Activities of Daily Living (IADLs). The IADLs children typically participate in include: care of others such as babysitting siblings or other children, pet care, which may involve walking, feeding, and grooming an animal, use of the phone or other electronic communication devices, moving throughout the community, money management, health management and maintenance, which may include eating a healthy diet, exercising, avoiding drugs and alcohol, and getting enough sleep, home maintenance (chores), meal preparation and clean up, safety procedures such as wearing seatbelts, bike helmets, and also knowing how to recognize potentially unsafe situations, and shopping (AOTA, 2002). Although the rate and quality of participation in the above tasks may differ from their adult counterpart, a child's participation in IADL responsibilities plays an important role in supporting cognitive, social emotional, and even physical growth and development. Successful participation in IADLs may enhance a child's sense of self-esteem and provide a foundation for later independent (as indicated) living. *An important note*: like ADLs, IADLs are culturally bound. While children from certain cultural backgrounds may be encouraged to achieve a high level of independence, others may not. Before implementing a program to enhance IADL skills, it is critically important for the OT practitioner to communicate with the family/caregivers, in order to support and respect their wishes and beliefs.

CARE OF OTHERS AND CARE OF PETS

For some adolescents, care for younger siblings and care of the family pets may be one of their various roles and responsibilities within the family. In addition, babysitting may also be seen as a common job for adolescents and requires acquisition of many of the IADL skills discussed in the following sections.

COMMUNICATION DEVICE USE

Communication devices refer to devices used to send or receive information (AOTA, 2002). Devices that may be used include computers, augmentative communication devices, emergency systems, telephones, and devices for the deaf and blind (please refer to Chapter 23: An Overview of Assistive Technology). In almost every school district and other clinical setting across the United States, computers are a commonly used learning tool, and for some children, an alternative method for effective communication within the classroom. Further, augmentative communication devices such as high and low technology communication boards are widely used with children with multiple handicapping conditions to enhance and facilitate communication skills. The OT practitioner may work side by side with speech language pathologists to determine the optimal fit of the specific communication device. The OT practitioner may assist in the implementation of augmentative communication devices by assessing the child's physical and cognitive abilities, and if the child is wheelchair bound, the OT practitioner may also assess how to attach or position the device.

The OT practitioner may also work with the child on enhancing telephone skills and may recommend specific telephones to maximize independence. There are many different types of telephones available that may meet various needs, such as preprogrammed or voice activated for children with cognitive impairment, large numbers or Braille for the visually impaired, and cordless for the physically impaired, to name just a few.

COMMUNITY MOBILITY

Community mobility refers to the ability to safely maneuver within the community, and may include the use of public or private transportation. Many activities that a child participates in require the ability to make use of transportation, such as going to school, sporting events, after school activities, and social activities. The OT practitioner has an important role in assessing the child's functional community mobility skills and goals. Specific issues regarding community mobility may include determining whether a child is able to use maps or schedules to take a bus, taxi, or subway. If that is the case, are they able to understand and use tokens or money to ride a bus, taxi, or subway? Community mobility also entails access; can a child maneuver in and out of community transportation, can he/she travel throughout the community, be it on foot, or in a wheelchair? Community mobility training for children with visual impairment may include environmental modification such as increasing contrast, use of visual aids, and orientation and mobility training.

FINANCIAL MANAGEMENT

A child or adolescent's participation in financial management may range from paying for meals at school to maintaining a bank account. The OT practitioner must consider the child or adolescent's ability to identify, handle, and manage money in order to best facilitate successful financial management.

HEALTH MANAGEMENT AND MAINTENANCE

The AOTA (2002) identifies health management and maintenance activities as those activities that promote health and wellness such as, adhering to a predetermined pattern of medication management, engaging in a regular exercise program, proper nutrition, and maintaining a healthy body image. Consider the teenager with a dysmorphic sense of self, or anorexia. The goal of treatment would be to improve self esteem, develop healthy eating patterns, develop positive self image and be able to maintain and manage a healthy lifestyle.

The health and education team collaborate on the plan for medication management. It is important that team members are aware of the medications taken by children as side effects may affect their overall performance. The health care and/or education team is also an important go between for the physician in terms of reporting back on the effect of certain medications.

HOME ESTABLISHMENT AND MANAGEMENT

If we all think back to our roles and responsibilities as children growing up in a family, we can probably remember what our chores were. These chores were an important part of developing our sense of responsibilities as a family member. Chores are a normal part of childhood, and may include making our beds, clearing the dishes, or putting away the laundry.

MEAL PREPARATION AND CLEANUP

A child's participation in meal preparation and cleanup may vary. Culture or family values may determine the level of participation in meal preparation and clean up for a child. As many children have dual working parents or single parents, increased job responsibilities may be left to the child (please refer to Chapter 9: Interacting With Families). A child may be responsible for preparing meals for themselves or even their siblings.

Questions that the OT practitioner might consider when working with a child on the IADL task of meal preparation and clean up include:

1. Is it safe for the child to complete these activities?
2. Does the child make good food selection choices?
3. Based on the availability of food, are the meals healthy and well balanced?
4. Is the child safe with use of cooking utensils and appliances?
5. When considering meals provided at a child's school, is he/she able to open containers or prepare food such as sandwich or salad?

Perhaps most importantly, before undertaking working with a child on meal preparation and clean up, the OT practitioner must consider the family values and cultural practices. In some cultures, independence in meal preparation and clean up may *not* be a valued skill.

SAFETY PROCEDURES AND EMERGENCY RESPONSE

Safety procedures and emergency response activities refer to a child's ability to respond to emergency situations in an appropriate manner or having the awareness to remain safe in his/her environment (AOTA, 2002). The OT practitioner must look at the child's ability to use *environmental control units* (ECU's) or other communication systems. Can the child anticipate and respond to emergency situations? Can the child communicate his/her needs either through written, auditory, or other means? Is the child able to independently participate in school emergency drills? If not is there a plan in place for this child to be attended to in either simulated or real emergency situations?

SHOPPING

A child or adolescent's level of participation in shopping may differ significantly from that of an adult. However, no matter what the situation, the ability to manage money or participate in the activity is important. The OT practitioner must consider the child's ability to identify, handle, and manage money in a safe and responsible manner. For example, consider an adolescent girl with cognitive impairment being invited to the mall with her peer group. When working in a situation such as this, the OT practitioner should consider issues like; is she able to manage her money? Is she able to make responsible choices with her money? Is this a safe and appropriate activity for her? And, is there anything that the OT/OTA can do to facilitate her independence and safety in this activity?

Summary

This chapter examined the ADL and IADL tasks typically associated with childhood. Making use of compensation techniques, adapted equipment, and environmental adaptations were discussed in terms of helping children with special needs become as independent as possible with self-care tasks. As a child's family, culture, socioeconomic status, cognitive level, and functioning level are all factors that ultimately impact participation in ADLs and IADLs, when working in pediatrics, always remember that each child is unique, and must be treated as such.

Case Study

Joey is a 10-year-old boy with Down syndrome. He ambulates independently with a wheeled walker. However, Joey is slightly unstable when standing without assistance. Joey wants to be more like his older brother. For Joey, this means wanting to take showers instead of baths, and to be able to take them without the help of his mom or dad. Joey's mom has many concerns about this, mainly for Joey's safety. She would like to see Joey be able to shower independently, but knows that since he has difficulty maintaining his balance and requires minimal assistance with washing his body and washing/rinsing his hair she would prefer to see Joey have the option to sit when showering.

Based on the above information, how would you answer the following questions?

- What modifications should be made to the shower?

- What adapted equipment would help Joey become independent in showering?

- How would you go about teaching Joey how to use the adapted equipment?

- What safety issues would be raised and how would you address them, such as water temperature, skid mats, and so on?

Application Activities

1. Plan a "Disability Day." Complete a self-care task as if you have a disability. Have a discussion group following the activities to talk about how you felt doing the task and ways to make that task easier.

2. Pair up and practice using adapted equipment such as sock aides, dressing sticks, reachers, and button hooks.

3. Prepare a brief case study about a fictitious child with self care needs. Make enough photocopies of each case study to provide one to each student. Split into groups and present list practical treatment ideas based on the case study and discuss.

4. Fabricate adaptive devices/equipment that address a specific ADL or IADL task, such as dressing boards.

References

American Occupational Therapy Association. (2002). Occupational therapy practice framework: Domain and process. *American Journal of Occupational Therapy, 56,* 609-639.

Adler, C., Tipton-Burton, M., & Lehman, R., (1998). Wheelchairs and wheelchair mobility, functional mobility and transfer training, and ambulation aids. In M. Early (Ed.), *Physical dysfunction practice skills for the occupational therapy assistant.* St. Louis: Mosby, 276- 296.

Borel, R. (1994). Shoetying made easy. *OT Week,* January, 19.

Dunn, W. (2000). *Best practice occupational therapy: In community service with children and families.* Thorofare, NJ: SLACK Incorporated.

Egan, M. (1992). Steps to shoe tying success. *OT Week,* September, 20-21.

Jones, L., & Machover, P. (2000). Occupational performance areas: daily living and work and productive activities. In J. Solomon (Ed.). *Pediatric skills for occupational therapy assistants.* St. Louis: Mosby, 211-283.

Orelove, F., & Sobsey, D. (1996). *Educating children with multiple disabilities: A transdisciplinary approach* (3rd ed). Baltimore, MD: Paul H. Brookes.

Pedretti, L., & Umphred, D. (1998) Teaching and learning in occupational therapy. In M. Early (Ed.). *Physical dysfunction practice skills for the occupational therapy assistant.* St. Louis, MO: Mosby, 225-236.

Shepherd J. (2001). Self-care and adaptations for independent living. In J. Case-Smith (Ed.). *Occupational therapy for children* (4th ed.) (pp. 461-503). St. Louis, MO: Mosby.

Shepherd, J., Procter, S., & Coley, I., (1996). Self-care and adaptations for independent living. In J. Case-Smith, A. Allen, & P. Pratt, (Eds). *Occupational therapy for children* (3rd ed). 461-503. St. Louis, MO: Mosby.

Visual Perceptual Dysfunction and Low Vision Rehabilitation

Jennifer Kaldenberg, MSA, OTR/L, CLVT

Chapter Objectives

- Provide an introduction to the visual system.
- Describe the development of vision and visual perceptual skills in children.
- Identify common visual and visual perceptual disorders of childhood.
- Identify common assessment tools used by occupational therapy practitioners in the evaluation of children.
- Describe occupational therapy intervention for specific visual deficits.

Introduction

Vision is a complex sensory system. It provides information about our world and assists individuals in adapting to changes within it. Vision is not just what we see; vision contributes to posture, motor control, communication, cognition, and emotion (Hyvarinen, 1995; Warren, 1994). Children with visual dysfunction experience difficulty with many activities including activities of daily living (ADLs), reading, writing, and play activities. Given the impact that vision has on a child's function and development, occupational therapy practitioners have an important role in the evaluation and treatment of visual dysfunction. This chapter will provide the occupational therapy practitioner a brief review of the visual system, an overview of common visual and visual perceptual disorders seen in childhood, and a guide to evaluation and treatment methods.

Anatomy of the Eye and Visual System

In order to understand dysfunction and appropriate intervention techniques, it is important to be aware of the basic anatomy and function of the eye and visual system (Figure 16-1). The eye functions by bringing light to the retina in order to form an image. This light is transmitted and focused on the retina by the cornea and lens. The cornea is a clear structure through which we see. It plays an important role in focusing and refracting light. The lens is located just behind the iris and assists in bringing light into sharp focus. Located behind the cornea is the iris, the colored portion of the eye. It contains muscles, which open or close the pupil in response to the brightness of light. The light must then pass through the vitreous in order to form the image on the retina. The vitreous is a gel like substance that fills much of the interior of the eye. Due to the way light is refracted onto the retina, the resulting image is upside-down (American Academy of Ophthalmology [AAO], 2001) (Figure 16-2). Once the retina receives light rays from the front of the eye, it is then processed and converted into electrical impulses. The impulses are brought to the brain by the optic nerve and then interpreted as we see our environment, in an upright position (AAO, 2001; The Association for Retinopathy of Prematurity and Related Diseases [ROPARD], 2000).

The eye contains three layers: the sclera, choroid, and retina. The sclera is a white, elastic layer that assists in the stability of the eye. The choroid, a vascular layer located between the sclera and retina nourishes the outer portions of the retina. The thin layer lining the inside of the eye is the retina. The retina is comprised of two types of receptor cells,

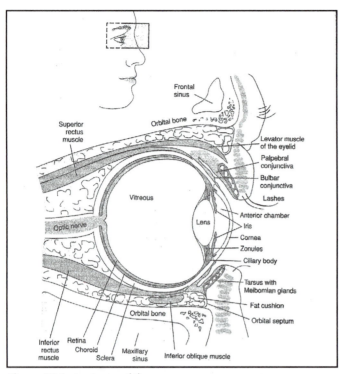

Figure 16-1. Anatomy of the eye.

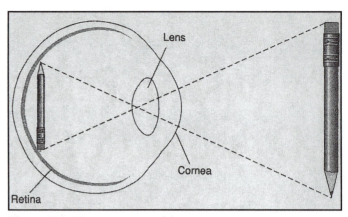

Figure 16-2. How we see an object.

rods and cones. The rods are responsible for night vision, and the cones for color vision. There are a few parts of the retina that have special function. The macula is responsible for central vision and the fovea centralis is the point of best visual acuity.

We have two vision pathways. The peripheral system provides us with general information about our environment. The second system the central system provides detailed information about our environment, including detail and color. When we are born, the only functioning system is the peripheral, yet by 6 months of age, the central system begins to develop. In order to function efficiently in life tasks, the developing child must integrate both systems (Dickson, 2001; Warren, 1994).

Development

At birth, the visual system is immature. The visual pathway and gross anatomical structures are basically developed by 24 weeks gestation, but continue to mature through 6 months of age (Glass, 1993). At birth, children have primary visual fixation and tracking abilities and the acuity to see approximately the distance from the mother's breast to her face (Glass, 1993). Developmentally, "Visual acuity increases rapidly in the first 4 months of life and stabilizes between 2 and 5 years of age. Specifically:

- At 4 weeks, visual acuity is 20/1200
- At 17 weeks, it is 20/200

- At 1 year, it is 20/60
- At 2 years, it is 20/30 (Todd & Tsurumi, 1993, p. 23).

Visual acuity is reported to reach optimal functioning at 18 years of age, and begins to decline thereafter (Schneck, 2001).

Researchers indicate that by 2 months of age, a child's accommodation and convergence (the ability to bring eyes together to focus on an object at near), and oculomotor systems are established (Bouska, Kauffman, & Marcus, 1990). At 5 years of age, maximum accommodation is reached, so that the normally developing child is able to focus for a set period of time from a fixed distance from the object. Tracking skills develop in a sequential pattern from horizontal to vertical, diagonal, and then circular orientations. Based on acquisition of these visual milestones, by kindergarten age, a normally developing child is generally able to focus on the chalkboard and scan his or her environment (Schneck, 2001).

Theories of Visual Function

The following theories attempt to explain how children and adults learn to adapt or use their visual function. These theories assist occupational therapy practitioners in providing the most useful and appropriate evaluation and treatment to meet the needs of the individual child.

WARREN'S HIERARCHY OF VISUAL PERCEPTUAL SKILL DEVELOPMENT

Mary Warren described the development of visual perception as a spiral, such that visual skills interact with one another, with each building upon the previous (Figure 16-3a). In the Warren hierarchy, each level is dependent upon the development of the skills that preceded it. Based on a spiral development pattern, if there is dysfunction in the

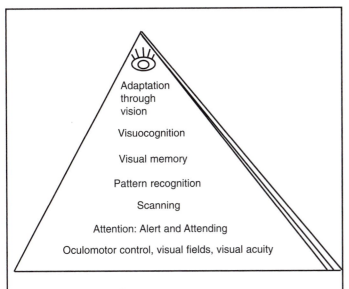

Figure 16-3a. Hierarchy of visual perceptual skill development. Reprinted with permission from Mary Warren.

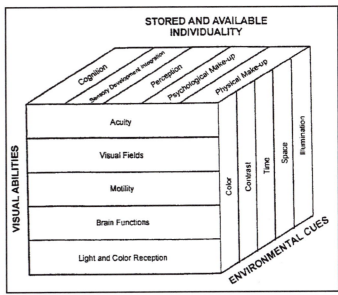

Figure 16-3b. Model of visual functioning. Reprinted with permission from Corn, A. Using technology to enhance cues for children with low vision. *Teaching Exceptional Children, 35*(2), 36-42.

lower levels, higher-level skills will also be impaired. It is important to note that the majority of visual perceptual deficits are found in foundational skills, which include oculomotor control, visual field, and visual acuity (Warren, 1994). These skills are needed in order to form a visual image. Oculomotor control is the ability to control eye movements. Visual field is the area perceived when looking straight ahead (Hyvarinen, 1995), while visual acuity refers to the clarity of the object we perceive. These skills must be integrated in order to proceed to the next higher level of the spiral, which is visual attention, the ability to attend to a stimulus and perceive its detail.

The next skill level is visual scanning, the ability to move the eyes from one object to another. Other terms that may be used interchangeably with visual scanning include saccadic eye movements and visual pursuit. Visual scanning requires the ability to disengage the gaze from one object onto another. The typical scanning pattern in western culture orients from left to right and from top to bottom.

Reflections for the OTA

Individuals whose first language is not read or written from left to right, and top to bottom may have learned a different scanning pattern, which should not be interpreted as abnormal.

Pattern recognition follows scanning in the hierarchy. Pattern recognition is the ability to identify and define features that make an object, an object. Pattern recognition assists in the ability to recognize, match, and categorize objects. This skill is dependent upon a child's ability to scan.

Visual memory is the next skill on the hierarchy, and is the ability to store a visual image of what is perceived.

The top of the hierarchy or most mature visual skill is visuo-cognition, "the ability to mentally manipulate visual information and integrate it with other information in order to solve problems, formulate plans, and make decisions" (Warren, 1994, p. 2). Visuo-cognition provides the basis for classroom learning, and is developed from all previous skills in the hierarchy. Visuo-cognitive skills include, form constancy, visual closure, figure ground, and spatial perception (Warren & Powel, 1998; Warren, 1994). These will be discussed further in the treatment portion of this chapter.

Reflections for the OTA

A child with decreased visual acuity or a limited visual field will have difficulty with visuo-cognitive skills, unless provided compensatory strategies or treatment.

CORN'S THEORY OF LOW VISION

Corn presented a theory of low vision. She proposed that children use three components for visual function (Figure 16-3b). The three components include visual abilities, environmental cues, and stored and available individuality (Corn & Koenig, 1996). For the child to have visual function all components must be minimally functioning. According to Corn, the components of visual ability include visual acuity, visual field, motility (eye movement), brain function and light and color reception, similar to the foundational skills included in Warren's hierarchy. The environmental cues include color, contrast, time, space, and illumination. The

Table 16-1

Symptom Questionnaire: Children

Patient's Full Name:

DOB __/__/__   Date __/__/__   Age _____

Please place a check mark next to any problem that seems to occur often for this child.

Signs of Eye Teaming Problems
Covers or closes one eye when reading
Rubs eyes
Child complains of eyestrain
Child complains of headaches
Child complains of double vision
Child complains of words moving on the page
Inattentive
Poor reading comprehension
Loses place

Signs of Focusing Problems
Child complains of blurred vision
Child complains of blurred vision when looking
   from desk to board
Child complains of eyestrain
Child complains of headaches
Rubs eyes
Inattentive
Poor reading comprehension
Is tired at the end of the day
Holds things very close

Signs of Tracking Problems
Loses place often
Must use finger or guide to keep place
Skips lines and words often
Poor reading comprehension
Short attention span

Signs of Visual Processing Disorders
Trouble learning left from right
Reverses letters and numbers
Mistakes words with similar beginnings
Cannot recognize the same word repeated on a page
Trouble learning basic math concepts of size, magnitude
Poor reading comprehension
Poor recall of visually presented material
Trouble with spelling and sight vocabulary
Sloppy writing skills
Trouble copying from board to book
Erases excessively
Can respond orally but not in writing
Seems to know material but does poorly on written tests

From Scheiman, M. (2002). *Understanding and managing vision deficits: A guide for occupational therapists.* (2nd ed.). Thorofare, NJ: SLACK Incorporated. Reprinted with permission.

---

final component is stored and available individuality; this includes cognition, sensory development integration, perception, psychological make up and physical make up. If a child has decreased visual abilities such as decreased visual acuity, increasing the number of environmental cues may increase the child's ability to function visually.

Reflections for the OTA

For example, a child with 20/100 vision who is working on reading in the classroom, may have improved function given increased illumination, and increased contrast in the printed material. By using additional components and compensating, the child may be able to enhance visual functioning.

Many children with visual deficits will be directly referred to occupational therapy services, while others due to missed or slow diagnosis; may silently struggle through the educational system. There are many signs or red flags that may alert teachers and parents to early diagnosis of visual deficits in children (Scheiman, 2001; Todd & Tsurumi, 1993). These red flags (Table 16-1) may assist in the early detection of childhood visual and visual perceptual dysfunction. When these red flags are observed the child should

be evaluated by the vision team, which may consist of optometrists, ophthalmologists, low vision instructors, orientation and mobility specialists, mental health practitioners, teachers, occupational therapy practitioners, and other professionals as needed. The assessment must look at the whole child, as vision affects all aspects of a child's life. Each member of the team provides important information to develop a treatment plan that will best meet the child's needs.

Goals of Occupational Therapy Intervention

1. To evaluate the functional status of the child (in conjunction with the supervising OTR), with regards to visual perceptual skills, ocular motility, visual system, and functional status at home or in the classroom.

2. To assess the impact of visual dysfunction on learning, play and ADLs.

3. To provide developmentally appropriate low vision and/or visual perceptual intervention to improve the child's visual function.

Table 16-2
Assessment Tools

Assessment Tool	Year	Visual or Visual Perceptual Skills Assessed
Motor Free Visual Perceptual Test (MVPT), (Colarusso & Hamill, 1996)	1996	Spatial relations, visual discrimination, figure ground, visual closure, visual memory
Bruininks Oseretsky Test of Motor Proficiency, Bruininks, R. H. (Bruininks, 1978)	1978	Visual motor control
Jordan Left Right Reversal Test (Jordan, 1990)	1990	Right left orientation, position in space, visual reversal
Visual Skills Appraisal (VSA), Richard, R., et al. (Richards, Oppenheim, & Getman, 1990)	1984	Pursuit, scanning, aligning, locating, eye hand coordination, fixation unity
Test of Visual Perceptual Skills Non Motor (TVPS), (Gardner, 1997)		Visual discrimination, visual memory, visual spatial relations, form constancy, visual memory, figure ground, visual closure
Developmental Test of Visual Perception 2nd Edition (DTVP-2), (Hammill, Pearson, and Voress, 1993)	1993	Eye hand coordination, position in space, copying, figure ground, spatial relations, visual closure, visual motor speed, form constancy
The Developmental Test of Visual Motor Integration (VMI), Beery, K. E. & Buktenica, N.A. (Beery & Buktenica, 1997)	1997	Visual motor integration
Test of Visual Motor Skills (TVMS) Gardner, M. F. (Gardner, 1986)	1986	Visual motor integration
Southern California Sensory Integration Test, (Ayres, 1972)	1972	Visual perceptual sub-tests include: figure ground, position in space, spatial relations, right left discrimination

4. To educate the child, family, and team on visual impairment and provide recommendations for treatment and carryover.

5. In conjunction with the supervising OTR, to provide appropriate referral/ recommendations.

Visual and Visual Perceptual Disorders, Evaluation, and Treatment Methods

The following section provides a brief description of common visual and visual perceptual disorders/ dysfunction and their functional impact on the child. It also provides information regarding common evaluation tools and treatment methods. As this is not meant to be an all-inclusive guide to the evaluation and treatment of visual and visual perceptual disorders, the interested reader is encouraged to pursue further reading (Table 16-2).

RETINOPATHY OF PREMATURITY

Retinopathy of Prematurity (ROP) is one of the most common visual disorders seen in children. As discussed in the development of the eye, the retina and visual system are not fully mature until 40 weeks gestation, yet continues to develop until 6 months of age. ROP occurs in many preterm infants and is the leading cause of blindness in preterm children. In many cases, ROP is associated with severe central nervous system (CNS) damage such as periventricular leukomalacia (Schneck, 2001; ROPARD, 2000). In ROP, the vessels of the eye begin to turn from the retina toward the center of the eye. Many children have laser surgery and other procedures to stop the blood vessels from pulling on the retina. ROP may lead to varying visual disabilities such as visual field loss, decreased visual acuity, loss of binocular (bilateral) vision, visual perceptual dysfunction, and blindness.

Functional Impact

Children with ROP will have varying degrees of dysfunction, ranging from no functional limitation, to complete blindness. Many children will have impaired visual acuity, which magnification may correct. ROP may limit functional performance skills associated with self-care, play, and education. Others with ROP may experience varying degrees of functional impact based on visual field impairments, visual perceptual problems, or complete blindness.

Evaluation

Evaluation is completed through a comprehensive visual assessment including visual acuity, visual field, visual perception, and observation of a child's environment and functional skills.

Treatment Methods

Treatment methods are directed at the identified problem(s). These will be discussed in the following treatment sections.

ALBINISM

Albinism is an inherited disorder in which there is a reduction or absence of melanin pigment in the skin, hair, eye and retina. Visual symptoms include reduced visual acuity, photophobia, nystagmus and strabismus (also refer to disorders of binocular vision and strabismus) (Amos, 1987, Alexander, 1995).

Functional Impact

Children with albinism will have varying degrees of dysfunction, ranging from mild low vision to legal blindness, with visual acuity ranging from 20/60 to 20/400. Children with albinism may struggle with performance skills associated with self-care, play and education.

Evaluation

Evaluation is completed through a comprehensive visual assessment including visual acuity, contrast sensitivity, binocular vision, visual perception, and observation of functional skills and a child's environment.

Treatment Methods

Treatment methods are directed at the identified problem(s). These will be discussed in the following treatment sections.

OCULOMOTOR CONTROL

Oculomotor control is the ability to control eye movements. A common impairment of oculomotor control is nystagmus. Often associated with CNS damage, nystagmus is nonvoluntary, jerky movement of an eye or eyes (Schneck, 2001). Nystagmus makes directing visual gaze a difficult task.

Functional Impact

Children may have slow or inaccurate eye movement as the head may move instead of the eyes, which may then interfere with reading. Children with nystagmus may experience frequent loss of place with reading, writing, and *copying* tasks, and may demonstrate poor eye contact. With nystagmus, the visual image may also be blurry.

Evaluation

Evaluation may be through observation, optometry assessment, eye *dominance* tests, contrast sensitivity tests, visual perceptual testing such as the Visual Skills Appraisal (VSA) and finding null point position.

Treatment Methods

Based on the significance of the dysfunction, treatment will vary. Treatment may include surgery or dispensing of prescription lenses; both of which are completed by optometry or ophthalmology practitioners. Other treatment may include such things as sensory integration therapy, target activities involving moving the visual stimuli from close to far away, ball activities, proper positioning techniques (Diamant, 2000), matching, and dot-to-dot activity sheets.

DISORDERS OF BINOCULAR VISION

Disorders of binocular vision may include strabismus (esotropia, exotropia), convergence insufficiency (difficulty converging the eyes for near tasks), and deficits of stereopsis (vision of three-dimension) (Scheiman, 1997). Strabismus is one of the most common visual disorders seen in children; especially esotropia, the tendency for the eyes to turn in, and exotropia, the tendency for the eyes to turn out (Cotter & Franz, 1997).

Functional Impact

Children may experience double vision, headache, fatigue, difficulty attending to task, difficulty with eye hand coordination tasks, and difficulty with reading and writing tasks. Children with binocular vision problems may experience frequent loss of place with reading, writing, and copying tasks, and may demonstrate poor eye contact. Children with strabismus may also struggle with the cosmetic appearance of the eye/s.

Evaluation

Evaluation may be through observation, optometry assessment, eye dominance tests, stereopsis testing, and visual perceptual testing.

Treatment Methods

Based on the significance of the dysfunction, treatment will vary. Treatment may include surgery, dispensing of prescription lenses, prisms or occlusion, all of which are completed by optometry or ophthalmology practitioners. Other treatment may include environmental assessment, vision therapy, sensory integration therapy, gross and fine motor eye-hand coordination activities, and teaching compensatory strategies for reading and writing tasks.

VISUAL FIELD

Visual field is defined as the area that we see when we are looking straight-ahead (Hyvarinen, 1995). Normal visual field is 60 degrees upward, 60 degrees inward, 70 to 75 degrees downward, 100 to 110 degrees outward (Scheiman, 2001; Warren, 1994).

Functional Impact

Children with visual field deficits may have decreased or slow scanning and focusing abilities, they may miss visual details, and have difficulty with handwriting. They may have impaired mobility (such as on the playground or moving around in their own home), and miss environmental cues (such as changes in walking surface, walls, etc.).

Evaluation

Evaluation may include observation, nonstandardized assessments such as the H-Scan and line bisection test, and automated perimetry, a test of the entire visual field. An optometry practitioner generally administers automated perimetry. Due to age related decreased attention and comprehension abilities, automated perimetry is a difficult evaluation to use with young children.

Treatment Methods

Treatment methods may include education on compensatory strategies, environmental adaptation, use of and training with optical aids (such as prisms and mirrors), reading exercises, functional activities such as word searches, puzzles, board games, ball activities, computer activities, and cards.

VISUAL ACUITY

Visual acuity is the sharpness or clarity of vision based on what is determined to be normative (20/20) vision. Children with partial sight or sight that cannot be fully corrected with surgery or glasses are classified as low vision. Low vision can be categorized as mild impairment to near total blindness (Table 16-3).

Functional Impact

Three of the most common disorders of acuity are myopia, hyperopia, and astigmatism. Myopia is more commonly referred to as near sightedness, or difficulty seeing distances. This is observed in the classroom as difficulty seeing the chalkboard or watching television. Hyperopia or far-sightedness refers to difficulty seeing things at the near. Hyperopia appears as difficulty reading or completing paper and pencil tasks. Astigmatism is an uneven focus on the retina causing a blurred or partial image, leading to complaints of blurry vision at all distances (Scheiman, 2001).

Evaluation

Evaluation for visual acuity is generally completed by an optometrist or ophthalmologist. The most commonly used tool is the Snellen Chart. For the child with low vision, the Feinbloom chart for distance acuity and the Lighthouse Near Acuity Chart may be used. Evaluation provides the optometry practitioner an appropriate prescription for refraction to assist the child to maximize his or her vision. Contrast sensitivity tests may also be completed to determine how well children can see from high to low visual contrasts. This is important to understand because visual contrast influences how teachers, parents, and occupational therapy practitioners should best present information to a child with reduced contrast sensitivity. For example, using white on black vs. black on white handouts, or avoiding use of the chalkboard that has reduced contrast due to smudges and glare may improve the child's performance within class activities.

Treatment Methods

Treatment methods for visual acuity deficits are clearly defined for the occupational therapy practitioner. The role of the occupational therapy practitioner is not to prescribe, but to teach and encourage proper use of the optical aids, and to adapt the environment to maximize independence (Dickson, 2001). Magnifications for near vision include spectacle mounted reading lenses, telescopes, hand magnifiers, stand magnifiers, and electronic devices. Magnifications for distance include telescopes and electronic devices (Fraser, et al, 1997; Nelms, 2000; Riddering, 2001; Scheiman, 2001). When encouraging the proper use of optical aids, the occupational therapy practitioner must keep in mind the needs of the child, the available social supports, financial constraints, and what works best for him or her. Environmental adaptations include lighting, contrast, color, distance, size, and placement of materials or the child. Nonoptical aids may also be used such as writing guides, large faced clocks, large print books, or marking techniques (Figure 16-4).

VISUAL SCANNING

Visual scanning, saccadic eye movement, or visual pursuit is the ability to move one's eye/s from one object to another.

Functional Impact

A child with visual scanning deficits may miss or omit segments of his or her environment or academic assignments. This may affect a child's ability to complete all self-

Table 16-3

Visual Acuity

	Visual Acuity	Visual Field	Classification	Function
Normal to Near Normal Vision	20/15-20/60			No significant limitations. 20/50 near visual acuity is required to read newspaper sized print. Driving may be restricted at end range .
Moderate Impairment	<20/60-20/160		Low Vision Qualify for Special Education Assistance	Functions well with adaptations and aids. May require Orientation and Mobility (O&M) Instruction at end range.
Severe Impairment	<20/160-20/400	Less than or equal to 20 degrees of visual field	Low Vision–"Legal" Blindness–definitions may vary	Functional impairments even with aids. May require O&M instruction.
Profound Impairment	20/500-20/1000	Less than or equal to 10 degrees of visual field	Legal Blindness	Greater Functional impairments even with aids. Ability to read will be limited. O&M Instruction.
Near Total Impairment	<20/1000	Less than or equal to 5 degrees of visual field	Legal Blindness	Greater Functional impairments even with aids. Braille, books on tape. O&M Instruction.
Total Impairment	No light perception		Blindness	IMPAIRED Braille, books on tape. O&M Instruction.

Reprinted with permission from Colenbrander, 2002, ICD-9-CM, 2003.

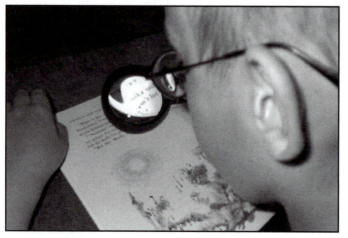

Figure 16-4. Child using magnifier.

care, play, and work skills. Visual scanning deficits may lead to missed details, decreased attention, and decreased ability to obtain information from the environment.

Evaluation

Evaluation may include optometry assessment, observation, structured scans such as the letter scan, mobility assessment, and visual perceptual testing such as the VSA.

Treatment Methods

Treatment methods should be presented in an organized manner, with emphasis placed on accuracy before increasing speed of scanning. Patterns should begin with large movements scanning left to right and then progressing to smaller movements. Prior to introducing binocular work, exercises should begin with one eye at a time. To isolate eye movement, head and neck motions should be avoided during scanning tasks. Functional activities may include matching, computer games, letter boards, community mobility, safety education, education on compensatory strategies (such as color coding or numbering beginning and endings of sentences and scanning strategies to effectively scan his/her environment with head movement), card activities, sorting, adapting or modifying the environment, such as position of chair in the classroom, and increasing contrast to increase a child's awareness of an objects beginning and end.

VISUAL ATTENTION

Visual attention is the ability to attend to an object and perceive its detail.

Functional Impact

Children with visual inattention may demonstrate difficulty maintaining attention to task and be distracted by their environment. They may experience challenges with detail and identifying the most important information from stories and tasks. Shifting focus from one task to another may also be difficult for these children.

Evaluation

Evaluation is commonly done through observation during functional tasks.

Treatment Methods

Treatment methods may include modifying or adapting the environment to increase or decrease arousal. It may also involve increasing or decreasing the amount of stimuli or task length. Activities may include eye-hand coordination activities, copying tasks, computer games, visual scanning (in an organized manner), word searches, matching activities, teaching compensatory strategies such as finger pointing and marking the beginning and end of assignments, and use of multisensory input to compensate for visual inattention.

PATTERN RECOGNITION

Pattern recognition is the ability to identify and define features that make an object an object. For example:

```
LLLLLL        LLLLLL
L    L        L
LLLLLL        LLLL
L    L        L
LLLLLL        LLLLLL
```

Because of pattern recognition, we see the letters B E, but also identify the detail, which in this case is that the letter L makes up each letter (adapted from Warren, 1994). Pattern recognition assists in the ability to recognize, match, and categorize objects. Matching refers to the ability to identify

similar objects, and categorization is the ability to group items based on similarities and differences.

Functional Impact

Children may have difficulty recognizing, matching, and categorizing objects or information. Generally, children with pattern recognition difficulties struggle with all academic tasks. Pattern recognition is also necessary for visual memory.

Evaluation

Evaluation may be completed through observation, contrast sensitivity testing, the Motor-Free Visual Perceptual Test (MVPT), Developmental Test of Visual Perception (DTVP-2), and the Test of Visual Motor Skills (TVPS).

Treatment Methods

Treatment methods may include functional activities such as puzzles, drawing, painting, craft or art tasks, blocks, sorting and matching tasks, copying, computer activities, writing, and reading activities.

VISUAL MEMORY

Visual memory is the ability to store a visual image of what is perceived. For success in school, a child must be able to store and recall a visual image in order to apply it to learning.

Functional Impact

The child may be unable, or demonstrate inaccuracy in recalling or storing objects from memory. Children with visual memory difficulties may also have difficulty with academic tasks and play activities.

Evaluation

Evaluation may include use of the TVPS, Kaufman Assessment Battery for Children (KABC), MVPT, and/or the DTVP-2.

Treatment Methods

Treatment methods may include teaching compensatory strategies such as mnemonics, rehearsal, and imagery (Todd & Tsurumi, 1993), planning and sequencing tasks, such as the game Connect Four™ (Hasbro, East Longmeadow, MA), card activities, and copying. Any educational task may require modification, including changing the amount of information to be recalled, the time requirements, how the information is provided, and/or the sequence of the task.

VISUO-COGNITION

Visuo-cognition is the ability to use visual information to solve problems, plan, and make decisions (Warren, 1994). Visuo-cognition provides the basis for all classroom learn-

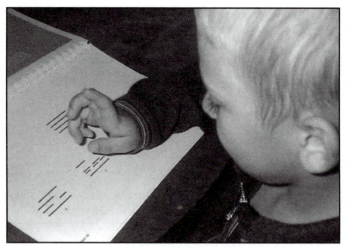

Figure 16-5. Child completing MVPT.

ing, and builds on all previous visual perceptual skills. Visuo-cognitive skills include, form constancy, visual closure, figure ground, and spatial perception (position in space and depth perception).

FORM CONSTANCY

Form constancy is the ability to identify an object based on its form, even when it varies in size or position.

Functional Impact

Form constancy may impair a child's ability to read or identify printed versus cursive writing. Children with form constancy problems will have difficulty identifying subtle variations in form or may confuse similar objects. Identifying errors in assignments such as writing will also be difficult for children with form constancy problems.

Evaluation

Evaluation may involve administration of the MVPT, DTVP-2, and the TVPS (Figure 16-5).

Treatment Methods

Treatment methods may include writing exercises, chalkboard activities, parquetry, sorting activities, computer games, paper pencil tasks, matching activities, and scanning activities that require the child to identify similar shapes or letters.

VISUAL CLOSURE

Visual closure is the ability to recognize an object in its incomplete form.

Functional Impact

Due to the inability to anticipate a visual form or word, difficulty with visual closure may slow the processing of visual information. The child may demonstrate errors in identifying objects, signs, or written information presented in incomplete form.

Evaluation

Evaluation may include the use of the MVPT, DTP-2, TVPS, and Contrast Sensitivity Tests.

Treatment Methods

Treatment methods may include puzzles, word searches, parquetry, block designs, or visual-motor tasks oriented in different planes or distances.

FIGURE GROUND

Figure ground is the ability to identify the foreground from the background.

Functional Impact

Children may have difficulty copying figures and writing. Difficulty with figure ground may also interfere with the completion of mathematical equations. Children with figure ground problems may experience difficulty with sorting, and identifying specific objects when placed among other similar or dissimilar objects.

Evaluation

Evaluation may include use of the DTVP-2, MVPT, and the Ayres Figure Ground Subtest of the Southern California Sensory Integration Test (SIPT).

Treatment Methods

Treatment methods may include increasing contrast (black and white is optimal), teaching scanning techniques to identify key points of information, bean bag activities with targets, color code information to increase the child's awareness of figure ground, and sorting and matching activities.

POSITION IN SPACE

Position in space is the awareness of the position of an object in relationship to one's self (laterality) and other objects (directionality).

Functional Impact

Position in space is essential for reading and writing skills. Children with position in space difficulties often struggle with these tasks. Children with position in space problems may also have impaired safety awareness or decreased sense of personal space. The concepts of directionality such as in, out, or on top of may also be diminished.

Evaluation

Evaluation may be completed through the Ayres Position in Space Sub-Test of the Southern California Sensory Integration Test, DTVP-2, TVPS, and Jordan Left Right Reversal Test.

Treatment Methods

Treatment methods may include chalkboard activities, writing exercises, adaptation or modification of the environment (such as marking the floor for child's place in line), writing tablets with color coded lines for beginning and ending of letters, games such as Simon Says (laterality), treasure hunt, and map activities.

DEPTH PERCEPTION

Depth perception is the ability to identify the distance from one's self and an object.

Functional Impact

A child with depth perception difficulties may experience impaired mobility and safety with such things as changes in walking surfaces or stairways. Depth perception difficulties may impact a child's performance in physical education with such tasks as catching a ball, or walking on a balance beam. Mathematical concepts, such as geometry, may also be difficult for children with depth perception difficulties. Additionally, children with depth perception difficulties may experience challenges with all aspects of self-care and play.

Evaluation

Evaluation may be completed through observation, DTVP-2, TVPS, and functional mobility assessments.

Treatment Methods

Treatment methods may include increasing contrast, adapting or modifying the environment by marking the top and bottom step with a high contrast color to promote increase awareness, paper, pencil, and cutting tasks, ball toss and catching activities, eye hand coordination tasks, compensatory strategies, and community mobility tasks.

Summary

Vision contributes to communication, postural control, and mobility (Warren, 1994). As the majority of communication is nonverbal, the child who misses visual detail may also miss important information within a conversation. As occupational therapy practitioners, it is important to make others aware of this discontinuity and provide the child with

visual challenges increased verbal information. In addition, vision also provides an individual the ability to anticipate and adapt to changes within the environment. When vision is compromised, the child may demonstrate postural insecurity and impaired mobility (Warren, 1994). The child may move slowly or bump into things. The child may have to adjust his or her head to put an object into view, which may then cause the child to make postural adjustments in order to maintain balance. When a child has difficulty with depth perception, visual acuity, or binocularity, the environment becomes very difficult to predict, causing the child to become insecure and less likely to explore without correction or other sensory input (Corn & Koenig, 1996). Awareness of how vision affects the child's function, and provision of appropriate compensatory and educational carry-over strategies to the child, the family, and team members is critical.

Based on treatment methods, the occupational therapy practitioner must consider the goals of treatment and the interest and needs of the child. The occupational therapy practitioner must also adapt or modify the environment to maximize the child's function. Potential adaptations could include examination of lighting, positioning of the child in regards to desk placement, distance from chalkboard and light source, and assessment of obstacles present in the child's environment. For example, illumination is optimal if directed over the child's shoulders on to the work surface. Children should not face windows, as this increases glare. The child's environment should be assessed to keep it free from obstacles or hazards. Further, the child's placement within the classroom must be based on the nature of the specific visual or visual perceptual deficits. For instance, to optimize the child's performance a child with visual acuity problems should be placed in the front row. Every child with visual perception difficulties presents with individual challenges, and as such, must receive individualized attention in developing the most functional environment possible.

To maximize the child's performance, the occupational therapy practitioner must look for carryover of therapeutic effect. This can be completed through educational means directed toward a child's awareness of his or her abilities and limitations, and how the limitations may affect his/her performance. In addition, the family and rehabilitation or educational team needs to be made cognizant of a child's specific deficits and recommendations for carryover.

This chapter provided the occupational therapy practitioner with a brief discussion of the visual system, an overview of common visual and visual perceptual disorders identified in childhood, and a guide to the evaluation and treatment of children with visual and visual perceptual dysfunction. As discussed, vision has a significant impact on a child's function and development. Occupational therapy practitioners have an important role in the evaluation and treatment of visual dysfunction. Continued research and technology continue to shape and mold the occupational therapy practitioner's role.

Case Study

Tyler is a 6-year-old entering the first grade. He was born at 26 weeks gestation and has bilateral retinopathy of prematurity. He has light perception in the right eye and 20/200 uncorrected, 20/80 corrected visual acuity in the left eye. Tyler is currently struggling with reading and writing tasks.

DISCUSSION QUESTIONS

1. What visual and visual perceptual skills could be impaired?

2. What recommendations would you make to assist Tyler with these skills?

3. How would you modify or adapt the environment to maximize Tyler's performance?

Application Activities

1. Produce or fabricate one developmentally appropriate activities for each visual skill discussed in this chapter.

2. Prepare a list of other team members who may be appropriate for providing additional services for children with visual skills deficits.

References

Alexander, K. L. (1995). *The Lippincott manual of primary eye care.* Philadelphia, PA: J. B. Lippincott Company, pp. 453-454.

American Academy of Ophthalmology (AAO). (2001). [On-line] Available: www.eyenet.org

Amos, J. F. (1987). *Diagnosis and management in vision care.* Boston, MA: Butterworth-Heinemann, pp. 276-272.

Ayres, A. J. (1972). *The Southern California sensory integration test.* Los Angeles, CA: Western Psychological Services.

Beery, K. E., & Buktenica, N. A. (1997). *The developmental test of visual motor integration, examiner's manual.* Cleveland, OH: Modern Curriculum Press.

Bouska, M. J., Kauffman, N. A., & Marcus, S. E. (1990). Disorders of the visual perception system. In D. Umphred (Ed.), *Neurological rehabilitation* (2nd ed.). pp. 522-585. St. Louis, MO: Mosby.

Bruininks, R. H. (1978). *Bruininks-Oseretsky test of motor proficiency, examiner's manual.* Circle Pines, MN: American Guidance Service.

Cassel, G. H., Billig, M. D., & Randall, H. G. (1998). *The eye book: Complete guide to eye disorders and health.* Baltimore: The Johns Hopkins University Press.

Colarusso, R., & Hammill, D. (1996). *Motor free visual perceptual test, examiner's manual.* Novato, CA: Academic Therapy Publications, Inc.

Colenbrander, A. (2002). *Visual standards-aspects and ranges of vision loss.* Sydney: International Council of Ophthalmology.

Corn, A. L., & Koenig, A. J. (1996) Perspectives on low vision. In A.L Corn & A. J Koenig (Eds.), *Foundations of low vision clinical and functional perspectives* (pp. 3-25). New York, NY: AFB Press.

Cotter, S. A. & Frantz, K. A. (1997). Strabismus: Detection, diagnosis & classification. In B. D. Moore (Ed.), *Eye care for infants and young children.* Boston, MA: Butterworth-Heinemann, 123-154.

Diamant, R. (2000). Partnering with parents: Guidelines for positioning and play. *OT Practice,* 15-18.

Dickson, P. (2001). Paul Dickson's family vision care center, Hamilton, New Zealand. [On-line] Available: www.vision-care.co.nz/who.html/

Downing-Baum, S. (1995). Exercises in pediatric vision therapy. *OT Week,* 20-23.

Fraser, K. E., et al. (1997). *Optometric clinical practice guidelines: Care of the patient with low vision.* St. Louis, MO: American Optometric Association.

Gardner, M. F. (1997). *The developmental test of visual perceptual skills (non-motor), examiner's manual.* Burlington, CA: Psychological and Educational Publications.

Gardner, M. F. (1986). *Test of visual motor skills, examiner's manual.* San Francisco, CA: Children's Hospital of San Francisco.

Glass, P. (1993). Development of visual function in preterm infants: Implication for early intervention. *Infants and Young Children, 6*(1), 11-20.

Hammill, D. D., Pearson, N. A., & Voress, J. K. (1993). *Developmental test of visual perception, examiner's manual* (2nd ed.). Austin, TX: Pro-ed.

Hyvarinen, L. (1995). Considerations in evaluation and treatment of the child with low vision. *American Journal of Occupational Therapy, 49*(9), 891-897.

International Classification of Diseases, 9th Revision-Clinical Modification (ICD-9-CM). (2003). Los Angeles, Practice Management Information Corporation, 256-258.

Jordan, B. T. (1990). *Jordan left right reversal test, examiner's manual* (3rd ed.). Novato, CA: Academic Therapy Publications, Inc.

Moore, B. D. (1987). *Eye care for infants and young children.* Boston, MA: Butterworth-Heineman.

Nelms, A. C. (2000). New vision. *OT Practice,* 14-18.

Richards, R., Oppenheim, G., & Getman, G. N. (1984). *Visual skills appraisal, examiner's manual.* Novato, CA: Academic Therapy Publications, Inc.

Riddering, A. (2001). Geriatric low-vision rehab: An introduction. *OT Practice,* 17-22.

Scheiman, M. (2002). *Understanding and managing vision deficits: A guide for occupational therapists* (2nd ed.). Thorofare, NJ: SLACK Incorporated.

Schneck, C. M. (2001). Visual perception. In J. Case-Smith (Ed.), *Occupational therapy for children* (pp. 382-412). St. Louis, MO: Mosby.

St. Luke's Cataract & Laser Institute. (2000). [On-line] Available: www.stlukeseye.com.

The Association for Retinopathy of Prematurity and Related Diseases. (2000). [On-line] Available: www.ropard.org.

Todd, V., & Tsurumi, K. (1993). *A second look: "Visual perceptual disorders" in children.* Conference conducted at Woodbridge, NJ.

Warren, M., & Powel, S. (1998). Treatment of visual deficits. In M. B. Early (Ed.), *Physical dysfunction practice skills for the occupational therapy assistant* (pp. 397-409). St. Louis, MO: Mosby.

Warren, M. (1994). *Evaluation and treatment of visual perceptual dysfunction.* Rocky Mount, NC: Advanced Rehabilitation Institutes. Presentation conducted in Boston.

Warren, M. (1993). A hierarchical model for evaluation and treatment of visual perceptual dysfunction in adult acquired brain injury. Part 1. *American Journal of Occupational Therapy, 47,* 42-54.

17

HAND DEVELOPMENT

Sandra J. Edwards, MA, OTR, FAOTA
Jenna D. McCoy-Powlen, MS, OTR/L
Donna Buckland Gallen, MS, OTR/L

Chapter Objectives

- Provide an overview of relationship of hand skills to cognition, language development, trunk control, visual motor coordination, and sensory function.
- Describe typical development of hand reflexes that impact grasp and the development of reach, grasp, release, bilateral skills, in-hand manipulation skills, and hand dominance.
- Explain application activities for treatment of hand skills.

Introduction

The study of the development of hand skills is fascinating and important for occupational therapy (OT) practitioners in order to understand and effectively treat children. Children's primary occupations of play, work, and self-care all depend on adequate hand skills. The development of cognition, language and communication, trunk strength, motor skills, visual motor, and sensory function are also dependent on hand skills because hands are used to explore and learn about the environment. For instance, through exploration of new toys and objects, hands help children develop cognitive skills, and through gestures, help children communicate and interact with others. Through visually guided reach, grasp, pointing, and eventually, manipulation, children develop and refine precise motor skills of the hands. Children also use their hands to experience a variety of sensations, such as the weight, shape, texture, and sound of various objects, and to develop peer relationships, such as engaging in a shared game of stacking blocks or playing a board game. This chapter offers insights into how hand skills develop and help children successfully interact with their environment.

Hand Skills and Cognition

The abundance of information the hands take in about the properties of objects aids in cognitive development. An infant with limited opportunity to explore objects has less opportunity to learn about the properties of objects, which may in turn have a negative impact on his/her cognitive development (Ruff, McCarton, Kurtzberg, & Vaughan, 1984).

Hand Skills and Language Development

Hand skills and language development are connected in a number of ways. Infants may gesture and communicate with their hands before speaking more than a few words. This is because hand skills develop before small movements of the tongue necessary for speaking. The hands also help with language development by exploring the environment and gaining information about the objects one encounters. Ruff (1984) speculates that infants and children categorize objects while exploring them, thus affecting early language development.

Hand Skills and Trunk Control and Motor Development

Postural control or trunk control is important for creating a stable base for the hands and arms. Motor skills involve upper and lower limb coordination, which requires movement of large and small muscles. The large muscle movements are called gross motor skills (such as creeping and walking) and the fine movements are called fine motor skills (such as picking up a bead and writing). Large movements of the shoulder develop before fine hand movements. For instance, at 6 months, children can feed themselves using a whole hand grasp, and by 2 years, improved precision and control enable rotation of the forearm to scoop with a spoon held in the hand. OT practitioners offer activities that provide an opportunity to use the hands and body, and to assist with the development of manipulation skills.

Hand Skills and Visual Motor Development

"Vision is an important motivator that leads the hand into space and serves to facilitate grasp and manipulation" (Pehoski, 1995, p. 140). The first stage of visually guided reaching or eye-hand coordination is typically seen around 2 to 3 months when an infant starts to visually inspect his/her own hand, and is followed by visually guided swiping. Around 4 months, an infant begins to use vision to assist in the exploration of objects rather then the hand and mouth and by 5 months, using the hands to inspect an object is so dependent upon vision that if vision is occluded, inspection of the object is highly diminished (Rochat, 1989). Eye hand coordination is necessary for mastery of most occupations of childhood such as feeding, writing, dressing, using a computer, and playing sports.

Hand Skills and Sensory Functions

Infants use a number of techniques to explore toys, beginning with using the hand to bring toys to the mouth. An infant's hand begins to take on a larger role in exploring objects around the 4th month. At this age, the infant begins to finger objects, which is the first way of providing information about object properties using the hand. This milestone is seen as the first differentiation between the hands two basic functions: grasping and exploration (Rochat, 1989). Up until this point, the hand was only used for grasping. As an infant develops, the exploration of objects changes depending on the texture, shape, or property of the object (Ruff, 1984). This sensory information guides the hand to precisely grasp an object, while providing information such as position, dimension, weight, and force needed to secure the object (Edwards, Buckland, & McCoy-Powlen, 2002).

Typical Progression of Hand Skills

It is important to understand that every infant and child develops at his or her own pace, therefore the information provided below should be used as a general guide for the developing child. This information may be used to help ascertain if an infant is developing new skills, which are important for planning appropriate treatment. Further, *dynamical theory* asserts that infants and children do not always develop skills in the typical sequential pattern. For instance an infant may not hold a bottle at the expected age if the opportunity to learn this skill was never offered. Therefore it is important to look at many factors when planning effective treatment.

The development of grasp and release is a gradual process that is observed as the infant grows. In fact, the development of grasp starts long before an infant reaches for a toy. At birth, the infant lacks volitional control over the body. Instead, reflexes control the newborn's movements, which automatically occur when the baby is moved in a certain manner. As the infant develops, reflexive behavior changes, and with these changes the infant begins the developmental journey toward purposeful hand use. Please refer to the Developmental Milestones Chart in the back of the book for more information.

Reflexes

At birth, the infant has fisted hands, flexed elbows, and adducted shoulders. The infant's movements are controlled by reflexive behaviors. The development of voluntary grasp is related to the automatic grasping reflexes (*traction response*, grasp reflex, *instinctive grasp reaction*), and their equilibrium with the *avoiding response*. The asymmetrical tonic neck reflex (ATNR) also plays a role in this process. The emergence and integration of these reflexes, along with the infant's interaction with the environment plays a vital role in the acquisition of hand skills (Edwards et al., 2002). Table 17-1 shows a more detailed discussion of these reflexes and their influence on the development of hand skills. Also, please refer to the Major Infant Reflexes Chart found in the Appendices.

Reaching

As previously discussed, flexor patterns predominate an infant's first posture, with reflexive patterns dominating

Table 17-1
Reflexes

Reflex	Emergence	Integration	How to Elicit and What To Observe	Influence on Hand Development
Asymmetrical tonic neck reflex (ATNR)	Present at birth	4-6 months of age	Turning the infant's head to the left or right leads to lateral extension of arm and leg on head/face side and contralateral flexion of other arm and leg	The presence of the ATNR encourages hand regard on the side of arm extension. When the infant begins to swipe at objects, it is with this extended arm that these movements occur.
Traction response	Present at birth	2-5 months of age	Pulling the infant's arm into shoulder flexion leads to flexion of all the joints of the arm including the shoulder, elbow, wrist, and fingers.	An integrated traction response is necessary for reaching with an open hand in order to grasp. A persistence of this reflex will inhibit reach, grasp, and object exploration.
Avoiding response	Soon after birth	6 months of age	Light contact to the back of the hand leads to hand and arm withdrawal from the stimulus (Ammon & Etzel, 1977).	The avoiding response helps to offset the grasp reflex by assisting with release of an object.
Grasp reflex	As the traction response begins to fade	6-9 months of age	Pressure to the palm elicits finger flexion and adduction.	Enables the infant to grasp objects, and over time, becomes more purposeful and less reflexive. As the grasp reflex develops, if only one finger is stimulated, isolated flexion of that finger is observed, a precursor to voluntary fin ger individuation.
Instinctive grasp response reaction	After the grasp reflex emerges	10 months of age	A light contact stimulus to the hand leads to grasp.	Helps adjust hand position according to the position of the object to be grasped.

movement patterns. Arms are held close to the body with the hands fisted and thumbs close to the palm of the hand. Initially the infant's arms move in an asymmetrical pattern, yet in time, he/she will move an arm toward an object held near the hand. Table 17-2 describes the typical progression of the development of reach skills.

Grasp

The development of grasp skills begins with the involuntary grasp reflex and in time, progress to precise and refined voluntary movements of the fingers. Table 17-3 describes the typical progression of the development of grasp skills.

Release

As previously stated, the development of release is progressive. Unlike grasp development, development of release does not have specific names given to each stage, but specific developmental advancements can be noted. Similar to grasp development, the need for external support is necessary when the infant is learning a new release skill, but as the hand becomes more stable, the need for external support fades. The need for external support ebbs and flows as the infant begins to practice a new grasp or release pattern. Table 17-4 describes the typical pattern of the acquisition of release skills.

Bilateral Manipulation

The ability to bring the hands to midline at approximately 3 months is the first step towards bilateral hand use. By 5 months, the infant is able to demonstrate a crude transfer of an object between hands (Case-Smith, 1995). An example of this would be a toy pulled out of the holding hand by the receiving hand. These first transfers are often accidental, but as bilateral skills continue to emerge, transferring objects

Table 17-2

Development of Reach Skills

Age	Pattern
Birth to 3 months	Often an infant's first attempts at reach are when positioned in supine. These first attempts are described as more of a swiping motion, in which the infant will look toward an object and attempt to contact it with a full arm movement and closed fist (Gilfoyle, Grady, & Moore, 1990). Placing an infant in the prone position helps to develop the strength in the upper body needed for reaching. Initially the infant rests on the head, arms, and shoulders when placed in the prone position, but as strength improves, begins to raise the head to visually explore the environment.
3 months	In supine, the infant begins to direct arm movements, first to one side or the other, and then towards midline. The infant is unable to grasp the object due to the reflexive fisted hand position. The infant also begins to raise the upper trunk while propped on forearms.
5 months	Bringing an object and trapping it against the body at midline develops. The infant uses both hands to secure the object, but since the object is held against the body, it is not actually grasped. As the infant develops, the arms and hands begin to move farther away from the body and begin to reach and grasp objects, but the approach of the reach is not always direct. Frequently the infant will need to correct or redirect the angle of the reach to actually grasp the desired object. With practice and increased strength, the infant begins to shift weight to one side and reach for a desired toy (i.e., reaches for a desired toy with the left arm while shifting weight to the right). Yet, the hands initially remain fisted, so the object is actually moved toward the body and not grasped, leading to many unsuccessful attempts at obtaining the toy.
6 months	When in a supine position, the infant can reach toward and grasp an object using a wide circular approach; redirection is often necessary. Soon, the infant is able to reach for and grasp objects with a direct approach. Reach continues to develop in prone, so that the infant successfully reaches and grasps a desired object when weight shift to the side occurs.
7 months	The infant will soon assume and maintain a hands and knees position and with practice and increased strength, will shift weight in this position so that reaching and grasping for a desired object while supporting body weight on the knees and opposite hand is possible.

from hand to hand becomes more purposeful (Gilfoyle et al., 1990). Once hand-to-hand transfer has developed, an infant may passively hold the object with one hand while the other hand explores its contours.

By 7 months, the infant uses bilateral hand movements to manipulate objects. The two hands work together so that one hand stabilizes an object while the other hand pokes or fingers the object. After 7 months, infants are able to manipulate an object held in each hand at the same time, like banging two blocks together (Case-Smith, 1995). It is important to note during the observation of this activity that banging two blocks together involves the movement of both hands/arm. Holding a block passively in one hand while banging it with a block held in the other hand is a more primitive developmental skill than banging blocks together with active movement of both arms. Typically around 8 to 9 months, after banging two toys together, the infant starts to experiment with clapping the hands together (Folio & Fewell, 1983).

Between 12 months and 2 years, the toddler makes great developmental strides in the control needed for bimanual skills (Bruner, in Pehoski, 1995). Bimanual hand use is seen when both hands perform complementary actions at the same time. Speed, accuracy, and dexterity of these skills improve. Complexity of motor patterns also increases. By 15 months, a toddler begins to use one arm to stabilize an object while the other manipulates it. These skills enable the toddler to perform activities such as stabilizing a bowl while using a spoon to self-feed or scribbling with a crayon while stabilizing the paper (Case-Smith, 1995).

Between 18 months and 2 years, the ability to use both hands together in a complementary action is also developing (Gilfoyle et al., 1990). This action occurs when both hands are actively manipulating at the same time. An example of this skill is stringing beads. When a child is performing this activity, one hand is holding the bead while the other must grasp and maneuver the string through the bead. Then, the bead must be transferred between the two hands to complete the action. This activity requires complementary hand movements. This skill is typically not attained until the second birthday, and is necessary for some activities of daily living, such as pulling up pants or socks (Pehoski, 1995). This is an important developmental milestone because to accomplish this, the toddler must be able to motor plan two different but complementary actions with the hands. The ability to use both hands in a complementary action continues to be expanded and refined as the child continues to develop, becoming more complex, skilled, and smooth over the years.

Table 17-3

Development of Grasp Skills

	Age Ranges	Arm Position	Observable Form and Function
Reflex Squeeze	around the 4th month	The infant's hand extends beyond the desired object (Halverson, 1931) and upon contact pulls the object toward the body (Gilfoyle et al., 1990)	The infant is unable to manipulate the object, but rather holds the object against the body, and eventually involuntarily drops the object. At this stage, grasp remains reflexive and is initiated by touching or moving an object through the palm (Case-Smith, 1995).
Crude Palmar Grasp	4th to 5th month	The infant reaches for an object and upon contact, simultaneous flexion of all fingers press the object firmly against the heel of the hand. The thumb does not play a role in pressing the object into the palm (Case-Smith, 1995).	The infant's forearm must be supported while grasping the object, but once grasped, the infant is able to bring the object to midline for exploration. This grasp is clumsy and often unsuccessful (Case-Smith & Bigsby, 2000). This grasp is adapted from scratching, which is the alternating pattern between flexion and extension when the fingers come in contact with a surface. Scratching is often seen when an infant is in the prone on elbows position.
Palmar Grasp	5th to 6th month	"This grasp is characterized by the child putting the pronated hand down on the object, the fingers flex simultaneously around the object to secure it in the midsection of the palm" (Edwards et al., 2002, p. 48).	Every object is held in the palm of the hand regardless of size; therefore, small objects are often lost in the palm (Gilfoyle et al., 1990).
Radial Palmar Grasp (Figure 17-1)	6th to 7th month	The index and middle fingers flex around the object as the the thumb begins to assist the fingers with pressing the object into the palm. The thumb becomes more active as the grasp matures (Case-Smith, 1995). The ring and little finger (ulnar digits) flex into the palm to provide stability for the radial side of the hand.	This is a significant development for the infant as this digit differentiation is used throughout life to provide strength and stability to the hand during grasp.

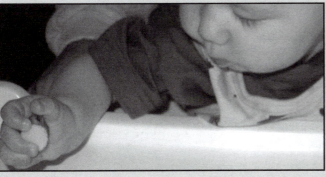

Figure 17-1. Reprinted from Edwards, S., Buckland, D., & McCoy-Powlen, J. (2002). *Developmental & functional hand grasps*. Thorofare, NJ: SLACK Incorporated. Used with permission.

Raking Grasp	7th to 8th month	The hand is held in a rake like position, with the fingers flexed at the IP joints; the arm moves as a unit to "rake" the object into the palm (Bruni, 1998).	This grasp is not always successful and stabilization of the arm may be necessary to actually grasp the object. Infants typically use this grasp to rake small pieces of food into their palms off the highchair tray.

<u>Table 17-3 (continued)</u>
Development of Grasp Skills

	Age Ranges	*Arm Position*	*Observable Form and Function*
Radial Digital Grasp (Figure 17-2)	8th to 9th month	When the forearm is held in a neutral position, the infant is now able to grasp an object with the fingers rather than having it locked in the palm of the hand. The object is held proximal to the pads of the radial fingers; but the infant lacks the control and stability to hold the object at the fingertips. The ulnar digits are flexed into the palm for stability.	A gap now exists between the object and the palm (Edwards, et al., 2002), which differentiates this grasp from the radial palmar grasp. Now that the object is out of the palm, the infant can begin to manipulate the object. The thumb is beginning to oppose the radial fingers. Opposition, or rotation of the thumb toward the other fingers, is significant for the developing child as it provides the opportunity to use precision grasping. The differentiation of the two sides of the hand allows the infant to grasp two small objects at the same time, such as holding two small cubes, one pressed against the palm by the little and ring finger and another help by the radial digits. The neutral forearm position enables increased visual regard for objects, which in turn allows the infant to better direct the grasp.

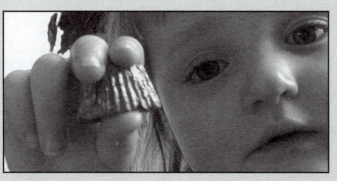

Figure 17-2. Reprinted from Edwards, S., Buckland, D., & McCoy-Powlen, J. (2002). *Developmental & functional hand grasps*. Thorofare, NJ: SLACK Incorporated. Used with permission.

Developmental Scissors Grasp	8th to 9th month	This grasp is characterized by securing an object between the adducted thumb and radial side of the flexed index finger (Edwards et al., 2002). The thumb is not opposed but instead traps the object against the index finger by adduction, which precludes object manipulation.	This grasp was named scissors closure by Castner (1932) because the movement of the thumb being drawn to the index finger is similar to the motion of scissors opening and closing.
Inferior Pincer Grasp (Figure 17-3)	8th to 9th month	"This grasp is characterized by thumb adduction and emerging opposition to secure the object against the extended index finger" (Edwards et al., 2002, p. 53). The object is not yet held at the fingertips. The precision needed for a fingertip grasp has not yet developed at this age. The ulnar three digits are flexed into the palm for support and stability.	The independent movement of the index finger is necessary for more precise patterns of grasp. Index finger probing, when an infant uses an index finger to poke and explore and object, is a precursor to this grasp (Gilfoyle et al., 1990). The independent movement of the index finger is necessary for more precise patterns of grasp.

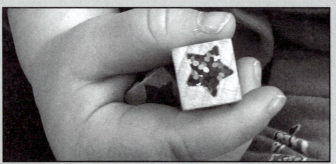

Figure 17-3. Reprinted from Edwards, S., Buckland, D., & McCoy-Powlen, J. (2002). *Developmental & functional hand grasps*. Thorofare, NJ: SLACK Incorporated. Used with permission.

Table 17-3 (continued)

Development of Grasp Skills

	Age Ranges	*Arm Position*	*Observable Form and Function*
Three Jaw Chuck (Figure 17-4)	10th to 11th month	Characterized by thumb opposition to the index and middle fingers. The object continues to be held at the finger and thumb pads as opposed to the fingertips.	The ulnar two digits do not participate in grasping the object but instead provide stability to the radial side of the hand. This grasp is the infant's first use of the tripod posture, which is used for holding a spoon and using a pencil (Edwards et al., 2002). The pads of the fingers and thumb secure the object instead of the radial digits flexing around the object (Halverson, 1931).

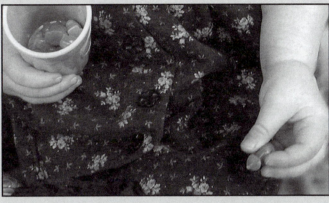

Figure 17-4. Reprinted from Edwards, S., Buckland, D., & McCoy-Powlen, J. (2002). *Developmental & functional hand grasps*. Thorofare, NJ: SLACK Incorporated. Used with permission.

Pincer Grasp	10th to12th month	The thumb is opposed and the object continues to be held at the pad of the finger. The ulnar digits are flexed into the palm.	Holding an object between the thumb and index or middle finger characterizes this grasp. Minimal arm support is needed for the child to pick up the object.
Neat Pincer Grasp (Figure 17-5)	10th to 12th month	Securing an object between the opposed thumb and the finger-tip of the index or middle finger characterizes this grasp. When the opposed thumb and index fingertip are touching, the web space between the two should look like an O (giving the OK sign).	The ability to position and maintain a desired degree of flexion and extension of the finger and thumb allow for precise fingertip control. At this point in development, the infant does not need external support for successful grasp. The forearm is in a neutral position increasing visual regard.

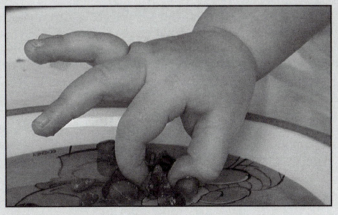

Figure 17-5. Reprinted from Edwards, S., Buckland, D., & McCoy-Powlen, J. (2002). *Developmental & functional hand grasps*. Thorofare, NJ: SLACK Incorporated. Used with permission.

Table 17-4

Development of Release Skills

Age	Observable Patterns
Birth to 4 months	Grasp and release is reflexive and is controlled by either fully flexed or fully extended fingers. Infants will briefly hold onto an object placed in the hand. The grasp reflex facilitates flexion and the avoiding response facilitates finger extension (Gilfoyle et al., 1990). If the grasp reflex is stimulated, the fingers will be tightly flexed around the object until the hand touches a surface and elicits the avoiding response and the object is dropped or released
By 4 months	The infant begins to bring hands to both midline and to mouth. Mouthing objects assists with early release patterns as the mouth acts as a stabilizer. Initially, releasing a larger sized object from one hand to the other is not smooth as the object is actually pulled from the holding hand by the receiving hand, which is stabilizing the object for transfer (Gilfoyle et al., 1990).
By 7 months	An infant can transfer a small cube smoothly between the hands. It is around this age that the infant begins to fling objects off of a supporting surface such as a highchair by using full arm and finger extension. As the infant develops, the flinging motion is no longer needed, but the fingers continue to fully extend, thus limiting accuracy with release.
By 9 months	Release becomes more refined, the infant is able to release a cube into a large container and transfer a small pea sized object between the hands (Erhardt, 1994). Up until this age, the child was unable to transfer a small object between the hands.
By 12 months	The infant is able to precisely release cubes into a small container (Erhardt, 1994). As the infant develops increased control over finger extension, graded extension of the fingers during release is observed. The infant may continue to rely on external support to the forearm and wrist for graded extension of the fingers or may use pressure on an object to assist with release.
By 15 months	The infant demonstrates increased precision by releasing a small object into a small container (Erhardt, 1994). Over the next few years, increased control over the release of objects as demonstrated by graded extension and precise release will develop.

In-Hand Manipulation

In-hand manipulation refers to adjustment of a toy or object in one hand in order to place, use, or let go of it. These processes occur in the hand without contact with the table, and are categorized into patterns of translation, shift, and rotation (Exner, 1992). These basic patterns of in-hand manipulation coupled with dexterity and motor control are important ingredients for successfully carrying out childhood occupations such as fastening and unfastening clothing, using utensils, picking up coins, using school tools, and playing games.

A child typically acquires control of the hand, fingers, and thumb during the first 12 months of life by using isolated finger movement as well as the finger tips to oppose with the rotated thumb for grasping (Edwards et al., 2002). However, to manipulate objects they must continue to refine these skills for the next several years. From 2-6 years, development of these skills are practiced and honed into functional movement. First, the *extrinsic muscles* of the arm as well as bilateral hand movements enable the child to begin to manipulate objects. For instance, a child may transfer a pop bead from the left to the right hand in order to reposi-

tion it for putting together two pop beads. After the extrinsic muscles and bilateral manipulation develops, the child progresses to using the *intrinsic muscles* of the hand. This involves using one hand to manipulate objects such as repositioning a bead in order to string it. Acquisition of proficient in-hand manipulation skills is enhanced, in part, through ample practice opportunities.

While several researchers have defined in-hand manipulation, Exner's (1990) has had the most significant clinical relevance to the practice of occupational therapy.

These definitions are as follows:

1. *Finger-to palm translation*: moving an object from the finger pads to the palm of the hand. Finger to palm translation occurs when a child picks up a piece of candy with the tips of fingers and hides it by moving it to the palm.

2. *Palm-to finger translation*: moving an object from the palm to the finger pads. Palm to finger translation occurs when a child holds a small object in the palm and moves it from the palm to the distal surface of the *radial* fingers.

3. *Shift*: using the finger pads to produce a slight linear adjustment of the object. Shift occurs when a child

Early Intervention - Key for proper grasp - which is better for endurance!

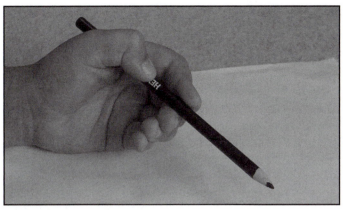

Figure 17-6a. Note how the fingers "walk" down the shaft of the pencil in this example of shift.

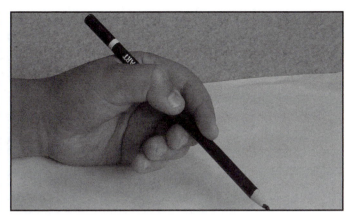

Figure 17-6b.

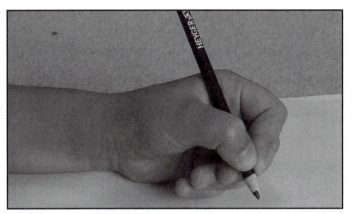

Figure 17-6c.

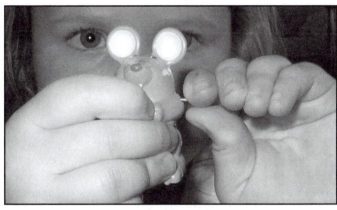

Figure 17-7. This is an example of how a child might use simple rotation to wind a toy (turning less than 180°).

holds a crayon at the midshaft and inches the fingers down the crayon in order to position it to prepare to draw and write (Figures 17-6a through c).

4. *Simple rotation*: rotating an object by using the thumb in *opposition* to the fingers, the fingers usually act as a unit and the object is usually rotated less than 180°. Simple rotation occurs when a child uses all the fingers to partially unscrew a jar lind or wind a toy (turning it less than 180°) (Figure 17-7).

5. *Complex rotation*: moving an object between 180° and 360° by using differentiation of finger movements and active thumb movements. Complex rotation occurs when a child is writing and needs to flip-turn the pencil to erase, and the pencil is rotated 180° (Figures 17-8a through c).

As previously discussed, hand skills require proximal stability for distal mobility. This principle is illustrated while observing the stability in proximal joints during skilled hand movements such as in-hand manipulation. In addition to the stability of the proximal joints, the proper positioning of the wrist and forearm is necessary for skilled finger move-

ments. The forearm may be positioned in supination, pronation, or in neutral. Wrist stability is also important as it positions and steadies the hand for grasp and helps provide the necessary positioning for the fingers to manipulate objects in the hand. As skilled movements improve, using a precision grasp, which depends on thumb opposition to contact the pads of the fingers in order to hold objects is possible (see Table 17-3).

The hand arches and the separation of the hand into the skill (radial) and stability (*ulnar*) side is important for in-hand manipulation. The arches provide both stability (*transverse* [proximal] *carpal arch*) and mobility (*transverse* [distal] *metacarpal arch*) for the fingers during manipulation tasks (please refer to Chapter 24: Orthotics). Separation of the two sides of the hand is also essential for skilled in-hand manipulation. Typically, separation of the hand and finger is observed around 6 to 7 months. This separation designates the radial side of the hand (thumb, index, and middle fingers) as the skill side of the hand and the ulnar side (ring and index fingers) as the power side (Case-Smith, 1995). Hand side separation, along with the development of the arches of the hand, support later tool use, such as proficient writing

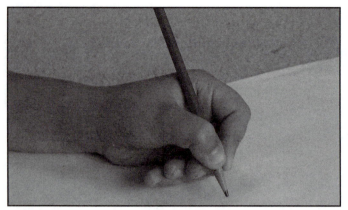

Figure 17-8a. Observe how this child uses *complex rotation* to turn the pencil from tip to eraser (turning between 180° to 360°).

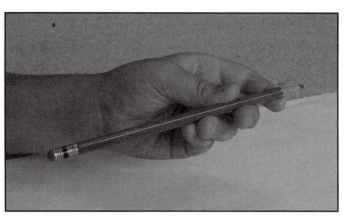

Figure 17-8b.

with a pencil. Table 17-5 presents a checklist of typical in hand manipulation problems and Table 17-6 describes the approximate age levels for the acquisition of in- hand manipulation skills.

Hand Dominance

Hand dominance is defined as consistent use of one hand for finer manipulative skills while the other (non-dominant) hand stabilizes and positions objects in order to maximize efficiency (Levine, 1991). Murray (1995) indicates that by age 3, most children have established a dominant hand, which, barring accident or injury, remains constant throughout life. If an infant under the age of 2 consistently uses one hand, this may indicate a weakness on the opposite side and further evaluation may be necessary. Certain activities such as cutting and writing require use of a dominant hand, while other activities such as carrying, grasping, and reaching are not clear indicators of dominance (Heinlein, in Erhardt, 1994).

Hand Skills and Play

Bundy (2002) defines play as an activity that occurs between a child and the environment, is intrinsically motivated, internally controlled, and includes freedom of the imagination. Play is a child's primary occupation. Through play, children gain an understanding of the world and competence in interacting with it (Knox 1997). Play is also the medium through which children socialize with their peers. When children play, they create and explore various situations and learn about their environment. Children learn about their environment, in part, through use of their hands during what is known as object manipulation activities.

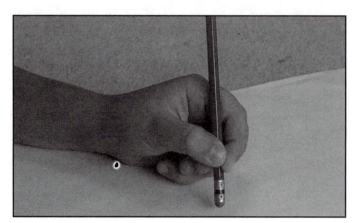

Figure 17-8c.

Facilitation of Hand Skills

The ability to manipulate objects with skill and precision takes years to master, yet its developmental course begins long before an infant first reaches for a toy. This is because reach and grasp involve much more than arms and hands. They involve the integration of postural stability with the voluntary control of these extremities. For the infant, postural stability and coordinated reach and grasp develop in a complementary pattern and can be facilitated by both fine and gross motor activities. Table 17-7 outlines treatment activities that, based on demonstrated competency and state and facility guidelines, the occupational therapy assistant (OTA) can incorporate into therapy sessions in order to facilitate development of hand skills.

Table 17-5

Checklist for Treatment and Documentation of In-Hand Manipulation Problems

__ 1. Can maintain forearm in mid-ranges
__ 2. Good wrist stabilization
__ 3. Hands are coordinated with each other
__ 4. Finger flexion for grasp well balanced
__ 5. Cups hand by using arches to accommodate objects of various sizes
__ 6. Can identify fingers and move them independently
__ 7. Can identify size and/or weight of objects in hand
__ 8. Precision grasp is developing and being used in treatment
   a. Thumb opposition and rotation
   b. Tactile or proprioceptive awareness of fingers
   c. Good balance of extensors/flexors (co-contraction)
__ 9. Intrinsic muscles are well developed and used for precision grasps

---

Table 17-6

Approximate Age Levels for Acquisition of In-Hand Manipulation Skills

Translation
finger to palm	1.5-2.0 years
palm to finger	2.0-2.5 years

Shift
with bulky object	2.0-2.5 years
turning pages of book	3.0-3.5 years
shift of writing tool	4.0-5.0 years

Rotation
simple rotation of jar lid	2.0-2.5 years
simple rotation of wind up toy	3.5-4.0 years
complex rotation of writing tool	5.0-5.5 years

Modified from Pehoski, C. (1995). Object manipulation in infants and children. In *Hand function in the child* (p. 144). St. Louis, MO: Mosby Year-Book; and Exner, C. E. (1990). In hand manipulation skills in normal children: A pilot study. *OT Practice, 4,* 68.

worker hand / helper hand

Table 17-7

Facilitating Hand Skills: An OT Practitioner's Guide to Treatment Strategies

Skill	Purpose	Treatment Strategies
Prone	Activities that strengthen the postural (neck, shoulder, and trunk) muscles are important for later hand use.	• This position is often one that infants find difficult to tolerate. This is because flexor tone predominates in infancy and a prone position requires using the extensor musculature, which are comparatively weaker, to lift the head and body against gravity. During the first month of life, this position can be gradually introduced by placing the infant across an adult's thighs for a few moments, as tolerated. • As most infants seek out close physical contact, placing the infant in prone on the parent/caregiver's chest while lying on the floor or bed is another way to improve the infant's tolerance of this position. • OTA or parent/caregiver may lie face to face with the infant, or put a mirror or other visually interesting toys in front of him/her during this "tummy time." • Periodically and firmly placing a hand on the infant's buttocks encourages lifting the head against gravity (Parks, 1986), because pressure on the buttocks provide a point of stability which helps facilitate extension of the neck and trunk. • Later, as the infant grows stronger, he can be placed in prone on the floor. To help maintain this position, putting a small rolled up towel under the infant's chest with elbows placed in front of the roll is often effective. • With practice, by placing some weight on his/her forearms when in a prone position, the infant eventually begins to lift the chest up and turn the head from side to side. As strength and stability increase in this propped on elbows position, the OTA can encourage the infant to continue to lift the chest and begin to bear weight on the hands by placing toys at a higher eye level (Parks, 1986).
Supine/Sidelying	To encourage reach and exploration in these positions. Sidelying facilitates bringing the hands to midline and allows the infant to reach and grasp without gravity.	• Placing small rolled towels behind the infant's shoulders while in supine provides additional shoulder stability and encourages forward reach. • Having an infant play under a stationary mini gym, holding a toy above him/her, or encouraging exploration of an OTA or caregiver's face encourages this forward reaching pattern. • Place small rolled towels behind the infant's back while in sidelying (for additional support) and place toys within his/her reach to explore.
Preparing to Creep and Creeping	Creeping helps strengthen the trunk and upper extremities, normalize the flexor tone in the hand, provide tactile input to the hand, and plays a role in development of the hand arches. Creeping also provides opportunities for infants to independently explore their environment. Spending time in the prone position strengthens the proximal upper extremity muscles that are important for creeping, and infants who spend time in this position may be better prepared to creep.	• Once proximal strength and stability is established, infants begin to reach for objects when in a prone position. This early upper extremity weight shifting from side to side also helps the infant prepare for commando crawling and creeping. • To encourage reaching in prone, which involves weight shifting from side to side in order to free up an arm, offering the infant toys in front and to each side of his/her body provides opportunities to reach in all planes.
Sitting	Provides the first opportunity to explore the world from an upright position.	• Before the infant is able to independently sit and explore toys, placing the infant inside a soft, crescent-shaped pillow may facilitate sitting. This pillow supports the lower trunk, thus leaving the upper trunk and arms free to reach to objects placed around him/her. • Sitting in a high chair for short periods of time provides another way to play in supported sitting. If the high chair does not provide adequate lateral or side support, placing rolled towels on the sides of the chair may be helpful.

Table 17-7 (continued)

Facilitating Hand Skills: An OT Practitioner's Guide to Treatment Strategies

Skill	Purpose	Treatment Strategies
Object Manipulation	To learn about the properties of an object through touch.	• Offering a variety of textured toys encourages fingering behaviors and toys with varying shapes elicit mouthing and transferring (Ruff, 1984). Keep in mind that large objects require grasp with the whole hand, but small objects such as raisins or cereal encourage the use of the fingers in grasp.
Hand Regard	Awareness of the hands is essential for any purposeful movement of the hands.	• Facilitate through various sensory activities such as massage, finger and hand naming, play songs and games, playing touch games with using various textures, and tying a ribbon with a secured bell around wrist (Parks, 1986).
Midline Skills	The ability to bring the hands to midline, and eventually crossing the midline is important in that it facilitates transfer of objects and is a sign of neurological wellness.	• Play pat-a-cake or other hand/finger play games, placing his/her hands on the bottle during feeding, through massage, patting and by stroking the hands while at midline during play or when in the bathtub. • Position your face (or encourage the parent/caregiver to do so) within the infant's reach and encourage him/her to touch and explore it with both hands. This helps facilitate development of midline skills (Parks, 1986). • To prepare for bringing hands and toys/objects to midline in play, the first step is to encourage an infant to hold objects in each hand. Offering one toy to each hand can facilitate this skill. When the infant is able to hold a toy in each hand, using a hand over hand approach, show how to bang the toys together. It is beneficial to start this activity with bigger objects that are easy to hold, and then move to holding smaller ones (Parks, 1986).
Reach	Helps infants obtain and explore objects in their environments.	• Offer toys placed a few inches away from the hand instead of placing in the infant's hand. • Try tapping the infant's hand with a toy and gently guiding the arm so the toy is within reach (Parks, 1986). • Toys such as mobiles and busy boxes are often stimulating and encourage spontaneous reaching. Tabletop mazes (three-dimensional mazes in which beads are run along the paths of the wires) also facilitate reach as well as shoulder development.
Release Skills	An essential part of object manipulation that enables the infant to transfer, turn over, and drop an object during exploration.	• Initiate release by touching the back of the infant's hand or the tips of the fingers. • Make a game out of handing objects back and forth to the infant or dropping them in a container and listening for a sound.
Separation of the 2 sides of the hand	Separation designates the radial side of the hand (thumb, index, and middle fingers) as the skill side of the hand and the ulnar side (ring and index fingers) as the power side (Case-Smith, 1995). This is an important milestone because it is with the skill side of the hand that the most precise object manipulation occurs and with the radials side that object stability occurs.	• Finger feeding and placing small edibles into miniature muffin tins or empty egg cartons (Parks, 1986). • Encourage play with toys that have buttons to press or small knobs and dials to turn. • An older child might enjoy picking up a designated number of coins or bingo/poker chips all at one time and then placing them in a piggy bank or other slotted container one at a time.
Index Finger	Isolation of the index finger is a fundamental component of mature prehension patterns (Gilfoyle et al., 1990).	• Introduce activities that involve poking with the index finger such as pressing on piano keys, placing individual fingers into pegboard holes, or into boxes with holes punched into them, and toys that have buttons or dials to activate. • Draw in trays of sand, salt, and flour, finger paint with yogurt, and point to pictures of body parts (Parks, 1986).

Table 17-7 (continued)

Facilitating Hand Skills: An OT Practitioner's Guide to Treatment Strategies

Skill	Purpose	Treatment Strategies
Grasp with Digits	As children develop greater distal motor control and precision, they begin to use the radial digits instead of the palm of the hand to secure an object.	• Offering an object so that only a small part of it is exposed requires the child to grasp with only the radial fingers and thumb. • When seated in a high chair or other chair with a tray, offering a few small pieces rather than a large scoop of food at a time may also encourage use of the radial fingers rather than the whole hand to grasp the food. • Providing objects that encourage use of the thumb in opposition to the fingers in grasp such as when picking up a teething biscuit, a piece of crumpled paper, a firm gelatin square, or a small ball (Parks, 1986) also aid in development of more precise grasp skills. • For the older child, playing with stamp sets (with small handles) and dispensing colorful water from eye droppers encourage the use of the radial digits. • Table games such as Lite Brite®, Battleship, Kerplunk®, Mastermind for Kids®, and Don't Spill the Beans® encourage an older child to use the radial fingers and thumb to manipulate the game pieces. • For older children who persist in holding a writing tool with the palm or whole hand, providing 1-inch pieces of crayons or pencils also helps to facilitate radial side digital grasp skills.
Bilateral Hand Skills	Significantly expands the toddler's capacity to explore the environment, which is fundamental to enhancing cognitive and perceptual development.	• Provide toys that can be held two hands at the same time, such as a teddy bear, or toys such as a toy key ring or a long handled rattle that can easily be transferred from one hand to the other. • Smearing foods such as yogurt or pudding on one hand to encourage exploration of the material by the other hand is another fun way to enhance bilateral hand skills. • Stringing beads, empty spools of thread, and ring shaped cereal onto chenille sticks or sturdy string, and fastening and pulling apart pop beads also facilitate bilateral hand use. One hand manipulates the bead and the other stabilizes the chenille stick, string, or other pop bead. Keep in mind that larger beads require use of a whole hand grasp, which requires minimal skill, while manipulating smaller beads requires a grasp using only the fingers, which requires greater skill and precision. • For the older child, playing with a Mr. Potato Head® toy requires stabilization with one hand while the other snaps each play piece into place and is an enjoyable way to support bilateral hand use.
In-Hand Manipulation	In-hand manipulation tasks require precise movement patterns of the hands. In-hand manipulation involves elements of finger to palm translation, palm to finger translation, simple and complex rotation, and shift, which are important in order to carry out such childhood occupations as fastening and unfastening clothes, using utensils, using school tools, picking up coins, and playing games.	• Play the squirrel game by offering small objects such as raisins or cereal for children to pick up one by one and store in the same hand. As this skill improves, introduce palm to finger translation by encouraging children to then drop the stored objects in the palm one by one into a container. • For the older child, playing the game Mancala® encourages both palm to finger and finger to palm translation as the game pieces are moved along the playing board. • Simple rotation skills can be addressed by having children open and close jars or bottles with screw-on lids. To encourage complex rotation, introduce markers with a stamp on one end and a felt-tipped pen on the other, and encourage children to switch between the stamp and the marker end without help from the other hand. • Activities involving Play-Doh®, clay, or therapy putty can also be used to encourage simple rotation, complex rotation, and shift. Have children rest their elbow(s) on a table top at a 90°+ angle and make balls using only the fingers of one hand. To increase the challenge, encourage children to make balls using the fingers of both hands at the same time. • Card games that require turning such as Memory® or Go Fish encourage shift skills.

Lite Brite®, Battleship®, Mr. Potato Head®, Play Doh®, Don't Spill the Beans®, and Memory® are registered trademarks of Hasbro (East Longmeadow, MA). Kerplunk® is a registered trademark of Mattel (El Segundo, CA). Mastermind for Kids® and Mancala for Kids® are registered trademarks of Pressman Toy (New Brunswick, NJ).

Summary

The typical sequence of development of basic reach, grasp, and manipulation has been presented. These hand skills are an instrumental part of successful engagement in all occupations of childhood. The OTA plays an important role in helping to facilitate the development of children's hand skills.

Case Study

Tom is 3 years old and has Down syndrome. He is social and likes to smile and talk with other children. His fine motor skills are on the 2 year old level according to the OT's report. His is demonstrating over extension of the fingers during release. He uses a pincer grasp when picking up a 1-inch block, he uses bilateral manipulation to change the position of and explore objects. He has some thumb rotation, but uses a lot of thumb adduction. He brings his thumb to the middle finger at the middle phalanx rarely bringing his thumb and index finger together to grasp an object.

Discussion Questions

1. What aspects of reach, grasp, release, and manipulation would you address in treatment?
2. Design the first three sessions of activities and explain how you would present them to the child.

Application Activities

1. Visit a toy store and analyze the characteristics of different toys.
2. Prepare a birthday list of toys for parents to refer to that can be used to develop children's hand skills. Be ready to discuss the reasons for choosing the toys you did.

References

Ammon, J. E., & Etzel, M. E. (1977). Sensorimotor organization in reach and prehension a developmental model. *Physical Therapy, 57*, 7-14.

Bruni, M. (1998). *Fine motor skills in children with Down syndrome: A guide for parents and professionals*. Bethesda MD: Woodbine House.

Bundy, A. C. (2002). Play theory and sensory integration. In C. Bundy, C. Lane, & E Murray (Eds.), *Sensory integration theory and practice* (pp. 227-239). Philadelphia, PA: F.A. Davis Company

Case-Smith, J., & Bigsby, R. (2000). *Posture and fine motor assessment in fine infants*. Tucson, AZ: Therapy Skill Builders.

Case-Smith, J. (1995). Grasp, release, and bimanual skills in the first two years of life. In A. Henderson & C. Pehoski (Eds.), *Hand function in the child* (pp. 113-135). St. Louis, MO: Mosby.

Castner, B. M. (1932). The development of fine prehension in infancy. *Genetic Psychology Monographs, 12*, 105-193.

Edwards, S. J., Buckland, D. B., & McCoy-Powlen, J. D. (2002). *Developmental and functional hand grasps*. Thorofare, NJ: SLACK Incorporated.

Erhardt, R. P. (1994). *Developmental hand dysfunction: Theory, assessment and treatment*. Tucson, AZ: Therapy Skill Builders.

Exner, C. E. (1992). In-hand manipulation skills. In J. Case-Smith & C. Pehoski (Eds.), *Development of hand skills in the child* (pp. 35-46). Bethesda, MD: American Occupational Therapy Association.

Exner, C. E. (1990). In-hand manipulation skills in normal young children: A pilot study. *Occupational Therapy Practice, 1*, 63-72.

Folio, M. R., & Fewell, R. R. (1983). *Peabody developmental motor scales and activity cards*. Chicago: Riverside Publishing Company.

Gilfoyle, E. M., Grady, A. P., & Moore, J. C. (1990). *Children adapt* (2nd ed.). Thorofare, NJ: SLACK Incorporated.

Halverson, H. M. (1931). An experimental study of prehension in infants by means of systematic cinema records. *Genetic Psychology Monographs, 10*, 107-286.

Knox, S. (1997). Development and current use of the knox preschool play scale. In D. Parnjam & L. Fazio (Eds). *Play in occupational therapy for children* (pp. 35-66). St Louis, MO: Mosby.

Levine, K. J. (1991). *Fine motor dysfunction therapeutic strategies in the classroom*. San Antonio TX: Therapy Skill Builders.

Murray, E. A. (1995). Hand preference and its development. In A. Henderson & C. Pehoski (Eds.), *Hand function in the child* (pp. 154-163). St. Louis, MO: Mosby, Inc.

Parks, S. (1986). *Make every step count: Birth to one year*. Palo Alto, CA: Vort Corporation.

Pehoski, C. (1995). Object manipulation in infants and children. In A. Henderson & C. Pehoski (Eds.), *Hand function in the child* (pp. 136-153). St. Louis, MO: Mosby, Inc.

Rochat, P. (1989). Object manipulation and exploration in 2 to 5 month old infants. *Developmental Psychology, 25*, 871-884.

Ruff, H. A. (1984). Infant's manipulative exploration of objects: Effects of age and object characteristics. *Developmental Psychology, 20*, 9-20.

Ruff, H., McCarton, C., Kurtzberg, D., & Vaughan, H. G. (1984). Preterm infants' manipulative exploration of objects. *Child Development, 55*, 1166-1173.

18

Handwriting

Linda Cammaroto, OTR/L

Chapter Objectives

- Understand the developmental progression of pre-writing and writing skills.
- Examine treatment strategies for enhancing underlying writing skills such as positioning, grasp alteration, and use of alternative writing paper.
- Explore age appropriate prewriting and writing activities to implement when working with children.

Introduction

One of the most important occupations of young school aged children is learning to write and communicate through written communication. This chapter explores the occupation of handwriting and ways in which the occupational therapy assistant (OTA), working under the supervision of an occupational therapist (OT) may help children with handwriting, and/or carry-out an occupational therapy handwriting intervention program.

Foundations of Handwriting

Hand Dominance

In preparation for using both hands separately and together, the typically developing child progresses through stages of unilateral and bilateral hand use, (Gesell & Amatruda, 1969). By using hands together and separately, the child learns which hand has better control for different activities. This exploration leads to the establishment of hand dominance, which appears to correlate with the development of the mature dynamic tripod *pencil grasp* pattern typically integrated between ages 4 and 6 (Amundson & Weil, 2001; Erhardt, 1994).

Activities to Encourage Dominance

1. *Hammering activities.* Turn empty egg cartons upside down. Have children hammer the eggcup sections using one hand and then the other. Save packing Styrofoam, cover with burlap, and use as a hammering table. Children can hammer golf tees into the Styrofoam with a small hammer or mallet.

2. *Bead stringing activities.* Bead stringing encourages children to select one hand to hold and one to manipulate. Tip: To encourage midline crossing put the beads on the left side if the child is using the right and vice versa.

3. *Using tweezers, tongs, or clothespins to pick up items* improves fine motor skills and encourages children to develop a preferred hand. Strawberry hullers are a good size for little hands. Clothespins are also very versatile and a favorite of young children. A good game involves rolling dice, and picking up the same number of small items with clothespins as the number on the dice shows and putting them in cups. To encourage midline crossing, place the cup on the opposite side from the hand a child typically uses.

Some children with handwriting problems may not have a preferred writing hand and frequently switch. With regard to hand switching, and through evaluation procedures completed by an OT, questions to be assessed may include, is the child switching hands because of fatigue? Is the child switching hands to avoid crossing the midline of the body? Does the child switch hands rather than reach across midline to color on the other side of the paper? Does the child reach across midline to pick up a small item to glue onto the paper? Can the child reach across midline twisting at the waist to retrieve an item that fell to the floor? The OTA may be asked to assist the OT by keeping a log of what hand the child uses for different activities.

PREWRITING

A child begins engaging in prewriting skill activities at around 18 months of age and continues to refine these skills until about age 6 (Klein, 1982; 1990). Before they can attain mastery over a pencil and begin to write children need to develop prewriting skills. Klein (1989) describes a sequence of developmental stages of prewriting skills. They include:

- The child mouths crayons or crinkles paper
- Bangs crayons on paper
- Scribbles randomly
- Scribbles spontaneously in a horizontal direction
- Scribbles spontaneously in a vertical direction
- Scribbles spontaneously in a circular direction
- Imitates a horizontal scribble
- Imitates a vertical direction
- Imitates a circular scribble
- Imitates a horizontal line
- Imitates a vertical line
- Imitates a circular line
- Copies a horizontal line
- Copies a vertical line
- Copies a circle
- Imitates a cross (pp. 11-17).

Prior to being ready to write, children must also recognize and attach meaning to number and letter symbols. In most public schools in the United States, number recognition is taught before letter recognition.

In addition to number and letter recognition, in order to be ready to learn to write, children must also demonstrate refined hand skills. The OTA, working as part of a team, helps to facilitate both number and letter recognition as well as refined hand skills. A multi-sensory approach to learning to write may be one effective means for young children to integrate and master these important skills (Amundson & Weil, 1996; p. 535). A multisensory approach involves using a variety of sensory experiences such as tactile, proprioceptive, kinesthetic, visual, auditory, olfactory and even gusta-

tory activities and instructional materials to enhance handwriting skills and learning. A few examples include:

- Tearing, crumpling, and gluing small pieces of tissue paper onto predrawn (oversized) letters or numbers. Remember to have the child start gluing at the top, and also work from left to right. Top to bottom and left to right orientation should always be encouraged when working on any prewriting or writing activity.

- Drawing letters or numbers with index finger in a tray of sand or shaving cream. Whipped cream and chocolate pudding may also be used, unless food allergies have been identified.

- Fanny books. Take a simple children's book (number, or letter books work well) apart. Laminate each page horizontally in a continuous roll with about a foot of laminating film between each page. Unroll the book in the classroom or hallway and have the child do sit-pull-throughs to "read" each page, resting his/her "fanny" on the clear portion of laminating film between each page.

Reflections for the OTA

How to do a Sit-Pull-Through:
Have the child sit long-legged on the floor with his/her hands placed on the floor at his/her sides. Fingers should be adducted and pointed away from the body. The thumbs should be abducted from the rest of the fingers to make an "L." This posture will encourage the child to take all of his weight on the heel of his/her hands. As he/she slides backwards, the web space expands, which helps develop thumb musculature necessary for handwriting. (Benbow, 2002).

While some children show an interest in formal writing by age 4 or 5 and have developed writing readiness skills, many others may not be ready until age 6. Lamme (1979) outlined six prerequisites that must be established prior to initiating formal handwriting instruction; 1) small muscle development, 2) eye-hand coordination, 3) utensil or tool manipulation (can the child cut a coil of play dough with a plastic knife, and eat with a spoon and fork?), 4) basic stroke formation such as circles and lines, 5) alphabet letter and number recognition, and 6) orientation to written language (pp. 20-27). Benbow, Hanft, and Marsh (1992) discussed four prewriting competencies necessary for formal handwriting instruction; dominant hand use, midline crossing with the dominant hand, proper posture and pencil grasp, and the ability to copy the first nine shapes of the Developmental Test of Visual-Motor Integration (VMI) (Beery & Bukenica, 1989); the vertical line, horizontal line, circle, cross, right oblique line, square, left oblique line, oblique cross, and triangle. While Beery (1989) suggests that formal

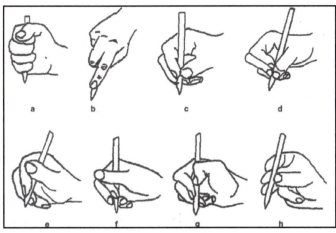

Figure 18-1. Typical development of pencil grasp: (a) palmar supinate grasp, (b) digital pronate grasp, (c) static or dynamic tripod grasp. Atypical pencil grasps: (d) quadrupod grasp, (e) lateral tripod grasp, (f) lateral quadrupod grasp, (g) tripod grasp without web space, (h) four finger with tips only grasp. Copyright 2001 by the American Occupational Therapy Association Inc. Reprinted with permission.

pencil and paper writing be postponed until the child can easily copy the oblique cross from the VMI, Weil and Amundson (1994) and Marr and Windsor (2001) suggest that most kindergarten children are ready for handwriting instruction in the latter half of the kindergarten year.

Reflections for the OTA

Common Terminology Associated With Handwriting:

Imitation: After watching someone model a drawn line, shape, form, letter, or word, the child tries to reproduce it. This skill comes first in learning to draw. When a child masters this skill he/she is ready to copy.

Copying: The ability to reproduce from a model such as copying from a book or board.

Automatic Writing: After mastering manuscript or cursive, the child becomes familiar enough with letter formation so as to be able to remember how to form the letter from memory.

Directionality: The ability to interpret right and left directions in space. It is important for the child to discriminate right from left, and to transfer this understanding to his/her body and to objects in space because it is the foundation upon which handwriting is built. In most western cultures, children must learn to move from left to right across the page, and to support this, must be taught to form manuscript letters from top to bottom and in a counterclockwise orientation. Being able form letters correctly is dependent, in part, on good directionality skills.

Holding the Pencil

HAND DEVELOPMENT

Recall from Chapter 17: Hand Development, the hand can be separated into two sides, the ulnar (little finger or power side) and radial (thumb or skill side). Benbow (2002) describes the early development of motoric separation as occurring when the baby crawls and bears weight on the ulnar side of the hand and carries toys with the radial side. As children develop, they begin to use the index and middle fingers in opposition to the thumb to do things like pick up small objects, pull on objects, and tear paper. The ring and little fingers provide support while the thumb, index, and middle fingers manipulate the object. These hand skills help form the motoric foundation for learning to write (please refer to the Developmental Milestones Chart at the end of the book).

DEVELOPMENT OF PENCIL GRASP

The developmental progression of pencil grasp (or hold) parallels the principles of physical development from proximal to distal, global to differentiated, and axial to appendicular (Erhardt, 1994). Erhardt (1994) described the normal progression of grasp from an immature pattern at 1 year to a mature, refined pattern by about age 6 (Figure 18-1). At about 15 months, a child's first grasp on a crayon or pencil is a palmar-supinate, a shoulder generated movement with hand fisted around the pencil in a "palm up" position (Figure 18-1a). At about 2 to 3 years of age, as shoulder stability develops and elbow mobility improves, the digital pronate grasp (Figure 18-1b) emerges. At around 3 years a child begins to use a static tripod grasp (Figure 18-1c). Motion continues to be generated mainly from the shoulder and elbow, and while for the first time limited wrist motion is contributing to the overall movement pattern, the arm still moves as a unit. Skilled use of the hand itself requires that the thumb be abducted, medially rotated, stable, and opposed to the index and middle fingers; all movement patterns necessary to hold a pencil in a mature way. Corresponding with improved distal fine motor control at about age 4, the dynamic tripod grasp (Figure 18-1c) emerges. The dynamic tripod becomes more refined between ages 4 and 6. Refinement of the dynamic tripod grasp coincides with improved shoulder, elbow, and wrist stabilization. With increased stability, the intrinsic muscles of the hand are readying to perform skilled and individuate movements necessary to manipulate a writing tool in an efficient way. With development of intrinsic hand musculature comes distal, differentiated, and appendicular control of the hand. At this stage in handwriting development, the child also learns to stabilize the writing hand by resting it on a desk or table top.

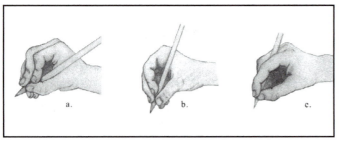

Figure 18-2. Mature efficient pencil grasps. a. Mature tripod, b. dynamic quadrupod, c. alternate pencil hold (Sassoon) (also called adapted (Benbow), D'Nealian (Thurber), Monk's hold (Admundson), and arthritic pen hold. Illustration by Jessica Cammaroto.

PENCIL POSITION

Reflections for the OTA

Try holding a pencil with your wrist in flexion. Is it difficult to hold? Now lift your hand as if to write in the air. Gravity will pull your wrist into extension, abduct the thumb, and place it in opposition, all positions necessary for proper pencil hold. Many OT practitioners find that having children do prewriting, writing, and fine motor work on an inclined plane or vertical surface (slant board, easel, chalkboard) helps strengthen the wrist extensor musculature necessary for proper pencil hold.

Working as a tripod, refined movement of the thumb, index, and middle fingers enable the child to carry out small and highly coordinated motions. A tripod grasp is achieved by holding a writing tool when the thumb and index finger are placed gently on either side of the pencil with the middle finger resting underneath, while the ring and little finger rest on the palm. To be able to make quick changes in direction, the index finger should be positioned slightly in front of the thumb. When the motion is generated from the hand, this grasp pattern is called the dynamic tripod, and as discussed above, typically emerges between ages 4 to 6. The tripod grasp keeps the web space open, thus allowing for the greatest possible movement between the thumb, index, and middle fingers when writing.

Reflections for the OTA

When the thumb is placed in front of the other digits, such as in a thumb wrap grasp, the child has less control over the pencil. He/she may develop a lump where the pencil presses down on the middle finger as the pressure from the thumb forces the index DIP up at a sharp angle (Sassoon, 1986) (refer to Figure 18-3).

Ideally, a left-handed child should hold the pencil with the first two fingers and thumb and point the pencil toward the left elbow. The right-handed child holds the pencil with

the first two fingers and thumb and points the pencil toward the right shoulder.

Because of the distal control it affords over the pencil, the dynamic tripod grasp with open web space is considered by many OT practitioners and teachers to be the optimal functional grasp for handwriting performance (Amundson & Weil, 2001; Amundson & Weill, 1996; Bonney, 1992; Tseng & Cermak, 1993). Alternatively, Dennis & Swinth (1999) point out that the dynamic tripod grasp is not the only functional grasp used by individuals demonstrating no apparent handwriting difficulties. Bergmann (1990) describes functional grasp patterns as those characterized by use of intrinsic hand musculature, dynamic wrist control, and distal finger control of the writing tool.

This information is important because a child needs a pencil hold that provides speed, legibility, is comfortable, and will not cause harm to the joints of the hand over time. If a pencil hold satisfies these criteria there is no need to change it (Benbow, 2002). For example, Sassoon (1993) describes an alternate pencil hold, sometimes called the D'Nealian grip, adapted grip, Monk's grip, or arthritis grip. Callewaert, a Belgian neurologist researched this pencil hold and found it a good grasp pattern to alleviate writer's cramp (Sassoon, 1999). This grasp pattern may also be a good option for children who hold their pencils very tightly with atypical placements of the fingers. Children using a fingertip hold, a very light hold on the pencil using just the tips of the fingers, with movement generated from the entire arm may also find the alternate pencil hold a more stable and efficient grasp pattern (Figure 18-2).

In Figure 18-2, pencil grasps are divided into mature and efficient pencil holds, which are presumed over time to work well for the child, and in Figure 18-3, atypical and inefficient pencil holds that are presumed to be detrimental for the child are illustrated. While an inefficient pencil grasp pattern can probably be changed at any point in an individual's life, it is often far more difficult to do so after second grade. Grasp patterns have become habitual and are difficult to alter, especially if the child is not motivated to do so. Therefore it is best practice to encourage use of a mature and efficient pencil grasp pattern before second grade (Amundson & Weil, 1996).

Moving On To Writing

LEARNING STYLES

With regard to handwriting, Olsen (1997) identifies three types of learners, the visual, the auditory and the tactile-kinesthetic. The visual learner benefits from instruction involving visual demonstration, models, and pictures. The auditory learner learns best from verbal directions, remembering stories, and verbal cues. The tactile and kinesthetic learner benefits from instruction involving tactile experi-

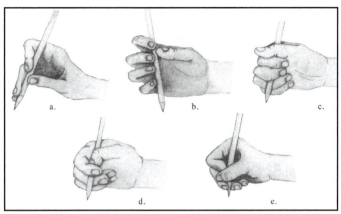

Figure 18-3. Atypical, inefficient pencil grasps. a. Index grasp: child tries to approximate the tripod but pencil is help stiffly and thumb does not move into full abduction and medial rotation to oppose the distal fingertip of the index. b. Fingertip grasp: four fingers and thumb with tips only used. This is an unstable, inefficient pencil hold. c. Interdigital brace: This is an inefficient pencil hold because it limits finger movement on the pencil. d. Thumb tuck (very commonly seen in regular classrooms): fingers cannot move as freely and cramping of the fingers may occur. e. Thumb wrap (very commonly seen in regular classrooms): the student has less control when the thumb is on top. This grasp may also lead to cramping of the hand, a bump on the middle finger from pressure, and awkward handwriting. Illustration by Jessica Cammaroto.

ences such as finger tracing, drawing letters in the air, and movement activities. A multisensory approach to learning handwriting supports use of visual, auditory, and kinesthetic stimuli, and helps support success with learning to write.

The following multi-sensory activities may help a child learn to form numbers and letters without having to think about them.

1. Air Writing: After watching how a letter or number is written on the blackboard, children silently talk themselves through the process, while drawing the letter in the air using index fingers and large arm movements.

2. Rainbow Writing: Children trace over a letter, number, or word on the blackboard several times using different colors of chalk. This activity helps to reinforce motor memory for letter production.

3. Tactile Writing: Tracing letters or numbers on carpet samples with the thumb tucked under the index and middle fingers while the other two fingers are bent into the palm provides tactile input and reinforces the separation between the power and skill sides of the hand. This tactile input also reinforces the motor memory of writing letters and numbers. Forming letters and numbers out of waxed string, Wikki Stix® (Omnicor, Inc., Phoenix, AZ), or chenille sticks also provide tactile input and reinforce motor memory for writing letters and numbers.

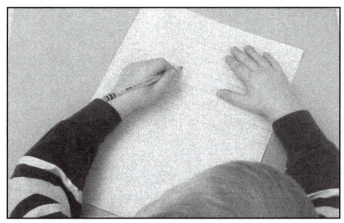

Figure 18-4. Left-handed paper position.

Working With Left-Handed Children

For manuscript writing, the lower right corner of the paper should point toward the left of the body's midline. For cursive, the lower right corner of the paper should point toward the body's midsection (Figure 18-4). *Note:* if the paper is slanted as if for a right-handed person, the child may then use a hook grasp. A hook grasp occurs when the child positions his/her hand above the paper line with the pencil tip toward the writing line. This is very uncomfortable and can become habitual. Children do this so they can see what they are writing. To prevent a hook grasp, have the child hold the left arm close to the body and keep the hand below the writing line. He/she will still be able to see what they are writing.

If the child is young, is motivated to change, and has the support of teachers and caregivers, it may be helpful for the OTA working under the supervision of the OT to address developing hand skills and try to switch the "hook" grasp to a more comfortable one. Changing any grip is difficult and frustrating for a child and should only be done with great care and understanding.

Some left-handed writers prefer their paper to be angled so that it is sideways on the writing surface. It may simply ease the pressure on the wrist and enable the child to see what he or she is writing. It is important to allow the child to select his or her own comfortable paper slant.

Keep in mind that the left-handed writer must push the pencil from the outside of the body towards the midline, while the right-handed writer pulls the pencil from the midline to the outside of the body. Left-handed writers may cross the T, A and H by pulling right to left (vs. the left to right direction used by the right-handed individual). If the left-handed writer finds it hard to push uphill to join to round letters, he or she may find it easier to lift the pen more often or frequently change hand position. It is important for the OT or OTA working under the supervision of the OT to sit beside the child and demonstrate or model with his or her

Figure 18-5. Elastic pencil holder.

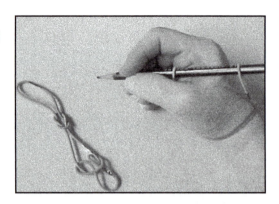

Figure 18-6. Small piece of crayon promotes tripod grasp.

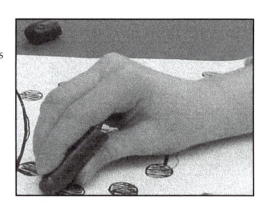

left hand, correct left-hand posture, positioning, and finger movements.

Reflections for the OTA

Felt tipped pens may be easier to use than a pencil. Using felt tipped pens also helps promote fluid writing.

PROSTHETIC DEVICES AND ADAPTED WRITING DEVICES

As previously mentioned, changing a pencil grasp is difficult and may be very stressful for the child. For this reason, attempting to change a pencil hold should be a team decision. It should also be done slowly and under the supervision of the OT. The best intervention is prevention; in preschool care should be taken to not introduce pencils until the child has developed the arches of the hand (please refer to Chapter 24: Orthotics). When a child uses a pencil grasp that may put him/her at risk for future hand problems, the OTA working under the supervision of the OT may recommend prosthetic and adapted writing devices. For a child with limited use of the writing hand, looping three small ponytail elastics together may provide a functional pencil holder. The center elastic slips over the wrist. The top elastic slips over the shaft of the pencil holding it in place in the web space. The bottom elastic slips under the pencil near the pencil point to hold the pencil in a tripod grip (Figure 18-5). The rubber band is a versatile, inexpensive way to help a child maintain a proper hold on a pencil. To use, slip the rubber band on the child's wrist. Place the pencil in his/her hand. Slip the rubber band up over the shaft of the pencil and it will automatically pull it into the web space. Placing a small item such as a tiny eraser in the palm under the pinky and ring finger encourages isolation of the two sides of the hand by keeping the ulnar side closed. Small bits of chalk and crayons are almost impossible to hold with an inefficient or immature grasp, thus encourage assumption of a tripod grip without any verbal or visual cues from an adult (Figure 18-6). The Handiwriter® (HandiThings, New Melle, MO) is a commercially available device that works similarly to the rubber band and eraser set up, as described above. Some other commercially available pencil grips (Figure 18-7) include the

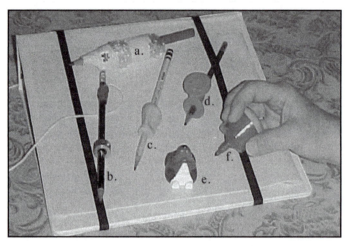

Figure 18-7. Three-ring binder slant-board with elastic bands to hold paper: a. built-up pencil; b. weighted pencil; c. The Pencil Grip® (Los Angeles, CA); d. The Start Right® Pencil Grip (Start Right Co., Middlesex, NJ); e. animal bulb marker.

Start Right® Pencil Grip (Start Right Co., Middlesex, NJ) (Figure 18-7d), The Pencil Grip® (The Pencil Grip Inc., Los Angeles, CA) (Figure 18-7c), and triangular grips.

COMPONENTS OF LEGIBLE HANDWRITING

Slant, proportion, spacing, size, and the ability to stay on the lines all influence handwriting legibility. The slant of a child's writing is determined by the paper position, the direction of the down strokes, and the shifting of the paper during writing. When letters have a consistent slant they are easier to read and look neater.

Reflections for the OTA

Generally speaking, vertical manuscript and vertical cursive writing programs may be easier for a child to learn, and further, Olsen (1997) suggests that the vertical format is developmentally easier than the slanted line to perceive and copy.

Correct spacing between letters and words also makes handwriting easier to read. Size and position on writing lines may also affect the appearance of a child's work. Some children have difficulty writing smaller and/or staying on the writing lines; letters float above the lines or dip below them.

Reflections for the OTA

Structuring a Writing Session:

1. Focus on the positives and give praise. Negative remarks will not support the aim of improving a child's handwriting performance.
2. Nothing is more demoralizing to a child than to see red marks on a paper. Ban red pens and pencils from your arsenal.
3. When employed in a school district, work with teachers to ensure carry over of the handwriting program and that children practice for short periods, and do so regularly.
4. Children may have a fear of failure and need to start their work at a point where they can be successful.

WORKING SURFACES

Years ago, school desks were made with inclined surfaces of about 20 degrees, an ideal position for handwriting tasks. In fact, and as previously discussed, using vertical work surfaces when working with children cannot be emphasized enough. Because the eyes and face are parallel with the surface, inclined desk surfaces or, alternatively, easels placed on flat desks facilitate optimal visual monitoring of reading and writing materials. Working at vertical surfaces also helps to develop arm and shoulder muscles (Myers, 1992). Another advantage of encouraging young children to do prewriting, writing, and fine motor activities on a vertical surface is that they may have weak wrist extensor muscles and so do writing and fine motor activities best when working on an inclined plane.

With a little thoughtful planning, an amazing number of prewriting, writing, and fine motor activities can be done in the vertical position. For instance, drawing on the chalkboard, painting at an easel, putting stickers on charts on the wall, using magnets or shapes on wall magnet boards, are all ways to aid the development of prewriting skills by helping to develop the hand and wrist positions necessary for handwriting (Myers, 1992).

TYPES OF PAPER

Some OT practitioners prefer certain paper options to others. Handwriting Without Tears© paper (Handwriting Without Tears, Inc., Potomac, MD) has two writing lines, a baseline, and a centerline. Primary Ready Write© paper (Pocket Full of Therapy, Morganville, NJ) has colored rule lines to assist with proper pencil placement for writing letters. Dark green top and light green centerlines indicate where to start the letter and a red bottom line indicates stop or caution before passing through to form a tail letter. Smart Start Writing Paper™ (Frog Street Press, Crandall, TX) has a blue top line with sun/cloud, a red dashed midline, and green (flower/grass) bottom line. This paper uses small icons to prompt the child to start at the sky and pull down to the ground when writing. Raised line paper has raised green lines. The raised line assists children by providing a physical bump to help "feel" where to stop. Puffy paint products can also be used to make raised line paper.

PAPER POSITION

The right-handed writer slants the paper with the lower left corner pointing toward him or her, on the right side of the body. The paper should be placed to his or her right side. The right-handed writer pulls the down strokes toward his or her midsection. The left-handed writer slants the paper with the lower right corner pointing toward him or her, with the paper placed on the left side of the body. This allows the arm to move freely while writing and prevents the child from twisting to see what he or she is writing. The left-handed writer pulls the down strokes toward his or her left elbow. Note: as previously stated, slant angle of paper described is a guide; children must find their own comfortable slant. For the child who has difficulty remembering to slant his or her paper, using tape to create a frame on the desk around each corner of the paper (do not tape the paper to the table) acts as a "guide" for paper placement.

Handwriting Letterform Programs

It is important to know and be familiar with what letterform programs are used in the school district, clinic, or other work environments, as well as by the supervising OT you are working with. Some commercially available letterform programs used today can be found in Appendix 18-2. Although all letter form programs share the common goal of providing an instructional curriculum for learning to write letters and numbers, the underlying philosophy and approach to instruction differ. Some OTs have developed an eclectic point of view regarding handwriting and letter formation, and, depending on the child's needs, use a variety of strategies and elements of more than one program. When working with children, becoming educated on various letterform programs is representative of best practice. Information and sample materials for various letter form programs are often available at little or no cost online.

Handwriting Interventions

POSTURE AND SEATING

Good posture contributes to efficient handwriting. An important first handwriting intervention involves selecting the correct size seat for the child. Ideally, the hips, knees, and ankles should be flexed at 90 degrees. A phonebook wrapped in duct tape and covered with non-slip sheeting material supports the feet so they do not dangle or slip from the footrest (Figure 18-8). Chairs with side supports or angled seat bottoms provide children with support and correct postural alignment so they are better able to sit upright to write, draw, and engage in other skilled hand movements. Inflatable or buckwheat hull filled seat cushion inserts encourage children to sit up straight by providing anterior pelvic tilt. Although these cushions are actually designed to offer slight movement and sensory stimulation for the child who tends to move about a lot, which may, in turn, promote better overall focus for seatwork, they also help to support good sitting posture. Use of T stools, and ball chairs also facilitate a more erect sitting position and help improve posture. Some children will need a seat belt to prevent them from falling out of their seat and injuring themselves. Documentation procedures regarding the need for a seatbelt must be followed according to school district or facility guidelines.

The desk height should be about 2 inches above slightly flexed elbows when the child is sitting upright. If the child is slumping forward, the desk might be too low; if the child is leaning back with his/her elbows raised up, the desk might be too high. The child should be encouraged to sit up tall, place both arms on the table, feet flat on the floor, with hips touching the back of the desk (please refer to Chapter 11: Positioning in Pediatrics: Making the Right Choices).

PREWRITING

As previously discussed, the best handwriting intervention is prevention. Putting pencils in little hands before they are ready may be one cause for the plethora of immature, inefficient, and atypical pencil holds seen in kindergarteners today. Instead, most 3- and 4-year olds are ready to engage in activities that develop hand arches and fine motor skills such as twisting, squeezing, pinching, pulling, stringing, and stacking. For the 4- to 5-year-old child who is eager to start to write, choosing a more age appropriate writing implement such as bulb crayons, large thick chalk, and animal shaped markers rather than the traditional pencil or crayon encourages the young child to develop the palmar arches while holding onto the writing device (see Figure 18-7e).

In preparation for learning to write, the preschool aged child should also be developing foundational trunk stability and generalized muscle tone, strength, and endurance, as well as basic directionality skills. Activities such as jumping, crawling, animal walks, building with large blocks, playing on playground equipment, shoveling sand, playing with clay, and finger plays are all age appropriate activities which help to develop the upper body, shoulder, arm, and wrist, and provide a good motoric foundation for learning to write. Directionality involves understanding and distinguishing right from left. By learning directionality skills through large body movement the child can later transfer this understand-

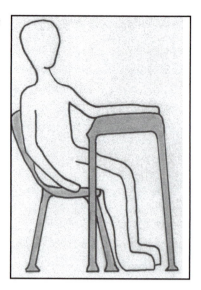

Figure 18-8. Correct posture at desk. Illustration by Jessica Cammaroto.

ing onto the paper to move from left to right across the page, and from left to right and top to bottom to form letters.

Reflections for the OTA

Letter reversals: Letter and numeral reversals are commonly seen with kindergarten, first, second, and even third grader's written work, though with decreasing frequency as the child gets older.

MAKING MODIFICATIONS

Children experiencing difficulty with writing may benefit from specific modifications. The OTA working under the supervising OT may determine what modifications might best meet a child's needs.

Modifications may include:
- Providing a slant board to position work sheets and workbooks at a more functional angle for the eyes.
- Encouraging a child to write legibly, but not to worry about the appearance of the written product during writing assignments for which the content material is the priority.
- When assignments are devoted to the mechanics of handwriting (penmanship), encourage child to check written work for errors by proofreading to see if incorrect letters were substituted and then completely erase the errors.
- If writing output is slow, uncoordinated, looks poorly formed, and recall of letter formation is difficult, consider reducing writing load requirements and instead, allowing more time to complete a shortened exercise.
- Allow child the opportunity to type assignments according to a predetermined schedule. This bypasses the need for recall of letter formation and enables the child to focus attention on other features of the activity, such as rules of punctuation and content.

Table 18-1

Addressing Common Handwriting Problems

Problem	Associated Symptoms	Treatment Strategies
Heavy Pencil Pressure	Tires easily Cramping of the hand· Tearing of the paper when writing Messy handwriting Potential sensory issues	Therapy putty warm up. Use of mouse pad under the paper, nonslip matting, or construction paper. Use a #3 pencil. Use Padded 3 ring binder. Ghost writing (write lightly on paper and then erase it).
Light Pencil Pressure	Weakness of hand musculature Poor finger dexterity Poor sensory awareness Finger tip grasp Light pencil hold	Cue child to push down harder on pencil when writing. Use carbon paper. Provide deep pressure input. Use short pencils or crayons. Put sandpaper under paper. Use markers versus crayons or pencils as lines are darker. Use #1 pencil. Wrap rubber band around pencil one-inch from point for optimal finger placement guide
Tremor	Need for increased sensory awareness	Use weighted pencils. China marker (wax pencil). Heavier pencil lead (i.e., #1).

Table 18-1 summarizes several handwriting problems that OT practitioners commonly encounter in their work with children.

Handwriting Evaluations

Standardized testing tools are valuable because they provide objective measures and quantitative scores, and can help an OT monitor a child's progress. (Campbell, 1989). There are several standardized tools that evaluate handwriting. These tests evaluate handwriting legibility by examining various components of handwriting such as speed, legibility, and specific visual perceptual skills. The purpose of handwriting evaluation is to determine the "whole picture" with regard to writing. Table 18-2 describes the features of several standardized handwriting evaluations (please refer to Chapter 8: An Overview of Developmental Assessments).

Some OTs do not use standardized handwriting evaluation tools, and instead, rely on clinical observation skills and an extensive background in working with children with handwriting problems. In this situation looking at work products as well as observation during writing assignments serves as a functional evaluation of the child's handwriting skills.

Observations may be done by the OT or, based on demonstrated competency and state and facility guidelines, an OTA. No matter what setting a child is seen in for handwriting based occupational therapy services, it is important to observe in the classroom environment, as the child may perform differently when working one on one with the OTA in a quiet room away from the distractions and the pressure of the classroom. In the classroom, the OTA observes functional elements such as posture and positioning, pencil grasp, head to table distance, attention to task, seating arrangement in the classroom (is the child facing the board or does he have to turn his head to see the board and teacher?), does the child remember instructions or require frequent prompts from the teacher, does the child appear to be fidgety and restless, and/or visually and auditorally distracted?

Summary

Handwriting is a complicated end product of many skills including good balance, trunk and upper body strength, endurance, bilateral coordination, motor planning, visual perception, hand dominance, eye-hand coordination, memory, tactile and kinesthetic sense, and attention. To support development of this important communication tool, a description of the foundations of handwriting and the components influencing the development of prewriting and writing skills was provided in this chapter. Strategies for helping children overcome common problems with handwriting were also addressed. While the OT and the OTA are not handwriting teachers, they have much to bring to the table to support the goal of developing sound handwriting skills.

> ## Table 18-2
> ## Standardized Handwriting Evaluations
>
> ### ETCH: Evaluation Tool of Children's Handwriting
>
> Susan Amundson, MS, OTR/L. Designed to assist in qualitatively measuring and documenting handwriting skills for manuscript and cursive writing. It is normed for children grades 1 to 6.
>
> ### Minnesota Handwriting Assessment
>
> Judith Reisman, Ph.D., OTR, FAOTA. Handwriting evaluation that addresses manuscript and D'Nealian print. It is normed for children in grades 1 and 2.
>
> ### Wold Sentence Copying Test
>
> Wold, Robert, OD. Used to determine if a child has the ability to rapidly and accurately copy a prewritten sentence located at the top of the testing protocol to the predrawn lines at the bottom of the protocol. It is normed for grades 2 to 8.

Case Study

David was first referred to OT at the age of 4 with reports of visual distractability, visual defensiveness, difficulty paying attention, difficulty coordinating hand movement with vision, and overall functioning at a 2- to 3-year-old level. Motor planning was poor and David had difficulty following directions related to movement in the classroom. He struggled with using scissors, drawing, coloring, managing dressing, zippers, and buttons. At the onset of OT services, David used a radial cross-palmar pencil grasp (1 year level). The first year of occupational therapy focused on developing prewriting skills. David was at the scribbling stage; the precursor of writing, which encourages the development of visually guided hand movements. Activities such as molding clay, playing in the sandbox, using large tweezers or tongs to pick up play dough or cotton balls, tearing and crumbling paper, finger painting, placing stickers on the backs of his hands, or placing ponytail holders and weighted bracelets on his wrists were introduced to develop hand regard, bilateral motor coordination, and body awareness. Small bits of crayon or chalk were used to write on vertical surfaces to encourage a more mature pencil hold, which he did upgrade to an index grasp (see Figures 18-3a and 18-9). Toward the end of the school year different pencil grips were tried, but David always managed to rearrange his fingers so that he could continue to use an index grasp on the pencil. To help him hold the pencil with a more mature and age appropriate grasp, an elastic band was wrapped around the base of the pencil to help him with finger placement. An elastic band was also placed on his wrist, and then slipped onto the shaft of the pencil to pull it down into the web space. All of these interventions ultimately proved to be unsuccessful in upgrading David's pencil grasp to a mature tripod pattern.

The following school year, David remained in preschool for the morning session, but attended afternoon kindergarten. The OTA adapted a pencil by wrapping packing foam around it (see Figure 18-7a). Two stickers were placed near the pencil point to guide correct finger placement. Initially, this seemed to help David, however, he would still revert to an index grasp. An index grasp is a difficult grasp to change. It is not a functional grasp pattern because of the limitations in speed it precludes. Therefore, before this pattern became habitual it seemed critical and timely to find a grasp for David that would be efficient for him in the academic years to come. The OT and OTA working with David decided to try implementing the alternate pencil hold (Figures 18-2c and 18-10). It took most of the kindergarten year for David to become used to this grasp. By the end of the school year he had become comfortable with the alternate grasp pattern and was using finger movement instead of elbow and shoulder movement to control the pencil (Figure 18-10).

DISCUSSION QUESTIONS

1. Did the OT and OTA work to upgrade David's pencil grasp using a multisensory approach? If so, what evidence is there for this?

2. How might the OT and OTA go about ensuring carryover of their efforts to both the classroom and home?

3. If you were to structure and plan one of David's early occupational therapy sessions, how might it have looked? What specific activities, and in what order might you introduce them? How about seating and positioning and environmental issues?

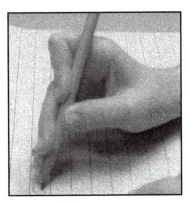

Figure 18-9. Index pencil grasp.

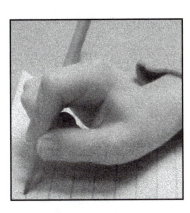

Figure 18-10. Alternate pencil grasp.

Application Activities

1. Examine classmates' pencil holds and different styles of handwriting. Collect a sample of handwriting from each student (no names) and note the differences in personal style and letter formation.

2. Examine classmates' hands to see if the various hand-holds have caused any joint deformities, calluses, or lumps

3. Prepare some materials for a hypothetical child "experiencing" handwriting difficulties.

4. Take turns demonstrating proper paper position, pencil hold, and sitting posture at desk.

References

Amundson, S. J., & Weil, M. (2001). Prewriting and handwriting skills. In J. Case-Smith (Ed.). *Occupational therapy for children* (4th ed.) (pp. 545-570). St. Louis, MO: Mosby.

Amundson, S. J., & Weil, M. (1996). Prewriting and handwriting skills. In J. Case-Smith, A. Allen, & P. N. Pratt (Eds), *Occupational therapy for children* (3rd ed., pp. 524-541). St. Louis: Mosby.

Amundson, S. J. (1998). TRICS For Written Communication, Pocket Full of Therapy. Homer, AK: OT Kids, Inc.

Benbow, M. (2002a). *Loops and other groups*. Tucson: Therapy Skill Builders.

Benbow, M. (2002b). Understanding the hand from the inside out. Handout distributed at a workshop, Sept. 2002.

Benbow, M. (1995). Principles and practices of teaching handwriting. In A. Henderson & C. Pehoski (Eds). *Hand function in the child: foundations for remediation* (pp. 255-281). St. Louis: Mosby.

Benbow, M., Hanft, B., & Marsh, D. (1992). Handwriting in the classroom: improving written communication. In C. B. Royeen (Ed.). *AOTA self-study series: Classroom applications for school-based practice* (pp. 1-60). Rockville, MD: American Occupational Therapy Association.

Beery, K. (1997). *The Beery-Buktenica developmental test of visual-motor integration* (3th ed.). Cleveland, OH: Modern Curriculum Press.

Bergmann, K. P. (1990). Incidence of atypical pencil grasps among nondysfunctional adults. *American Journal of Occupational Therapy, 44,* 736-740.

Erhardt, R. P. (1994), *Developmental hand dysfunction: Theory, Assessment, and treatment*. Tucson, AZ: Therapy Skill Builders.

Gesell, A., & Amatruda, C. S. (1969). *Developmental diagnosis* (2nd ed.). New York: Harper and Row.

Klein, M. D. (1982, 1990). *Pre-writing skills*, revised, *skill starters for motor development. A success learning program for teaching sequential pre-writing skills to preschool and developmentally delayed children*. Tucson, AZ: Communication Skill Builders, Inc.

Lamme, L. L. (1979). Handwriting in an early childhood curriculum. *Young Children, 35*(1), 20-27.

Lyle, J. (1976). Development of lateral consistency and its relation to reading and reversals. *Perceptual and Motor Skills, 43,*695-698.

Marr, D., & Windsor, M. M. (2001). Handwriting readiness: Locatives and visuomotor skills in the kindergarten year. *Early Childhood Research & Practice, 3*(1).

Marsh, D. (1992). *AOTA presents: Getting a grip on handwriting.* Rockville, MD: American Occupational Therapy Association.

Marsh, D. & Hanft, B. (1992). *Getting a grip on handwriting.* 30 minute videotape. American Occupational Therapy Association, Products Division.

Myers, C. A. (1992). Therapeutic fine-motor activities for preschoolers. In J. Case-Smith, C. Pehoski (Eds.), *Development of hand skills in the child*. Bethesda, MD: AOTA.

Olsen, J. Z. (1997). *Cursive teacher's guide*. Potomac, MD: Handwriting Without Tears, Inc.

Sassoon, R., Nimmo-Smith,I., & Wing, A. M. (1986). *An analysis of children's penholds, graphonomics: Contemporary research in handwriting,* Elsevier Science Publishers B.V. (North-Holland).

Sassoon, R. (1993). *The art and science of handwriting*. Bristol, England: *Intellect Books.*

Sassoon, R. (1999). *Handwriting of the twentieth century*. London: Routledge.

Schneck, C. (1991). Comparison of pencil grip patterns in first graders with good and poor writing skills. *American Journal of Occupational Therapy, 45,* 701-711.

School System Taskforce. (1989) *Guidelines for occupational therapy services in school systems*. Rockville, MD: AOTA.

Appendix 18-1

A Sample of Resources for the OTA

A Sense of Direction, Activities to Build Functional Directional Skills, Laura Sena. Addresses directional confusion by targeting concepts such as left/right, forward/backward, and up/down.

Action Alphabet: Sensorimotor Activities for Groups contains activities themed by alphabet letters such as finding objects hidden in a tray of sand, or games and activities, which start with the letter being learned.

Alphabatics, Catherine Rainey. Contains tactile, kinesthetic, and visual activities to teach children letter formation, promote perceptual orientation, and practice hand skills.

Callirobics, Liora Laufer. Preschool, manuscript and cursive preparation callirobics programs are available. These programs consist of handwriting exercises set to music.

Chalk-Board Fun, Laura Sena. Designed to help children develop a strong foundation for handwriting.

Correcting Reversals, Penny Groves. Contains over 40 reproducible pages of exercises to help children eliminate commonly reversed letters and numbers.

Development of Pre-Writing and Scissor Skills: A Visual Analysis, Kristen Johnson Levine. A video containing information about prewriting and scissors skills development.

Dysgraphia: Why Johnny Can't Write, 3rd ed., Diane Walton Cavey. Provides guidelines for recognizing dysgraphic children and explains their special writing needs.

Fingerplay Fun! by Rosemary Hfallum. Provides many fingerplay activities for children to enjoy.

Getting a Grip on Handwriting, a 30 minute videotape directed by Barbara Hanft and Dottie Marsch.

Getting to Know Myself, Hap Palmar. Music available on tape or CD.

Hands at Work and Play, Developing Fine Motor Skills at School and Home, Janice Miller Knight and Mary Jo Gilpin Decker. In addition to information on prewriting development and developing good habits for handwriting, this program includes reproducible masters, sensorimotor activities, and sample send-home parent letters.

Handwriting, Not Just in the Hands, Eileen Vreeland. Reviews current literature and research on handwriting skills, handwriting instruction, ergonomics of handwriting, informal assessment in the classroom and remedial and compensatory strategies with reproducible handouts. It has three complete inservice modules, each including instructor's notes, overheads, and participant handouts.

Learning in Motion, Patricia Angermeier, Joan Krzyzanowski, and Kristina Keller Moir. Contains movement activities in which children learn important prerequisites for later skill in handwriting (directionality, body awareness,). Also contains an index themed by letters of the alphabet and by month of the year and holidays.

Let's Do it- Write, Writing Readiness, Gail Kushnir. A workbook of prewriting activities and exercises focusing on development of eye-hand coordination and motor, sensory and cognitive skills, posture, cutting skills, pencil grasp, spatial orientation, and problem solving.

Pre-writing Skills Revised, Marsha Dunn Klein. A resource for the new OT; contains diagrams, developmental charts and checklists, prewriting activities, and adaptations and information on how to individualize a prewriting program.

Tool Chest: For Teachers, Parents & Students. A Handbook to Facilitate Self-Regulation, Diana Henry. This book contains activities for use at school and home for children aged 4 to 13.

Tricks For Written Communication, Techniques for Rebuilding and Improving Children's School Skills, Susan J. Amundson.

Write from the Start, Ion Teodorescu and Lois M. Addy. A two-book program for developing fine motor and perceptual skills needed for effective handwriting. The program contains exercises to develop the intrinsic muscles of the hand, and for gaining the control required to form the varied letter shapes. It also has activities to develop the perceptual skills required to orient letters and organize the writing page.

Appendix 18-2
A Sample of Instructional Handwriting Programs

Handwriting Without Tears, Jan Olsen. A prewriting readiness program, as well as a manuscript and cursive program.

Loops And Other Groups, Mary Benbow. A Zaner Bloser Kinesthetic Cursive writing program.

D'Nealian Handwriting Program, Donald Thurber. A continuous stroke manuscript and cursive writing program.

Zaner-Bloser Handwriting With a Simplified Alphabet, Clinton S. Hackney. Continuous stroke manuscript, with vertical alphabet and simplified cursive letterforms.

Getting it Write, LouAnne Audette and Anne Karson. A 6 week course for individuals or groups of 4-10 children, aged 6 to 12 years.

Let's Do It-Write: Writing Readiness Workbook, Gail Kushnir. Prewriting activities and exercises focusing on development of eye-hand coordination, and motor, sensory, and cognitive skills.

Big Strokes for Little Folks, Bonnie Levine Rubell. A developmental handwriting training program for children aged 5 to 9. Designed for children who already recognize most letters but have had limited success in learning to form them.

Hands at Work and Play, Developing Fine Motor Skills at School and Home, Janice Miller Knight and Mary Jo Gilpin Decker. Designed for the 5- to 7-year-old writer.

Helping Your Handwriting, Rosemary Sassoon. An Italics writing program; this book shows the student how to identify, understand, and correct personal handwriting problems.

Fluent Handwriting, Nan Jay Barchowsky. An Italics writing program.

Appendix 18-3

Games to Support Prewriting and Early Writing Skills for the Kindergarten Classroom

(Courtesy of Jackie Carey, OTA).
All of the following games were placed in a plastic container and following instruction to the teacher, were left in the kindergarten classroom for use in a fine motor center.

Paper Clip Race

Materials: Dice, box of large paper clips, and a playing card made from oaktag 12" x 4". Draw line down middle from top to bottom. Draw 15 lines across spaced from top to bottom. Number the boxes 1 to 15, from bottom to top with a star at the top. Laminate cards.
Procedure: Take turns rolling dice. Count out the paperclips for the number rolled on dice. Attach clips to game sheet. First to reach top is winner.

Twisted Pipes and Pipe Letters

Materials: Accordian Pipe®, tiny dice, cards (use regular 8 x 11 copy paper) with upper and lower case letters drawn on them with numbers and arrows for correct letter formation guides.
Procedure for Twisted Pipes: Roll die. Connect that many pipes. Twist them and connect ends.
Procedure for Pipe Letters: Put the procedures in same bag as Accordian Pipe® letters. Use same materials. Make letter or number of the week.

Do You Know Your Money?

Materials: Coin bank, plastic coins, and cards with a picture of a different coin on each.
Procedure: Place coins on table and put lid back on bank. Match the coins to the proper card. Count them as you put them in the bank.

How Much Money Can You Hold?

Materials: Plastic coins and coin bank, dice
Procedure: Spread money on table. Put lid back on can. Keep one hand behind back. Roll die. Pick up coins to match number on die using only one hand. Put coins in slot while one hand is still behind back.

Eraser Race

Materials: Small mini erasers, dice, tongs, disposable plastic cup with hole in bottom
Procedure: Spread out small erasers on table. Turn cup upside down. Roll dice. Put one hand behind back. Use tongs to place erasers in hole in cup. Repeat with other hand.

Feed the Alligator

Materials: Cotton balls, Alligator Snatcher®, large disposable cup with hole, paper plate
Procedure: Place plate on floor with cotton balls on it. Roll dice. Using alligator, pick up the cotton balls or colored pom-poms and place in cup.

Feed the Frog (variation on Feed the Alligator but use Crazy Clickers®).

Magic Writing

Materials: Erasable Highlighter Pen
Procedure: Draw some shapes with the yellow marker. Go over the line with the white side of the marker. Magic! Make sure tops are on when done (snap!)

Feed the Tennis Ball

Materials: Tennis ball with a slit cut out for mouth and two eyes drawn with marker, and buttons or small bingo chips.
Procedure: Squeeze ball to open mouth and feed chips.

Games to Support Prewriting and Early Writing Skills for the Kindergarten Classroom

Mini-Etch a Sketch®

Materials: Ohio Art Pocket Etch a Sketch® (Bryan, OH), oak tag cut into small cards with designs to copy drawn on them, such as a horizontal line, vertical line, cross, stairs, T, square, triangle, circle.
Procedure: Children copy the shapes on etch a sketch.

What's Missing?

Materials: Plastic Stringing Discs®
Procedure: Set comes with 21 pattern cards. The child has to duplicate the color pattern. At the end, they have to figure out how to repeat the pattern (what's missing).

Button Necklace

Materials: Soft thin foam sheets, and yarn. Cut foam sheets into squares and cut slits into them. Take a piece of yarn and tie a medium sized button to it. Tie another button to the other end. Make cards with patterns.
Procedure: Child has to slide the button through the hole in the foam squares. The child has to duplicate the color pattern. At the end, they have to figure out how to repeat the pattern.

Martian Popping Thing

Materials: Martian Popping® toy (Gag Works, Los Alamitos, CA), dice
Procedure: Roll dice. Squeeze the Martian the number of times rolled using first one hand and then the other.

Paperclip Game

Materials: Large and small paperclips, a laminated playing card 8" x 12." With marker, draw a line down the center of the card. Number 1 through 12 from top to bottom on each card and draw lines horizontally across and under each number.
Procedure: Child rolls the dice. Count and pick up number of paper clips rolled. Place paper clips on card. Next child rolls. First child to fill their side of the card wins.

Letter Wheel

Materials: Carbon paper and white paper cut into 4"x 6" pieces, tracing wheel.
Procedure: Put shiny side of carbon paper face down between two pieces of paper. Use wheel to trace over letters. Hold wheel like a piece of chalk with index finger on top.

Giant Stencils

Materials: Giant sized stencils and large pieces of construction paper.
Procedure: Lie on tummy on floor. Use one hand for drawing and other hand to hold stencil.

Eraser Race

Materials: Zoo Sticks® (available through TheraPro, Framingham, MA), mini erasers, tongs, small cup with hole in bottom, mini dice.
Procedure: Spread out erasers on table. Turn cup upside down. Roll die. Put one hand behind back. Use tongs to place erasers in hole. Use other hand.

Wikki Stix®

Materials: A handful of Wikki Stix® (Omnicor, Phoenix, AZ) dot to dot patterns, and a sheet of paper for letter of the week practice.

Remaining Bags

Other bags contained items that were self-explanatory. Items included: Short, fat, broken pieces of crayons to color with, wind-up toys, a magnetic tracing maze game, toys that vibrate when you pull the string, a sparkle wheel, dancing animals, Tornado Spinners®, Buzz Saws®, and Reptile "Buddies"®.

Chapter 19

EARLY INTERVENTION

Olga Baloueff, ScD, OTR/L, PT, BCP

Chapter Objectives

- Explain the meaning, rationale, and goals of early intervention.
- Understand current legislation governing the delivery of services to infants and toddlers with disabilities.
- Understand and discuss rationale for family-centered practice in early intervention.
- Describe the various aspects of service delivery proper to early intervention, such as Individualized Family Service Plan and natural environments.
- Explain the role of the occupational therapy practitioner in early intervention.

Introduction

Susie, Jack, and Jeff are beautiful triplets who were born 3 months prematurely at 28 weeks of gestation to first time parents. Two of the babies experienced a very stormy course of events in the Neonatal Intensive Care Unit (NICU). Susie and Jeff had a grade 1 bleed, pulmonary hypertension, and many other complications. The infants are now at home and their parents, although elated with having them, are overwhelmed with the daily routines of caring for three children, two of them still very fragile. They also have concerns regarding their feeding and the persistent crying, potential developmental delays, acquisition of motor milestones, and what the future holds for their family.

Pierre is a 22-month-old little boy who is the youngest of three children. At birth he was diagnosed with Down

Syndrome and a congenital heart defect. He lives with his siblings and his parents; the family recently immigrated to the US. Pierre is not yet walking or talking. He is a fussy eater who gets tired very easily. His parents and his two sisters are very involved in his care. They are looking for guidance on how best to help him in his development.

Sophia is a 19-month-old girl who was recently adopted from Eastern Europe. Her adoptive mother is a middle class, single professional who, at the moment, has taken a 6 months leave from her job. She reports that the orphanage in which the young child spent her early life was quite bleak and overcrowded. Although Sophia's mother does not have much experience with children, she is quite aware that her daughter is not developing at the same rate as other children her age. Sophia is also very slow to warm-up to her mother's affections. She is a fussy child with a poor appetite who does not play with toys, engages in self-rocking, and wakes up often during the night. Her mother is losing confidence in her ability to manage the day-to-day care of such a lovely but difficult child.

Joey is a 3-month-old boy, born to Gloria who is a 17-year-old young woman who dropped out of school in her senior in high school and has been trying to prepare for the GED exam. She lives with her mother and her two younger sisters in a small apartment. Joey is the product of an unexpected and unplanned pregnancy. Until she was 8 weeks pregnant, Gloria was actively using cocaine, valium, alcohol, and cigarettes. Upon discovering that she was pregnant, she tried to discontinue the use of drugs, but was not fully successful. Joey was born almost full term, but was small for gestational age. He spent a few days in the NICU, but shortly afterwards went home with his mother. He was a very difficult newborn, with a high-pitched cry and little ability to self-calm. He was jittery, and his knees and elbows were rubbed raw from his agitated movements. In addition, the muscles of his tiny legs were so stiff that it was difficult to straighten them when diapering him. Now, 3 months later, Joey is better, but he is still a very difficult child to care for. He gets easily over-aroused, and is a fussy eater. The pediatrician has concerns over his development and Gloria's ability to provide an environment supportive of her young son's development.

These stories are examples of young children and their families participating in early intervention programs. They receive services from a number of professionals with diverse disciplinary backgrounds, among them occupational therapy (OT) practitioners. These families represent a wide range of needs and come from various cultural and socioeconomic backgrounds.

Defining Early Intervention

Early intervention (EI) refers to federally supported developmental and community-based services for children with disabilities or developmental delays, ages zero to three. Services are multidisciplinary, and designed to enhance child development, minimize potential delays, remediate existing problems, prevent and limit further acquisition of additional disabilities, and promote adaptive family functioning (Hanson & Bruder, 2001; Simeonsson, 2002).

Federal Policy and Early Intervention Services

Federal legislations since 1975 have transformed the delivery of educational, health, and social services for children with disabilities and developmental deviations. The first of these public laws (PL), the Education of the Handicapped Act (EHA, PL 94-142) mandated that a free appropriate education be given in the least restrictive environment for all children with "handicaps" (terminology used at the time), age 5 through 21.

Knowledge about the influence of early childhood experiences and the importance of the family in children's development and school performance strongly influenced the next law, EHA Amendments, PL 99-457, passed in 1986. Part H of the law gave financial incentives to all states to plan, develop, and implement family-centered early intervention programs to provide for the needs of young children from birth to age three with disabilities and developmental deviations. It was left to each state to not only determine how to define and assess developmental delays but also to decide whether or not to serve young children who were at risk for such delays. This law opened the door for a wide range of children to be served and for the participation of a

variety of professional service providers, including OT practitioners (Hanson & Bruder, 2001). It also resulted in great variation from state to state in the implementation of services.

Since the passage of these two pioneering legislations, subsequent reauthorizations have been enacted (Baloueff & Cohn, 2003). The Individuals with Disabilities Education Act (IDEA) Amendments, PL 105-17, passed in 1997 addresses the continuum of services from birth to age 21 (Reinson, 2000). Part C of the law provides guidelines for EI services for infants and toddlers from birth to age three. It also defines EI as "developmental services that are provided: a) under public supervision; b) at no cost except where Federal or State law provides for a system of payments by families, including a schedule of sliding fees; c) designed to meet the developmental needs of an infant or toddler with a disability" (PL 105-17, sec. 632.4).

State requirements for EI implementation as mandated by PL 105-17 are listed in Table 19-1.

Early Intervention Goals

Table 19-2 lists the EI goals as stated in PL 105-17, Part C of IDEA Amendments of 1997.

To meet the EI goals, Simeonsson (2002) recommends an approach that:

- Recognizes the child's individual differences in terms of abilities and disabilities.
- Has a comprehensive focus encompassing the child's health, development, and well-being in assessment and intervention.
- Designs interventions that are personalized for the child and family as a unit.
- Implements intervention that involve families in a social and cultural context.
- Supports and complements the caregiving role of families.
- Takes child and family development into account as factors influencing intervention goals and outcomes.
- Provides for quality assurance in services to children and families (p. 6).

Rationale for Early Intervention

The first three years of life are times of enormous growth and development. Developmental theory and research, and practical applications with children who are at high risk for developmental deviations due to biological, social, and environmental conditions, all suggest that specific, targeted interventions conducted early have a good chance of success (Guralnick, 1997). Because the early years provide the

Table 19-1

Statewide Requirements for Early Intervention Services Implementation

It is up to each individual state to:

1. Define developmental delay.
2. Ensure availability of appropriate EI services to all infants and toddlers with disabilities and their families.
3. Provide timely, comprehensive multidisciplinary evaluation of the functioning of each infant and toddler with a disability and a family-directed identification of the family needs.
4. Establish a process for implementing the individualized family service plan (IFSP) that includes the coordination of services.
5. Develop a comprehensive child find system.
6. Create a public awareness program focusing on early identification of infants and toddlers with disabilities.
7. Create a central directory of information on EI services, resources, and experts available in the State, including research and demonstration projects being conducted in the State.
8. Design and implement a comprehensive system of personnel development, including the training of paraprofessionals and primary referral sources.
9. Establish and maintain policies and procedures for ensuring personnel standards.
10. Designate and establish a single line of responsibility in a lead agency for identifying and coordinating all available resources within the State from Federal, State, local, and private sources.
11. Establish a policy for contracting and coordinating services with local service providers to provide EI services in the State.
12. Develop procedures for securing timely reimbursements and funds.
13. Put procedural safeguards in place.
14. Design and implement a system for compiling data of EI services.
15. Establish a State interagency coordinating council (ICC) composed of parents, service providers, government officials and members of agencies of EI and preschool services, Head Start, child care, and health insurance. The ICC role is to advise and assist the lead agency in the administration and coordination of the EI system.
16. Develop policies and procedures to ensure that EI services for infants and toddlers are provided: a) in natural environments, and b) in a setting other than the natural environment only when EI services cannot be achieved satisfactorily in the natural environment.

(PL 105-17, Part C, sec. 635)

Table 19-2

Goals of Early Intervention Stated in IDEA Amendments of 1997, PL 105-17, Part C

The Congress finds that there is an urgent and substantial need:

1. To enhance the development of infants and toddlers with disabilities and to minimize their potential for developmental delay.
2. To reduce the educational costs to our society, including our Nation's schools, by minimizing the need for special education and related services after infants and toddlers with disabilities reach school age.
3. To minimize the likelihood of institutionalization of individuals with disabilities and maximize the potential for their independently living in society.
4. To enhance the capacity of families to meet the special needs of their infants and toddlers with disabilities.
5. To enhance the capacity of State and local agencies and service providers to identify, evaluate, and meet the needs of historically underrepresented populations, particularly minority, low-income, inner-city, and rural populations.

(sec. 631, a)

foundation for later adaptation, intervention during this time period offers the opportunity to alter not only the early experiences, but also the life trajectories of children (Farran, 2000; Ramey, Campbell & Blair, 1998; Wolery, 2000).

Research in the neurobiological, behavioral, and social sciences has stressed "...the importance of early experiences, as well as the inseparable and highly interactive influences of genetics and environment on the development of the brain and the unfolding of human behavior" (Shonkoff & Phillips, 2000, p. 283). The first three years of life often are referred to as a special "window of opportunity." Starting at conception, the brain develops at a remarkable pace through the first years of life (Blackman, 2002). Early brain development is characterized by the elaboration of many critical structures, increased myelinization of the pathways, and rapid proliferation of synaptic connections (Nelson, 2000). At the same time, these rapid periods of growth, especially in the fetal stage of development, make the infant's brain vulnerable to possible damage.

Nature and nurture are totally intertwined, and environmental influences both positive and negative affect brain development (Hawley & Gunner, 2000; Nelson, 2000; Shonkoff & Phillips, 2000). Brain development and function in early childhood are highly dependent on environmental experiences and relationships with caregivers (Fenichel, 2002; Shonkoff & Phillips, 2000). The brain continues to develop postnatally, and social experiences during this time help to wire both the structure and function of the brain (Blackman, 2002). The early care and nurture an infant receives affect the formation of neural pathways and have a long-lasting impact on how the infant develops, learns, and regulates emotions. Healthy early development depends on nurturing and dependable relationships (Shonkoff & Phillips, 2000). Traumatic experiences, however, can inhibit normal brain development and lead to serious emotional and developmental problems (Shonkoff & Phillips, 2000). The combination of socioeconomic disadvantages, such as family and neighborhood poverty, with a child's biological vulnerability at birth has been shown to have negative effects on the child's development (Fenichel, 2002). This is referred to as "double jeopardy". Significant parent mental health problems, substance abuse, and family violence impose heavy developmental burdens on young children (Shonkoff & Phillips, 2000) (please refer to Chapter 9: Interacting With Families).

Eligibility for Services: Population Served through EI

The population of children served by EI programs are infants or toddlers with disabilities. According to the law (PL 105-17, Part C, sec 632), disability "...means a child under 3 years of age who is experiencing developmental delays in one or more of the following areas: cognitive, physical, communication, social or emotional, and adaptive." It also includes young children who have a diagnosed physical or mental condition that has a high probability of resulting in developmental delay. At each state's discretion these services may also be extended to at-risk infants and toddlers who more than likely would experience substantial developmental delays unless they receive EI.

Each state is responsible for developing more specific definitions of developmental risk and delay, including criteria for determining eligibility for services for the infants, toddlers, and their families residing in that state (Widerstrom, 1997). They also must establish the appropriate diagnostic instruments and procedures to determine this eligibility. Thus, there may be great variations from state to state regarding the risk categories of children and their families served by EI as well as the extent of their developmental delays.

In general, there are three categories of risk for developmental delays: a) established risk; b) biological risk; and c) environmental risk (Reinson, 2000; Widerstrom, 1997). Children with established risks are those manifesting early-appearing atypical development due to a diagnosed physical or mental condition, which has a high probability of resulting in developmental delay. These conditions may include Down syndrome and other chromosomal abnormalities, metabolic disorders, and/or sensory impairments. Biological risks are conditions that make infants and toddlers more likely to acquire developmental delay than children without the condition (Widerstrom, 1997). Children born prematurely or prenatally exposed to drugs are examples of this category of risk. Finally, environmental risk, the less clearly defined category, refers to children who, although physically and mentally sound, may acquire developmental deviations due to depriving life experiences such as poor caregiving and family circumstances. Children living with parents who are experiencing poverty, violence, or substance abuse are more likely to fall into that category of risk.

These three categories of risk are not mutually exclusive, and many young children have a combination of risks for developmental deviations. For example, a child born early with a low birth weight to a teenage mother who has an addiction to drugs and a chaotic lifestyle that limits her ability to properly care for her infant is at greater risk for developmental deviations than a child born prematurely in a stable and nurturing family.

Service Delivery in Early Intervention

Part C of PL 105-17 provides guidelines for EI service delivery. The core components of these services are: a) family-centered and parental participation; b) multidisciplinary assessment; c) the individualized family service plan; d) service provision in natural environments.

Family-Centered Services and Parental Participation

Families are the primary social context in which children live and receive care and nurturing (Baloueff & Cohn, 2003). Every family, like every child, is to some extent unique. Families differ in many ways, including beliefs, habits, values, routines, racial and ethnic backgrounds, socioeconomic conditions and geographic location, and education. Family composition, coping styles, and the efforts involved in raising a child with a disability greatly affect family dynamics. EI services are different from any others in that they are family-centered, focusing not just on the child's needs but also on the family unit. Involvement of the family in all aspects of the services they receive is the "central tenet of early intervention programs" (Simeonsson, 2000, p. 7). These services must reflect respect, acceptance, and sensitivity to the cultural diversity of families.

Parents/caregivers hold a central importance in the health, well-being, and development of their infants and toddlers. Thus, the collaboration between professionals and parents is vitally important in planning and providing services for the child. In such a partnership, service providers are considered to be the technical experts with their knowledge and perspective on the child's condition and intervention strategies, and the parents are the experts on their child, their family, and their strengths, needs and values (Rosenbaum, King, Law, King, & Evans, 1998). Filer & Mahoney (1996) outline the key points of such partnership:

1. Parents having the opportunity to express their concerns and priorities to their early interventionists.

2. Providers listening to what parents are asking for, and being willing to respond to their requests.

3. Providers being able to communicate effectively with parents about the types of services they will provide, and how or why these services are likely to address parents' priorities (p. 23).

Addressing the family's expectations of the role of service providers in the care of their child, a parent writes: "To our family, service providers are our greatest resource who, after having given us all pertinent information must respect our ability to make decisions that will enhance our child's strengths" (Viscardis, 1998, p. 43).

Thus, the challenge for service providers in EI is to understand not only the principles of family-centered care but also to develop a spirit of collaboration with families and

skills in promoting parental participation (Baloueff & Cohn, 2003; Rosenbaum et al., 1998). Parents who report a high degree of satisfaction with the services they receive indicate that, "their families' choices and decisions are respected and that services are planned with families' scheduling needs in mind" (Viscardis, 1998, p. 49). These professionals will also acknowledge that, "they may provide only a portion of the service to a family and that in many cases there are other priorities in the family's life" (Viscardis, 1998, p. 49).

MULTIDISCIPLINARY ASSESSMENT

In young children all areas of development are interdependent. For example, taking turns in talking on the toy telephone or pointing to its picture in a book are indicators of cognitive, motor, and language skills. "Underlying all of this is the emotional capacity that enables children to relate to others and to organize their world" (Meisels & Atkins-Burnett, 2000, p. 232). Developmental gains or gaps in some areas affect development in others. The complexity and interrelationships of infants' and toddlers' needs cannot be fully addressed by a single discipline or outside of the family context. Children are viewed in the context of their families, and families in the context of the communities in which they live (Brown & Barrera, 1999).

In early intervention, assessments are a collaborative process between parents and a multidisciplinary team (Greenspan & Meisels, 1996; Mulligan, 2003). The developmental assessment is a "process designed to deepen understanding of a child's competencies and resources, and of the caregiving and learning environment most likely to help a child make fullest use of his or her developmental potential" (Greenspan & Meisels, 1996, p. 11). Throughout the assessment the parents' concerns, priorities, and resources are explored along with the supports and services necessary for meeting their children's needs. The child's relationship and interactions with his or her caregivers forms the cornerstone of the assessment process (Greenspan & Meisels, 1996; Meisels & Atkins-Burnett, 2000). The choice of developmental assessment varies from state to state, as the law only indicates that the child's developmental delays have to be "measured by appropriate, standardized developmental assessment tools" (Mulligan, 2003, p. 10).

Miller & Hanft (1998) offer the following guidelines for building an alliance with parents during their child's assessment:

1. Build a relationship with family members (p. 50).

2. Do more than a single standardized evaluation (p. 51).

3. Respect and rely on the parents' knowledge (p. 52).

4. View the child from a framework of competency embedded within a cultural context (p. 53).

5. Focus on the parents' questions, not your knowledge (p. 53).

THE INDIVIDUALIZED FAMILY SERVICE PLAN

A major requirement, and central to the delivery of family-centered services as outlined in Part C of PL 105-17, is the Individualized Family Service Plan (IFSP). Following the completion and results of the child's evaluation, the IFSP is developed collaboratively by a multidisciplinary team and the child's family members. This plan outlines in writing the services that will be put in place to address the child's developmental needs and the supports for the family/caregivers in meeting their child's needs (Sandall, 1997).

The IFSP has to be completed and signed within 45 days of the child's referral to the EI program and is updated at least every 6 months with an annual revision, following the child's developmental reassessment. Eight specific components to be included in the IFSP are mandated by law (Table 19-3). It is an outcome-based developmental care plan with specific goals and objectives, written in a language understandable to parents. The IFSP even contains parents' own words in sections relative to their concerns, and perceptions of their child's strengths and needs and desired outcomes. Through the IFSP, the intervention plan builds on the family strengths and needs and on the parents' hopes and aspirations for their child. Professionals developing this document must show respect and sensitivity to the family's beliefs, caregiving practices, and daily routines.

This document indicates the specific EI services (e. g., OT, PT, Speech, others) designed to meet the needs of the child and the family, along with the frequency, intensity, and method of service delivery. The IFSP also specifies the environment in which the services are to be provided (natural environment) and a statement of justification if these services are not delivered in the child's natural environment.

Unique to PL 105-17, in Part C is the identification and role of a service coordinator who is responsible for the IFSP implementation and coordination of services with other agencies and persons. Service coordination is an active and ongoing process throughout the entire duration of the recipient's EI services. The service coordinator is chosen from the profession most immediately relevant to the child's and family's/caregiver's needs. Occupational therapy practitioners are among EI professionals who can be designated as service coordinators (Case-Smith, 1998).

The last section of the IFSP contains the steps to be taken to support the transition of the child with a disability to preschool or other appropriate services. Required components of the IFSP are listed in Table 19-3.

SERVICE PROVISION IN NATURAL ENVIRONMENTS

A major component of Part C is the requirement for services to be delivered in natural environments (Hanson & Bruder, 2001). According to the law, natural environments means settings that are natural or normal for the child's age peers who have no disabilities. These settings are the places where young children live, play, and learn. The most natural environment for infants and toddlers is of course their home, but day care centers, parks, libraries, and neighborhood play groups are some examples of other places where young children go in their community. Not all of the EI services have to be provided at the same location and, as the child's and family's needs change, the settings may change as well (Hanson & Bruder, 2001). What constitutes a natural environment for each individual family is determined by that family in conjunction with their EI service coordinator and is documented in the IFSP. Thus, EI in natural environments occurs wherever a child and the family choose it to be (Hanft & Pilkington, 2000).

There are many benefits of delivering services in natural environments (Bruder & Hanson, 2001; Hanft & Pilkington, 2000; Pilkington & Malinowski, 2002). Children and families forge links within their communities and develop supports, which will make transition to preschool services easier when they reach the third birthday. Children with disabilities also benefit socially, cognitively, and emotionally from participating in activities with children without disabilities (Hanson & Bruder, 2001). According to Hanft & Pilkington (2000), there are several advantages for professionals working in natural environments, such as:

1. Enhanced relationships among family members and between therapists and parents;

2. Modeling and support to assist caregivers in their efforts to improve a child's performance; and

3. Improved capacity to assess a child's strengths and select meaningful outcomes. (p. 4)

By delivering services in natural environments, professionals have the opportunity to gain knowledge of the families' typical daily routines, beliefs, values, roles, and responsibilities regarding caregiving and raising a child with a disability (Case-Smith, 1998; Hanft & Pilkington, 2000; Hanson & Bruder, 2001). Follow-up on interventions are more likely to be carried out if they are part of the daily routines or are naturally occurring activities. For examples, activities to increase hand function and trunk balance can be carried out during bath time, diaper change, and sitting on the parent's lap. While playing in the bath or toddler pool, a child can more readily explore various textures and receive deep touch with a towel when coming out of the water.

Role of the Occupational Therapy Practitioner

According to PL 105-17, part C, occupational therapy (OT) is included among the developmental services offered

---

Table 19-3

Required Components of the Individualized Family Service Plan (IFSP)

The IFSP shall be in writing and contain the following (PL 105-17, Part C, sec. 636):

1. A statement of the infant's or toddler's present levels of physical development, cognitive development, communication development, social or emotional development, and adaptive development, based on objective criteria;
2. A statement of the family's resources, priorities, and concerns relating to enhancing the development of the family's infant or toddler with a disability;
3. A statement of the major outcomes expected to be achieved for the infant or toddler and the family, and the criteria, procedures, and timelines used to determine the degree to which progress toward achieving the outcomes is being made and whether modifications or revisions of the outcomes or services are necessary;
4. A statement of specific early intervention services necessary to meet the unique needs of the infant or toddler and the family, including the frequency, intensity, and methods of delivering services;
5. A statement of the natural environments in which early intervention services shall appropriately be provided, including a justification of the extent, if any, to which the services will not be provided in a natural environment;
6. The projected dates for initiation of services and the anticipated duration of the services;
7. The identification of the service coordinator from the profession most immediately relevant to the infant's or toddler's or family's needs (or who is otherwise qualified to carry out all applicable responsibilities under this part) who will be responsible for the implementation of the plan and coordination with other agencies and persons; and
8. The steps to be taken to support the transition of the toddler with a disability to preschool or other appropriate services.

---

in early intervention (Mulligan, 2003). Case-Smith (1998) has identified four overriding goals for OT intervention:

1. Promote change in the child's functional performance.
2. Reframe or redefine the child's behavior.
3. Assist the family and child to compensate for and adapt to the disability.
4. Support family members (p. 39).

Occupational therapy practitioners may be working in teams with other professionals during the child and family evaluation or the IFSP development. Occupational therapy can also stand alone as a service for IFSP implementation (Mellard, 2000). State and facility guidelines and demonstrated competence will dictate the specific role of the OTA in Early Intervention services.

The team approach is used widely in early intervention; interdisciplinary and transdisciplinary team models are the most common (Sandall, 1997; Stephens & Tauber, 1998). In the interdisciplinary model of interaction, professionals of various disciplines involved with the child collaborate with the family and each other in delivering services. This approach is built on the skills unique to each professional specialty. Decision making regarding the interpretation of the child's assessment, goal setting, and IFSP implementation is shared, and reflects the team's consensus. In the transdisciplinary approach, professionals cross the lines of their own traditional discipline and become more like generalists. One member of the team is designated to provide the intervention with the others serving as consultants. This approach gives parents and the child access to one person who consistently works with them and limits the number of professionals coming in and out of their lives.

"Implementation of this model requires role release, or the relinquishing of some or all of one professional's functions to another professional" (Stephens & Tauber, 2001, p. 714) (please refer to Chapter 4: Collaborative Models of Treatment).

Whatever the setting and the model of service delivery, OT practitioners work always in partnership with the child's parents, who are acknowledged as full members of the team. Yet, they also bring into the assessment and intervention processes "a unique understanding of the interdependence and relationship between the child's functional and developmental skills and of sensory perception, behavior, and neurodevelopmental processes" (Stephens & Tauber, 2001, p. 719).

Although the choice of assessments used by OT practitioners in EI may vary according to personal preferences and geographic location, several of them are frequently cited. To assess children's (birth to 3 years) sensory processing abilities, the Infant/Toddler Sensory Profile (Dunn, 2002) is given as a questionnaire to their caregivers. It assesses the child's general, auditory, visual, and vestibular processing from the caregiver's perception. The Peabody Developmental Motor Scales-II (Folio & Fewell, 2000) measures children's (1 to 84 months) gross-motor and fine-motor function. The Pediatric Evaluation of Disability Inventory (PEDI) is used to assess children's (6 months to 7 years) social function, self-care, and mobility (Haley, Coster, Ludlow, Haltiwanger & Andrellos, 1992). All three of these tests are standardized.

Additionally, non-standardized procedures are widely used, such as observations of children at play and in other activities in their natural environments, caregivers' interview, checklists, and questionnaires. Asking parents about their child's sleeping and eating patterns and daily routines is part of the assessment process (please refer to Chapter 8: An Overview of Developmental Assessments).

Summary

Services for infants and toddlers with disability and developmental deviations are mandated by PL 105-17, part C. The EI services are individualized, coordinated, family-focused, and delivered in natural environments. Occupational therapy practitioners have an essential role in EI, working in collaboration with parents and other professionals.

Case Study

BACKGROUND INFORMATION

Brenda is a 9-month-old (6.5 months corrected) little girl who was born very prematurely at 26.5 weeks of gestation, weighing 1.5 lbs. She spent 2.5 months in the NICU and suffered a very difficult perinatal course including being on a ventilator for quite some time. Brenda is the third child in her family and has two older sisters (10 and 8 years old). A year ago, shortly before her birth, the family moved to this new town because of her father's work. This has been particularly difficult on the family because they have not had the time to settle in this neighborhood and have no close relatives in the area. The mother was working part-time in a bank before the family's move, but is now staying at home.

Brenda is currently receiving EI services at home. The interdisciplinary team evaluated Brenda in the presence of her parents. It was found that she is a lovely little girl who is interested in her environment, smiles, sleeps though the night, and sits with support. She has low muscle tone in her trunk, does not yet roll over, and does not hold a rattle in her hand. She drinks from a bottle, but with poor lip control, and seems hypersensitive around her mouth. She likes to be held when wrapped in her baby blanket, but starts crying when her parents and her sisters bounce her up on their lap or gently tickle her. Her parents are eager to help her.

In the IFSP it was determined that an occupational therapy practitioner would visit Brenda weekly at home to help her and her family. Activities were designed to improve her motor and feeding skills and to normalize her sensori responses as well as provide support for the family, especially the mother. These activities are incorporated within the family's daily routines.

DISCUSSION QUESTIONS

1. What are the reasons for providing EI services to this family? What category of risks does this child fit in?
2. What skills and abilities do infants develop in the first year of life?
3. What is the difference between chronological and corrected age in children born prematurely?
4. What kind of activities would an occupational therapy practitioner use in addressing Brenda's motor, feeding, and sensori needs?

Application Activities

1. Visit an EI program in your community and compare experiences with classmates.
2. Interview an EI director or EI service provider and ask them about their roles and experiences.
3. Interview parents (friends, neighbors, etc.) about their child's birthing experience and about a typical day with their infant or toddler.
4. Explore various cultural practices regarding such as sleep environment, feeding, discipline, toileting, play.

References

Baloueff, O. & Cohn, E. S (2003). Introduction to the infant, child and adolescent population. In E. B. Crepeau, E. S. Cohn & B. A. Boyt Schell (Eds.). *Willard & Spackman's occupational therapy* (10th ed., pp. 691-698). Philadelphia: Lippincott Williams & Wilkins.

Blackman, J. A. (2002). Early intervention: A global perspective. *Infants & Young Children, 15*(2), 11-19.

Brown, W. & Barrera, I. (1999). Enduring problems in assessment: The persistent challenges of cultural dynamics and family issues. *Infants & Young Children, 12*(1), 34-42.

Case-Smith, J. (1998). Defining the early intervention process. In J. Case-Smith (Ed.), *Pediatric occupational therapy and early intervention* (pp. 27-48). Boston: Butterworth-Heinemann.

Dunn, W. (2002). *Infant/toddler sensory profile.* San Antonio, TX: Psychological Corporation.

Farran, D. C. (2000). Another decade of intervention for children who are low income or disabled: What do we know now? In J. P. Shonkoff & S. J. Meisels (Eds.), *Handbook of early childhood intervention* (2nd ed., pp. 510-548). New York: Cambridge University Press.

Fenichel, E. (2002). Have you read N to N yet? *Infants & Young Children, 14*(3), v-viii.

Filer, J. D. & Mahoney, G. J. (1996). Collaboration between families and early intervention service providers. *Infants & Young Children, 9*(2), 22-30.

Folio, M. R. & Fewell, R. R. (2000). *Peabody developmental motor scales* (2nd ed.). San Antonio, TX: Psychological Corporation.

Greenspan, S. I. & Meisels, S. J. (1996). Toward a new vision for the developmental assessment of infants and young children. In S. J. Meisels & Fenichel (Eds.). *New visions for the developmental assessment of infants and young children* (pp. 11-26). Washington, DC: Zero to Three.

Guralnick, M. J. (1997). *The effectiveness of early intervention.* Baltimore, MD: Paul H. Brookes.

Haley, S. M., Coster, W. J., Haltiwanger, J. T. & Andrellos, P. J. (1992). *Pediatric evaluation of disability inventory.* San Antonio, TX: Psychological Corporation.

Hanft, B. E. & Pilkington, K. D. (2000). Therapy in natural environments: The means or end goal for early intervention? *Infants & Young Children, 12*(4), 1-13.

Hanson, M. J. & Bruder, M. B. (2001). Early intervention: Promises to keep. *Infants & Young Children, 13*(3), 47-58.

Hawley, T. & Gunner, M. (2000). *Starting smart.* Washington, DC: Zero to Three, The Ounce of Prevention Fund.

Individuals with Disabilities Education Act (IDEA) Amendments of 1997 (Public Law 105-17), USC 1400. http://www.ideapractices.org 1997.

Meisels, S. J. & Atkins-Burnett, S. (2000). The elements of early childhood assessment. In J. P. Shonkoff & S. J. Meisels (Eds.). *Handbook of early childhood intervention* (2nd ed., pp. 231-257). New York: Cambridge University Press.

Mellard, E. (2000). Impact of federal policy on services for children and families in early intervention programs and public schools. In W. Dunn (Ed.). *Best practice occupational therapy: In community service with children and families* (pp. 147-156). Thorofare, NJ: SLACK Incorporated.

Miller, L. J. & Hanft, B. E. (1998). Building positive alliances: Partnerships with families as the cornerstone of developmental assessment. *Infants & Young Children, 11*(1), 49-60.

Mulligan, S. (2003). *Occupational therapy evaluation for children.* Philadelphia, PA: Lippincott Williams & Wilkins.

Nelson, C. A. (2000). The neurological bases of early intervention. In J. P. Shonkoff & S. J. Meisels (Eds.), *Handbook of early childhood intervention* (2nd ed., pp. 204-227. New York: Cambridge University Press.

Pilkington, K. O. & Malinowski, M. (2002). The natural environment II: Uncovering deeper responsibilities within relationship-based services. *Infants & Young Children, 15*(2), 78-84.

Ramey, C., Campbell, F., & Blair, C. (1998). Enhancing the life course for high-risk children. In J. Crane (Ed.). *Social programs that work* (pp. 184-199). New York: Russell Sage Foundation.

Reinson, C. (2000). A framework for the identification and evaluation of developmentally vulnerable children and their family members: Part II. *Developmental Disabilities Special Interest Section Quarterly, 23*(3), 1-3.

Rosenbaum, P., King, S., Law, M., King, G., & Evans, J. (1998). Family-centered service: A conceptual framework and research review. *Physical & Occupational Therapy in Pediatrics, 18*(1), 1-20.

Sandall, S. R. (1997). The individualized family service plan. In A. H. Widerstrom, B. A. Mowder, & S. R. Sandall (Eds.). *Infant development and risk: An introduction* (2nd ed., pp. 237-257). Baltimore: Paul H. Brookes.

Shonkoff, J. P. & Phillips, D. A. (Eds.) (2000). *From neurons to neighborhoods: The science of early childhood development.* Washington, DC: National Academy Press.

Simeonsson, R. J. (2000). Early childhood intervention: Toward a universal manifesto. *Infants & Young Children, 12*(3), 4-9.

Stephens, L. C. & Tauber, S. K. (2001). Early intervention. In J. Case-Smith (Ed.). *Occupational therapy for children* (4th ed., pp. 708-729). St. Louis, MO: Mosby.

Viscardis, L. (1998). The family-centered approach to providing services: A parent perspective. *Physical & Occupational Therapy in Pediatrics, 18*(1), 41-53.

Widerstrom, A. H. (1997). Newborns and infants at risk for or with disabilities. In A. H. Widerstrom, B. A. Mowder & S. R. Sandall (Eds.) *Infant development and risk: An introduction* (2nd ed., pp. 3-21). Baltimore: Paul H. Brookes.

Wolery, M. (2000). Behavioral and educational approaches to early intervention. In J. P. Shonkoff & S. J. Meisels (Eds.). *Handbook of early childhood intervention* (2nd ed., pp. 179-203). New York: Cambridge University Press.

20

PRESCHOOL AND SCHOOL-BASED THERAPY

DeLana Honaker, PhD, OTR, BCP

Chapter Objectives

- List legislations that influence special education and related services for children with special needs.
- Define key terms and acronyms used in legislation and services related to school-based practice.
- Define the role of occupational therapy in evaluation, developing individual education plans, and service provision in school-based practice.
- Identify mandated elements of an individualized education plan.
- Discuss models of service delivery in school-based practice.
- Discuss the role of occupational therapy in transition planning.
- Identify readiness skills and occupational activities that facilitate mastery of educational goals and objectives.

Origins of Occupational Therapy Services in Schools

HISTORY

Prior to early 1970s, children with special needs were enrolled in special schools at the parents' expense or in state-funded institutions, which may or may not have been in near proximity to the family's home, or simply were not enrolled, or even required to enroll in school. With the passage of Section 504 of the Rehabilitation Act in 1973 (Pub. L., 93-112), access to and accommodations for education and work for persons with a physical and/or mental disability changed significantly (Martin, 1997) and the influence of this act continues today through the Individuals with Disabilities Education Act (IDEA) (1997) (Pub. L. 105-117) and the Americans with Disabilities Act (ADA) (1990) (Pub. L.101-336). As a result, and as illustrated in Table 20-1, a child with a disability is very likely to benefit either actively or passively from all three acts during his/her lifespan.

In this scenario, Jason initially experiences IDEA Part C services as an infant born 6 weeks prematurely and with a possible diagnosis of cerebral palsy; upon evaluation and as part of his services in the early intervention program, Jason and his family receive consultations and direct services from occupational, physical and speech therapy as well as case management services from a social worker. When Jason turns 3, he is evaluated again and becomes eligible for IDEA Part B services as a student with an orthopedic impairment (at age two he was formally diagnosed with cerebral palsy, left hemiplegic type) and attends a preschool program specifically designed for children with disabilities in the local school district. In this classroom Jason has a special education teacher and teaching assistant and often spends his day at school playing with his peers, some of whom also have disabilities, learning pre-academic skills, and learning how to walk and dress himself. In this setting, Jason continues to receive direct and consultation occupational, physical, and speech therapy services. By the time Jason enters kindergarten, he is walking independently but still has some fine motor skill and speech articulation delays. Beginning with kindergarten, Jason is enrolled in general education

Table 20-1

Jason's Lifespan of Services

Jason's Lifespan	Actively Served By	Passively Served By
Infancy through age 2 years	IDEA '97 Part C	Americans with Disabilities Act (ADA) (1990)
3 years old to middle school	IDEA '97 Part B	
Middle school through high school	Section 504	
College	ADA	
Work	ADA	

classes with special education providing support on an inclusion and pull-out basis. Frequently, Jason is the only student with a physical impairment in his classes, although there are other children with learning differences in his classroom, and in his school. A special education teacher often comes in to work with Jason during certain classroom activities, yet other times he goes down to the special education teacher's classroom for individualized instruction. He continues to receive direct and consultation occupational therapy services to address written communication delays and direct and consultation speech therapy services to address articulation skills. At this stage of his academic career, Jason only receives consultation services from physical therapy; these consultation services are often with the physical education (PE) teacher, as both the PE teacher and the physical therapist discuss ways to adapt gym activities so that Jason can participate fully with his peers. As Jason grows older, he continues to make good progress in his classes, becomes more independent and/or uses adaptive strategies to complete all classroom tasks. As Jason becomes more independent and masters special and general education objectives, the occupational and speech therapists decrease the amounts of service provided to Jason, and eventually dismiss him from related services. By the time Jason enters middle school, he has mastered all special education objectives, is making excellent grades and no longer requires special education services, so is dismissed from special education. The Section 504 student support team in Jason's school meets to discuss possible accommodations Jason may require to continue to participate in his general education setting. Jason's teachers, parents and Jason, himself, discuss the need for additional time to walk to his classes and assistance with note taking as he is not always able to keep up with the pace of classroom lectures. Jason also asks about the requirements of the keyboarding class that he will take the following semester. As the student support team discusses these issues, they decide that Jason is eligible to receive the accommodations of additional time to travel within the school and note taking assistance under Section 504. In addition, the team decides to request an occupational therapy evaluation to determine what possible

accommodations may be required in order for Jason to complete his keyboarding class, a requirement for graduation. Upon the completion of the evaluation and based on the recommendations from the occupational therapist, the student support team meet again and add an accommodation that allows Jason to learn and use a one-handed typing program. Jason continues to make progress, graduates with his peers, and makes plans to attend college.

Throughout his childhood and adolescence, Jason and his family passively received ADA services in the form of community access. However upon entering college, the ADA becomes an active service. Prior to beginning college, Jason and his mother meet with the ADA compliance officer at his university to discuss possible accommodations. Jason's mother provides documentation regarding Jason's disability and the compliance officer arranges for Jason to have access to a first floor dormitory room, works with Jason in developing a course schedule that allows him plenty of time to get to his classes, and assists Jason in completing an application for a special parking permit that allows him to use the campus handicapped parking spaces. Over the years, Jason declares a major in information systems. The compliance officer contacts the state rehabilitation commission to evaluate Jason's technology needs necessary to his major. Jason eventually graduates with a degree in information systems and applies for several positions in various companies. After accepting a position with one company, reasonable accommodations are discussed during Jason's vetting and as part of his rights under ADA, he is again provided a designated parking place and adapted equipment for his computer workstation.

As you can see, a person with a disability continues to have full access to education and work throughout his lifetime under current legislations. At no other time in American history have there been as many opportunities for persons with disabilities to learn, to participate, to work, and to be self-sufficient.

Although this chapter primarily explores occupational therapy services provided under IDEA Part B, the basic origins of IDEA and evolving trends in education law, provide an important foundation to this discussion.

THE EVOLUTION OF IDEA

The predecessor of IDEA, the Education of the Handicapped Act (EHA) (1975) was enacted by Congress to specifically address the special education and related services for children with disabilities, particularly those in the public schools. The significance of this law was the mandate that all children ages 3 to 21 years with disabilities should receive free and appropriate public education (FAPE) regardless of the level or severity of their disability (Mehfound, 1998; American Occupational Therapy Association [AOTA], 1999a). With each reauthorization, IDEA has experienced changes beginning in 1978, and subsequently in 1986, 1990 and 1997, with significant changes occurring in 1990 and 1997. The Individuals with Disabilities Education Improvement Act of 2003 initiated the process to reauthorize IDEA again and on December 3, 2004, President Bush signed H.R. 1350, the Individuals with Disabilities Education Improvement Act of 2004. This is expected to take effect in July 2005. As this book is being published prior to publication of H.R. 1350 regulations and policies, only fundamental differences of the latest reauthorization of the IDEA are discussed in this chapter; check your state and local education agencies for the latest information and changes. To briefly summarize the changes in EHA/IDEA over the years, a discussion of trends in access, evaluation, accountability, and the role of occupational therapy in schools follows.

The issue of access encompasses the child with special needs attending a public school under EHA, to the child with special needs participating with nondisabled peers in the classroom under IDEA, to the child with special needs participating in all aspects of the general education curriculum, including state and district assessments under IDEA '97 (National Information Center for Children and Youth with Disabilities, [NICHCY], 1998). The Individuals with Disabilities Education Improvement Act of 2003 attempts to comply with the No Child Left Behind Act of 2001 (NCLB) by extending the issue of access to include school district accountability through assessment of *all* children, even those with significant disabilities. Does this mean the child with significant cognitive impairment will take a state assessment at his/her grade level in reading and writing? Probably not, but the state and district education agency will be obligated to develop and provide appropriate alternative assessments and to report the results of these assessments to parents/caregivers just as the state and districts are required to report the results of these assessments for the nondisabled child as mandated by NCLB. The key focus with regard to access is not only does the child with special needs have access to FAPE, but that FAPE includes *all* elements of education in the areas of assessment, participation, and learning.

A major trend guiding evaluations and reevaluations, as well as eligibility determination is the ever-increasing involvement of parents (or guardians/caregivers) in this process. Evaluation and reevaluation continues to drive all special education and related services in all reauthorizations of IDEA, supporting the need for well-educated, well-informed professionals to work with children with special needs (NICHCY, 1998; President's Commission on Excellence in Special Education [PCESE], 2002).

Accountability also became evident as issues related to the Individual Education Plan (IEP) became increasingly specific in IDEA '97 and is a critical component of H.R. 1350. Under the provisions of IDEA '97, the IEP must include measurable goals and objectives, evaluation methods to measure these outcomes, supplementary aids and services, modifications to the curriculum, frequency/location/duration of services, the influence of behavior on educational progress and communication accommodations (for students and/or parents with vision or hearing deficits or with limited English proficiency). In addition, IDEA '97 mandates that regular reports on the child's progress in general and special education be provided to the parents/caregivers at least as often as progress is reported for the nondisabled child, such as at the end of the district's grading periods (i.e., every 6 or 9 weeks, quarter or semester) (NICHCY, 1998). While the notion of regular reports on the child's progress in general and special education appears ideal, the reports have actually significantly increased the amount of documentation and paperwork for special education and related service providers. In an effort to reduce the burden of extra paperwork, H.R. 1350 attempts to eliminate the need for short-term objectives and benchmarks except for children "...who take the alternate assessment aligned to the alternate achievement standard" (Council for Exceptional Children, 2004). Therefore, some paperwork reduction is expected; however, final regulations as well as state interpretations and regulations may still require short-term objectives and/or benchmarks with less frequent reports of progress, such as quarterly reports rather than a report each grading period.

A further trend is the evolving role of related services under IDEA. While occupational therapy has always played an important role in EHA / IDEA in the form of related services to evaluate and support special education goals and objectives, the role becomes more secured and more specific in assistive technology, as a contributor in meetings to plan educational services, and in transition planning under IDEA '97 (NICHCY, 1998; NICHCY, 2001). The role of occupational therapy as well as other related services continues to evolve with H.R.1350; in particular related services may be provided as an early intervening service or as a preventative measure rather than only after the child experiences failure-to-make-progress (AOTA, 2004). This is a significant role change for occupational therapy in the schools and allows occupational therapists (OTs) and occupational therapy assistants (OTAs), depending upon state and facility guidelines, demonstrated competency, and working under the supervision of an OT, to be involved in and make programming suggestions for children at risk prior to eligibility for special education services.

IDEA '97

Over the years key components of EHA/IDEA have progressed from broadly defined services to specific services as defined by the nine parts of IDEA and then to consolidated services or the restructured four parts of IDEA '97. The four parts include:

PART A–GENERAL PROVISIONS

In this section of IDEA 97, issues are covered such as how IDEA '97 will be funded; the mandate to states to locate, evaluate, and provide services to all eligible children with disabilities; definitions of the 13 disability categories; and effective dates for the various parts of IDEA '97 are covered (AOTA, 1999a; Council for Exceptional Children, 1997).

PART B–ASSISTANCE FOR EDUCATION OF ALL CHILDREN WITH DISABILITIES

This section mandates that states locate, evaluate, and provide services to children with disabilities aged three years through 21 years; ensures that all children with disabilities are entitled to free and appropriate public education (FAPE), including special education and related services to meet their individualized educational needs; protects the rights of the children and their families; and ensures effectiveness of the efforts to educate children with disabilities (AOTA, 1999a; 34 C.F.R. §300.1).

PART C–INFANTS AND TODDLERS WITH DISABILITIES

Part C mandates that states locate, evaluate, and provide services to infants and toddlers aged 0-2 years, and their families. The focus of this part of IDEA '97 is to direct states "...to expand opportunities for children under 3 years of age who would be at risk of having substantial developmental delays if they did not receive early intervention services" (Council for Exceptional Children, 1997; 34 C.F.R., §303) (please refer to Chapter 19: Early Intervention).

PART D–NATIONAL ACTIVITIES TO IMPROVE EDUCATION OF CHILDREN WITH DISABILITIES

This section of IDEA '97 allows for the formation of discretionary programs or national efforts to improve education of children with disabilities. Grant funds are available to research the efficacy or improvement of services to children

with disabilities, and professional development, personnel preparation, technical assistance, support, and dissemination of information (Council for Exceptional Children, 1997).

As noted earlier, Part A of IDEA '97 defined 13 categories of disabilities and they are listed in Table 20-2 along with brief definitions.

It is expected that H.R. 1350 will retain current eligibility categories and definitions with the exception for Learning Disabilities. In recognition of the fact that current eligibility for LD is based on severe discrepancy between achievement and intellectual ability in basic reading, reading comprehension, written expression, oral expression, listening comprehension, math computation, and/or math reasoning, the severe discrepancy model may not be sensitive to identifying younger children with delays in these areas or children who are struggling to make academic progress but do not meet the eligibility for learning disabled. To that end, school districts may use alternate evaluation procedures such as documenting the child's ability to make progress using alternative research-based interventions or curricula to determine an LD eligibility (Council for Exceptional Children, 2004). Again, check with your local and state education agencies to learn how eligibilities will be determined in your district.

Part B: Assistance for Education of All Children With Disabilities

Delving into IDEA '97 Part B, common terms and acronyms and their definitions are critical to understanding the law. This section begins with a review of commonly used acronyms and then moves into a discussion of the structure of IDEA '97 and Section 504.

In addition to the acronyms used for eligibility categories, the following are often used in literature related to IDEA:

- IDEA: The 1990 reauthorization of the EHA.
- IDEA '97: Latest reauthorization of the Individuals with Disabilities Education Act.
- Section 504: Services provided under Section 504 of the Rehabilitation Act in 1973.
- LRE: Least restrictive environment.
- LEA: Local education agency—usually refers to the local school district.
- SEA: State education agency.
- Eligibility: Prior to specialized services beyond those afforded to any student, eligibility for these special services must be established through evaluation and the criteria set in IDEA Part A's Eligibility Categories.
- Modifications/Accommodations: Supplementary support and/or aids that will be provided to the student to

Table 20-2

Disabilities as Defined by IDEA '97

Disability & Acronym	*Definition*
Autism (AU)	A developmental disability significantly affecting verbal and nonverbal communication and social interaction that adversely affects educational performance.
Deaf-Blindness (DB)	Simultaneous hearing and visual impairments resulting in severe communication and other developmental and educational needs that cannot be accommodated in special education programs solely for children with deafness or children with blindness.
Emotional Disturbance (ED)	A condition exhibiting one or more of the following characteristics over a long period of time and to a marked degree: <ul><li>an inability to learn that cannot be explained by intellectual, sensory, or health factors</li><li>an inability to build or maintain satisfactory interpersonal relationships with peers and teachers</li><li>inappropriate types of behavior or feelings under normal circumstances</li><li>a general pervasive mood of unhappiness or depression</li><li>a tendency to develop physical symptoms or fears associated with personal or school problems</li></ul>
Hearing Impairment (Including Deafness) (D)	A hearing impairment so severe that a child is impaired in processing linguistic information through hearing, with or without amplification, that adversely affects a child's educational performance.
Mental Retardation (MR)	Significantly below average (generally 2 standard deviations below the mean) general intellectual functioning, existing at the same time with deficits in adaptive behavior.
Multiple Disabilities (MD)	Simultaneous impairments (such as mental retardation-blindness, mental retardation-orthopedic impairment, etc.), the combination of which causes such severe educational needs that they cannot be accommodated in a special education program solely for one of the impairments; an exception for this eligibility is deaf-blindness.
Orthopedic Impairment (OI)	Severe orthopedic impairment that adversely affects a child's educational performance. The term includes impairments caused by a congenital anomaly, impairments caused by disease, and impairments from other causes (i.e., cerebral palsy, amputations).
Other Health Impairment (OHI)	Having limited strength, vitality, or alertness, including a heightened alertness to environmental stimuli, that results in limited alertness with respect to the educational environment. Possible diagnoses that fall in this category include chronic or acute health problems such as asthma, attention deficit disorder or attention deficit hyperactivity disorder, diabetes, epilepsy, a heart condition, hemophilia, lead poisoning, leukemia, nephritis, rheumatic fever, and sickle cell anemia.
Specific Learning Disability (LD)	A disorder in one or more of the basic psychological processes involved in understanding or in using language, spoken or written, that may manifest itself in an imperfect ability to listen, think, speak, read, write, spell, or to do mathematical calculations. The term includes such conditions as perceptual disabilities, brain injury, minimal brain dysfunction, dyslexia, and developmental aphasia.
Speech or Language Impairment (SI)	A communication disorder such as stuttering, impaired articulation, a language impairment, or a voice impairment that adversely affects a child's educational performance.

Table 20-2 (continued)
Disabilities as Defined by IDEA '97

Disability & Acronym	Definition
Traumatic Brain Injury (TBI)	An acquired injury to the brain caused by an external physical force (i.e. open or closed head injury), resulting in total or partial functional disability and/or psychosocial impairment, that adversely affects a child's educational performance.
Visual Impairment (Including Blindness) (VI)	An impairment in vision that, even with correction, adversely affects a child's educational performance. The term includes both partial sight and blindness.

Adapted from Council for Exceptional Children (1997) Summary of the Individuals with Disabilities Education Act (IDEA) amendments of 1997.

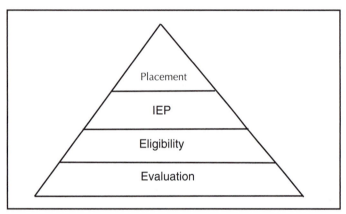

Figure 20-1. Structure of IDEA Part B.

assist in making educational progress. Modifications and accommodations cannot significantly change the curriculum; if the modifications or accommodations set forth are to the extent that the curriculum is different for the child with special needs, another curriculum should be considered as part of the IEP.

- IEP (Individual Education Plan): A written plan based on assessment results that is developed, reviewed, and revised in a meeting. This plan will be implemented for the student with special needs and includes, among other things, goals and objectives.

- IEP Meeting: A meeting, held at least annually, to review the results of the evaluation or reevaluation, to determine eligibility, to develop the IEP, and to dismiss a student from special education and related services.

- IEP Committee: Participants at the IEP meeting are often referred to as the IEP committee, and must include at minimum the parents/caregivers, an administrator, a general education teacher, special education teacher, and any other invited personnel/professionals (such as related services personnel).

- Due Process: A provision available to parents/caregivers and advocates against the LEA or an LEA against the parents for an administrative hearing before an impartial hearing officer (Dunn, 2000).

- Mediation: An alternative due process provision for the parents and LEA when in disagreement about a child's IEP (National Information Center for Children and Youth with Disabilities [NICHCY],1998).

- Special Education: Special education is additional instruction or special instruction that is required for a child to make progress. This is considered an instructional service for eligible students.

- Related Service: Related services are those services for eligible students who requires "...such developmental, corrective, and other supportive services as are required to assist a child with a disability to benefit from special education" (NICHCY, 2001; 34 C.F.R. §300.24[a]). Related services may include occupational therapy, physical therapy, speech therapy, music therapy (if not special instruction), psychological services, orientation and mobility specialists, recreation, including therapeutic recreation, counseling services, including rehabilitation counseling, orientation and mobility services, medical services for diagnostic or evaluation purposes, school health services, social work services in schools, parent counseling and training, and transportation (NICHCY, 2001).

THE STRUCTURE OF IDEA '97 PART B

Figure 20-1 illustrates the basic premises of IDEA '97 Part B, as well as the sequence of service delivery. Note that all services for children with disabilities begin with evaluation at the base of the pyramid. The next level is eligibility followed by IEP development and then placement. These structural elements are explored. The structure of Part B in H.R. 1350 is expected to remain essentially unchanged.

Evaluation-Based Services

Eligibility for all special education and related services, as well as preparation of the IEP is always based on evaluation. Once a child has been referred for special education and parents/caregivers have given consent to proceed, the LEA is required to evaluate the child within a reasonable amount of time (IDEA '97 suggests that a reasonable amount of time is 30 school days) and hold a meeting to review those results within another 30 days (34 C.F.R. §300). H.R. 1350 definitively establishes a 60 day timeline from receipt of parental consent to evaluate, unless the SEA has already established a timeline. In addition, under Part B of IDEA '97 the student must be reevaluated for eligibility at least once every 3 years; under H.R. 1350, reevaluations every 3 years will not be necessary if the LEA and parents are in agreement. Reevaluation may begin with a review of existing evaluation data on the student, and if it is determined to be sufficient information to make certain recommendations, additional testing or other evaluation procedures may not be necessary. The decision to not conduct additional testing may be particularly appropriate when a child has a chronic condition such as mental retardation, orthopedic impairment, or vision impairment, and no significant changes in the disability have occurred that may affect educational performance. However, if parents request that the reevaluation include additional testing, the LEA must conduct the testing. (NICHCY, 1998).

IDEA '97 requires the LEA to assess the child in all areas of suspected disability using a variety of technically sound, nondiscriminatory assessment instruments and strategies. Information from parents/caregivers that directly assists persons in determining eligibility and educational needs (Council for Exceptional Children, 1997; NICHCY, 2002) are necessary. These requirements suggest that multiple sources for assessment are preferred. A comprehensive evaluation should include at least some of the following: standardized tools, criterion-referenced tools, observations, interviews, inventories, scales, and portfolio review.

The role for occupational therapy in the evaluation process is primarily diagnostic, in which occupational therapy assessment results contribute to the overall picture of a child's abilities and differences in his/her educational setting. It is important to note that an occupational therapy assessment should not be conducted solely for the purpose of "eligibility for related services"; all children who are eligible for special education are also eligible for related services such as occupational therapy. However, the need for related services to meet educational objectives is up to the IEP team to determine, based on recommendations from related service providers. As part of a comprehensive evaluation, the student's cognitive, psychosocial, and sensory motor performance areas should be assessed. Depending on the suspected disability, many school psychologists and diagnosticians administer a battery of tests designed to cover all three performance areas, with emphasis either on cogni-

tion, psychosocial skills, or sensory motor skills. Additional in-depth information about a child's educational performance may be requested from professionals with additional expertise in a certain area. For example, for a child suspected of having autism and whose parents/caregivers reports significant sensory issues, an OT with additional expertise in sensory integration evaluation may be involved. For a child experiencing difficulty ambulating around the school campus, it would be appropriate to request a physical therapy evaluation. An evaluation for a child with moderate mental retardation who is having difficulties with self-help skills may also require additional assessment by the OT. In all of these examples, the related services personnel contribute to the child's overall evaluation, which in turn facilitates development of an appropriate IEP.

When IEP committee members recognize that the student's goals and objectives may require the additional expertise of an OT (or other service providers), the IEP committee may agree to request additional assessment and then meet again to review those results. At this second meeting, the related services provider may suggest additional goals and objectives for the IEP committee to consider, as well as make recommendations for related services to assist in implementing these goals and objectives.

Linking Assessment Results to Educational Performance

Most of us are aware of the statistical data of an assessment tool or the results in terms of standard and scaled scores, percentile ranks and age equivalence, but what do these scores have to do with classroom performance? In October 2001, the President's Commission on Excellence in Special Education was created. This commission held hearings and meetings throughout the United States to listen to the concerns about special education services from parents, teachers, administrators, and the public. As a result of these hearings, the Commission published a summary of findings, one of which stated that a "...need to improve the linkage between assessment and intervention" exists (PCESE, 2002). These findings imply two problems:

1. Special education staff do not appear to relate test results to educational performance.

2. Special education staff do not appear to use assessment information in planning individualized special education programming.

The OT practitioner's ability to understand assessment results in functional or educational terms is paramount to planning effective interventions or in the educational setting, effective IEPs. Therefore, a critical thinking process to determine the child's abilities and differences for diagnostic and eligibility purposes is necessary. An example of how the scores for a standardized test such as the Test of Visual Perceptual Skills-Revised (Gardner, 1996) may be interpret-

Table 20-3
Excerpt of Mark's Evaluation Report

The Test of Visual Perceptual Skills - Revised (Gardner, 1996) subtest results are reported in standard scores (85-115 is average range), scaled scores (8-12 is average range) and perceptual age (scores converted to age equivalence). Mark's scores were:

Subtest	Standard Score	Scale Score	Perceptual Age
Visual discrimination	87	7	6 years 7 months
Visual memory	59	2	4 years 7 months
Visual spatial relationships	104	11	8 years 7 months
Visual form constancy	79	6	4 years 10 months
Visual sequential memory	85	7	6 years 6 months
Visual figure-ground	77	5	5 years 1 month
Visual closure	80	6	5 years 11 months

Strengths:
According to these results, Mark's strength is in visual spatial relationships. In the classroom, these strengths would indicate that Mark is able to:
- note differences in similar shapes, letters, words, pictures
- recognize reversed letters and numbers in words.

Differences:
Mark's visual memory score is significantly below average and his visual discrimination, form constancy, sequential memory, figure ground and closure are slightly to moderately below average. In the classroom, Mark may have difficulties with:
- remembering picture, shape and letter formation.
- recognizing the same letter/word in different font/size such as this "A" is the same as this "a" or this "a" or that this "WORD" is the same as this "word" or this "word" is different from "WOOD."
- recalling (without visual structures) routines that occur during the school day such as P.E. comes before lunch and science is after break time.
- locating objects that may appear to be hidden among other items (ex: Where's Waldo™ or Highlights™ puzzles) or a desired item on crowded shelves or on "busy" boards.
- locating a particular word in text (i.e., vocabulary definitions or word search puzzles).
- reading quickly - because reading is mostly about reading a few letters and allowing our minds to 'fill-in-the-blanks", Mark's score on visual closure suggests that Mark may need to read each letter of each word carefully before being able to read the whole word. In reading assignments he may need to read once for content (decoding) and then re-read for content or comprehension, particularly in new materials/books.
- completing an art/science/social studies project without a completed model and step-by-step visual instructions.

Where's Waldo is a registered trademark of Candlewick Press, Cambridge, MA. Highlights is a registered trademark of Highlights, Columbus, OH.

ed and subsequently translated into a rationale for service provision are demonstrated in Table 20-3, which contains an excerpt from an evaluation report for Mark, an 8-year-old second grader who has been diagnosed as having Asperger's Syndrome (an Autism Spectrum Disorder); Mark has some difficulties with reading and written communication skills.

The functional implications are clearly stated in this excerpt and based on the presented information, goals and objectives, as well as possible modifications for the IEP are easily formulated.

Eligibility

Once an evaluation has been completed, the information must be discussed among the IEP committee, and eligibility for special education and related services be determined. As noted in the definition of terms, IDEA '97 considers general and special education, speech language pathology (if considered special instruction), adapted physical education, and vocational education as instructional services (NICHCY,

2000). Related services include:
- Occupational therapy
- Physical therapy
- Speech therapy
- Music therapy (if not special instruction)
- Psychological services
- Orientation and mobility specialists
- Recreation, including therapeutic recreation
- Counseling services, including rehabilitation counseling
- Orientation and mobility services
- Medical services for diagnostic or evaluation purposes
- School health services
- Social work services in schools
- Parent counseling and training
- Transportation (NICHCY, 2001).

IDEA '97 intended for related services to support instructional services, therefore services under IDEA '97 may be provided one of two ways:

1. The child may receive special education services (and no need for related services exists); or

2. The child may receive special education services along with related services to support the IEP.

This means that the child must qualify for special education before he can be considered for related services (AOTA, 1999a; Dunn, 2000; NICHCY, 2000).

As noted earlier, one of the significant differences between IDEA '97 and H.R. 1350 is availability of special education and related services. H.R. 1350 states that an LEA may spend up to 15% of IDEA funding to provide research-based interventions for children before eligibility for special education and related services (NICHY, 2004). Specifics on these prereferral services will be delineated in the regulations for H.R. 1350.

indirect

Eligibility for Section 504 Services

In contrast to IDEA '97, Section 504 eligibility is broader and more loosely defined. Section 504 determines a child to have a disability if they have a physical or mental impairment which substantially limits a major life activity (29 U.S.C., Section 706[8]). Physical or mental impairments may include impairments in learning, vision, hearing, or diseases such as diabetes, AIDS; or mental illness. Major life activities include: breathing, caring for oneself, hearing, learning, performing manual tasks, seeing, speaking, walking, or working (29 U.S.C., Section 706[8]). Eligibility for Section 504 in the schools is generally based on evaluation, and while no specifics are given in this code for timelines or an individualized plan, many LEAs will follow IDEA '97's lead and meet annually and make an accommodation plan (AOTA, 1999a). Designated members for this meeting are not stipulated, however best practice would suggest at least the parents/caregivers, a general education teacher, and an administrator participate in a Section 504 meeting.

Need for Occupational Therapy and Related Services Under IDEA '97

Once an evaluation has been completed, a series of questions may be asked to determine need for related services to assist a child in meeting his/her educational objectives. As noted earlier in this chapter, a child must first qualify for special education services and related service(s) which must be deemed necessary for the child to make progress in special education (NICHCY, 2000). Following up on Mark's test results and educational implications, Table 20-4 contains the eligibility questions that also appeared in Mark's evaluation report:

Answers to these questions clearly indicated a need for occupational therapy services to support Mark's IEP. With this information, the IEP committee is able to make well-informed decisions about provision of related services.

Occupational Therapy Services Under Section 504

The current standard for Section 504 eligibility is that the student must demonstrate a physical or mental disability that substantially affects a major life area. As noted earlier in this chapter, the disability categories are not specifically defined in Section 504, therefore occupational therapy's role may be critical in the determination of need for implementation of a Section 504 plan. As with any evaluation, best practice suggests that using a variety of assessment tools is invaluable in determining the child's disability, and its effect on learning. To assist the parent, teacher, and administrator in making an appropriate accommodations plan, similar guiding questions as discussed in the previous section may be helpful.

Zach, who has a diagnosis of dyslexia, was evaluated by occupational therapy for his written communication needs. To determine the educational need for occupational therapy services to facilitate Zach's educational program, the questions in Table 20-5 were considered.

As the testing results indicate, Zach has dyslexia, which appears to be affecting his ability to learn. Results of the occupational therapy evaluation also indicate that visual motor and handwriting skills are also limiting Zach's learning experience. Based on the results of this evaluation, the OT made recommendations to the parents, administrator, and teachers to assist Zach in meeting his educational objectives.

Direct !!

Developing the IEP

IEP: The IEP (noted as the second level on Figure 20-1) is the educational plan developed to meet a child's needs once eligibility for special education and related services is established. An IEP includes:

- Parental concerns.
- A statement of the specific communication needs of the child with vision deficits, hearing deficits, or of limited English proficiency.
- Results of the evaluation or reevaluation.
- Strengths and competencies of the child.

Table 20-4

Mark's Need for Related Services Questions

Is Mark eligible for special education services?	Yes	[X]
Eligibility: Autism; Speech Impairment	No	[ ]
The degree to which Mark's *motor planning* skills affect progress toward special education objectives:	Negligibly	[ ]
	Mildly	[ ]
	Moderately	[X]
	Significantly	[ ]
The degree to which Mark's *sensory modulation* skills affect progress toward special education objectives:.	Negligibly	[ ]
	Mildly	[ ]
	Moderately	[ ]
	Significantly	[X]
The degree to which Mark's *visual perceptual skills* affect progress toward special education objectives:	Negligibly	[ ]
	Mildly	[X]
	Moderately	[ ]
	Significantly	[ ]
The degree to which *handwriting skill* evaluation results affect progress toward special education objectives:	Negligibly	[ ]
	Mildly	[X]
	Moderately	[ ]
	Significantly	[ ]
Evaluation data indicates that this student needs *occupational therapy* to assist in meeting educational goals/objectives:	Yes	[X]
	No	[ ]

Table 20-5

Zach's Section 504 Eligibility Questions

Zach has a mental or physical impairment:	Yes	[X]
Dyslexia which affects the major life activity of Learning	No	[ ]
Is Zach making progress toward current general education goals? (answered by campus student support team)	Yes	[ ]
	No	[X]
Zach continues to have significant difficulties with reading and with handwriting legibility		
The degree to which Zach's visual motor/handwriting skills affect progress toward educational objectives:.	Negligibly	[ ]
	Mildly	[ ]
	Moderately	[ ]
	Substantially	[X]
The degree to which Zach's visual perceptual skills affect progress toward educational objectives:	Negligibly	[ ]
	Mildly	[ ]
	Moderately	[X]
	Substantially	[ ]

- A statement of the present levels of educational performance of the child.
- Annual goals, including benchmarks or short-term objectives, as well as the method(s) to measure goals and objectives.
- The special education and related services and supplementary aids and services to be provided to or on behalf of the child (including modifications).
- Anticipated frequency and location of services to be provided.
- The projected date for initiation and anticipated duration of services.
- The extent to which the child will be able to participate in general educational programs.
- Consideration of behavior issues.
- Report of progress toward special education goals and objectives (this report must be provided as often as progress is reported for the nondisabled child, i.e., the district's grading periods.
- Transitional needs for students age 14 and older.

As noted above, a meeting must be held to review the results of the evaluation or reevaluation and to develop the IEP. Typically these meetings are referred to as an IEP meeting.

IEP Meeting Process: Participants to the IEP meeting are often referred to as the IEP committee, and must include at minimum the parents, an administrator, a general education teacher and special education teacher, and any other invited personnel/professionals (such as related services personnel). As discussed earlier in this chapter, during the meeting, assessment results are reviewed and then the IEP committee makes the determination for eligibility. Once consensus is reached regarding eligibility, the committee develops goals and objectives. While drafting the goals and objectives, the IEP committee must also determine the necessary personnel to implement the goals and objectives. The final charge to the IEP committee is to determine placement. This last task is particularly important. According to NIHCY (1999),

The appropriate placement for a particular child with a disability cannot be determined until after decisions have been made about the child's needs and the services that the public agency will provide to meet those needs. These decisions must be made at the IEP meeting, and it would not be permissible first to place the child and then develop the IEP. Therefore, the IEP must be developed before placement (p. 15).

Occupational therapy may be involved in all elements of developing the IEP as listed above. The following section addresses the distinction of developing goals and objectives in school-based practice, report of progress toward special education goals and objectives, modifications/accommoda-

tions, consideration of behavior issues, and the transition needs for students age 14 and older, issues most commonly dealt with by the school based OT practitioner.

DEVELOPING GOALS AND OBJECTIVES FOR THE IEP

The same principles to developing measurable goals and objectives as discussed in Chapter 6: Documentation, can be applied in school-based settings, however under IDEA '97 these goals and objectives should focus primarily on the educational needs of the student. For example, an assessment indicates that Mary, who was referred for additional assessment by occupational therapy due to handwriting difficulties, also has proximal instability among other differences. Rather than write an objective to improve proximal stability, best practice under IDEA '97 would be to address Mary's educational need. In this scenario, an effective objective for the educational setting would be:

"Mary will write 2 sentences with appropriate letter formation, directionality, and spacing independently 4 out of 5 opportunities as measured by portfolio review."

While this objective does not directly address proximal instability, the therapy plan should include activities to address individual performance skills such as proximal instability. Success of these activities to improve proximal stability should become evident and are measured by the educational objective, or Mary's ability to write legibly.

Since the IEP committee should develop all goals and objectives, no goal and objectives should be discipline specific. In other words, all committee members develop goals and objectives. However due to the fact that it is acceptable for various committee members to write draft goals and objectives prior to the IEP meeting, a sense of "ownership" or belief that certain goals and objectives "belong" only to the resource teacher, or occupational therapist, or counselor may exist. Remember, all goals and objectives are part of the whole IEP and in the next level in the pyramid in Figure 20-1, the IEP committee is then charged to determine which professional(s) is best qualified to implement the goals and objectives. Frequently multiple members may be designated to implement specific goals and objectives, such as the resource teacher and occupational therapist, or the adaptive physical educational teacher and physical therapist.

REPORT OF PROGRESS TOWARD SPECIAL EDUCATION GOALS AND OBJECTIVES

In addition to annual meetings to discuss progress, reports on the child's progress on annual goals and objectives should be sent to the parents at the end of each grading period (i.e., each 6 or 9 weeks or each semester) as mandated by IDEA '97. As noted earlier in this chapter, H.R. 1350 recommends less frequent reports in an effort to reduce paperwork. If occupational therapy is noted as one of the implementers of a goal and/or objective, the OTA's role in this process may include providing accurate documentation of therapy intervention sessions and offering verbal reports of the child's progress.

MODIFICATIONS/ACCOMMODATIONS

After reviewing evaluation results, two possible scenarios may result. A child may demonstrate the need for some type of occupational therapy intervention, but not to the extent that a goal may be necessary. Alternatively, the need for occupational therapy services is significant but cannot be addressed by an occupational therapy specific goal. For example a student with special needs may have received long-term and intensive instruction and therapy services to address handwriting legibility but has only made limited progress. Rather than continue to write goals and objectives to address this performance skill, a modification such as reduced written work or an accommodation such as access to a computer for written assignments may be considered.

CONSIDERATION OF BEHAVIOR ISSUES

A significant change in IDEA '97 is the notion that a child's behavior must be considered when preparing the IEP (Warger, 1999), as behavior may significantly affect a child's educational progress. Occupational therapy, with its grounding in psychosocial theory may provide invaluable assistance to the IEP committee in planning an appropriate IEP. To determine if a child's behavior may adversely be affecting his educational performance, the IEP committee and the OT and may consider the following questions:

- Does the child need to learn and/or use new behaviors, skills, and/or strategies?

- Does the child demonstrate behaviors that are unsafe and/or that significantly interfere with the learning environment?

- Does the child's current presenting behavior require a behavior intervention plan?

- Is the child routinely removed from the general education classroom because of inappropriate behavior?

- Is the child's behavior related to, or a manifestation of, a disability? (Council for Exceptional Children, 1997)

If the answer to any of the questions is yes, as part of the IEP process, the committee first determines the present level of educational performance and then develops annual goals and short-term objectives or benchmarks to address specific behavioral concerns. The behavioral plan set forth in the IEP includes clearly identified rules, expectations, and procedures, as well as clearly defined reinforcements and consequences to assist the student in learning to manage his own behavior (Council for Exceptional Children, 1997).

TRANSITION NEEDS FOR STUDENTS WITH DISABILITIES

Although children with special needs will experience many transitions during their educational career; two specific transitions addressed as part of the services offered by Part B of IDEA '97 are especially significant. The initial transition period occurs as a child who received Part C (Infants And Toddlers With Disabilities) services moves to Part B services. In this transition, the focus of services moves from a family-centered model to an educational model. While the family's concerns and goals continue to be addressed, under the educational model the focus is now on the child's pre-academic and academic skills, as well as preparation for the transition to post-secondary education and/or vocation upon graduation and community participation (34 C.F.R. §300.29). One of the significant changes in H.R. 1350 will be the option of SEAs to join with Part C agencies to offer an extension of Part C services to families with children with special needs until the child enters or is eligible to enter kindergarten in the LEA (NICHCY, 2004). Through this option, families will be given the opportunity to continue the IFSP and family-centered services for the child from birth to 6 years of age, rather than transition to educational model services at age 3.

In addition to considering the transitional needs that occur upon entering Part B services, the IEP committee must also consider the transitional needs and services for children eligible for special education and related services aged 14 and older. H.R. 1350 changes the requirement to consider transitional needs and planning to the age of 16 years (NICHCY, 2004). These transitional services are based on the child's needs and take into account personal preferences and interests, which may include, "instruction, community experiences, the development of employment and other postschool adult living objectives, and (if appropriate) the acquisition of daily living skills and functional vocational assessment" (NICHCY, 1999, p. 13).

As part of the transition services, the IEP committee may invite community agency representatives to gather and collaboratively discuss the student's options following graduation (such as additional education, a vocation, and/or community involvement). Community representatives include designated personnel from state vocational guidance/counseling services, assisted living facilities, post secondary agencies such as a local technical school or college/university, mental health/retardation agencies, and the social security administration. After this collaborative meeting, a child may be evaluated to determine current competencies and progress, results of which are then used, in part, to develop a plan to reach the mutually determined outcomes.

The OT practitioner may be involved in transition planning as part of the process of evaluation for the child's needs

Table 20-6
Continuum Questions

Length of Service (LOS)

Less than 1 year	1	2	3	4	5	More than 1 year

Frequency

Less often	1	2	3	4	5	More often

Duration

Less time	1	2	3	4	5	More time

Intensity

Low (1-2 activities)	1	2	3	4	5	High (several activities)

Consult/Direct

Consult	1	2	3	4	5	Direct

and services. Inherent in the nature of occupational therapy and relative to the occupational roles of work, play and/or self-help, the OT practitioner may provide invaluable assistance to the IEP committee in developing an effective transition plan, and if determined by the IEP committee, provide services to assist the child in the transitional process.

Determining Services

The highest level of the pyramid in Figure 20-1 is determining placement, and part of placement includes determining services. Upon consensus of the IEP, members of the committee must review the recommendations of the various evaluators and/or providers to determine what services, if any, are necessary to implement the IEP. Based on assessment results, the OT may recommend direct or consultative related services. How does the therapist determine the frequency, duration, intensity, and method of services? Consideration of all the possible options of service delivery that best meets the child's needs is necessary, and since all services are individualized, extraneous considerations such as the current personnel, current caseload size, schedules or personal preferences cannot be factored in this decision process. This is a difficult concept for many OT practitioners to embrace; however it is up to the LEA rather than the related services providers to provide the necessary personnel to implement the IEP. The OT must consider only what services are necessary in order for the child to make progress. In many instances, only consultative services may be needed; in other instances, direct services or even a collaborative

model may be more appropriate. So how does the school based OT therapist determine the frequency, duration, intensity, and method of services? A series of questions may be asked.

1. How much time is necessary to meet the IEP goals? (less than a year, more than a year)?

2. Is consistent, regular intervention (such as weekly intervention) required more than an intensive intervention (every day for 2 to 3 weeks with follow up consult)?

3. How long should therapy sessions be (several short session or fewer longer sessions)?

4. How intense should therapy sessions be (1 to 2 activities or several activities)?

A strategy to assist in this decision-making process is to answer a series of continuum questions such as the ones listed in Table 20-6.

After considering the child's IEP goals and objectives, completing the continuum may proceed as follows.

An IEP for a third grade student with Down syndrome (with moderate mental retardation and difficulties sequencing) is in a self-contained classroom and participates in general education fine arts classes. The following recommendations may be derived from completing the continuum above:

- LOS – (5) suggesting that not all the IEP annual goals and objectives will be met within the year.

- Frequency – (4) suggesting at least a weekly intervention schedule.

- Duration – (2) suggesting short therapy sessions, maybe 20 minutes.

- Intensity – (2) suggesting 2 to 4 activities per session (due to the student's limited attention span).
- Consult/Direct – (3) suggesting a mostly equal balance of direct sessions with the student and consultative sessions with the teacher/paraprofessionals (for reinforcement of the direct session success).

Therefore in this example, the recommendations may consist of: three weekly consultation sessions for 20 minutes with student's teacher and three weekly direct sessions for 20 minutes with the student. Each therapy session will include at least 2 to 4 sequenced activities.

A consideration in service delivery is environment. Does the child attend general education or a self-contained class the majority of the time? As IDEA '97 emphasizes providing special needs children with access to general education, another factor to consider is staff-to-student ratio. For a child in a small classroom environment with low student-to-staff ratio, the need for related services may not be as great as the student in a larger classroom with higher student to staff ratio, as the teacher in the smaller classroom setting can offer individualized services on a more consistent basis. A student in general education may require more direct services as he/she may require additional individualized services to make progress. The student in the more restricted environment may only require consult services to the teacher, who can then implement the individualized services.

Up to this point, evaluations, eligibility, development of the IEP, and placement in school-based services have been discussed. Special topics related to school-based practice such as role delineations between the OT and OTA in the schools and therapy planning strategies are explored next.

Role Delineations in Schools

JOB DESCRIPTIONS

One of the first places an OT or OTA should look at in determining occupational therapy's role in an LEA is the written job description. Ideally these job descriptions should be based on current state licensure rules and take into account the educational model focus of the school district. Please also refer to *Guide for Supervision of Occupational Therapy Personnel* (AOTA, 1999). Listed in Table 20-7 is a sample job description written by the author of this chapter for the Lubbock Independent School District in Lubbock, Texas (Table 20-8).

Many of duties of the OT and OTA are very similar, yet there are clear role distinctions that require an interpretative factor such as writing the student's initial evaluation, writing goals and objectives for the IEP committee's consideration, updating progress on the goals and objectives, and 3 year re-evaluations as provided by the OT. Occupational therapy

assistants provide invaluable assistance by helping with screening and evaluation duties such as conducting standardized assessments, classroom observations, as dictated by state and facility guidelines and established competencies, documentation of intervention sessions, and verbal or written observations of the student's skills and performance.

ADDITIONAL ROLES

Within the role of service provider the OT and OTA may provide direct and consultation/monitoring services. As a consultant, the OT and OTA address:

1. Student-centered consultations (SC)
2. Classroom-centered consultations (CC)
3. Building consultation (BC)
4. School/program-centered (which includes in-services, trainings for parents, teachers, paraprofessionals and administrators) (PC)

In student-centered consultations, the OT practitioner problem solves with parents and school personnel for an identified student; these problem-solving sessions will typically address an issue from the IEP. In classroom-centered consultations, the OT practitioner typically works with the teacher and paraprofessional(s) on problem-solving issues for the entire classroom. Building consultations may include addressing building modifications such as access issues, or being available to other staff in the building for problem-solving sessions. In the last type of consultation, school/program-centered, the OT practitioner may lead in-services for staff/administration, or provide trainings for parents about a particular topic.

Examples of these roles can be found in Table 20-9. Note that the acronyms in parentheses refer to the various roles that the OTA fulfills.

Obviously the typical day for an OTA is full of direct and consult services as well as other unexpected duties.

Therapy Planning And Activities

Students are in school about 35 hours a week (roughly 7 hours per day). Many related services are provided for 30 to 60 minutes a week, which means that related services consume 3% of a student's time at school. The typical caseload for an OT practitioner ranges from 30 to 60 students with the majority seen weekly or in other words, one student is equivalent to 1.5 to 3% of an OT practitioner's caseload. A concerned OT practitioner may wonder "Just how effective is that 3% going to be in making substantial changes in this student?" This section presents strategies that enable the OT and OTA to combine the needs of the students with the reality of school-based practice.

Table 20-7

Job Description for the Occupational Therapist

Lubbock Independent School District

Job Description

Name: **Soc. Sec. No.**:
                                                        Length of Contract:
                                                        Schedule:

Job Title: Occupational Therapist
Department/School: Special Education Department
Reports To: Director of Special Education
Supervises: Occupational Therapy Assistants

Qualifications:
- Must be initially certified in accordance to guidelines established by the National Board for Certification in Occupational Therapy (NBCOT)
- Hold a valid, regular, or provisional license to practice occupational therapy in the state of Texas.

Job Goal: The role of the occupational therapist is to provide assessment, consultation and service to identified special education students with needs in the areas of fine motor, oral motor, environmental adaptations, sensory-motor processing and functional classroom tasks.

Major Duties:
The duties of an occupational therapist will be to:
- Screen and evaluate children referred for occupational therapy evaluation
- Serve as a member of the admission, dismissal and review (ARD) committee [name of the IEP committee]
- Write interdisciplinary individualized education plans (IEPs)
- Develop therapy service plans

Service delivery models include direct therapy, consult services and collaboration in the areas of:
1. Improving motor skills necessary for interaction with the environment ranging from mobility to manipulation of objects to handwriting.
2. Improving the student's ability to receive, process, and use sensory information (including visual perceptual skills) allowing for more environmental interaction.
3. Promote development of motor skills, reduce effects of motor dysfunction and prevent deformity, which limits function.
4. Improve self-care skills (feeding, dressing, grooming and toileting) through use of adapted equipment and strategies to compensate for disability.
5. Increase movement available at all joints to allow for better positioning during activities and rest as well as allow for more functional use of arms, legs and head for educational tasks/activities.
6. Support or increase a student's ability to function within the classroom and make adaptations necessary within the classroom to allow the child to function more efficiently and effectively.

OTs supervising OTA's responsibilities include:
1. The OTR shall delegate responsibilities to the OTA that are within the scope of the OTA's training and competence.
2. Provide a minimum of eight hours of supervision per month for full time OTAs as documented on the OTA Supervision Log according to guidelines set by the Texas Occupational Therapy Board of Examiners (TBOTE). The number of hours beyond the minimum of eight hours per month for supervision shall be dependent upon the OT's and OTA's collaborative determination of the OTA's competency level, setting and caseload.
3. The OT is responsible for determining if a physician's referral is required for occupational therapy evaluation or intervention.
4. A OTA may initiate the screening process and collect information for the OT's review in preparation for evaluation/evaluation.
5. The OT is responsible for completing the student evaluation/evaluation. The supervising OT may delegate any evaluative task to a OTA that the OT and OTA agree is within the competency level of that OTA.

Table 20-7 (continued)

Job Description for the Occupational Therapist

6. The OT is responsible for developing and modifying the student's IEP and therapy services plan. The therapy services plan must include the following components:
   a. Goals and objectives or benchmarks
   b. Interventions/modalities
   c. Frequency and duration
   d. The OTA must follow the IEP and therapy services plan and cannot make any modifications without approval (either verbal or written) by the supervising OT.
7. The supervising OT has overall responsibility for providing the supervision necessary to protect the health and welfare of the student receiving services by a OTA. However, this does not absolve the OTA from his/her professional responsibilities.
8. The supervising OT is responsible for writing the student's initial evaluation, IEP updates, and 3 year Re-evaluations as these documents require an interpretive element that can only be determined by the OT.
9. Due to the interpretative factor or the need to evaluate a student's progress each six-weeks, the OT is responsible for updating IEPs each six-weeks and annually to evaluate the need for services. This type of evaluation may consist of a review of the daily documentation and/or observations and/or information from the 3 year Re-evaluation.
10. The supervising OT, along with the OTA, is responsible for co-signing all documentation by the OTA that becomes part of the student's permanent record.

Reprinted with permission from the Lubbock Independent School District, Lubbock, TX.

Table 20-8

Job Description for the Occupational Therapy Assistant

Lubbock Independent School District

Job Description

Name: **Soc. Sec. No.**:
                                                       Length of Contract:
                                                       Schedule:

Job Title: Occupational Therapy Assistant
Department/School: Special Education Department
Reports To: Director of Special Education, Occupational Therapist
Supervises: Not applicable

Qualifications:
- Must be initially certified in accordance to guidelines established by the National Board for Certification in Occupational Therapy (NBCOT)
- Hold a valid, regular, or provisional license to practice occupational therapy in the state of Texas, and is required to be under general supervision of an OT.

Job Goal: The role of the occupational therapy assistant is to provide assessment, consultation, and service to identified special education students with needs in the areas of fine motor, oral motor, environmental adaptations, sensory-motor processing and functional classroom tasks.

Major Duties:
The duties of an OTA will be to:
1. Represent the supervising OT in the IEP committee by reading the evaluation and/or presenting draft IEP objectives; however no changes can be made without verbal or written approval by the supervising OT.
2. Improving motor skills necessary for interaction with the environment ranging from mobility to manipulation of objects to skills required for written communication.
3. Improving the student's ability to receive, process, and use sensory information (including visual perceptual skills) allowing for more environmental interaction.
4. Promote development of motor skills, reduce effects of motor dysfunction and prevent deformity, which limits function.
5. Improve self-care skills (feeding, dressing, grooming and toileting) through use of adapted equipment and strategies to compensate for disability.

Table 20-8 (continued)

Job Description for the Occupational Therapy Assistant

6. Increase movement available at all joints to allow for better positioning during activities and rest as well as allow for more functional use of arms, legs and head for educational tasks/activities.
7. Support or increase a student's ability to function within the classroom and make adaptations necessary within the classroom to allow the child to function more efficiently and effectively.

Supervision of OTAs:

An OTA shall provide occupational therapy services only under the general supervision of a licensed OT. The OTA's responsibilities will include:

1. Maintaining the OTA Supervision Log - providing a copy to both the supervising OTs, facility (LISD) and to the Texas Occupational Therapy Board of Examiners (TBOTE) annually.
2. Ensure that all documentation prepared by the OTA that becomes part of the student's permanent record is co-signed by the supervising OTs.
3. Maintain consistent, regular contact with the supervising OTs, either by face to face meetings at the school, by telephone, written report or conference.
4. Completion of regular progress notes (i.e.: daily documentation) and other documentation as assigned by the supervising OT.

Reprinted with permission from the Lubbock Independent School District, Lubbock, TX.

Table 20-9

A Day in the Life of an Occupational Therapy Assistant in School-Based Practice

Time	Services	Additional Notes
Night before	Talk by phone with Amy (supervising OT) about kids to see the next day and what goals to address.	
8:00am	Arrive at Washington Elementary, gather therapy items from car, sign-in in the office, make copies as requested by the OT.	Secretary says that all rooms are full but I can use the assistant principal's office (which was formerly a storage closet). Kensey with nurse; will join us if she feels better.
8:15am	Find and pick up Tony and Kensey.	
8:18am	Direct services with Tony.	Worked on handwriting objectives.
8:50am	Send Tony back to his classroom; find and pick up Lacy and Isaiah.	
8:55am	Direct services with Lacy and Isaiah.	
9:20am	Kensey shows up halfway through session; get Kensey started on activity.	
9:22am	Walk Lacy and Isaiah back to class; go to pick up Kanisha but she is absent.	Kanisha's teacher asks me to come back during lunch break because she needs to ask me a question.
9:25am	Continue direct services with Kensey.	
9:50am	Send Kensey back to class, jot down notes, clean up, sign out and leave.	
9:55am	Get in car, drive to Lincoln elementary for 10:00 group.	
10:05am	Arrive, sign-in in the office.	
10:07am	Go into supported education classroom to work with Amy (OT) in group cooking activity (CC).	Worked with all 9 students; 5 are "officially" on the OT caseload.
10:30am	Clean up after group, go to parent room and prepare for next student.	
10:35am	Chantal arrives; work with her on activity.	
11:05am	Finish/clean up with Chantal, send her back to class, then write notes on Chantal and Supported Ed. group kids.	
11:30am	Sign out and leave for lunch; eat lunch in car, driving back to Washington Elementary.	
11:45am	Consulted with Kanisha's teacher; teacher is concerned that Kanisha is having difficulties with reading; asks what she needs do in class to help Kanisha (SC).	Suggest Kanisha's teacher try colored transparencies (will bring next week after talking with supervising OT) and to try a "window" card.
11:50am	While talking with Kanisha's teacher, the other 1st grade teacher asks where to get raised line paper as she would like to try it for some of her students who having some difficulties with writing the 'tails' on letters below the line (BC).	Will send several sheets of raised line paper to other 1st grade teacher in campus mail.

Table 20-9 (continued)

A Day in the Life of an Occupational Therapy Assistant in School-Based Practice

11:55am	Make small window card in teacher workroom and then take it to Kanisha's teacher.	Index card with small window cut in it to isolate individual words in text.
12:00pm	Drive over to Grant elementary; drop off seat cushion, pick up raised line paper, consult with Philip (Lead OT) about next week's schedule, walk down to office to send raised line paper (along with order form for more paper) to Washington Elementary teacher by campus mail.	OT classroom where supplies are kept.
12:30pm	Leave for Kennedy Elementary	
12:40pm	Arrive, sign-in in the office, go to set up in the Speech Therapy office, talk with Jesse (supervising OT) about which students need to be seen and what goals to work on.	
12:55pm	Pick up Brandy and Laura.	
1:00pm	Direct services with Brandy and Laura; get started on activity.	
1:30pm	Send Brandy and Laura back to class and pick up Chris.	
1:35pm	Direct services with Chris; get started on activity.	
2:05pm	Send Chris back to class and pick up Jonathan and Jordan.	
2:10pm	Direct services with Chris; get started on activity; Jesse returns from group session.	
2:20pm	Jesse begins to work with Chris; walk down to office answer page from office.	Principal introduces me to Laura's parent who asks about some handwriting activities to work on at home.
2:30pm	Check with Jesse about making copies of hand strengthening and in-hand manipulation exercises to send home to Laura's parent (PC).	Make copies of handouts and demonstrate exercises to parent.
2:50pm	Clean up, begin writing daily notes on kids seen today.	

Time	Services	Additional notes
3:10pm	Sign out, drive back to Grant Elementary.	
3:20pm	Arrive for bi-monthly OT staff meetings.	Make copies of handouts for the staff for Philip.
3:30pm	Meeting begins.	Offer to coordinate meal schedule for one of the OTs out on maternity leave.
4:45pm	Meeting ends; meet with Amy about kids and their goals for the next day.	
5:00pm	Continue writing daily documentation notes.	
5:30pm	Finish notes, go pick up my own kids from daycare.	
7:30pm	Amy calls and wants to make some minor changes to plan tomorrow.	
7:35pm	Finish call.	

Adapted from schedules of Sheila Joy, COTA and Teresa Alford, COTA. Names of children served were changed as were school names for confidentiality purposes.

THERAPY AS AN EDUCATIONAL TECHNIQUE

A scenario: A great number of students who have handwriting goals are seen for direct services by occupational therapy. Tom, a third grader in general education classes qualified for special education as a student with a learning disability. The IEP committee also noted that Tom had difficulties with written communication skills and asked that the OT to complete an evaluation. The OTA administered standardized visual motor and visual perceptual tests (which were interpreted by the supervising OT) to Tom while the OT met with Tom's teachers, looked at handwriting samples, and completed the Evaluation of Children's Handwriting (ETCH) (Admundson, 1995). Partial results of Tom's assessment indicated that he had trouble with:

- Visual form constancy
- Hand strength
- Letter formation
- Letter directionality

Table 20-10

Readiness Skills and Occupational Activities

Readiness Skills

Skill-based activities that prepare the child for occupational activities.

Includes preparatory techniques, instruction or assistive devices.

Techniques based on theory that can be implemented and supervised by classroom staff:

- Sensory integration
- Biomechanical
- Neurodevelopmental theory
- Visual perception
- Coping

Instruction:

- Inservice training on particular topic related to a student's education
- Individual consultation with teacher/paraprofessional/ parents

Assistive devices:

- Assistive technology
- Environmental modifications or accommodations

Occupational Activities

Tasks or activities related to the occupational role—that of a student in an educational setting.

Are the activities that require the expertise and guidance of occupational therapy to facilitate the adaptation process.

Occupational activities are:

- Active
- Meaningful
- Process oriented with products or results
- Facilitates the internal adaptation process

What we do with kids best!

- Craft activities
- Play activities
- Education-based activities
- Individualized interventions
- Therapeutic use of self

The IEP committee reviewed the evaluation results and accepted suggested goals to address handwriting deficits and recommendations for weekly direct services. The OT and OTA then developed a therapy services plan incorporating therapy putty-type readiness exercises to address hand strength as well as use of a new handwriting curriculum into Tom's program. As time went by, the OT and OTA discussed the effectiveness of doing hand strengthening exercises once a week during occupational therapy services. During these discussions, the OT and OTA began to problem solve about how the hand strengthening exercises could be implemented on a more regular basis. One suggestion from the OTA was for Tom to do the exercises daily during class announcements and agenda development, a 10 minute period in the classroom program when the teacher reviewed the schedule and objectives for the day. It was determined that the OTA would prepare a one-page handout of illustrated exercises for Tom to follow each day as well as gather the necessary supplies to implement this activity. The OT discussed this plan with the classroom teacher, who was receptive and willing to give the program a try. About mid-way through the school year, the OT and OTA discussed the fact that Tom had met all his goals and objectives regarding written communication. The OTA also shared with the OT comments from the teacher that Tom's handwriting was more legible and that the teacher had no difficulties with reading Tom's written work. The OT requested an IEP meeting and a mutual decision was made by the committee to dismiss Tom from occupational therapy services.

In this scenario, readiness and occupational activities were used and ultimately led to good progress for Tom, so much so, that he no longer required occupational therapy as a related service. The use of readiness skills and occupational activities in this format is based on the theory of Occupational Adaptation (Schkade & Schultz, 1992; Schkade & McClung, 2001; Schultz & Schkade, 1992).

Reflections for the OTA

Readiness skills are skill-based activities that prepare the child for occupational activities and include preparatory techniques, instruction or assistive devices. Occupational activities are tasks or activities related to the occupational role - in this case, that of a student in an educational setting.

Table 20-10 illustrates the distinctions between readiness skills and occupational activities in an educational setting.

To develop a therapy services plan that incorporates readiness skills and occupational activities, evaluation results and goals and objectives must first be considered. Once the evaluation results and goals and objectives have been reviewed, an analysis of the readiness skills and occupational activities needed to meet the goals and objectives should be prepared. Table 20-11 begins with a format that assists in the analysis.

This set of goal and objectives addresses handwriting issues. Based on this information, a readiness program may

Table 20-11

Evaluation Summary

Name/Age:	John Smith	8 yrs
School/Teacher:	Washington Elementary	Davenport
Classroom / Grade:	General Ed	3rd
Eligibility/Services (Occupational Environment):	Learning Disabled Goes to resource classroom - 90 minutes weekly	
Presenting Problem(s) (Reason for referral):	Illegible handwriting Difficulties with reading	
Evaluation Tools:	ETCH Teacher report Observations	TVPS-R Class work folder review
Strengths:	Beginning to write cursive letters with fair legibility Average or mildly below average in visual discrimination, spatial relations, sequential memory, closure Good speller	
Differences:	Poor hand strength (affecting handwriting endurance) Poor in-hand manipulation (affect handwriting legibility) Poor directionality Poor form constancy (affecting reading & handwriting) Poor figure ground (affects reading, copying skills)	
Recommendation(s):	OT direct 4 times per 6 weeks; 30 minutes direct OT consultation 1 time per 6 weeks to address readiness skills Occupational readiness activities daily - 15 minutes: (supervised by campus staff; OT consults to develop 6 wks lesson plans for readiness activities)	
IEP goals and objectives to address:	Goal: Improve from 71% to 85% handwriting legibility or better as measured by the Objective Scoring Procedures for Student's Handwriting Objective: Write up to 4 complete sentences imitating a sample (i.e. copying from the board or over head, passage from book) with at least 85% legibility as measured by portfolio review. Objective: Write spelling words and definitions independently with 85% legibility as measured by weekly spelling tests.	

be developed to address hand strength and letter formation skills, while occupational activities may be developed to address typical classroom activities. In Table 20-12, a sample therapy services plan for a six weeks grading period is listed:

The hand strengthening exercises and daily handwriting practice are implemented on a daily basis in the resource classroom and supervised by the resource teacher. During occupational therapy sessions, the OT and OTA use a variety of typical activities that are meaningful and fun for the child.

Summary

In this chapter, key legislations, IDEA '97 and Section 504, which drive special education and related services for children with special needs were discussed. IDEA '97 Part C provides services for infants and toddlers with disabilities and at the age of three Part B services begin and remain in effect through age 21. In Part B services, the related service of occupational therapy serves may serve dual roles, diagnostic and to determine eligibility, in the evaluation phase of services. In the next phase of services, occupational therapy may draft goals and objectives that form the foundation of an individualized educational plan as well as provide input

---

Table 20-12

Sample Therapy Services Plan

Readiness Skills	Implementer	Occupational Activities	Implementer
1. Hand strengthening readiness program 15 minutes daily theraputty exercises.	Resource teacher	Introduce new handwriting curriculum.	OT
		Write Valentine's Day cards (copying short poems).	OTA
		Work on spelling/ vocabulary homework.	OT
2. Daily practice session using handwriting curriculum booklet		Handwriting bingo game.	OTA
		Consultation with classroom and resource teachers.	OT and OTA

---

for transition planning. Service provision in school-based practice includes both direct and consult models and are individualized to meet the educational needs of the student.

Case Study

For this case study, refer to Table 20-13. After reading Cassie's evaluation summary, answer the following questions.

DISCUSSION QUESTIONS

1. Develop at least one readiness program and list several occupational activities that may be used to facilitate progress in Cassie's educational goals.

2. Develop an observation checklist that will allow school staff to measure Cassie's progress in IEP objectives.

3. If Cassie met the IEP objectives, what might be the next step or direction in her occupational and education services?

Application Activities

1. What are children doing in schools today? What skills are they expected to know in kindergarten, 3rd grade, and 8th grade? When should a student be expected to know the alphabet, the multiplication table, to locate the capital of France on a map? Each state education agency (SEA) lists its current educational curriculum on its website. For this activity:

- Choose one of the following educational skills and go surfing the web to find out when a student is expected to know that skill in your home state.

- Discuss the importance of this particular skill in everyday terms and everyday living.

- Discuss how occupational therapy might assist a student in learning this skill.

Educational Skills

a. Write the alphabet.

b. Begin to share and cooperate with others in group activities.

c. Begin to practice self-help skills (e.g., zipping, buttoning).

d. Recognize that print represents spoken language and conveys meaning such as his/her own name and signs such as Exit and Danger.

e. Identify cells as structures containing genetic material.

f. Understand literary terms by distinguishing between the roles of the author and illustrator such as the author writes the story and the illustrator draws the pictures.

g. Use alphabetical order to locate information.

h. Use text organizers, including headings, graphic features, and tables of contents, to locate and organize information.

i. Interpret important events and ideas gleaned from maps, charts, graphics, video segments or technology presentations.

j. Clarify and support spoken ideas with evidence, elaborations, and examples.

Table 20-13
Evaluation Summary for Cassie

Name/Age:	Cassie Phillips	9 yrs
School/Teacher:	Jefferson Elementary	Jamieson
Classroom / Grade:	Self-contained life skils classroom	Preschool
Eligibility/Services (Occupational Environment):	Orthopedic Impairment (Cerebral Palsy)	
Presenting Problem(s) (Reason for referral):	Difficulties with feeding self Difficulties with drinking from a cup	
Evaluation Tools:	Oral/Motor Feeding Scales Teacher report Observations	Informal manual muscle test Range of motion measurements
Strengths:	Finger feeds independently; beginning to use a spoon. Passive range of motion in hand/wrist within functional limits.	Demonstrates good sucking from a straw skills.
Differences:	ATNR still present—interfering with feeding in midline and bringing utensils to mouth. Tongue thrust present while drinking from a cup. Poor directionality	Fluctuating tone hand flexion and extension—interfering with hand closure on utensils. Moderate limited functional range of motion in wrist.
Recommendation(s):	OT direct 4 times per 6 weeks; 30 minutes direct OT consultation 1 time per 6 weeks to address readiness skills. Occupational readiness activities daily - 15 minutes: (supervised by campus staff; OT consults to develop 6 wks lesson plans for readiness activities).	
IEP goals and objectives to address:	Goal: Improve in feeding skills from minimum assistance to independence after set-up (of tray, utensils, and drinking cup) in self-feeding skills as documented in classroom observation checklist. Objective: Student will scoop and feed self from a spoon independently 70% of the meal as measured by classroom documentation. Objective: Student will drink independently from an adapted cup with no liquid loss as measured by teacher report.	

k. Proofread his/her own writing and that of others.

l. Use the distinguishing characteristics of various written forms such as essays, scientific reports, speeches, and memoranda.

m. Identify circles, triangles, and rectangles, including squares, and describe the shape of balls, boxes, cans, and cones.

n. Use patterns to develop strategies to remember basic addition facts.

o. Evaluate the impact of research on scientific thought, society, and the environment.

p. Identify patterns in related multiplication and division sentences (fact families) such as 2 x 3 = 6, 3 x 2 = 6, 6/2 = 3, 6/3 = 2.

q. Use models to relate decimals to fractions that name tenths, hundredths, and thousandths.

r. Use tables of related number pairs to make line graphs.

s. Estimate answers and use formulas to solve application problems involving surface area and volume.

t. Identifies and sketches graphs of parent functions, including linear ($y = x$), quadratic ($y = x2$), square root ($y = Ö\ x$), inverse ($y = 1/x$), exponential ($y = a^x$), and logarithmic ($y = \log_a x$) functions identifies and applies patterns from right triangles to solve problems, including special right triangles (45-45-90 and 30-60-90) and triangles whose sides are Pythagorean triples.

u. Evaluate role conflicts and methods of resolution that may occur among individuals and groups.

v. Use conic sections to model motion, such as the graph of velocity vs. position of a pendulum and motions of planets.

w. The value of a collection of coins and bills.

x. Use amortization models to investigate automobile financing and compare buying and leasing a vehicle.

y. Collect information using tools including hand lenses, clocks, computers, thermometers, and balances.

z. Make wise choices in the use and conservation of resources and the disposal or recycling of materials.

aa. Describe the structure and parts of an atom.

bb. Compare the arrangement of atoms in molecules, ionic crystals, polymers, and metallic substances.

cc. Explain the distribution of different types of climate in terms of patterns of temperature, wind, and precipitation and the factors that influence climate regions such as elevation, latitude, location near warm and cold ocean currents, position on a continent, and mountain barriers.

dd. Identify the approximate mass, size, motion, temperature, structure, and composition of the sun.

ee. Describe various beliefs, customs, and traditions of families and explain their importance.

ff. Explain how geographic factors have influenced the location of economic activities.

gg. Support a point of view on a social studies issue or event.

hh. Analyze the contributions of people of various racial, ethnic, and religious groups to our national identity.

2. You are the OTA working at an elementary school campus that has pre-kindergarten classrooms, a self-contained classroom for students with modified academic expectations and general education classrooms for students in kindergarten through 6th grade. Review the IEP goals and objectives for John and Cassie (illustrated in Tables 20-11 and 13). To meet John and Cassie's educational needs, plan appropriate occupational activities. In this assignment, what occupational activities would you plan? Plan at least three occupational activities for each objective and discuss how they relate to the student's educational needs.

References

Admundson, S. J. (1995). *Evaluation tool of children's handwriting.* Homer, AK: O.T. KIDS, Inc.

American Occupational Therapy Association. (1999a). *Occupational therapy services for children and youth under the Individuals with Disabilities Education Act.* (2nd ed.). Bethesda, MD: Author.

American Occupational Therapy Association. (1999b). Guide for Supervision of Occupational Therapy Personnel in the Delivery of Occupational Therapy Services. *American Journal of Occupational Therapy, 53,* 592-594.

Individuals With Disabilities Education Improvement Act Of 2003. Retrieved June 27, 2004 from

http://www.aota.org/members/area1/links/link70.asp?PLACE=/members/area1/links/link70.asp

Brigance, A. (1999). *Brigance diagnostic inventory of early development* (2nd ed.). North Billerica, MA; Curriculum Associates, Inc.

Council for exceptional children. (2004). *The new IDEA: CEC's summary of significant issues.* Retrieved December 23, 2004 from http://www.cec.sped.org/pp/IDEA 120204.pdf

Council for exceptional children. (1997). *Summary of the Individuals with Disabilities Education Act (IDEA) amendments of 1997(H.R. 5) (S. 717).* Retrieved February 3, 2003 from http://www.cec.sped.org/pp/idea-a.htm#1a

Dunn, W. (2000). *Best practice occupational therapy: In community service with children and families.* Thorofare, NJ; SLACK Incorporated.

Individuals with Disabilities Education Act, 20 U.S.C. Chapter 33 (EDLAW, 1997).

Gardner, M. (1996). *Test of Visual Perceptual Skills (n-m) - Revised.* Hydesville, CA; Psychological and Educational Publications, Inc.

Martin, J.L. (1997). *Brief overview of main 1997 IDEA amendments* (1997). Retrieved February 1, 2003, from

http://www.504idea.org/Reauth_.pdf

Mehfound, K. S. (1998). *The new IDEA: IEP development. School law in review 1998.* Alexandria, VA: National School Board Association Council of School Attorneys.

National Information Center for Children and Youth with Disabilities. (1998). *The IDEA amendments of 1997.* Washington, D.C.: Author.

National Information Center for Children and Youth with Disabilities. (1999). *Individualized education programs* (4th ed.). Washington, D.C.: Author.

National Information Center for Children and Youth with Disabilities. (2000). *Questions and answers about IDEA* (2nd ed.). Washington, D.C.: Author.

National Information Center for Children and Youth with Disabilities. (2001). *Related services* (2nd ed.). Washington, D.C.: Author.

National Information Center for Children and Youth with Disabilities. (2002). *General information about disabilities: Disabilities that qualify infants, toddlers, children, and youth for services under the IDEA.* Washington, D.C.: Author.

National Information Center for Children and Youth with Disabilities. (2004). IDEA 2004 summary. Retrieved December 23, 2004 from http:\\www.nichcy.org/reauth/2004IDEAsummary-12.04.doc

President's Commission on Excellence in Special Education (2002). *A New era: Revitalizing special education for children and their families*. Retrieved February 1, 2003 from http://www.ed.gov/inits/commissions-boards/whspecialeducation/reports.html

Schkade, J. K. & McClung, M. (2001). *Occupational adaptation in practice: Concepts and cases*. Thorofare, NJ: SLACK Incorporated.

Schkade, J. K. & Schultz, S. (1992). Occupational adaptation: Toward a holistic approach to contemporary practice. Part 1. *American Journal of Occupational Therapy, 49*, 829-838.

Schultz, S. & Schkade, J. K. (1992). Occupational adaptation: Toward a holistic approach to contemporary practice. Part II. *American Journal of Occupational Therapy, 49*, 829-838.

Warger, C. (1999). *New IDEA '97 requirements: Factors to consider in developing an IEP*. Retrieved February 5, 2003 from
http://ericec.org/digests/e578.html

PEDIATRIC SERVICE DELIVERY IN HOSPITALS, OUTPATIENT CLINICS, HOME HEALTH, HOSPICE, AND PRIVATE CLINICAL PRACTICE

Tara J. Glennon, EdD, OTR/L, BCP, FAOTA

Chapter Objectives

- Compare and contrast the role of the Occupational Therapy Assistant in the pediatric medical model practice settings discussed in this chapter.
- Understand the specialized nature of occupational therapy services in the NICU.
- Identify the varying roles of the occupational therapy practitioner within a hospital-based model.
- Appreciate the philosophical intricacies of the pediatric hospice setting.
- Recognize the pros and cons of working within the pediatric home-health model of service delivery.

Introduction

There are a wide variety of pediatric settings open to occupational therapy practitioners. Because of the many available options, occupational therapy practitioners need to be aware of the wide range of systems dictating how we function when working in pediatric settings. The philosophy, objectives, governance, rules, regulations, procedures, and unspoken expectations or standards of each system impact the scope of occupational therapy practice.

Within this chapter, the primary focus is on the role of the occupational therapy practitioner in the medical model of service delivery. However, based on each practice setting or environment and its individual system(s), how this model is implemented will vary. For example, a palliative care system in a hospice facility drives different support plans than a private practice facility. In order to deliver what is considered "best practice" within a specific practice environment, the occupational therapy assistant (OTA) needs to appreciate how the system and occupational therapy fit together. When these two components are congruent or even complimentary, occupational therapy practitioners may have maximum impact on the quality of a child's life. When opposing philosophies, objectives, and values are a reality, ineffective intervention plans and limited availability of therapy department resources will most likely result. For these reasons, the OTA should take care to choose an employment site that is congruent with his or her background, knowledge level, and professional desires.

Medical Model

Historically, the medical model focused on diagnostic testing of underlying functions that contributed to a presenting problem. Environmental conditions that interfered with function were not an issue. Fortunately, the characteristics of the medical model have expanded, and with the introduction of the World Health Organization's International Classification of Functioning, Disability and Health (ICF) (2001), today, disability is looked at very differently. No longer is a person categorized as disabled simply because there is a known diagnosis. The *Occupational Therapy Practice Framework: Domain and Process* (American Occupational Therapy Association [AOTA], 2002b) expands on the ICF concept of a more holistic view of disability by encouraging occupational therapy (OT) practitioners to address a variety of variables that are either facilitators or barriers to function and participation. Despite these changes, the medical model system remains somewhat rigid. This is not to say that personnel involved in the medical model will not continue to expand their theoretical and practical approach to service delivery. Providing adequate documentation that not only records service delivery, but also educates those within the medical model system, including the funding agencies (insurance companies), regarding the relevancy of pediatric occupational therapy services is necessary. All practitioners must remember that it is the funding agency that drives the system (for additional reimbursement issues, please refer to Chapter 6: Documentation). Within the pediatric realm, in order for an insurance company to financially support medically based services, documentation that services are medically necessary is required. This substantiation, including diagnostic testing that documents both a functional concern and the client factor(s) at issue, is required before services can be authorized for payment. This is a critical point from which the occupational therapist (OT) and OTA need to coordinate all evaluative information, determine expected goal outcomes, and identify appropriate intervention strategies. Once services have been authorized, ongoing documentation needs to be completed based on the requirements of the funding source (please refer to Chapter 6: Documentation for additional information).

Within the medical model, one can quickly identify the team's quarterback, the physician. While some state licensure laws do not require a physician's order for occupational therapy intervention, it is still required for insurance reimbursement. As with any team, ongoing communication and collaboration is essential (please refer to Chapter 4: Collaborative Models of Treatment). Within the medical model, this communication can mean the difference between a child obtaining funding for occupational therapy or not. If the therapy goals and objectives do not clearly match the medical and rehabilitative concerns identified by the physician, occupational therapy services may be denied. In specialized children's hospitals where there are many specialists working to meet specific pediatric issues, effective communication will also avoid any duplication of services or inadvertent "stepping on toes". While stepping on a team member's toes can be managed in face-to-face communications, insurance company denials for duplication of

services may be an administrative nightmare. The amount of time and paperwork required in order to appeal an insurance company denial cannot be underestimated. Communication and collaboration, therefore, are not only the key to effective service delivery, but to the financial viability of the agency attempting to support children and their families.

To summarize, OT practitioners must be aware of and implement the necessary components for "best practice" children's services. Based on the configuration of the team, responsibilities for intervention or support might change depending on each team member's area of specialty and training. Team collaboration and communication are essential in order to ensure that the child and family/caregiver's needs are comprehensively addressed.

Practice Environments

HOSPITAL-BASED SERVICES

There are a wide-range of therapeutic services offered to children within a hospital-based setting, and several factors determine the length of stay available to children. These include funding sources, primarily insurance considerations, as well as the hospital's accrediting agency. In addition, the occupational therapy department, considered one of the rehabilitation departments, is often in close proximity to the physical therapy and speech language departments. As these three disciplines are typically involved in the child's care, consistent and ongoing communication can be facilitated, because close proximity of the departments helps to ensure that a child and his/her family/caregiver's needs are met in the most comprehensive manner possible.

The OTA may wish to investigate how an individual hospital functions prior to accepting employment to determine if the hospital's philosophy and procedures match his/her internal strengths. Within the hospital setting, OT practitioners typically share an office space and frequently provide therapeutic support in the same treatment area. As a result, interaction between the OT and OTA can be facilitated simply by the physical parameters of the hospital.

Inpatient Status

A child admitted to the hospital is in a very unique situation. Most typically developing children never see the inside of a hospital, never mind have it be a place to eat, sleep, play, and socialize. As a result, the experience itself must be factored into the occupational therapy intervention plan. The type of hospital is also an important factor in developing an occupational therapy intervention plan. A children's wing on a general hospital might function very differently from a specialized children's hospital. In a general hospital, it is common for OT practitioners to rotate through the various units or programs, so care tends to be more generalized in nature. Conversely, in a hospital specifically designed for children, the level of expertise is more consistent with the specific needs of each department.

In either general or specialized hospital situations, the role of the OTA is an integral part of the therapeutic process. State licensure laws, the OTA's skill level, demands of the job, and the needs of the client will determine the level of specific supervision and interaction by the OT during each phase of the therapeutic process (AOTA, 2002a). Based on these parameters, within the evaluation sequence, the OTA's role is well-defined. This includes implementing standardized assessments that he or she is trained and deemed competent to complete, obtaining objective data via task analysis, and communicating this information effectively to the OT. Once the information is coordinated, processed, and analyzed by the OT, the intervention plan can be created. While the OT is ultimately responsible for the intervention plan, if the OTA is to be involved in the implementation of a treatment plan, then the OTA may also be included in the development and modification of that plan (AOTA, 2002a). The OTA also has a responsibility to contribute to monitoring therapy progress and communicating that information back to the supervising OT, as well as playing a critical part in finding community resources near the child's home in order to provide ongoing or more frequent intervention following discharge.

There are a wide variety of situations that might bring a child into the hospital for more than an acute condition. These include premature or medically complicated births, failure to thrive, cerebral palsy, juvenile rheumatoid arthritis, spina bifida, a muscle disease, orthopedic conditions, craniofacial concerns, cystic fibrosis, childhood cancer, pediatric AIDS, spinal cord injury, or near drowning (please refer to Chapter 11: Diagnoses Commonly Associated With Childhood). In addition to longer-term hospital stays, several diagnoses require intermittent hospitalizations that call upon the in-hospital OT practitioners to implement and carry over interventions that the child might have been receiving in their home community. Some examples include the child with spina bifida coming in to learn self-catheterization techniques; a child with cerebral palsy scheduled for a tendon release; or a child with a spinal cord injury having an issue with decubiti. There is also the possibility that a child lives in such a rural area that community services are not readily available. In these situations, a child may be admitted to the hospital for a short period of time in order to receive a comprehensive medical and therapeutic work-up.

Outpatient Clinics

In order to follow-up or monitor a child's progress following hospital discharge, many hospitals also operate outpatient therapy clinics. Children are seen on a one-time or routinely scheduled basis in order to monitor, assess, follow-up on a procedure that may have been completed on an in-patient status, or consult on a specific issue. For example,

consider the case of a baby born prematurely with a heart defect. Once the baby is medically cleared to go home, a six-month follow-up appointment might be made with the feeding clinic, the motor team, or to set up a developmental assessment. Outpatient clinics are designed to ensure that the baby is progressing in a typical manner or to offer continued assistance to the baby's community team of therapists.

The regional children's hospital might also offer follow-up or specialized support clinics for children with diagnoses such as cerebral palsy, a muscle disease, spina bifida, orthopedic or splinting concerns, diabetes, or post surgery. For many families who were not part of the hospital system as an in-patient, access to these specialized services are a source for a second opinion, comprehensive assessment, or to offer support to the local team of medical or educational therapists. Due to the fact that these clinics require and focus on assessment and preparation of intervention plans that follow the child back home or to the local OT, this is not often a work site well suited for an OTA.

Neonatal Intensive Care Unit (NICU)

Technological advancements in the 1970s created a new reality for pediatric clinicians, the survival of premature infants and babies with complex medical concerns. While NICU practice began showing rapid growth in the 1980s, Vergara (2002) emphasizes that occupational therapy practice has yet to "reach consensus about some fundamental principles and concepts" (p. 8). It is clear that babies born prematurely or those with complex medical issues require intense developmental and environmental support. Likewise, psychosocial support for the family/caregivers is also critically important.

The *Occupational Therapy Practice Framework: Domain and Process* (AOTA, 2002b) attempts to integrate our professional direction into a traditional medical model of care. It should be emphasized that the NICU is not a traditional medical model. Rather, it encompasses sophisticated medical procedures, technology, and terminology specific to neonatology. The specific level of expertise required to address neonatal client factors and environmental modifications associated with these children is profound. As a result, when working in the NICU, the OT must proficiently incorporate these daily realities with theoretical models and framework conceptualizations of occupational therapy practice.

The level of expertise, advanced training, and theoretical knowledge required to work within a NICU cannot be underestimated. These sites rarely allow fieldwork experiences for the OT student, and very rarely employ an OTA. According to AOTA's 2000 Member Compensation Survey (2001), 0.0% of the responding OTAs worked in the NICU in both 1997 and 2000. For OTs, less that 1% of the responding therapists listed this environment as the primary work area during these same years. As core concepts of how occupational therapy services are to be best used in the

NICU continue to be debated, and the conceptualization of what occupational therapy practice should entail is yet to be clearly defined, the role of the OTA in the NICU is not yet defined.

The life-threatening nature of this work environment emphasizes the level of expertise expected of all medical team members. For instance, Sweeney and Chandler (1990) documented that insufficient experience and training increases the risks to medically fragile neonates. Therefore, if the OTA has an aspiration to work within this specific setting, an extreme amount of focused effort would be required beyond entry-level practice in order to achieve this goal.

HOSPICE

The American Occupational Therapy Association's position on the profession's role within the hospice model is documented in the *Occupational Therapy Practice Framework: Domain and Process* (AOTA, 2002b). This document emphasizes the unique role of OT practitioners in supporting the desire of a person with a terminal illness to engage in meaningful activities. However, as the introduction section of this chapter outlined, each working environment has its own "system" that dictates how personnel support the client. Knowing the system, and matching one's personal characteristics with the philosophy of the agency is never more important than within the hospice model. An organization committed to providing support and care for persons in the last phases of disease will require that all personnel support its mission and principles. As a result, OT practitioners need to have personal awareness and a deep understanding of the meaning of occupation within the model of hospice care (AOTA, 2002b). Having a role on a team working to prepare a child, and the family/caregivers, as he or she physically and mentally approaches death speaks for itself. For this reason, knowing one's own personal strengths, limitations, and coping skills are important when working in a hospice setting.

The second major factor for the OTA to appreciate when working in a hospice is that within this environment, one must have the ability to be flexible with a predetermined support plan. For example, suppose part of the occupational therapy plan calls for participation in a self-care task in order to restore a sense of control. For a teenage girl, an age appropriate task might be to braid her hair. When the OTA arrives for the morning session, the girl is quite fatigued from another medical procedure. Although hair braiding might have been the focus of the session allocated for her morning routine, a quick adjustment needs to occur. Perhaps this might be the time for a non-physically demanding photo album activity, which is also an age appropriate part of her occupational therapy plan. The OTA working in the hospice environment must be intricately linked with the OT in order to skillfully manage and be comfortable with the requirements of making, at any given moment, last minute adjustments based on the status of the child.

In hospice work, it is important that OT practitioners support the child's ability to engage in a meaningful life, but also to remember that this is not a rehabilitative or restorative model of service delivery. For example, OT practitioners must offer and suggest sitting or reclining positions that allow the child to explore, engage, and interact, but are not so taxing that it eliminates the possibility of further participation in daily tasks. Occupational therapy practitioners must also provide adaptive equipment so that the child has control over play and mealtime activities without expending so much energy that quality of the rest of their day is compromised. In hospice care, providing a comfortable life is equally as important as fostering functional independence, and must be factored into the plan of occupational therapy support.

In the hospice environment, providing outlets for communication as well as the child's ability to express thoughts, ideas, and emotions are critical. Remember that children are not always able to express themselves in the same way as adults. In many instances, providing a play-based outlet to encourage communication is an appropriate intervention strategy. Although the therapeutic relationship is interactive, for the child's benefit the OT practitioner must guide the relationship with a sense of dignity and empathy. While in many medical models the tone of the therapeutic relationship is set by the OT practitioner, in the hospice setting the OTA must skillfully read the child's cues and in doing so, help to nurture the relationship. Additionally, while unconditional acceptance is an essential aspect of any therapeutic relationship, the relationship with a child who is dying is unique. Again, the child's communications might not be carried out in verbal terms. For example, he or she may illustrate the level of coping by crying, sleeping, expressing anger, or asking questions. As a result, *all* staff working in a hospice must be watchful of what the child is trying to communicate through interactions and, more specifically in terms of occupational therapy, through play.

HOME HEALTH

There are several presenting circumstances in which a child's occupational therapy services are most appropriately delivered in the home. For example, a child with medical issues who cannot safely tolerate center-based or school-based programs; a medically fragile child who is not easily or safely transported to a center-based or school-based program; or a child who performs better given the familiarity of the home environment might all be better served through home health services. Incorporating rehabilitative needs, maintaining health and function, and training the family/caregivers while working within the home environment is quite a challenge. For the OTA, the ability to effectively communicate with the family/caregivers is extremely important (please refer to Chapter 9: Interacting With Families).

Jose Gonzalez

The OTA's ability to task analyze will support home based intervention. The ability to analyze real situations and everyday activities allows the OTA to incorporate the household resources to support the child. For example, the use of the child's own Boppy® (Boppy Company, Golden, CO) pillow as a means of supporting a functional sitting posture during play would be more appropriate than ordering a therapeutic seating device. Another unique facet of delivering occupational therapy services is managing siblings who also want to play with the "bag of tricks" and toys that you bring to each therapy session. Incorporating the family into the delivery of services is critical, whether it is the sibling or the parent/caregiver. One word of caution, however, pertains to the close personal relationship that may develop between the OTA and the parent/caregiver during the treatment process. It is important to communicate all appropriate information to the OT supervisor and to be clear with the parent/caregiver that all therapeutically relevant information will be shared. Based on these potentially difficult issues, it is often advantageous for the OT supervisor to make intermittent visits to the home as a point of contact, to have the ability to adjust the program as necessary, and to offer support to the treating OTA.

In home health care, facilitating consistent and ongoing communication between team members who do not often see each other is a situation that needs to be managed proactively. For instance, each team member needs to make a consistent commitment to attend full medical team meetings. These meetings are typically organized by the coordinating agency and often occur at the agency's office versus the client's home. On occasion, the coordinating agency will not hold case management meetings frequently enough for team members to share ongoing information about the child. In this case, a communication notebook and information binder may be kept in the child's home. The communication notebook provides each team member a consistent and time efficient method of sharing information with other team members. Intervention strategies, instruction sheets, or home program suggestions can also be added to the information binder as they are implemented in the home. This system allows each team member to be aware of what information the family is receiving from the other professionals. The communication notebook and information binder is an accessible means to gain insight into team member's interventions and allows all practitioners to alter, augment, modify, or expand his or her own intervention plan accordingly.

PRIVATE CLINICAL PRACTICE

By now you are aware that children are not just miniature adults, thus specific treatment approaches need to be meaningful and directed to the child. Within a private practice setting, this approach needs to be clearly articulated to the parent/caregiver. Consumers of private practitioners may often access these services in order to "get the expert, " and as such, the OT practitioner must live up to these expecta-

tions. Further, parents who philosophically adhere to the medical system may believe in "the magic pill" or procedure to fix the child, may question the relevancy of the treatment approaches that are being implemented in a private practice setting. As a result, this may be a tricky situation for the OTA. This is not because the actual implementation of therapy is difficult, but because the demands regarding clear and informed communication are very high. If the insurance company has denied medical necessity, and the parents are paying out of pocket for services, the ability to clearly articulate the rationale for intervention strategies is hugely important.

To further the idea of therapeutic relevancy discussed above, Hinojosa and Kramer (1993) talk about two reasons why pediatric occupational therapy intervention might not always appear "therapeutic." First, the intervention is focused on, and uses, routine daily activities. In addition, because intervention with children is activity oriented and often uses play, the casual observer might feel that anyone could simply "play" with the child. The ability to readily explain the complexity of the activity, the theoretical underpinnings, and the rationale for the specifically chosen task, is critical. Providing clear communication assists the parents/caregivers to understand that the systematic, yet flexible, step-by-step intervention approaches are designed to reach identified outcomes, as articulated in the goals and objectives portion of the documentation procedures (for additional information, please refer to Chapter 6: Documentation). The change or outcome that is brought about by the intervention strategies support the child's ability to participate in tasks previously identified by the parent/caregiver as difficult for the child. For these reasons, when working in private clinical practice the intricate working relationship between the OT and OTA needs to be perfected. Often, this synchrony is as crucial as the focus of intervention itself.

Depending on the organizational structure of the agency and with reference to team models, each private practice functions differently. For example, the practice may offer a variety of services for a child, including occupational therapy, physical therapy, speech, or social work, or may only offer occupational therapy. When the practice offers a variety of services, team coordination is facilitated by the physical parameters. When only occupational therapy services are offered, the OT staff must make clear and distinctive efforts to coordinate services with the child's other private service providers.

Summary

This chapter illustrated the varying models of medical service delivery for the pediatric client. While the basics of pediatric occupational therapy intervention remain consistent, the environmental context dictates how the services are implemented. Additionally, *Occupational Therapy Practice Framework: Domain and Process* (AOTA, 2002b) has expanded the components to be considered and accounted for within the intervention process. For these reasons, collaboration between the OT and OTA is crucial in order to implement best practice. Although the NICU and outpatient specialty clinic in a hospital would not be available to the entry-level OTA, hospital inpatient, private practice, hospice, and home health are appropriate employment contexts for the OTA.

Case Study

The intricacies of how the medical model operates in a variety of settings can be illustrated by the story of Kenny, an 8-year-old boy who fell out of a tree. Kenny was admitted to the regional medical facility for acute medical management. At that time, the role of the occupational therapy was limited, as life-sustaining supports were the focus. When Kenny was diagnosed as having an acquired head injury, he was transferred to the hospital's rehabilitation unit. The physiatrist or neurologist ran weekly case management meetings where all rehabilitative team members shared status, progress, goals, plan for treatment, and expected outcomes. Traditional rehabilitative roles were evident, and occupational therapy was responsible for daily living and self-care limitations, feeding, motor skills, and cognitive concerns. The team on the rehabilitation unit also included a cognitive therapist, vocation rehabilitation specialist, and life skills professionals. Unfortunately, based on Kenny's age, some of these services were not appropriate. The OT practitioners, as professionally obligated, addressed the developmentally necessary social, emotional, and family needs. While this occurred as a natural course of treatment, there were no "codes" on the rehabilitation billing ticket for this type of intervention.

Kenny was ultimately transferred to a children's rehabilitation hospital in an adjoining state. In this facility, the medical model expanded as appropriate for children's services. The team now included a play therapist, educational team, therapeutic recreational specialist, and life skills staff. Based on this new team configuration and areas of specialty available to the child and family, the role of occupational therapy was adjusted.

DISCUSSION QUESTIONS

1. How would the roles of the OT and OTA change throughout Kenny's different hospitalizations?

2. What type of service delivery model best describes Kenny's stays in both the regional medical facility and the children's rehabilitation hospital?

3. Based on the information presented in Chapter 20: Preschool and School-Based Therapy, what additional components of Kenny's therapeutic intervention would be expected by the educational team in the specialized children's rehabilitation hospital?

4. As Kenny's specialized rehabilitation is occurring in another state, investigate what housing resources might be available to the family through not-for-profit organizations.

Application Activities

1. Review the documentation from your own personal insurance carrier in order to determine the reimbursement policy related to occupational therapy services.

2. Call your insurance carrier and ask how you should proceed if you want to get occupational therapy services for your child. Ask what is necessary, what you should get from your doctor, and which local in-network agency offers pediatric services.

3. Verify the requirements of your own state as to whether or not a physician's referral is required in order for a client to access occupational therapy services. You can call the State Department of Health, the occupational therapy licensure department, or look up the licensure law on your state's governmental website.

References

American Occupational Therapy Association. (2001). *2000 Member Compensation Survey*. Bethesda, MD: Author.

American Occupational Therapy Association. (2002a). Guide for supervision of occupational therapy personnel in the delivery of occupational therapy services. In *The reference manual of the official documents of the American Occupational Therapy Association* (pp. 161-166). Bethesda, MD: Author.

American Occupational Therapy Association. (2002b). Occupational therapy practice framework: Domain and process. *American Journal of Occupational Therapy, 56*, 609-639.

Hasselkus, B. R., & Jacques, N. D. (2002). Occupational therapy and hospice. In *The reference manual of the official documents of the American Occupational Therapy Association* (pp. 365-369). Bethesda, MD: American Occupational Therapy Association, Inc.

Hinojosa, J., & Kramer, P. (1993). From frames of reference to actual intervention. In P. Kramer & J. Hinojosa (Eds.). *Frames of reference for pediatric occupational therapy* (pp. 439-454). Baltimore: Williams & Wilkins.

Sweeney, J. K., & Chandler, L. S. (1990). Neonatal physical therapy: Medical risks and professional education. *Infants and Young Children, 2*, 59-68.

Vergara, E. R. (2002). Enhancing occupational performance in infants. *OT Practice, 7*(12), 8-13.

World Health Organization. (2001). *International classification of functioning, disability and health* (ICF). Geneva, Switzerland: Author.

Pediatric Psychosocial Therapy

Joylynn Holladay, MS, OTR/L

Chapter Objectives

- Understand the different types of psychosocial disorders and their impact on areas of occupation.
- Describe the contexts in which psychosocial occupational therapy services are delivered.
- Define and delineate the role of the occupational therapy assistant and the role of the occupational therapist in the delivery of services.
- Identify strategies and activities used by occupational therapy assistants when working with children with psychosocial disorders.

Introduction

The burden of suffering experienced by children with mental health needs and their families has created a health crisis in this country. Growing numbers of children are suffering needlessly because their emotional, behavioral, and developmental needs are not being met by those very institutions, which were explicitly created to take care of them (Excerpted from Surgeon General Report on Children's Mental Health, Jan. 2001).

Within any given year, one in five children experience psychosocial problems serious enough to warrant psychiatric diagnosis (Lahey et al., 1996). One in ten children experience significant functional impairment as a result of psychosocial disturbance, affecting performance at home, school, or the community. Left untreated, mental illness can lead to school failure and dropout, family conflict, substance abuse, violence, or suicide.

Despite the prevalence of childhood mental illness, current research shows a disarmingly high rate of unmet need among children requiring psychosocial intervention. One study found that only 21% of children ages 6-17 identified as having mental health issues received the proper assistance, leaving an estimated 7.5 million children without the necessary care (Kataoka, Zhang, & Wells, 2002). This disparity in services disproportionately affects minorities, uninsured children, and preschoolers (Kataoka, Zhang, & Wells, 2002).

Stigma associated with mental illness including blame placed on family parenting patterns, fragmented services, and treatment limitations placed on mental health insurance coverage are just a few of the reasons why psychosocial needs of children and their families frequently go unaddressed. Lack of both public and professional awareness continues to contribute to the pervasive attitudinal bias surrounding mental health issues. Stigmatization leads to distrust, stereotyping, and avoidance of individuals diagnosed with mental illness (Penn & Martin, 1998) and is evident in our view and treatment of mental health issues. Advances in neuroscience have shown mental illnesses to be legitimate medical disorders of the brain. Despite these advances, in effect many health plans penalize individuals seeking mental health care by imposing co-payments, deductibles or limits on outpatient visits that are more restrictive than those placed on physical illness. Parents and children facing mental health problems are often made to feel guilty or embarrassed, and are therefore reluctant to seek help (Pavuluri, Luk & McGee, 1996).

As health care providers, occupational therapists (OTs) and occupational therapy assistants (OTAs) may play an essential role in the early identification and treatment of childhood psychosocial disorders in numerous settings. Yet,

---

Table 22-1

Psychosocial Core of Occupational Therapy—Key Concepts

- Influenced by the philosophy and practices of the Moral Treatment Movement of the late 1700s, a movement that stressed the value of human relationships, harmonious environment, and the importance of daily, purposeful activity in restoring and maintaining mental and physical health.
- Emphasis on the "critical importance of 'doing'" in developing self-competency and fulfilling social membership.
- Therapeutic engagement of the individual's motivations to participate in desired activities that minimize disability and encourage adaptive responses.
- Disability and illness elicit a variety of psychosocial responses on the part of the individual and their family.
- Interpersonal dynamic of all helping professions is characterized by the therapeutic extension and use of the self.
- Psychosocial dimensions of human performance are fundamental in all aspects of occupational therapy across settings.
- All specialty areas are grounded in the core psychosocial concepts.
- The specialty area of mental health also incorporates expert knowledge of how psychopathologies impact the individual's ability to cope and manage daily occupational roles.

Adapted from American Occupational Therapy Association & Fidler, G.S. (1997). The psychosocial core of occupational therapy position paper. *American Journal of Occupational Therapy, 51*(10), 868-869.

---

too often OT practitioners focus on motor skills at the expense of psychosocial and behavioral skills (referred to as communication/interaction skills and process skills under the *Occupational Therapy Practice Framework*) (AOTA, 2002). This is in part due to reimbursement regulations (Schultz, 1992) and setting constraints. Additionally, many OT practitioners are unaware of their potential for affecting positive change in the psychosocial realm, mistakenly assuming they are under qualified or need to be in a mental health setting to address these needs. Far be it from the case; occupational therapy is a discipline historically rooted in psychosocial principles, stressing a holistic approach to treatment regardless of diagnosis or setting. Table 22-1 outlines the Psychosocial Core of Occupational Therapy adopted by the Representative Assembly of the American Occupational Therapy Association in 1995.

Chronic illness and disability, whether it is of a physical or psychological nature, has an effect on the child's psychosocial functioning (Fidler, 1997). For example, a child with Spina Bifida may feel isolated by his/her condition, and may therefore be reluctant or even refuse to participate in social activities. Likewise, a child with an anxiety disorder may also show signs of social withdrawal due to increased feelings of fear and apprehension. In treating the whole child, the pediatric OT practitioners must take into account all factors affecting occupational performance in order to facilitate adaptive responses and enable the child to fully participate in his/her environmental contexts.

Population Identified

The concept of pediatric psychosocial dysfunction is a fairly new one. It was not until the late nineteenth century that scientists recognized childhood mental illness, and even then incidences were thought to be identical to adult forms. Because children are often unable to articulate the complexity of what they are feeling or going through, psychosocial disturbance often manifests itself behaviorally. Familiarization with symptoms of pediatric psychosocial disturbance is necessary to assist the OT in the screening and detection of psychosocial problems, and ensure that children receive the appropriate services. For instance, presence of self-destructive behaviors including substance abuse and suicidal ideation requires immediate professional attention. Other questions to take into account when deciding if a child should be referred for a psychiatric evaluation include:

1. How long have these symptoms been occurring?
2. If these symptoms are recent, have there been any obvious precipitating factors, such as a recent move, or parental discord?
3. Are these symptoms affecting performance in school, social relationships, or home life?
4. Has there been a sudden change in the child's personality or a sudden regression of skill level?
5. Does the child have a family history of mental illness or learning disability?

The following discussion is not meant to be an exhaustive overview of the myriad of psychosocial disorders. Rather, it focuses on those conditions most prevalent to the pediatric population. It includes conventional mental illness diagnoses as well as other disorders that affect psychosocial and emotional functioning. Particular emphasis will be given to the unique presentation of symptoms across developmental stages, especially infancy and early childhood. Information presented here is taken from the *Diagnostic and Statistical Manual of Mental Disorders*, Fourth Edition, Text revision (DSM-IV TR) (APA, 2000) and the *Diagnostic Classification* of *Mental Health and Developmental Disorders of Infancy and Early Childhood* (DC: 0-3) (Zero to Three, 1994). Given the overlap of symptomology and *comorbidity* among these conditions, it is important for the OT practitioner to focus on the impact that various symptoms have on the child's occupational performance rather than on the diagnosis itself.

ANXIETY DISORDERS

Affecting an estimated 13% of children ages 9 to 17 (Shaffer, Fisher, Dulcan et al., 1996), anxiety disorders are among the most common mental health problems of childhood and adolescence. Anxiety disorders are characterized by excessive feelings of worry, apprehension, fear, and distress to the point of interfering with the individual's day-to-day functioning. Scientists have proposed several potential causes of anxiety disorder, including the hypersecretion of stress hormones, and the imbalance of serotonin and GABA, both inhibitory *neurotransmitters* that quiet the stress response (Rush et al., 1998). Nearly half of all children with anxiety disorders also have a coexistent mental or behavioral disorder such as depression, or ADHD (Center for Mental Health Services, 1998). Research also points to a correlation between sensory processing difficulties and the development of anxiety disorders (Williamson & Anzaolne, 2001; DeGangi & Breinbauer, 1997). For example, infants often use social referencing, the ability to read the emotional expressions and cues of familiar individuals to self-regulate and explore new environments (Walker-Andrews, 1998). However, an eighteen month old with visual processing challenges may have difficulty scanning and locating his or her caregiver across space, thus causing feelings of undue distress and anxiety. This emotional anxiety may cause the child to become dysregulated and cling to his or her caregiver instead of engaging in spontaneous exploration of his or her environment. Without proper identification of the underlying sensory processing difficulty, the child's distress response may develop into or be inappropriately recognized as an anxiety disorder. Left untreated, anxiety disorders may lead to poor school attendance, low self-esteem, inadequate interpersonal skills, alcohol or other substance abuse, and difficulty adjusting. Table 22-2 is a select list and description of anxiety disorders.

MOOD DISORDERS

Mood disorders are defined by periods of depression, sometimes alternating with periods of elevated mood (APA, 2000). Diagnosis of mood disorders in children is problematic as many researchers feel the current diagnostic criteria does not adequately take into account the heterogeneous expression of depressive and manic symptoms across developmental stages (Brown, 1996). Research points to an imbalance of neurotransmitters, mainly serotonin and norepinephrine; genetic predisposition; and stressful life events as possible contributing factors to the development of mood

disorders (U.S. Public Health Service, 1999). Among both children and adolescents, depressive disorders confer an increased risk for illness and interpersonal and psychosocial difficulties that persist long after the depressive episode is resolved; with adolescents there is also an increased risk for substance abuse and suicidal behavior. Without treatment, episodes of mania and depression may last anywhere between 6 months and a year with an increased recurrence rate through adulthood. Each new episode confers additional risks of chronicity, disability, and suicide.

Major Depressive Disorder

Studies indicate that approximately 1% of preschoolers, 2% of school aged children, and 5% to 8% of adolescents suffer from major depression (Jellinek & Snydor, 1998). Childhood depression is associated not only with continued episodes of major depression into adulthood, but also with future onsets of bipolar disorder, conduct disorder, substance abuse, and suicide (Harrington, 2001). Risk factors include family history of depression, particularly maternal depression (Beardslee, Versage, & Gladstone, 1998); chronic physical illness such as diabetes, asthma, or cancer; poverty; and negative life events such as divorce and peer rejection.

Symptoms of depression in toddlers and preschool aged children include lethargy, disruption in feeding and sleeping patterns, sad or expressionless faces, irritability, and decreased affective responsivity (Carlson & Kashani, 1988). The elementary school aged child suffering from major depression may exhibit prolonged unhappiness, decreased socialization, sleep problems, poor school performance, accident proneness, phobias, separation anxiety, and attention-seeking behaviors (Carlson & Kashani, 1988; Edelsohn, Ialongo, Werthamer-Lars, Crockett, & Kellam, 1992). Depressed adolescents experience similar *somatic* complaints and social withdrawal; they also report more concerns about the future, pessimism, feelings of worthlessness, and apathy (Weiss, Weisz, Politano et al., 1992).

Bipolar Disorder

The lifetime prevalence of bipolar disorder in adults ranges from 0.6% to 1.1%, with the peak onset occurring between the ages of 15 to 19 (McClellan & Werry, 1997). Although once considered rare in the pre-pubertal population, researchers speculate as many as 1 million children suffer from the disorder (Kluger & Song, 2002). Bipolar disorder appears to have a strong familial component. When one parent has bipolar disorder, the risk to each child is estimated to be 15% to 30%; the risk increases to 50% to 75% when both parents are bipolar (Depression and Bipolar Support Alliance, 2002).

Bipolar disorder consists of cycles of deep depression and excessive euphoria, interspersed by normal periods of behavior (APA, 2000). Unlike adults with bipolar disorder, children under the age of nine do not typically experience

Table 22-2
Anxiety Disorders

	Generalized Anxiety Disorder (GAD)	Separation Anxiety Disorder	Post Traumatic Stress Disorder (PTSD)	Social Phobia or Anxiety	Obsessive Compulsive Disorder (OCD)
Symptoms	• Extreme, unrealistic worry pertaining to all situations. • Complaints of somatic ailments that have no physical basis • Need continuous reassurance about their performance and anxieties.	• Developmentally inappropriate distress when separated from parent. • Clingy behavior when around parent. • Difficulty falling asleep, nightmares, symptoms of depression such as apathy and withdrawal.	• Ongoing emotional distress resulting from the experience of a catastrophic event. • Re-experiences the event through strong memories, flashbacks, nightmares, or play. • Hypervigilance, exaggerated startle response, acting younger than their age, problems maintaining relationships, lack of concentration.	• Constant fear of being embarrassed in social situations. Palpitations, tremors, sweating, flushing, diarrhea, upset stomach. • May result in full-blown panic attack. May have tantrums, cry, freeze, or stay close to familiar adults.	• Presence of repetitive, time-consuming obsessions or compulsive behaviors that cause distress and/or impairment. Attempts to displace obsessions through ritualistic patterns of behavior.
Incidence	• Lifetime prevalence estimated at 5% among general population.	• Occurs in approx. 4% of children ages 7 to 9	Lifetime prevalence estimated at 1 to 14% among general population.	• Lifetime prevalence estimated at 3 to 13% • More common among females	• Occurs in approx .2 to .8% of children and up to 2% of adolescents.
Impact on Daily Functioning	• Affects child's ability to independently participate in home, school, and play. • Transitions and novelty are especially hard. • Child often requires a lot of verbal preparation and adult facilitation to complete simple tasks, especially novel ones.	• Affects all aspects of the child's life, esp. school and play. • Disturbances in sleep and depressive symptoms may lead to decrease physical energy, further impairing daily functioning • Adverse affect on parent-child interactions as parent becomes frustrated by child's over-dependence	• Affects all aspects of the child's life. • Lack of concentration may lead to poor school performance. • May become socially withdrawn, refusing to play with friends. • Routine avoidance of reminders of the event may disrupt daily functioning (e.g., child may refuse to go to school after witnessing an act of school violence).	• Affects school performance, play and social skills. • Fear of social situations may lead to school absenteeism or selective mutism. • Child may have difficulty making friends due to fear of rejection.	• Affects all aspects of the child's life. • Ritualistic behaviors interfere with the child's ability to perform basic tasks. • Inability for the child to "control" his/her behavior may lead to feelings of shame, further interfering with daily functioning.

Adapted from US Department of Health and Human Services.

Table 22-3

Behavioral Signs of Autism

- The child does not respond to his/her name.
- The child cannot explain what he/she wants.
- Language skills or speech are delayed.
- The child doesn't follow directions.
- The child seems to hear sometimes, but not others.
- The child doesn't point or wave bye-bye.
- The child used to say a few words or babble, but now he/she doesn't.
- The child throws intense or violent tantrums.
- The child has odd movement patterns.
- The child is hyperactive, uncooperative, or oppositional.
- The child doesn't know how to play with toys.
- The child doesn't smile when smiled at.
- The child has poor eye contact.
- The child gets "stuck" on things over and over and can't move on to other things.
- The child seems to prefer to play alone.
- The child gets things for him/herself only.
- The child is very independent for his/her age.
- The child seems to be in his/her "own world."
- The child seems to tune people out.
- The child is not interested in other children.
- The child walks on his/her toes.
- The child shows unusual attachments to toys, objects, or schedules (i.e., always holding a string or having to put socks on before pants).
- Child spends a lot of time lining things up or putting things in a certain order.

Adapted from National Institute of Child Health and Human Development.

---

classic manic symptoms of elation and grandiosity. Instead, the child may appear irritable, have motor agitation, or display prolonged, explosive temper tantrums. Another key feature of childhood bipolar disorder is the presence of rapid-cycling, continuous, or ultradian cycles of mood (Papolos, 1999). Children with bipolar disorder experience rapid and dramatic shifts in mood and energy, going from giddy and silly at one moment to hostile and belligerent the next. These mood swings may be set off by disruption to their sleep cycle or by caffeine consumption. There also appears to be overlap between symptoms of bipolar disorder, ADHD, and conduct disorder (Papolos, 1999). Some researchers feel this overlap may account for the under-detection and misdiagnosis of bipolar disorder. A child or adolescent who appears to be depressed and exhibits ADHD-like symptoms that are very severe, with excessive temper outbursts and mood changes, should be evaluated by a qualified professional.

PERVASIVE DEVELOPMENTAL DISORDER

Also known as autistic spectrum disorders, this category refers to a group of disorders characterized by delays in social relationships and communication. Autism is the best known and the most common Pervasive Developmental Disorder (PDD). Other disorders classified under this category include Asperger's syndrome, childhood disintegrative disorder, Rett's disorder, and PDD-not otherwise specified.

This group of disorders is four times more common in boys than girls. Although no national studies have been conducted, regional studies conducted by the Centers for Disease Control indicate that autism occurs in as many as 4 out of every 1000 children in certain areas of the country (1998). The disorder is marked by qualitative impairment in social interactions, communication, and/or the presence of restrictive, repetitive patterns of behaviors, interest, or activities (APA, 2000). Autism is also associated with severe sensory processing difficulties. For example, children with autism may present with movement seeking or movement avoiding behaviors, tactile defensiveness, delays in auditory processing, and severe motor planning deficits. Symptoms of autism appear before the age of three and generally last throughout a person's life. Behaviors that may signify autism include the absence of babbling and cooing by 12 months; lack of gestural communication (e.g., point, wave grasp) by 12 months; and lack of spontaneous two word utterances by 24 months (Table 22-3). PDD is believed to be the product of a confluence of genetic, neurological, and environmental factors. Brain abnormalities, food allergies, excessive amounts of yeast in the digestive tract, and exposure to environmental toxins such as mercury have all been sited as possible causes (Autism Society of America). Early identification and intervention of PDD has been linked to improved outcomes, including decreased negative and self-harming behaviors, increased development of functional skills, and increased

---

Table 22-4
Symptoms of Attention and Hyperactivity/Impulsivity

Inattention

Easily distracted by irrelevant sights and sounds
Failing to pay attention to details
Making careless mistakes
Difficulty following instructions
Losing and forgetting things needed for a task
Reluctance to engage in tasks requiring sustained
mental activity
Does not listen when spoken to directly
Difficulty organizing tasks and activities

Hyperactivity/Impulsivity

Feeling restless, fidgeting with hands or feet, squirming in seat
Difficulty remaining seated when required to do so
Talks excessively
Difficulty playing quietly
Always "on the go"
Blurting out answers before hearing the whole question
Difficulty waiting in line for a turn
Often interrupts or intrudes on others

From American Psychiatric Association (2000). *Diagnostic and Statistical Manual of Mental Disorders*, Fourth Edition, Text revision (2000). Washington, DC: APA.

---

communication skills and IQ (Baird et al., 2001) (please refer to Chapter 10: Diagnoses Commonly Associated With Childhood).

DISRUPTIVE BEHAVIOR DISORDERS

The presence of disruptive behaviors is the most common reason children are referred for mental health services. Disruptive behaviors are persistent patterns of behavior that usually incite adult authority figures or peers to respond with anger, impatience, punishment, or avoidance (Halgin & Whitbourne, 1994). This constellation of disorders also includes attention deficit/hyperactivity disorder, oppositional defiant disorder, and conduct disorder. Children with these disorders may be impulsive, argumentative, aggressive, or anti-social. Children with disruptive behavior disorders including ADHD, who do not receive proper treatment are at increased risk for medical and social problems including reckless driving, drug and alcohol abuse, smoking, academic failure, difficulty in forming relationships, trouble with the law, and symptoms of depression and anxiety (US Department of Health and Human Services, 1999).

Attention Deficit/Hyperactivity Disorder

Children with this disorder may display developmentally inappropriate levels of inattention; hyperactivity and impulsivity; or both (APA, 2000). Table 22-4 details symptoms of inattention and hyperactivity. In order for a diagnosis of Attention Deficit/Hyperactivity Disorder (ADHD) to be made, symptoms must be causing difficulties in two or more of the following settings: home, school, work, and/or social relationships (APA, 2000). Symptoms of inattention may continue through adolescence, whereas symptoms of hyperactivity and impulsivity tend to subside with age.

ADHD affects an estimated 3 to 7 out of every 100 school-aged children, occurring in boys four times more often than girls (Ross & Ross, 1982). Much of the research on the causality of ADHD has focused on the "dopamine hypothesis", which suggests that stimulants that increase the availability of this neurotransmitter appear to alleviate symptoms of inattention (USDHHS, 1999). Like many other psychopathologies, ADHD appears to run in families; approximately 50% of parents who had ADHD have children with the disorder. Disorders that commonly co-occur with ADHD are learning disabilities, major depressive disorder, anxiety, oppositional defiant disorder, SMD (sensory modulation dysfunction), or conduct disorder (please refer to Chapter 10: Diagnoses Commonly Associated With Childhood).

Oppositional Defiant Disorder

Marked by a consistent pattern of defiance, disobedience, and hostility towards various authority figures, children with Oppositional Defiant Disorder (ODD) display openly aggressive behavior as well as a tendency to bother and irritate others (APA, 2000). They also are quick to temper, act out, appear angry and resentful, and often blame others for their mistakes. ODD occurs more often in prepubertal boys, but after puberty the rates in both genders are equal (USDHHS, 1999). Parental marital discord, disrupted child-care, and inconsistent, unsupervised child rearing may contribute to the future development of ODD. These children may constantly fight and argue, actively defy rules laid down by adults, or deliberately annoy others. Sensory integration difficulties may also accompany this disorder. For example, the child may be oversensitive to loud noises causing him or her to lash out at others.

Conduct Disorder

Behaviors of conduct disorder (CD) fall outside the realm of what is considered socially acceptable, and may include: bullying, physical assault, destruction of property, theft, sexual coercion, and cruelty towards animals (APA, 2000). A diagnosis of CD is not dependent on a single display of such behavior, but rather a repetitive disregard of social rules and the rights of others. Depending on how CD is defined, it affects anywhere from 1% to 4% of the population (Shaffer, Fisher, Dulcan, et al., 1996). Children with early onset CD, i.e., diagnosed before age 10, have a greater risk for developing adult anti-social personality disorder (APA, 2000). Social risk factors include early maternal rejection, separation from parents with no adequate alternative caregiver available, early institutionalization, family neglect, abuse or violence, parents' psychiatric illness, parental marital discord, large family size, crowding, and poverty (Loeber & Stouthamer-Loeber, 1986).

ATTACHMENT DISORDERS

The connection forged between the infant and his/her primary caregiver (usually the mother) during the first year is crucial to normal development (Ainsworth, Blehar, Waters, & Wall, 1978; Bowlby, 1988). In a healthy, secure attachment relationship, the caregiver learns to fulfill the infant's physical, emotional, and psychological needs by interpreting his/her signals. For example, if an infant is crying from hunger, the caregiver will respond by feeding him/her. As the infant's needs are met on a consistent basis, he/she learns to trust the caregiver and views the external world as predictable, something he/she can control (Erikson, 1963; 1982). As this trust is established, the relationship between caregiver and infant evolves. The caregiver not only responds to her growing infant's needs, but now also sets limitations on her infant's behavior. For example, when the infant starts crying to be held, the caregiver may wait a few minutes and use affect or gestures to help regulate the infant before picking him or her up. This early attachment lays the foundation for future relationship development, moral conscience development, logical thinking, and the ability to cope with stress. Failure to form a secure attachment relationship with a primary caregiver may lead to attachment disorders, and may also play a role in the onset of oppositional defiant disorder and conduct disorder (please refer to Chapter 9: Working With Families).

Reactive attachment disorder (RAD), beginning before age 5 (APA, 2000), is defined by markedly disturbed and developmentally inappropriate social relatedness in most contexts. The DSM-IV TR (2000) recognizes two distinct manifestations of this disorder, the Inhibited Type and the Disinhibited Type. Inhibited RAD is distinguished from the Disinhibited Type by the presence of avoidant behaviors. The child is unable to initiate, form, and sustain lasting social attachments, and in fact, eschews affection. In Disinhibited RAD, the child forms indiscriminate and inap-

propriate attachments. For instance, the child may show excessive fondness to complete strangers. A diagnosis of this disorder is based on family history and specific observable behavior indicative of RAD. Clinical presentation of RAD includes compulsive lying, stealing, speech and language delays, lack of remorse, learning delays, poor impulse control, fascination with violence, indiscriminate displays of affection towards strangers, and hoarding or hiding food. Without treatment, RAD may lead to decreased self-esteem, the development of antisocial attitudes, and behavioral and academic problems in school.

RELATIONSHIP DISORDERS

Healthy infant growth and development occurs in the context of an emotionally sensitive, responsive, and involved infant-caregiver relationship. Prominent psychoanalyst D.W. Winnicott underscored the importance of this relationship when he noted that there is no such thing as an infant, only an infant and someone else (1965). When working with a pediatric population, OT practitioners need to be acutely aware of the relationship between child-caregiver interactions and adaptive and maladaptive emotional and behavioral patterns of response (Zero to Three, 1994) (please refer to Chapter 9: Working with Families). Axis II of the DC:0-3 (Zero to Three, 1994) is used to diagnose significant relationship difficulties. The criteria for determining whether a relationship disorder exists include behavioral quality of the interaction, affective tone, and psychological involvement. Table 22-5 lists four selected relationship disorders identified by DC:0-3 (Zero to Three, 1994) along with key features of each.

REGULATORY DISORDERS

According to Walker (2000), self-regulation "refers to the brain's ability to organize sensation in order to calm oneself, to delay gratification, and to tolerate change" (p. H-1). Infants with regulatory disorders may experience disturbances in sleeping and eating patterns, display high levels of irritability, inattention, inability to self-calm, difficulty with transitions, and sensory processing deficits (Zero to Three, 1994). As children grow older they may exhibit difficulties with gestural communication, affective expression, reciprocal play, and social interaction (DeGangi & Breinbauer, 1997). These children may display under (hypo) or over (hyper) reactivity to sensory input including auditory, tactile, visual, and vestibular stimulation (please refer to Chapter 12: Introduction to Sensory Integration). The DC:0-3 (Zero to Three, 1994) identifies four types of regulatory disorders: hypersensitive, under-reactive, motorically disorganized, and other. Regulatory disorders have been associated with future development of disruptive behavioral disorders including ADHD, sensory integration dysfunction (DSI), depression, aggressive behaviors, and learning disabilities (Walker, 2000).

Table 22-5

Relationship Disorders

	Overinvolved	Underinvolved	Anxious/Tense	Angry/Hostile
Behavioral Quality Parent	• Often interferes with infant's goals or desires. • Makes developmentally inappropriate demands.	• Insensitive or unresponsive to infant's cues. • Ignores, rejects, or fails to comfort infant. • Does not adequately protect infant from sources of physical or emotional harm. • Little eye contact or physical intimacy noted during infant-parent interactions.	• Extremely sensitive to infant's cues. • Expresses frequent concerns over the infant's well-being. • Physically awkward when holding infant (e.g., afraid of hurting the infant). • Poor fit between parent's and infant's activity level or temperament.	• Insensitive to the infant's cues. • Physical handling of the infant is abrupt. • May tease the infant.
Behavioral Quality Infant/Child	• May appear unfocused. • May display submissive or conversely defiant behaviors.	• May appear physically or psychologically uncared for (e.g., wears dirty clothing, lack of regular medical care). • May present with motor and language deficits due to lack of nurturing environment.	• May be very compliant or anxious around parent. • May excessively cling to parent. • Anxiety may interfere with developmental progress.	• May exhibit defiant behavior around parent. • May appear frightened. • May appear overly demanding.
Affective Tone Parent	• May have periods of anxiety, depression, or anger resulting in inconsistent infant-parent interactions.	• Constricted, withdrawn. • Flattened affect. • Lack of pleasure during interactions with infant.	• Anxiety evidenced through vocal quality, facial expressions. • Overreacts to child.	• Hostile. • Lack of enjoyment.
Affective Tone Infant/Child	• May passively or actively display anger and whine.	• Withdrawn, sad. • Lack of pleasure during interactions with parent.	• Anxious. • Overreacts to parent, leading to escalating interactions and dysregulation.	• Withdrawn. • Angry. • Affect may be constricted.

Adapted from DC:0-3.

SENSORY MODULATION DYSFUNCTION

In their research, Miller and colleagues (2001) described sensory modulation dysfunction (SMD) as a "problem in regulating and organizing the degree, intensity, and nature of responses to sensory input in a graded manner" (p. 57). Behavioral symptoms of SMD include sensation seeking or avoiding patterns, distractibility, disorganization, impulsivity, and hyperactivity (Miller et al, 2001). Current literature suggests that SMD is a syndrome that may occur with other disorders such as ADHD, anxiety disorders, PDD, or as a separate condition (Miller, Reisman, McIntosh, et al., 2001).

DEVELOPMENTAL COORDINATION DISORDER

Developmental Coordination Disorder (DCD) is a term introduced in 1994 by the American Psychiatric Association and the World Health Organization to diagnose children with significant impairment in the development of motor coordination. Also known as developmental dyspraxia, children with this condition display difficulties conceptualizing, planning, and/or executing motor sequences (Ayres, 1972). An estimated six percent of children aged 5 to 11 have some degree of DCD (APA, 2000). Children may exhibit delays in achieving motor milestone acquisition, appear clumsy, and have poor handwriting. DCD may co-occur with other disorders including ADHD, learning disability, DSI, and PDD. Frustration over the inability to perform basic tasks such as buttoning a shirt or catching a ball may result in low self-esteem and avoidance of activities requiring motor demands such as recess or gym.

LEARNING DISABILITY

As reported by the US Department of Education (2001), half of all children receiving special education services under the Individual with Disabilities Education Act (IDEA) have a learning disability. Under the IDEA, a learning disability is defined as:

A disorder in one or more of the basic psychological processes involved in understanding or in using language, spoken or written, that may manifest itself in an imperfect ability to listen, think, speak, read, write, or do mathematical calculations, including conditions such as perceptual disabilities, brain injury, minimal brain dysfunction, dyslexia, and developmental aphasia (34 Code of Federal Regulations §300.7(c)(10)

Gone untreated, learning disability may affect a child's school performance as well as his/her functioning at home and among peers. Early signs of learning disability in preschoolers include poor coordination and spatial skills, over or under-reactivity to sensory stimuli, decreased fine motor skills, and difficulty remembering what they see, especially sequences and patterns. A child may feel frustrated that she/he is unable to master skills that come easily to other classmates, possibly leading to feelings of self-worthlessness and anger (please refer to Chapter 10: Diagnoses Commonly Associated With Childhood).

EATING DISORDERS

Eating disorders constitute a very real and serious medical condition characterized by severe disturbances in eating patterns. The three main types of eating disorders are anorexia nervosa, bulimia nervosa, and binge eating. Individuals with anorexia nervosa are unwilling or unable to maintain a normal body weight; are intensely afraid of gaining weight; and have a significantly distorted perception of the size and shape of their body (APA, 2000). Bulimia nervosa is a condition involving binge eating followed by recurrent use of inappropriate compensatory behaviors to prevent weight gain such as self-induced vomiting, or misuse of laxatives, enemas, diuretics, and other medications (APA, 2000). Binge eating is a newly recognized condition in which the individual engages in episodic, uncontrolled food consumption, but does not engage in compensatory behaviors (Devlin, 1996). Disproportionately affecting females, eating disorders typically arise during adolescence. Eating disorders often co-occur with major depressive disorder, anxiety disorders, and substance abuse (APA, 2000).

Without treatment, these disorders may lead to serious medial complications, and even death.

The DSM-IV TR (APA, 2000) and the DC:0-3 (Zero to Three, 1994) also identify three eating and feeding disorders displayed during infancy and early childhood. Feeding disorder of infancy and early childhood is diagnosed when the child fails to eat properly resulting in either weight loss or failure to gain weight (APA, 2000). Children with pica persistently eat inedible, nonnutritive substances such as dirt, sand, paint, and clay. Rumination disorder includes the repeated and voluntary regurgitation, re-chewing, and re-swallowing of food. Possible causes of eating and feeding disorders include poor caregiving, neglect, lack of stimulation, or sensory processing difficulties. For example, infants with disorders of sensory integration may have decreased tongue awareness interfering with the mechanics of sucking (Genna, 2001). They may also present with oral tactile defensiveness and consequently may find certain textures aversive.

Models Associated With Psychosocial Treatment

DIRECT SERVICES

Direct services involve hands-on interaction with the child and family either one-on-one or in a group. Direct services are considered when the OT practitioner is the only one with the knowledge and skill necessary to safely provide intervention; and when ongoing evaluation and assessment is needed to carry out a treatment plan. Direct psychosocial therapy includes the application of skill-based techniques such as sensory integration, the Developmental Individual-difference Relationship-based or DIR/Floor time approach, task analysis, and teaching the child coping and anger management skills. These techniques require constant analysis of the child's responses and adaptation of selected techniques used (Dunn & DeGangi, 1992) in order to ensure effectiveness.

INDIRECT SERVICES

Indirect services may involve teaching, consulting with and/or directly supervising adults in the child's life such as teachers, paraprofessionals or family members carry out therapeutically appropriate activities. For example, an OT practitioner may train teachers and classroom aids on how to implement a sensory diet to help the child remain regulated throughout the day. The OT practitioner may also act as a consultant, sharing and discussing possible solutions and environmental adaptations to assist family, teachers, and other professionals working with the child. Best practice under this model includes the ongoing training, monitoring,

Table 22-6
Systems of Care

	Chronic and Severe Disturbance	Early Intervention	Prevention
Community Resources	Emergency/Crisis Treatment In-patient hospitalization Long-term therapy Probation/Incarceration Residential Care	Family support Early home visitation programs Screening programs Parent training	Prenatal care Immunizations Recreation and enrichment Child abuse education Public safety and awareness
School Resources	Special education services Comprehensive school based mental health programs Alternative schools	Early Intervention services Head Start programs Early screening programs	General health education Substance abuse education Support for transitions Conflict resolution

supervision, evaluation, and upgrading of programs and strategies in place in order to ensure that the child's functional needs are being met.

CASE MANAGEMENT

According to the AOTA (1991), OT practitioners are uniquely qualified to act as case managers, using skills in functional assessment, task analysis, intervention planning, and implementation. They also possess a working knowledge of related professional and community supports to coordinate appropriate services for the child and family. Given the impact of psychosocial dysfunction on occupational performance, OT practitioners are especially effective when serving as case managers for the mental health population. Responsibilities include psychosocial assessment, referral to and coordination of community resources including support groups, and development of a comprehensive service plan in collaboration with the child and family.

Settings

SYSTEM OF CARE

Systems of care refer to a spectrum of community based mental health services that are organized into a coordinated network to meet the multiple and changing psychosocial needs of children and adolescents (Stroul & Friedman, 1986). Systems of care are guided by the following core values and principles:
1. Services are driven by the needs and preferences of the child and family.

2. Family involvement and partnership with service providers is integrated into all aspects of service planning and delivery.

3. Services are provided in an individualized, coordinated manner and emphasize treatment in the least restrictive, most appropriate setting.

4. All services offered are sensitive and responsive to the child and family's unique cultural needs and community-specific characteristics.

5. Ongoing evaluation and accountability is expected throughout the process.

Systems of care are designed to increase interagency collaboration, reduce the use of costly inpatient and residential treatment facilities, increase family satisfaction with services, and improve child outcomes in areas of school attendance and law enforcement contacts. A fully implemented system of care includes treatment for chronic and severe psychosocial disturbance, as well as services aimed at early intervention and prevention (Table 22-6). The following discussion focuses on early intervention and school services as these areas offer unique opportunities for prevention and treatment of children with psychosocial disorders. Federal and State legislation mandates the provision of occupational therapy services to children with disabilities through early intervention programs and the school in accordance with the Individuals with Disabilities Education Act (IDEA) (1997) and the Rehabilitation Act (1973) (please refer to Chapter 20: Preschool and School-Based Therapy). Payment for services may also be out of pocket or through insurance. The Early and Periodic Screening, Diagnosis and Treatment (EPDST) program established by Medicaid authorizes that all medically necessary services including mental health care needs be provided to eligible children under the age of 21. Medicaid is a jointly funded, federal-state health insurance program for certain low-income and needy people.

EARLY INTERVENTION AND HEAD START PROGRAMS

Under part C of the IDEA, infants and toddlers ages zero to 2 with established physical or mental diagnoses or demonstrated developmental delays are eligible for family-centered early intervention (EI) services delivered in the child's natural setting (e.g., home, daycare, playground, etc.). Additionally, some states may offer services to children at risk for developmental delays in the absence of intervention. Risk factors may be either biological, such as low birth weight or pre-natal exposure to alcohol; or environmental, such as living in poverty, neglect, exposure to traumatic events, and having a parent with a mental illness.

Children who have a parent with a mental illness, especially depression, are at risk for development of emotional or behavioral difficulties. Parents with depression may be emotionally withdrawn and nonresponsive, lacking in physical and mental energy, thus contributing to poor child supervision. Infants of depressed parents may also receive lower amounts of stimulation (e.g., flattened affect, lack of eye contact and engagement) leading to possible learning and behavioral problems (Radke-Yarrow, Nottleman, Martinez, Fox, & Belmont, 1992).

The first 3 years of life represent a time of unprecedented brain growth and development. Early experiences are critical for forming new neural connections, strengthening existing ones, and organizing synaptic pathways for learning, emotion, and behavior (Schor, 1999). Neuroplasticity is much greater during the first couple of years of life, suggesting that intervention during this critical period may be more effective and possibly brain changing (Blair, 2001). EI and Zero to Three programs are thus intended to capitalize on this "window of opportunity" in order to prevent and augment developmental delays and psychosocial disorders (please refer to Chapter 19: Early Intervention).

Head Start programs operate under federally funded grants and also target high-risk infants and children ages zero to 5. Head Start programs mainly serve those from low-income households. Studies have consistently linked poverty to higher levels of psychological distress and poorer mental health (Adler, Boyce, Chesney, et al., 1994; Eaton & Muntaner, 1999). Head Start services are aimed at fostering healthy physical, cognitive, and social development; and enabling parents to become better caregivers and active participants in their child's education and learning.

Occupational therapy practitioners working in EI and Head Start settings may play a key role in the prevention of psychosocial disorders. More specifically, the OT practitioner is uniquely qualified to recognize regulatory disorders, facilitate positive child-caregiver interactive patterns, and train caregivers in the use of sensory rich activities to encourage the infant's exploration of the environment. The OT practitioner may provide appropriate stress and anger management techniques to caregivers with mental illness to help reduce direct and indirect harmful effects on the child.

SCHOOL

Part B of the IDEA allots funding for occupational therapy services to children with disabilities. Under the IDEA, disability encompasses serious emotional disturbance, autism, and specific learning disabilities in addition to physical impairments. Amended and passed into law in 1997, the IDEA-R extended the definition of disability to include children aged 3 to 9 experiencing developmental delays defined by each state in one or more of the following areas: physical, cognitive, communication, social/emotional, or adaptive development, and therefore require special education and related services including occupational therapy (IDEA-R, 1997). Children who do not qualify for special education services, but have a physical or mental impairment that is hindering performance in a regular classroom, may be eligible to receive occupational therapy under Section 504 of the Rehabilitation Act. School districts may also be reimbursed through Medicaid (please refer to Chapter 20: Preschool and School-Based Therapy).

Under the IDEA-R, there is increased emphasis on educating the child with disabilities among age related peers in a regular classroom setting. Accordingly, the child's individual education plan (IEP) team includes both special and regular education teachers. Another change is the added focus on behavioral problems that may be impeding the child's ability to learn. The OT practitioner may add to the effectiveness of the IEP evaluation process by assessing the impact of problem behaviors on academic performance and social relationships. This may be done through observation, interview, and formal assessment. Functional Behavioral Assessment (FBA) is a process of gathering information in the context in which problem behaviors occur. By identifying biological, social, affective, and environment factors that contribute to problem behaviors, the OT can develop a plan that: 1) eliminates opportunities for problem behaviors; and 2) teaches and supports replacement behaviors. Given the profession's focus on function-based and psychosocial-based approaches, conducting FBAs seems like a natural extension of the OT's responsibilities. The OTA who demonstrates service competency may assist in administering FBAs under the supervision of an OT. Even if the child does not present with problem behaviors or a mental health disorder, the OT practitioner should always take into account psychosocial functioning and its impact on the child's self-esteem, academic performance, and peer-peer interactions.

In addition to those services provided under the IDEA-R, there has been a push to move school programs towards a

Table 22-7
Screening Tools

Title	Purpose and Age Range	Administration Time
Ages and Stages Questionnaire (ASQ)	Parent completed questionnaire designed to screen for developmental delays for children ages 4 months to 60 months	10-15 minutes for parent to complete 2-3 minutes for tester to score
Beck Depression Inventory	Self-reporting inventory measuring characteristic symptoms and attitudes of depression; appropriate for adolescents and adults with a fifth to sixth grade reading comprehension	10 minutes for client to complete
Children's Depression Scale (CDS) Family Psychosocial Screening	Assesses parent risk factors for child behavioral problems including history of child abuse, parental substance abuse, and maternal depression	10 minutes for parent to complete
Infant/Toddler Checklist for Language and Communication	Parent completed checklist designed to screen for children at risk for developmental delays ages 6 months to 24 months	10 minutes for parent to complete
Parents Evaluation of Developmental Status (PEDS)	Parent completed questionnaire that screens for developmental and behavioral problems for children ages birth to eight years	1-2 minutes to administer and score
Temperament and Behavioral Scales (TABS)	Screens for self-regulation and temperament problems in children ages 11 to 71 months	5 minutes for parent to complete

system of care. As schools offer a logical setting for both the early identification and treatment of children with psychosocial disorders, they can play a crucial role in systems of care. For instance, through partnerships between school districts and community mental health agencies, expanded school mental health (ESMH) programs provide comprehensive mental health services, including prevention, assessment, case management, and intervention services to identified children in both general and special education (Weist, 1997). ESMH programs may include screening youth early for mental health problems; individual, group and family counseling; referral of youth for more intensive services; addressing "school-wide" issues such as violence; and providing educational materials and consultative services to teachers and parents. Preliminary data indicate that ESMH programs remove barriers to student learning; improve attendance, grades, and behavior; and help reduce school costs (Weist, 2001). Presently, ESMH programs exist in less than 10% of all school nation-wide (Brenner, Martindayle, & Weist, 2001). Regardless of whether or not an ESMH program is in place, school-based OT practitioners can still incorporate principles of this framework to ensure that the mental health needs of all students are being met.

Occupational Therapy Process

The OT is responsible for all aspects of service delivery regardless of setting. The OTA may deliver services only under the supervision of an OT and in accordance with state and facility guidelines. Please refer to AOTA's *Roles and Responsibilities of the Occupational Therapist and the Occupational Therapy Assistant During the Delivery of Occupational Therapy Services* (2002).

SCREENING

The screening process may be used to assess the presence of risk factors or symptoms that may indicate a medical or mental health condition, or to determine the need for further evaluation and intervention. Screening may include a chart review, medical and developmental history, parent or teacher interview, observation, and the use of quick assessment tools. Mental health screening tools are usually short questionnaires or checklists of behavioral and emotional symptoms that may indicate the presence of either psychosocial or occupational disturbance. Both OTs and OTAs may administer screenings, but it is the OT's responsibility to interpret the findings. Tables 22-7 and 22-8 list some of

Table 22-8

Other Assessments

Title	*Purpose and Population*
Adolescent Coping Scale	Assesses a broad range of coping strategies in children between the ages of 12-18.
Child Development Inventory (CDI)	Parent questionnaire that measures child development including strengths and delays; ages 15 months to 6 years.
Infant-Toddler Sensory Profile	Caregiver completed questionnaire used to assess sensory processing difficulties in children ages birth to 36 months.
Miller Assessment of Preschoolers (MAP)	Evaluates young children for mild to moderate developmental delays.
Occupational Therapy Psychosocial Assessment of Learning	Observational assessment tool that evaluates the elementary student's volition, habituation, and environmental fit within the classroom setting.
Pediatric Evaluation of Disability Inventory (PEDI)	Assesses key functional capabilities in areas of self-care, mobility, and social function in children between the ages of 6 months to 7 years.
Pediatric Volitional Questionnaire (PVQ)	Play-based observational assessment designed to assess the child's volition.
Piers-Harris Children's Self-Concept Scale	Self-report instrument that assesses how children and adolescents feel about themselves in areas of physical appearance, popularity, happiness, anxiety, and intellectual status.
Sensory Profile	Caregiver completed questionnaire used to assess sensory processing difficulties in children ages 3-10.
Vineland Adaptive Behavior Scales	Parent or caregiver interview based survey; evaluates the child's personal and social skills between the ages of birth and 18 years.

the common mental health screening tools used with the pediatric population. Mental health screens do not have any diagnostic value and should not take the place of a comprehensive psychiatric evaluation.

EVALUATION

A comprehensive evaluation identifies the child's specific wants and needs, and determine those factors that are preventing or limiting a child from fully engaging in desired and expected occupational areas (AOTA, 2002). The evaluation process is a collaborative effort between the OT and the child and family. The *Occupational Therapy Practice Framework* divides the evaluation process into two steps (AOTA, 2002). The initial step of the process is the compilation of an occupational profile that describes the child's occupational history, patterns of daily living, interests, values, and priorities (AOTA, 2002). The second step is the analysis of occupational performance (AOTA, 2002). Using various methods of assessment, the OT examines performance skills and patterns, context, client factors, and activity demands that may be influencing occupational functioning. Once service competency has been established, and based on state and facility guidelines, the supervising OT may delegate several evaluative tasks to the OTA including chart

review, interview, structured observation, and administration of standardized assessments (AOTA, 1998).

Information can be gathered through first-person interview if the child is old enough and deemed an accurate self-reporter. More than likely, information will come from third-party interviews with caregivers, teachers and other professionals working with the child, and/or a medical chart review. In general, the OTA should inquire about family context (e.g., how many siblings, who the primary caregiver is, etc.), medical history and diagnosis if applicable, and the child's strengths, and areas of concern. Knowledge of any medications the child may be taking is also crucial as many prescribed drugs may have residual effects on behavior. Table 22-9 provides an example of an initial parent interview.

When examining performance in various areas of occupation, the OTA needs to look at both performance skills and patterns. The existence of maladaptive patterns in one occupational area may interfere with functioning in another area. For example, many of the disorders discussed in this chapter have symptoms such as disrupted feeding and sleeping patterns. Lack of proper nutrition and sleep may lead to increased irritability and trouble concentrating which may subsequently have an adverse effect on school performance.

Table 22-9

Sample Questionnaire

Initial Parent Interview

Medical History
Is your child on any medications? Any special diet?
Has your child ever had an EEG?
Does your child have any allergies?
Is there a family history of depression, autism, or any other psychosocial disorders?
What other medical services and/or therapies does your child receive?

Pregnancy and Development
Did you carry your child to full-term?
Age when your child reached the following milestones: crawling, walking, first words, etc.
Does your child have any aversions to particular foods, textures, noises, etc.?
Does your child seek certain input, like deep pressure, movement, etc.?

Family Background
Parent's names
Siblings/ages and names

Behavior/Temperament
Describe your child's general disposition: for example, anxious, laid back, withdrawn, happy, sad.
How does your child deal with transitions and novelty?
How long does it take your child to recover from a tantrum?
What types of things appear to help your child self-calm when he or she is overly upset?

School Performance
What school does your child attend?
What grade is he or she in?
Does your child receive any special education services?
Does your child ever complain of not being able to concentrate in school?
Does your child have any difficulties with handwriting? Any other subjects?
Does your child complete work hastily, overlooking obvious errors?
Does your child seem to like school?
Describe your child's learning style: for example, "fast learner," visual versus auditory.

Activities of Daily Living
Describe a typical day for your child.
Does your child have any trouble sleeping?
Is your child responsible for any chores?
Does it take your child longer than usual to complete self-care routines?
Does your child complete self-care tasks and chores thoroughly? (e.g., Does the child remember to tuck the front and back of his or her shirt in? Are the clothes properly oriented?
Does your child need to be reminded a lot to do his or her chores?

Social-Emotional
Describe your child's play at home. Does your child prefer to play by him or herself? Does he or she get "stuck" on certain toys or themes?
Does your child prefer physical play over pretend play?
Does your child have any favorite toys or game?
Describe your child's play with other peers:
• sharing
• turn taking
• following rules
• leader versus follower
Does your child display any aggressive behaviors towards parents, siblings, or other peers (e.g., hitting, throwing toys, biting, screaming loudly)?

Sleep deprivation may also trigger a manic episode in children with bipolar disorder. Questions to consider are:

1. Does the child sleep through the night?
2. Does the child appear well rested following a night's sleep?
3. Does the child have difficulty concentrating?
4. Is the child making appropriate weight gains?
5. Has the child had a decrease in appetite?

When working with this population, the OTA may find it advisable to incorporate naturalistic observation in order to accurately gauge the child's abilities. For example, a child with an anxiety disorder may perform well in a clinic setting where everything is structured, sensory input is controlled, activities are graded to his or her skill level, and he or she knows what to expect at all times. However when the same child is placed in a school environment or a social setting where things are unpredictable, he or she may be flooded with feelings or emotional distress, thus limiting his or her participation in these contexts. Observing the child's performance within their natural environments rather than relying on second-hand report may help the OT practitioner come up with more appropriate suggestions and modifications to facilitate maximal independence.

As stated earlier, it is not uncommon for children with psychosocial disorders to have accompanying or underlying sensory integration challenges. There are a variety of checklists and questionnaires available to provide the OT practitioner with an accurate sensory profile of the child (see Table 22-8). Information from sensory checklists can be used to guide sensory diet activities.

When working with infants and young children, the OT should consider assessing the child-caregiver relationship. The Functional Emotional Assessment Scale (FEAS) (Greenspan, DeGangi, & Wieder, 2001) assesses the child's functional emotional and social capacities in the context of the relationship with the caregiver (White, 2002). The FEAS was designed for children who are experiencing regulatory disorders, attachment disorders, PDD, or socio-environmental challenges including poverty, or who have a caregiver with a mental illness. The FEAS assesses the child and caregiver in six different areas during symbolic, tactile, and movement-based play. The six areas correspond to the child's functional emotional developmental capacities expounded upon by the Developmental, Individual Differences, Relationship Based or DIR model (see intervention approaches for more information on the DIR model). The child and caregiver are scored on each individual item as follows: zero (0) if the behavior was not present or only observed briefly, one (1) if the behavior was present some of the time, or two (2) if the behavior is robust and consistently present. The total score for each item will determine if the child and caregiver are functioning in the normal, at risk, or deficient range. Table 22-8 outlines other selected assessments that may be helpful with this particular population.

GOAL SETTING AND DOCUMENTATION

Evaluation findings and the expressed needs and desires of the child and family determine therapy goals. The OT is responsible for developing an intervention plan including long-term goals and objectives, frequency and duration of services, and the child's needs. The *Standards of Practice for Occupational Therapy* (AOTA, 1998) state that goals should be:

- Clear—Written in easy to understand language so as to avoid confusion.
- Measurable—Includes what the child should be able to do as a result of therapy, the conditions under which the goal will be met, and the criteria used to determine if the child has successfully reached the goal (Mager, 1975).
- Behavioral—Outcome is a specified action stated in terms of explicit and observable action verbs.
- Functional—Clearly related to the child's ability to function and participate in his or her respected environments.
- Contextually relevant—Should include the dynamic and unique contexts of each individual child (Dunn, 1998).
- Appropriate to the child's needs, desires, and expected outcomes.

Refer to Table 22-10 for specific examples of goals used with this population.

Intervention Strategies

ENVIRONMENTAL ADAPTATIONS AND TASK ANALYSIS

The primary goal of occupational therapy across all populations is to facilitate active participation in every facet of life (AOTA, 2002). Often times this entails modifying the child's environment, activity demands, or performance patterns in accordance with the child's individual needs. For the child with ADHD, this may include seating the child up front near the blackboard or accommodating him or her with a study area with reduced stimuli and student traffic. Similarly, an organized study area at home with minimum distractions should also be provided.

Children with psychosocial disorders often demonstrate deficits in motor planning and executive functioning affecting their ability to plan, organize, and manage time and

---

Table 22-10

Sample Goals

Sensory Processing
A. Will verbally request sensory breaks as needed during the school day in order to maintain optimal attention and arousal for learning.
B. Will use a variety of adaptive strategies (e.g., proprioceptive input, sensory breaks, fidget toys, visual schedule) to maintain regulation and internally control anxiety given minimal adult support.
C. Will transition between math class and lunch room without becoming overwhelmed or dysregulated given environmental supports including visual schedule, consistent structure, and use of social story with minimal adult support.

Organization and Motor Planning
A. Will complete morning ADL routine including gathering items and clean-up using visual supports (e.g., checklist) for thoroughness.
B. Will set-up materials required for a 4 step art project, complete project, and clean-up workspace using adaptive strategies for sequencing and staying focused.

Behavioral-Social
A. Will verbally request assistance from another peer (e.g., asking peer to pass an item) using increased volume and establishing eye contact during art class 2/3 opportunities given minimal adult facilitation.
B. Will play a board game with another peer for a 10 minute period demonstrating the ability to follow directions, take turns, and sustain mutual engagement given minimal adult support and use of behavioral strategies to enforce positive behaviors.
C. Will verbally name three coping skill strategies and demonstrate at least one of them during group session.

---

space (Blondis, Snow, Roizen, Opacich, & Accardo, 1993). Working memory is an aspect of executive functioning that refers to the ability to hold information in one's mind while processing and manipulating it. Children with impaired working memory may have difficulty performing simple tasks such as brushing their teeth because they are unable to process and organize the steps of the task. The OTA can modify the activity demands by having the necessary materials set up, thereby eliminating extra steps. Another strategy is the use of external aids such as visual schedules, step-by-step written instructions, and checklists. To further increase the child's independence, he or she can plan out and write the steps involved in the task and then cross off each step as it is completed. As many children with impaired working memory also possess poor auditory processing, visual supports or gestural cues may be preferable to verbal cueing. Visual supports may also be used to decrease anxiety and ease transitions as when a child is given a visual representation of what is expected.

SENSORY INTEGRATION

Psychosocial deficits are manifested behaviorally. It is suggested that observable behaviors such as difficulty paying attention and aggressive outbursts may be due to decreased arousal or poor sensory modulation (Parham & Mailloux, 1996; Miller et al., 2001). Sensory integration (SI) treatment involves the remediation of underlying sensory processing difficulties by imposing controlled, sensory input on the child in order to elicit an adaptive response (Ayres,

1972). This model also incorporates the use of environmental adaptations to support the child's sensory needs. Please refer to Chapter 12 for an overview of sensory integration theory.

Williamson and Anzalone identify the four A's associated with sensory processing: arousal, attention, affect, and action (2001). Regulation in each of these processes contributes to behavioral organization. Arousal describes a state of alertness, wakefulness, or readiness controlled by nervous system activity. An optimal level of arousal is needed for meaningful interactions with our surrounding environment and learning to occur (Hanrahan, 2000). An OT may develop a sensory diet to calm a hyper-aroused system or stimulate a hypo-aroused system that is administered in a prescribed manner. For a hypo-aroused child with high sensory threshold, this may include bouncing him or her on a therapy ball, jumping on a trampoline, or providing a crunchy snack. The application of proprioceptive or deep pressure input may help calm and organize the hyper-aroused child with low threshold response. The OTA, depending on demonstrated competency, and state and facility guidelines, may be asked to tailor a sensory diet for both school and home use. Another effective tool used to support arousal is the Alert Program (Williams & Shellenberger, 1996). This program helps children learn to recognize, monitor, and change their level of alertness appropriate to the social situation.

Attention is the ability to focus selectively on a desired stimulus or task (Schaff & Anzalone, 2001). Attention involves a strong visual component, one needs to be able to visually fixate and shift focus between targets. Behaviorally, in Western cultures, we typically determine if someone is paying attention by his or her ability to maintain eye contact. A child who has difficulty shifting focus or who presents with poor occulo-motor control may appear distractible as his or her gaze will often shift and wander elsewhere. The OTA may remediate visual processing deficits through the use of visual-perceptual exercises such as the Flow or the Infinity Walk. The Flow (Professional Development Programs & PDP Products, Stillwater, MN) consists of a clear bag with handles on either end that can be filled with water. The child swings the bag back and forth across his/her body or in a figure eight motion while simultaneously rotating his/her head from right to left (over the shoulder). The OT practitioner stands behind the child and holds up a piece of paper with pictures or random letters and numbers. The child identifies the object that the OT practitioner is pointing to while looking over his/her shoulder. A variety of motor exercises can be performed to increase bilateral coordination, timing, and separation of the head from the body, an essential skill for the visual tracking and fixation of an object. The Infinity Walk is an exercise where the child walks in a figure eight pattern while simultaneously looking off at a 90 degree angle and performing a variety of graded challenges (Sunbeck, 1996). This may include following the path while reading the names of pictures off a card. This activity encourages the child to maintain visual fixation while the body is still moving. Referral to a developmental optometrist may also be recommended if the visual-perceptual deficit is impacting daily functioning.

Affect refers to the emotional component of behavior (Schaff & Anzalone, 2001). Affect provides meaning to actions, symbols, and social interactions. Children with sensory processing challenges may have difficulty engaging in higher level thinking and processing emotional information (Greenspan & Wieder, 1998). The child with tactile defensiveness may interpret someone lightly brushing up against them as noxious and threatening, eliciting an emotional response that is not appropriate to the situation. The Wilbarger Touch-Pressure Protocol may be used to help desensitize the tactilely defensive child. Beanbag tapping is another sensory strategy used to treat sensory defensiveness by systematically providing deep pressure input to various parts of the body. The Wilbarger Protocol and beanbag tapping may help increase the child's sense of self-control and body awareness, making the surrounding environment less fearful.

The term action encompasses motoric abilities and praxis, which is also referred to as *motor planning* (Schaff & Anzalone, 2001). Motor planning involves having an idea about what to do, planning an action, and executing the action (Ayres, 1985). We use knowledge of past experiences and sensory information to plan a new action. Motor planning is integral to the learning process. Children with motor planning deficits may perform tasks slowly or avoid them completely. They often require longer exposure to a new activity in order to learn it. By presenting the child with novel motor challenges graded to meet his or her skill level, and improving overall sensory processing, the OTA may help increase the child's motor planning abilities. Providing the child with a visual model or demonstration that he or she can imitate may also be helpful when working on motor planning skills.

DIR/FLOOR TIME

The Developmental, Individual Difference, Relationship (DIR) model developed by Greenspan (Greenspan & Wieder, 1998) is an intervention approach that emphasizes the child's functional-emotional developmental level; individual differences in sensory processing, modulation, muscle tone, and motor planning and sequencing; and relationships and interactions with others. The six functional-emotional developmental levels are: 1) regulation and interest in the world, 2) engagement, 3) intentional two-way communication, 4) complex problem-solving interactions, 5) elaborating ideas, and 6) building bridges between ideas. These emotional capacities lay the foundation for future learning and are the basis for further emotional, cognitive, motor, language, and social development (Greenspan & Wieder, 1998). The DIR model advocates a floor time approach whereby the child is presented with opportunities to master these emotional milestones through playful and dynamic interaction (Greenspan & Wieder, 1998). The therapist or parent working with the child actively follows his or her lead, challenging him or her to engage in two-person interactions (Greenspan, & Wieder, 1998).

The floor time approach may be used in conjunction with other intervention strategies such as sensory integration or behavior management. Table 22-11 provides a case study illustrating how floor time principles can be incorporated into OT sessions.

Notice how the OTA meets Jamie at his level, incorporating his interests and unique sensory profile to beckon him into a state of shared attention and engagement, moving up to two-way purposeful interactions. The OTA squeezes the play dough against Jamie's nose, providing him with an enjoyable form of sensory input and also keeping him engaged. The OTA also limits her use of verbal cues and language due to his poor auditory processing skills and instead uses gestures and affect to communicate. Rather than directing Jamie to get the play dough on top of the slide, the OTA allows him to initiate climbing the slide. When she loses him briefly in the transition to the slide, she regains his attention by rolling the play dough down the slide. The OTA has turned Jamie's initial perseverative and isolative play into an extended two-person interaction.

The floor time approach is not limited to children with autistic spectrum or communication disorders, but can be

Table 22-11

Case Study: Jamie—Illustration of the Use of DIR/Floor Time Approach

Jamie is a 5-year-old boy with autism. He presents with severe motor planning deficits, tactile defensiveness, impaired auditory processing, low tone, and under-reactivity to movement and deep pressure input. His mother describes him as being predictable and liking structure to the point of being inflexible and rigid. Jamie comes into the therapy room and notices a box of play dough. He begins taking off the lids of the containers, removing the play dough to examine it, and then replacing it. All the while he is completely oblivious to the OTA's presence. Building on his interest, the OTA takes play dough from one of the containers and places it on her head, thus encouraging Jamie to notice her and engage in the purposeful action of reaching for the play dough and putting it back in the container. The OTA extends the interaction further and takes the play dough and this time presses it against his nose. Jamie looks at the OTA and smiles. The OTA then takes the play dough containers and places them on top of a slide. She shrugs her shoulders in an exaggerated manner and asks Jamie what they should do. Jamie climbs the ladder to the slide and resumes removing the lids. The OTA removes the play dough and rolls it down the slide and exclaims "Crash" when the play dough hits the bottom. Again Jamie looks at his OTA and smiles. This time he takes the play dough and rolls it down the slide. They continue to take turns rolling the balls of play dough down the slide until they are all gone. The OTA asks Jamie, "Now what?" accompanying the language with a gestural cue. Jamie slides down the slide and begins to gather the balls of play dough. He attempts to roll them up the slide. He begins to laugh when the play dough rolls back down. The OTA exclaims, "Wow, that looks like fun," and joins Jamie in his new game as they take turns.

Table 22-12

Social Story Components

Type of Sentence	Definition	Example
Descriptive	Truthful, fact-based statements.	My name is Bobby. I attend the after school club on Tuesdays and Thursdays. At the club, the children get to play in the gym, then its circle time. During circle time Ms. J. reads a story.
Perspective	Statements that refer to or describe a person's internal state (i.e., thoughts, feelings, beliefs, opinions, motivation, etc).	Some of the other kids seem excited when they get to hear a story. Ms. J. likes it when we sit quietly and listen to the story.
Directive	Identify a suggested response to a situation.	I will try to sit quietly during circle time.
Affirmative	Express a commonly shared value or opinion within a given culture. Most effective when immediately following a descriptive, perspective, or directive sentence.	It is important to pay attention when Ms. J. is talking.

used to treat and facilitate social emotional development across all populations. Children with psychosocial difficulties often have difficulty reading social cues, leading to states of heightened anxiety or inappropriate responses. Creating high affect interactions improves the child's ability to process emotional information, improve social-emotional skills, and learning. Symbolic play may also be incorporated to further expand the child's interaction and communication as well as increase initiative, flexibility, problem solving, abstract thinking, and motor planning.

SOCIAL STORIES

A social story is a short story describing a situation, concept, or social skill that is relevant to that specific individual (Gray, 2002). Although originally developed for individuals with autistic spectrum disorders, social stories are compatible with any disorder that results in an impaired ability to interpret social situations (Schoonover, 2002). A social story is usually told in first person narrative in the present tense. It provides as much information as possible about a certain situation in order to better prepare the child to face and act appropriately during that situation. Social stories involve specific components. There are four types of sentences used in social stories: descriptive, directive, perspective, and affirmative (Table 22-12). For every one directive sentence, there should be two to five descriptive, perspective, and/or affirmative sentences. Other guidelines for social stories include: 1) use of positive language and positively stated behaviors; 2) avoid using absolute language, replace "I will" with "I will try," replace "always" with "usually," etc. in case things do not go as planned; and 3) customize the story according to the needs, learning style, and motivation of the child (Gray, 2002). Social stories can be adapted to include illustrations, symbols, or story boxes. The social story should be implemented in a calm, relaxing environment with minimum distractions and read in a reassuring, comforting voice. Social stories may be reviewed once a day or prior to the targeted situation. Social stories can be faded by allowing a longer time to pass between review sessions, or by rewriting the story to exclude directive sentences or changing them into partial sentences (e.g., "My little brother will probably feel _____, if I share my toys with him") to encourage the child to recall the information (Gray, 2002).

GROUP SESSIONS

Group participation allows the OTA to observe deficits that may not be seen during individual sessions. Groups also provide the child with the opportunity to experience positive peer-peer interactions. There are several types of groups. Sensory motor groups incorporate sensory rich activities and gross motor challenges to support increased sensory processing and modulation, body awareness, motor planning, age-appropriate interactive play, and social negotiation. The use of physical movement and activity helps relieve tension and can serve as a medium for emotional expression. The experience of being in a peer group may motivate the child to partake in activities that he or she usually avoids. Additionally, giving the child the opportunity to master physical challenges may lead to improved self-esteem and confidence.

Task oriented groups are designed to help members strengthen ego skills and minimize defense mechanisms. Targeted outcomes include improvements in reality testing and thought processes, increased sense of self (body image, self-esteem, and self-concept), increased sense of self-control, and acquisition of healthy coping strategies (Cole, 1999). The task provides the backdrop for discussion and problem-solving to occur. Examples include cooking groups, arts and crafts groups, and group field trips. Tasks can be graded to meet the skill level of the children in the group. For instance, the OT practitioner leading the group may need to provide more structure and assistance to lower functioning groups.

Psychoeducational groups may be appropriate for higher functioning adolescents experiencing psychosocial disturbance. The psychoeducational approach involves a strong didactic component. Information or skills are taught through short lecture, written material, demonstration, and hands on experience. Topics include assertiveness training, social and leisure skill development, and stress management. The OTA takes a more directive role in this type of group, employing cognitive behavioral principles (see section on cognitive behavioral approaches).

MUSIC AND LISTENING THERAPY

Music has long been associated with numerous beneficial physiological and psychological changes including faster healing time, improved immune response, increased endurance, decreased blood pressure and pulse rate, reduced anxiety, and improved emotional state (Boughton, 2001). Further, sustained positive emotion following a fulfilling exposure to music has been correlated with increases in cognitive flexibility, problem solving, and decision making (Staw, Sutton, & Pelled, 1994). Because of its ability to affect emotional changes, music may be a powerful tool when working with children experiencing psychosocial disturbances. Slower paced music with a consistent and predictable rhythm typically has a calming effect, while upbeat and quick paced music is generally alerting and facilitates movement and expression.

Several listening programs incorporate electronically altered music to facilitate improved sensory modulation, auditory processing, language, and affective response and engagement. Modulated music refers to music that has been processed using an alternating high and low pas filter, thus creating a contrast between the high and low end of the sound frequencies. Spectral activation is a type of gating of the higher spectral portions of the audio range. The Therapeutic Listening® program (Therapeutic Resources, Inc., Madison, WI) uses sound based technologies in conjunction with sensory integrative treatment techniques. Positive results of the Therapeutic Listening® program include increased organization of behavior, attention, greater emotional expressiveness, and emergence of praxis (Frick & Hacker, 2001). Regardless of whether or not a specific protocol is chosen, music can still be incorporated into treatment sessions. Good clinical judgment based on the child's needs and challenges guides the selection of listening program and choice of music.

BEHAVIOR MODIFICATION

Behavior can be understood using the ABC model: A=Antecedent, B=Behavior, and C=Consequence. The antecedent is the event that precedes an action. Behavior is the observable and measurable response to the event. Consequence refers to the events occurring after the behavior is exhibited. Behavior modification techniques manipulate antecedents and consequences to encourage desirable behaviors while deterring negative ones. Reinforcement is anything that increases the frequency or strengthens a behavior (Table 22-13). Positive reinforcement increases the frequency of a behavior through the contingent presentation of something desirable to the individual. Negative reinforcement increases the frequency of a behavior through the contingent removal of something undesirable. Reinforcement, as opposed to disciplinary measures, appears to be more effective in managing inappropriate behaviors in children with oppositional defiant disorder and conduct disorder.

Table 22-13

Reinforcers

Type	Description and Example
Natural Reinforcement	Results directly from the appropriate behavior, e.g., playing appropriately with peers will lead to more invitations to join such activities.
Social Reinforcers	Socially mediated actions of other people that strengthen behaviors, e.g., verbal and written praise, expressions of approval (clapping, smiling, nodding your head).
Activity Reinforcers	Allowing the child to participate in preferred activities, e.g., providing 5 minutes of free time or computer time after finishing a task.
Tangible Reinforcers	Includes food and objects as rewards for behavior, e.g., candy, stickers, toys, etc.

Punishment decreases the frequency of a behavior through the contingent application of an aversive stimulus. Types of punishments include time outs, reprimands, response cost (withdrawing a previously earned reward), restitution (the child has to return the environment to the state it was in before the misbehavior occurred), and positive practice (having the child repeat the action; this time doing it correctly). In order to be successful, reinforcement and punishment need to be applied in a consistent and timely manner.

In a token economy system, children earn points or tokens for socially appropriate and desired behaviors. These points may be exchanged for preferred activities, objects, or privileges. When implementing a token economy, the OTA needs to identify specific behavioral goals and assign point or token values to each goal. Next, the OTA should determine time intervals for assessment. In the beginning, it may be necessary to reward every instance of desired behavior. As time progresses the OTA may move to fixed time intervals. One of the key elements in a token economy is the selection of motivating rewards. The OTA may also help set up a token economy system for home or classroom use.

A contingency or behavioral contract is an agreement between the practitioner and child that clearly and explicitly states expectations and consequences of behavior. The OTA may work with the child to construct a contract, identifying specified behavior, conditions of the contract (when will it be in effect, what setting, etc), criteria for completion, and appropriate reinforcers. The contract should be signed and dated by both the practitioner and child. In both token economy systems and contingency contracts the identified goal should be an attainable behavior. Successful completion of the goal instills the child with a sense of personal satisfaction that serves as a positive reinforcer.

Modeling involves purposefully exhibiting specific behaviors to be imitated by others. According to Bandura (1986), the individual is motivated to reproduce those behaviors that have been observed to have positive conse-

quences. For example, during a group session, the OTA notices two of the children sharing crayons. The OTA brings this behavior to the groups attention and says, "That's really nice sharing. Good job." She smiles at them and gives them each a sticker. Seeing these two members of the group being rewarded and verbally praised for sharing serves as motivation for the other children to reproduce the behavior. The OTA constantly models positive behaviors during individual interactions with children. This may involve acting calmly during new activities and transitions to help ease a child's anxiety.

Children who are older or higher functioning can learn to self-monitor their behavior. Take for example a child who has difficulty waiting his or her turn. The child may carry around a note card with the words "Wait and count to ten," and refer to it as necessary. Similarly, a child may become overly frustrated and exhibit aggressive behaviors. On the child's desk, two pictures visually depicting "a little" and "a lot" can be taped to his or her desk. The child refers to these pictures to self-monitor frustration level and self-initiate strategies to improve regulation when necessary.

COGNITIVE-BEHAVIORAL THERAPY

The main premise of cognitive behavioral theory is that overt behavior is mediated by cognitive events. Accordingly, individuals can change behavior by influencing or altering cognitive events. Strategies are aimed at identifying, challenging, and ultimately changing maladaptive cognitions. For example, a child experiencing depression and having difficulties in math class may think, "I'm too stupid to ever get the answer right." As a result of this cognitive distortion, the child may engage in disruptive behaviors during math time, making inappropriate noises, or yelling out silly words. These behaviors are reinforced by the negative attention the child receives (e.g., laughter from his or her peers, increased attention from the teacher). Thus maladaptive behaviors have a learned component as well.

Table 22-14

Abdominal Breathing Exercise

- Lie down on a mat or carpeted floor with a pillow propped underneath your head and your knees bent.
- Close your eyes and rest your hands gently on your abdomen just below your rib cage.
- Inhale deeply and slowly though your nose as your abdomen expands.
- After you have taken a full breath, pause for a moment and then exhale slowly with your lips pursed, your abdomen contracting back to its starting position.
- Concentrate on your breathing. Take deep, full breaths. Feel your hands rise and fall as you inhale and exhale. Feel your body relax as your exhale. Imagine your arms and legs going limp like a rag doll.
- To help pace your breathing, count to four on each inhale and exhale.
- Continue with abdominal breathing for 5 minutes.

Cognitive restructuring is the process of questioning negative thought patterns and beliefs and changing them to truthful, positive ones. The OTA may assist older children and adolescents in identifying cognitive distortions. Another strategy involves challenging the child's negative perception by pointing to anecdotal evidence. For the child who believes he or she is too stupid to do anything right, the OTA may cite examples of the child succeeding at something. The next step is replacing the negative perception with a positive one. "I'm too stupid" could become "It's hard for me, but I'll keep trying."

Exposure-based training assumes that an individual's anxiety will decrease with systematic and repeated encounters with the feared situation or stimuli (Hope, 1996). Exposure training should be graded, that is the child should begin with situations that produce low-levels of anxiety and work up from there. Imaginal exposure involves having the child visualize a situation that causes distress. The OTA may also stage the feared situation through role-playing or in-session exposure. For the child with social phobia who is too afraid to initiate conversation with unfamiliar people, in-session exposure may involve having the child ask another therapist to borrow a piece of equipment or toy. Exposure training may be combined with social stories and cognitive restructuring techniques.

The Socratic Method is a teaching technique designed to encourage increased problem-solving and insight. When a child presents with inappropriate behaviors, it is common for OT practitioners to respond by redirecting the child as to what to do. Instead, in the Socratic method the OTA needs to help the child identify and initiate appropriate solutions. If a child throws a toy, rather than saying, "You're not supposed to throw things," inquire as to why he or she threw the toy. If a child appears dysregulated, ask him or her, "What do you think you need to do when you feel this way?" Eventually, the child may be able to internalize this method of questioning and use it as a way to self-monitor behavior.

Assertiveness and social skills training focus on improving the child's communication skills. It includes anger-management, understanding and reading nonverbal cues, and

learning ways to positively interact with peers. The child may use role-playing to practice new behaviors, improve perspective taking, increase self-confidence, and decrease anxiety by anticipating the consequences of a situation. Role-playing may also help the child generalize responses. Providing the child with appropriate feedback is also an important element of assertiveness training. Other activities include having the child keep a journal, and giving homework assignments. Homework may include worksheets describing hypothetical situations that require a response. Or, assertiveness and social skills training may involve an actual activity, like asking a friend to come over and watch television.

Relaxation training helps the child learn to reduce feelings of anxiety and stress. Benefits of relaxation include increased concentration, improved sleep habits, and protection against the physiological responses of stress (Jones & Heymen, 2002). The use of controlled breathing is one of the most effective relaxation techniques. This can be as simple as teaching the child to take slow, deep breaths. Table 22-14 outlines the steps of an abdominal breathing exercise that may be useful for older children experiencing anxiety. Abdominal breathing can also be paired with guided imagery techniques. Guided imagery involves assisting the child in imagining positive emotional states and responses. This may be done through the use of verbal prompts, scripted narratives, or music.

CAREGIVER TRAINING

Throughout the occupational therapy process, the OT practitioner should provide constant family and caregiver education on the child's condition and its impact on daily functioning. This information should be relayed in an easy to understand manner. The OTA may be asked to create and instruct the family on a home program as an adjunct to individual therapy, or initiate caregiver training as part of a consultative model. This may include instruction on sensory diet activities or behavior modification techniques.

Ineffective parent-child interactions can exacerbate behavioral problems and maladaptive responses. Training the parent and/or caregivers on how to encourage and sustain positive interactions with their child is therefore an important component of intervention. This may include directly coaching the parent on floor time principles when playing with his or her child. Another method involves videotaping the parent interacting with the child. The OT practitioner can review the tape with the parent and offer feedback.

Theraplay® (Theraplay Institute, Wilmette, IL) is a play-based treatment method that attempts to replicate the joy and pleasure experienced in a natural, healthy parent-infant relationship (Jernberg & Booth, 1999). Treatment typically involves the physical, active play seen in early parent-infant interactions as opposed to symbolic or pretend play. Theraplay® emphasizes the use of nurturing touch. As the first form of communication between infant and parent, touch is critical for developing and maintaining secure and loving attachments. The Theraplay® approach places the caregiver or therapist firmly in charge. The Theraplay® therapist is responsible for structuring the environment to meet the individual needs of the child, engaging the child by providing enticing activities, nurturing the child through touch and other comforting activities, and providing challenges to facilitate increased confidence. Parents are actively involved in treatment sessions as observers and co-therapists, learning ways to continue fostering positive parent-child interactions.

NEURONET

The NeuroNet program is "designed to automate the basic perceptual-motor skills of balance, hand movements and speech which are the essential components of many daily behaviors" (Rowe, 2002). In laymen's terms, the NeuroNet program is for children who cannot walk, chew gum, and carry on a conversation at the same time. Children with psychosocial disorders often display deficits in organizational skills, timing, and multi-tasking. Performing several simple tasks at once (low-level multitasking) is effortful, requiring constant thought. As a result, the child's movements may appear uncoordinated and clumsy. The child may require increased time to perform basic skills, and have difficulty with academic learning. Feelings of frustration and inadequacy may in turn lead to behavioral problems. The NeuroNet program incorporates rhythmic movements calibrated against gravity to integrate the motor, perception, and cognition (Rowe, 2002). The following is an example of an activity: The child sits on a therapy ball with his or her hips and knees at a ninety degree angle with feet firmly planted on the ground. The OTA holds up a piece of paper with the word "orange." The child bounces up and down to an external rhythm, clapping his or hands to knees, and reading the word aloud five times. A child with organizational or multi-tasking deficits may be able to perform all of these tasks

individually. When combined, the child may have trouble grading the bouncing movements against gravity, losing his or her balance with his or her feet coming off the floor. The bilateral clapping of hands to knees may be uneven, with one hand hitting first and then the other. When reading the word aloud they may say it too many or too few times.

Summary

Psychosocial disorders may have a deleterious effect on a child's ability to engage in age-appropriate and adaptive behaviors in the home, school, and play setting. The presence of isolative or disruptive behaviors may further lead to strained interactions between the child and caregiver. Rather than addressing the cause of the behavior, teachers and parents may incorporate unsuccessful disciplinary measures. The OT practitioner who is knowledgeable in pediatric psychosocial disorders plays an invaluable role in being able to identify those sensory, cognitive, and psychosocial deficits impeding the child from meaningfully interaction with his or her environment. The OT practitioner may incorporate a variety of intervention approaches designed to facilitate increased engagement, regulation, attention, organization, and problem solving.

Case Study

Case study can be found in Table 22-11.

DISCUSSION QUESTIONS

1. What underlying deficits are being addressed during this session?

2. What do you think would have happened if the OTA removed the container of play dough out of Jamie's line of vision and redirected him to another activity? How would the interaction be different?

Application Activities

Have the class divide into groups of 3 to 4 and discuss the following scenarios.

1. Brandon is a 6-year-old boy diagnosed with ADHD, oppositional-defiant disorder and SMD (sensory modulation dysfunction). He is "always on the go," unable to remain seated and always seeking sensory input, particularly proprioceptive and vestibular movement. Both Brandon's parents and teacher report that he frequently spits, sometimes even at students. During a group led occupational therapy session, the OTA

explicitly told Brandon that there was to be no spitting during the activity, or he would be sent to a time out. Brandon responded by promptly spitting at the little boy sitting next to him. Brainstorm various intervention approaches and strategies that may be used to help eliminate or control this problem behavior.

2. Peter is a 9-year-old boy with Asperger's syndrome. He presents with auditory processing deficits and is especially sensitive to loud noise. He is tactilely defensive and is averse to unexpected touch. He becomes quite anxious and upset during recess time. He often stands off by himself and avoids the other students. Recently, Peter asked his teacher if he could stay inside at his desk during recess time. Following the guidelines outlined by Carol Gray, construct a social story entitled "Recess Time," classifying each sentence used. Describe at least two other intervention approaches and strategies that may be used to help Peter participate in recess.

3. Danielle is a 5-year-old girl diagnosed with an attachment disorder. She was adopted when she was 13 months old from a Chinese orphanage. She presents with low tone, atypical movement patterns and delays in speech. She still speaks in "baby talk" and acts younger than her age. Her parents describe her as "demanding," noting that she will throw "spectacular temper tantrums" when she doesn't get what she wants. Her parents note that her younger sibling and other peers Danielle's age do not like playing with her because she always breaks their toys. Compare and contrast the DIR/Floor time approach with the Theraplay® model for use with a child with attachment disorder. What are the benefits of each? Drawbacks?

References

Adler, N. E., Boyce, T., Chesney, M. A., Cohen, S., Folkman, S., Kahn, R. L., & Syme, S. L. (1994). Socioeconomic status and health: The challenge of the gradient. *American Psychologist, 49*, 15-24.

Ainsworth, M. D., Blehar, M. C., Waters, E., & Wall, S. (1978). *Patterns of attachment: A psychological study of the strange situation.* Hillsdale, NJ: Lawrence Erlbaum Associates.

American Occupational Therapy Association (2002). *Roles and responsibilities of the occupational therapist and the occupational therapy assistant during the delivery of occupational therapy services.* Retrieved November 13, 2002 from
http://www.aota.org/members/area2/docs/rrota.pdf

American Occupational Therapy Association (1991). *The occupational therapist as case manager.* Retrieved October 12, 2002 from http://www.aota.org/members/area6/links/link39c2.asp?PLACE=/members/area6/links/link39c2.asp

American Occupational Therapy Association (1998). *Standards of practice for occupational therapy.* Retrieved November 13, 2002 from http://www.aota.org/general/otsp.asp

American Psychiatric Association (2000). *Diagnostic and statistical manual of mental disorders* (4th ed., Text rev.). Washington, DC: American Psychiatric Association.

Autism Society of America (n.d.). *What causes autism?* Retrieved September 14, 2002 from
http://www.autism-society.org/site/PageServer?pagename=autismcauses

Ayres, A. J. (1972). *Sensory integration and learning disorders.* Los Angeles, CA: Western Psychological Services.

Ayres, A. J. (1985). *Developmental dyspraxia and adult-onset apraxia.* Torrance, CA: Sensory Integration International.

Baird, G., Charman, T., Baron-Cohen, S., Swettenham, J., Wheelwright, S., & Drew. A. (2000). A screening instrument for autism at 18 months of age: a 6-year follow up study. *Journal of the American Academy of Child and Adolescent Psychiatry, 39,* 694-702.

Bandura, A. (1986). *Social foundations of thought and action.* Englewood Cliffs, NJ: Prentice-Hall.

Beardslee, W. R., Versage, E. M., & Gladstone, T. R. G. (1998). Children of affectively ill parents: A review of the past 10 years. *Journal of the American Academy of Child and Adolescent Psychiatry, 37*(11), 1134-1141.

Blair, K. (2001, March). Recognizing psychopathology in early childhood. *Neuropsychiatry Reviews, 2*(2). Retrieved from http://www.neuropsychiatryreviews.com/mar01/npr_mar01_psycho.html

Blondis, T. A., Snow, J. H., Roizen, N. J., Opacich, K. J, & Accardo, P. J. Early maturation of motor delayed children at school age. *Journal of Child Neurology, 8,* 323-329.

Boughton, B. (2001, January). Music's balm. *In Touch, 3*(1). Retrieved from http://www.intouchlive.com/home/frames.htm?http://www.intouchlive.com/journals/intouch/i0101c.htm&3

Bowlby, J. (1988). *A secure base: Parent-child attachment and healthy human development.* New York: Basic Books.

Brener, N. D., Martindale, J., & Weist, M. D. (2001). Mental health and social services: Results from the School Health Policies and Programs Study 2000. *Journal of School Health, 71,* 305-312. University of Maryland School of Medicine.

Brown, A. (1996). *Mood disorders in children and adolescents.* National Alliance for Research on Schizophrenia and Depression Research Newsletter. Retrieved on October 1, 2002, from
http://www.narsad.org/pub/archchildmood.html

Carlson, G. A., & Kashani, J. H. (1988). Phenomenology of major depression from childhood through adulthood: Analysis of three studies. *American Journal of Psychology, 145,*1222-1225.

Centers for Disease Control and Prevention (2000). *Prevalence of Autism in Brick Township, New Jersey 1998: Community Report.* Retrieved on August 25, 2002 from http://www.cdc.gov/ncbddd/dd/

Center for Mental Health Services (1998). *Anxiety disorders in children and adolescents.* Retrieved August 20, 2002 from the Center for Mental Health Services, A Component of the Substance Abuse and Mental Health Services Administration website:
http://www.mentalhealth.org/publications/allpubs/CA-0007/default.asp

Cole, M. (1998). *Group dynamics in occupational therapy* (2nd ed.). Thorofare, NJ: SLACK Incorporated.

DeGangi, G. A., & Breinbauer, C. (1997). The symptomatology of infants and toddlers with regulatory disorders. *Journal of Developmental and Learning Disorders, 1*(1), 183-215.

Depression and Bipolar Support Alliance (n.d.). *Bipolar disorder.* Retrieved August 20, 2002 from:
http://www.dbsalliance.org/info/bipolar.html

Devlin, M. J. (1996). Assessment and treatment of binge-eating disorder. *Psychiatric Clinics of North America, 19,* 761-772.

Dunn, W. (1998). Person-centered and contextually relevant evaluation. In J. Hinojosa and P. Kramer, *Evaluation: Obtaining and interpreting data.* (pp. 47-76). Bethesda: AOTA.

Dunn, W. (2000). *Best practice occupational therapy: In community service with children and families.* Thorofare, NJ: SLACK Incorporated.

Dunn, W. & DeGangi, G (1992). Sensory integration and neurodevelopmental treatment for educational programming. In C. Royeen (Ed.). *AOTA self study series: Classroom applications for school based practice.* Rockville, MD: American Occupational Therapy Association.

Eaton, W. W., & Muntaner, C. (1999). Socioeconomic stratification and mental disorder. In A. V. Horwitz & T. K. Scheid (Eds.), *A handbook for the study of mental health: Social contexts, theories, and systems* (pp. 259-283). New York: Cambridge University Press.

Edelsohn, G., Ialongo, N., Werthamer-Larsson, L., Crockett, L., & Kellam, S. (1992). Self-reported depressive symptoms in first grade children: Developmentally transient phenomena? *Journal of the American Academy of Child and Adolescent Psychiatry, 31,* 282-290.

Erikson, E. (1963). *Childhood and society.* New York: W.W. Norton Company.

Erikson, E. (1982). *The life cycle completed.* New York: W.W. Norton Company.

Fidler, G. (1997). The psychosocial core of occupational therapy position paper. *American Journal of Occupational Therapy, 51,* (10), 868-869.

Frick, S., & Hacker, C. (2001). *Listening with the whole body.* Madison: Vital Links.

Gray, C. (2002). *The social story guidelines.* Retrieved from the Gray Center for Social Learning and Understanding website on November 12, 2002 from:

http://www.thegraycenter.org/Social_Stories.htm

Genna, C. W. (2001). Tactile defensiveness and other sensory modulation difficulties. *Leaven, 37*(3), 51-53.

Greenspan, S. I., DeGangi, G. A., & Wieder, S. (2001). *Functional emotional assessment scale.*

Greenspan, S. I., & Wieder, S. (1998). *The child with special needs: Encouraging intellectual and emotional growth.* Reading, MA: Perseus Books.

Halgin, R. P., & Whitbourne, S. K. (1994). *Abnormal psychology: The human experience of psychological disorders.* Orlando: Harcourt Brace & Co.

Hanrahan, S. (2000, November/December). *How the arousal level of your child affects learning.* Autism Society of Southeastern Wisconsin Newsletter. Retrieved from:

http://www.asw4autism.org/ASSEW/news1100.htm

Harrington, R. C. (2001). Childhood depression and conduct disorder: Different routes to the same outcome? *Archives of General Psychiatry, 58,* 237-240.

Individuals with Disabilities Education Act, Pub. L. 105-17, 34 U.S.C., section 300 et. seq. (1999).

Individuals with Disabilities Education Act, Pub. L. 105-17, 34 C.F.R., section 307.7 (10) (1999).

Jellinek, M. S., & Snyder, J. B. (1998). Depression and suicide in children and adolescents. *Pediatrics in Review, 19*(8), 255-64.

Jernberg, M., & Booth, P. (1999). *Theraplay: Helping parents and children build better relationships through attachment-based play* (2nd ed.). San Francisco: Jossey-Bass.

Jones, K. R., & Heymen, S. (2002). Using relaxation: Coping with functional gastrointestinal disorders. Retrieved November 22, 2002 from: http://www.med.unc.edu/wrkunits/2depts/medicine/fgidc/relax.htm

Kataoka, S. H., Zhang, L., & Wells, K. B. (2002). Unmet need for mental health care among US children: Variation by ethnicity and insurance status. *American Journal of Psychiatry, 159,* 1548-1555.

Kluger, J., & Song, S. (2002, August 19). Young and bipolar. *Time, 160*(8), 38-46, 51.

Lahey, B., Flagg, E., Bird, H., Schwab-Stone, M., Canino, G., Dulcan, M., Leaf, P., Davies, M., Brogan, D., Bourdon, K., Howitz, S., Rubio-Stipec, M., Freeman, D., Lichtman, J., Shaffer, D., Goodman, S., Narrow, W., Weissman, M., Kandel, D., Jensen, P., Richters, J., & Regier, D. (1996). The NIMH methods for the epidemiology of child and adolescent mental disorders (MECA) study: Background and methodology. *Journal of the American Academy of Child and Adolescent Psychiatry, 35,* 855-864.

Loeber, R., & Stouthamer-Loeber, M. (1986). Family factors as correlates and predictors of juvenile conduct problems and delinquency. In M. Tonry & N. Morris (Eds.), *Crime and justice* (Vol. 7). Chicago: University of Chicago Press.

Mager, R. F. 1962, 1975. *Preparing instructional objectives* (2nd Ed.). Belmont, CA: Fearon Publishers, Inc.

McClellan, J., & Werry, J. (1997). Practical parameters for the assessment and treatment of children and adolescents with bipolar disorder. *Journal of the American Academy of Child and Adolescent Psychiatry, 36*(l),138-157.

Miller, L. J., Reisman, J. E., McIntosh, D. N., & Simon, J. (2001). An ecological model of sensory modulation: Performance of children with fragile X syndrome, autistic disorder, attention-deficit/hyperactivity disorder, and sensory modulation dysfunction. In S. S. Roley, E. I. Blanche, & R. C. Schaaf, *Understanding the nature of sensory integration with diverse populations* (pp. 57-82). San Antonio, TX: Harcourt Health Sciences Company.

Papolos, D. F. (1999). *The bipolar child.* New York: Broadway Books.

Parham, L. D., & Mailloux, Z. (1996). Sensory integration. In J. Case-Smith, A.S. Allen, & P.N.Pratt, (Eds.). *Occupational therapy for children* (3rd ed) (pp. 307-356). St. Louis, MO: Mosby.

Pavuluri, M. N., Luk, S. L., & McGee, R. (1996). Help-seeking for behavior problems by parents of preschool children: A community study. *Journal of the American Academy of Child and Adolescent Psychiatry, 35,* 215-222.

Penn, D. L., & Martin, J. (1998). The stigma of severe mental illness: Some potential solutions for a recalcitrant problem. *Psychiatric Quarterly, 69,* 235-247.

Radke-Yarrow, M., Nottleman, F., Martinez, P., Fox, M. F., & Belmont, B. (1992). Young children of affectively ill parents: A longitudinal study of psychosocial development. *Journal of the American Academy of Child and Adolescent Psychiatry, 31,* 68-71.

Rehabilitation Act, Pub. L. No. 93-112, 29 U.S.C. section 701 (1973).

Ross, D. M., & Ross, S. A. (1982). *Hyperactivity: Current issues, research, and theory.* New York: Wiley.

Rowe, N. W. (2002). *What is neuronet therapy?* Retrieved November 22, 2002 from: http://www.neuronetonline.com

Rush, A. J., Stewart, R. S., Garver, D. L., & Waller, D. A. (1998). Neurobiological bases for psychiatric disorders. In R. N. Rosenberg & D. E. Pleasure (Eds.), *Comprehensive neurology* (2nd ed., pp. 555-603). New York: John Wiley and Sons.

Schaff, R. C., & Anzalone, M. E. (2001). Sensory integration with high-risk infants and young children. In S. S. Roley, E. I. Blanche, & R. C. Schaaf, *Understanding the nature of sensory integration with diverse populations* (pp. 275-311). San Antonio, TX: Harcourt Health Sciences Company.

Schoonover, J. (2002). A cool tool for school. *ADVANCE for Occupational Therapy, 18*(21), 9.

Schultz, S. (1992). School-based occupational therapy for students with behavioral disorders. *Occupational Therapy in Health Care, 8,* 173-196.

Schor, E. (1999). *Caring for your school-aged child: Ages 5 to 12.* Washington, DC: American Academy of Pediatrics.

Shaffer, D., Fisher, P., Dulcan, M., Davies, M., Piacentini, J., Schwab-Stone, M., Lahey, B., Bourdon, K., Jensen, P., Bird, H., & Canino, G. R. D. (1996). The second version of the NIMH diagnostic interview schedule for children (DISC-2). *Journal of the American Academy of Child and Adolescent Psychiatry, 35,* 865-877.

Staw, B., Sutton, R., & Pelled, L. (1994). Employee positive emotion and favorable outcomes in the workplace. *Organization Science, 5,* 51-71.

Stroul, B., & Friedman, R. M. (1986). *A system of care for children and youth with severe emotional disturbances* (Revised Ed.). Washington, DC: Georgetown University of Child Development, CASSP Technical Assistance Center.

Sunbeck, D. (1996). *Infinity walk: Preparing your mind to learn* (2nd ed.). Torrance, CA: Jalmer Press.

US Department of Education (2001). *Twenty-third annual report to congress on the implementation of the individuals with disabilities act.* Retrieved October 15, 2002 from Office of Special Education Programs website:

http://www.ed.gov/offices/OSERS/OSEP/Products/OSEP2001AnlRpt/

US Department of Health and Human Services (1999). *Mental health: A report of the surgeon general.* Retrieved on August 25, 2002, from Office of the Surgeon General website:

http://www.surgeongeneral.gov/library/mentalhealth/home.html

Walker-Andrews, A. S. (1998). Emotions and social development: Infants' recognition of emotions in others. *Pediatrics, 102,* 1268-1271.

Walker, K. (2000). *Self-regulation and sensory processing for learning, attention, and attachment.* Retrieved September 21, 2002, from http://www.myflorida.com/myflorida/government/governorinitiatives/schoolreadiness/pdf/appendixH.pdf

Weiss, B., Weisz, J., Politano, M., Carey, M. P., Nelson, W., & Finch, A. J. (1992). Relations among self-reported depressive symptoms in clinic referred children versus adolescents. *Journal of Abnormal Psychology, 101,* 391-397.

Weist, M. D. (1997). Expanded school mental health services: A national movement in progress. In T. H. Ollendick & R. J. Prinz (Eds.), *Advances in Clinical Child Psychology,* Volume 19 (pp. 319-352). New York: Plenum Press.

Weist, M. D. (2001). Promoting the mental health of our nation's youth through school-based programs. Retrieved October 15, 2002, from the American Psychological Association website:

http://www.apa.org/ppo/issues/pweist601.html

White, R. (2002). *Sensory organization and the developmental, individual-difference, relationship-based (DIR) model.* Bethesda, MD: Interdisciplinary Council on Developmental & Learning Disorders.

Williams, M. S., & Shellenberger, S. (1996). *How does your engine run? A leader's guide to the alert program for self regulation.* Albuquerque, NM: TherapyWorks, Inc.

Williamson, G. G., & Anzalone, M. E. (2001). *Helping infants and young children interact with their environment: Improving sensory integration and self-regulation.* Washington, DC: Zero to Three.

Winnicott, D. W. (1965) *The family and individual development.* London: Tavistock Publications.

Zero to Three (1994). *Diagnostic classification of mental health and developmental disorders of infancy and early childhood.* Washington, DC: Zero to Three.

23

AN OVERVIEW OF ASSISTIVE TECHNOLOGY

David L. Lee, MS, OTR/L

Chapter Objectives

- Define assistive technology within the scope of pediatric occupational therapy.
- Describe the purpose of assistive technology in the therapeutic treatment of children with disabilities.
- Identify basic assistive technology services and devices, and their appropriate funding sources.
- Understand the occupational therapy assistant's role in using appropriate assistive technology as an integral part of occupational therapy treatment.

Introduction

Technology, the pervasive catchphrase of the 21st century, impacts nearly every aspect of society today. As we journey through this technological and information era, the ever-increasing use and reliance on technology to complete functional tasks in the workplace, home, and community increases almost exponentially as newer and more efficient technology are constantly being introduced in the marketplace. From an occupational therapy perspective, linking technology to therapy, such as using computers and electronic augmentative/alternative communication boards (AACs) to enhance functional communication, or using adaptive toy switches to promote child's play participation, is commonly referred to as assistive technology, while the device itself is referred to as an assistive device or adaptive equipment.

The purpose of this chapter is to provide an introduction to the principles and concepts of pediatric-based assistive technology, give an overview of the occupational therapy (OT) practitioner's role in the assistive technology treatment continuum (i.e., planning, implementation, and family/caregiver training), and provide information on current funding, legislation, and documentation issues relating to assistive technology within the scope of pediatric occupational therapy.

Discussion and Rationale

Since the 1980s, assistive technology has gained acceptance by healthcare professionals, and has become a major feature in the treatment process. This widespread acceptance was in part due to the introduction of the 1988 Technology Related Assistance for Individuals with Disabilities Act ("The Tech Act"; PL 100-407), defining assistive technology as assistive technology services, and assistive technology devices. Assistive technology is often referred to as or called adaptive technology, adaptive equipment, adaptive devices, or rehabilitation engineering. An assistive technology service is defined as, "any service that directly assists an individual with a disability in the selection, acquisition, or use of an assistive technology device" (AOTA, 1999; AMA, 1996; Cook & Hussey, 2002, p. 5; Jacobs, 1999). Provision of assistive technology services follow the traditional occupational therapy process, from evaluation, treatment/intervention, implementation, and discharge, to follow-up, family/caregiver training, and continuing education. An assistive technology device is defined as, "any item, piece of equipment, or product system, whether acquired commercially off the shelf, modified, or customized, that is used to increase, maintain, or improve functional capabilities of individuals with disabilities" (AOTA, 1999; AMA, 1996; Cook & Hussey, 2002, p. 5; Jacobs, 1999). Assistive technology may also be used for prevention of further disability, remediation, augmentation of current function, or substitution for a disability, or decreased function (AMA, 1996). An assistive device is an adaptation of a common object designed for more efficient completion of self-care, leisure/recreation, or communication activities. Given these definitions, assistive technology is very broad in its scope, includes a wide range of applications and devices, and is characterized by a wide spectrum of services available today. In fact, over 3.1 million Americans with a physical impairment used assistive technology in 1990 (LaPlant, Hendershot, & Moss, 1992). In 1992, approximately 4 million children and adolescents (6.1% of U.S. population) under the age of 18 had identified disabilities (Wenger, Kaye, & LaPlante, 1996), and approximately 7.4 million Americans used assistive technology due to mobility impairments in 1994 (National Center for Health Statistics, 2002). With over 4.7 million children under the age of 18, or 6.7% of all children identified as having activity limitations (Kraus, Stoddard, & Gilmartin, 1996), the National Center for Education Statistics reported in 2001 that at the national level, depending on the type of disability, 55 to 64% of schools serving students with disabilities provided assistive or adaptive hardware, and 39 to 56% provided assistive or adaptive software (NCES, 2001). Thus, the number of children using assistive technology is growing, and modern pediatric OT practitioners need to be aware and knowledgeable of the dynamic field of assistive technology for the successful treatment of children with disabilities.

Pediatric OT practitioners primarily concern themselves with helping children function to the best of their abilities within their natural environments. When indicated, assistive technology is used to enhance development and to maximize potential and mastery when interacting with the human and non-human environment (Kramer & Hinojosa, 1999). The human environment includes the people with whom a child interacts with on a daily basis, even just for a moment. The nonhuman environment includes everything else that a child comes in contact with that is not human, from toys to pets, to televisions and computers. It is important to realize that the human and non-human environment constantly changes for a child, as he or she grows from exploring the world from the floor level to a standing level, or from a home setting to a school environment. Thus, as a child's awareness and interaction with the human and non-human environments changes with varying physical environments, he or she learns to adapt to different surroundings (Kramer & Hinojosa, 1999). Assistive technology may be a vital component in the occupational therapy service and treatment process. The rationale for using assistive technology in occupational therapy treatment is that it must be functional and goal-oriented. Within the scope of pediatric occupational therapy, use of assistive devices play an important role in promoting development by enhancing a child's participation and functional outcomes within the occupational performance areas of activities of daily living (ADLs), instrumental activities of daily living (IADLs), work, education, leisure, play, and social participation (AOTA, 2002). Assistive technology, when designed and used appropriately, assists with improving quality of life, and ultimately restores a child's sense of self-esteem through independent or improved functional performance.

Assistive devices also help the child to practice specific or general skills by imitating the therapist's hands and movements, usually in a static manner, to enhance functional independence and skill development. Assistive technology may provide children with dynamic responses, such as visual (i.e., red/green lights, blinking lights), auditory (i.e., beeps), or verbal (i.e., word vocalizations) cues. For example, Sheldon, who is hungry and wants to eat an apple, may use an electronic communication board with pictures of food and simple verbal commands to communicate with his parents/caregivers by pressing the "hungry" button, which vocalizes, "I am hungry". Sheldon then proceeds to press the "apple" button and the board will vocalize, "apple", indicating that he is hungry and wants to eat an apple.

The High Tech Versus Low Tech Debate

Assistive technology is commonly divided into two major categories: high tech and low tech. High technology devices are characterized as having an electronic component, are generally more expensive than low tech devices, and due to a varying level of internal device complexity, require programming and training for the family/caregivers in order for the child to take full advantage of the assistive device. High tech devices are generally used for play and leisure activities, communication, or environmental control. Examples of high tech devices are electronic augmentative/alternative communication (AAC) boards or computers, electric wheelchairs, and environmental control units (ECUs). Robotic devices, another example of a high tech device, have been gaining popularity for use with enhancing functional independence (i.e., feeding, grooming) for children, as well as for play/leisure pursuits (Cook & Hussey, 2002; Kramer & Hinojosa, 1999).

Low technology devices, as compared to high tech devices, are usually less expensive, are nonelectronic, require little or no training to use, and provide ideal functional solutions for children with disabilities. Examples of low-technology devices include activities of daily living

Table 23-1

Considering the Need for Assistive Technology

Factors	Description	Questions to Consider
1. Purpose	The meaningfulness and purposefulness of the assistive device.	• Why are you using this recommended item? • Is this device meaningful and/or purposeful to the child? • Will this device serve more than one purpose?
2. Design	The functionality, usability, and safety of the assistive device.	• Is it functional, given the environment of the child? • Is it attractive? • Is it both functional and attractive? • Will the child be embarrassed to use the device with his or her peers? • Is this device culturally acceptable to the child and his or her family/caregivers?
3. Cost	The affordability, cost-effectiveness, and any maintenance of the assistive device.	• Is the device fully funded (federal, state, or private funds)? • Is the item covered by child's insurance plan? If not, what percentage is covered? • If not covered, can the family/caregiver afford the item? What is maximum amount of money the family/caregiver is willing to spend? • If not covered, will it be practicable and/or reasonable for the OT practitioner to build or construct the device rather than purchasing it? • Which option is more cost-effective? • Are there local organizations or sponsorships willing to fund or donate used devices? • Who can repair or replace the item if the device becomes inoperative? Is there a local vendor or repair shop nearby? Can the family/caregiver be educated to make simple adjustments or repairs? • How do you clean the device?

(ADL) aids, such as buttonhooks, adaptive forks and spoons, and paper communication boards. Low tech aids often work more effectively than high tech devices because of lower cost, generally less maintenance, and family/caregiver training. Sometimes the appropriate assistive device may be a combination of both a high tech and low tech device, depending on the child's functional status, the family/caregiver support system, and their collective goals. As a rule of thumb, when choosing the appropriate assistive device for a child, a high technology solution should be avoided when a low tech device can just as easily be used.

Reflections for the OTA

Never implement a high tech solution to solve a low tech problem.

Planning and Implementation of Assistive Technology

The assistive technology team may consist solely of, or include a combination of OT practitioners, special education teachers, rehabilitation engineer/technologists, nurses,

physicians, prosthetists/orthotists, durable medical equipment (DME) vendors, and the caregivers/family members. All members of the team may participate and contribute to the evaluation/assessment of a child's need for assistive technology. For the OT practitioner, the salient issues surrounding the planning and implementation of assistive technology includes examining the purposefulness and meaningfulness of an assistive device to the child, examining issues and barriers to progress, and evaluating the environments in which the child participates on a daily basis. When selecting an appropriate assistive device to facilitate childhood occupations, it must be purposeful, meaningful, and involve interaction with the environment such that it can be comfortable and motivating for the child.

When planning, implementing, and choosing the appropriate device for a child there are several major factors to consider. They include 1) the purpose and meaning of the assistive device, 2) the design, which includes the usability characteristics of the device, and 3) the cost, which includes the price of the device and any subsequent costs for the care/maintenance of the product or assistive device (see table below) (AMA; 1996; Cook & Hussey, 2002; Ryan, 1996; Trombly, 1995) (Table 23-1).

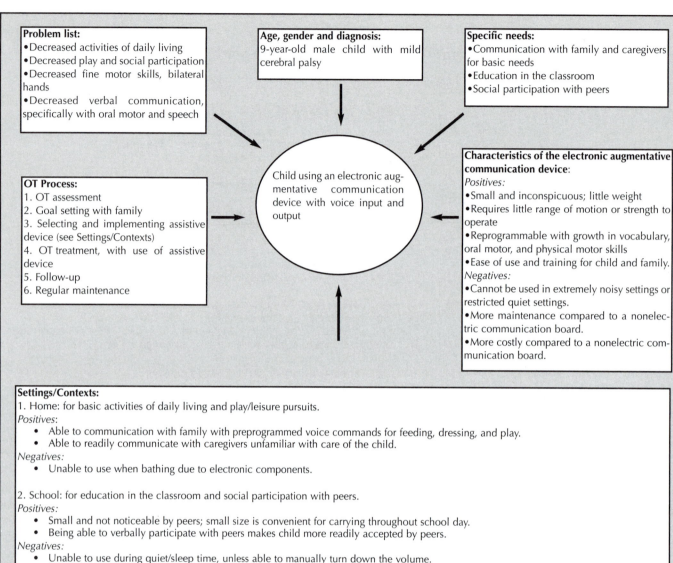

Figure 23-1. The context within various factors of assistive technology implementation.

Assistive Technology in Context

When designing or purchasing an assistive device, the setting in which it will be used is an important consideration to take into account because an assistive device used in one setting may not be appropriate for another. For example, an electronic communication board with voice input and output used in the privacy of child's home may not be appropriate in a noisy community setting as the child's voice may not be detected by the computer, or in a quiet context (i.e., library, movie theatre) where the child's voice would disturb other people (Figure 23-1).

Given the child's salient occupations of play, leisure, and education, assistive technology is most commonly used within the school, home, and community. In the school setting, assistive devices typically include devices or equipment to increase mobility, learning, and socialization in the classroom, such as mouthsticks, communication aids (i.e., AAC aids), switches, computers, pointers, mobility and positioning devices, and organizational and time management aids to enhance learning. In the home settings, assistive technology typically consists of assistive ADL devices for self care, environmental control units for mastering environmental challenges, computers for play, leisure, and educational pursuits, and communication devices to enhance functional communication with peers and family/caregivers. In the community setting, assistive technology is commonly used to support leisure and entertainment pursuits such as socializing with peers with use of a communication board or eating meals at a restaurant with use of adaptive utensils. For community mobility, a child with functional mobility or endurance issues may use a power wheelchair for shopping or traveling.

The Occupational Therapy Framework: Domain and Processes (2002) identifies seven primary contexts that influence the performance of the child: social, cultural, physical, personal, temporal, virtual, and spiritual. Each will be discussed with regard to assistive technology.

The *social* context, an extremely important factor in the application of assistive technology, encompasses societal norms that influence a child's self-esteem. Children with disabilities can be stigmatized and labeled as 'different' for using assistive technology. Relative to social norms, the OT practitioner should balance choosing devices that are not only functional, but also socially acceptable, in terms of what is considered "normal" or expected for the child and parents/caregivers in their particular society.

Related to the social context is the *cultural* context, which includes beliefs and values of the child and his or her family/caregivers. It is important to consider the cultural context when selecting and implementing assistive technology. Differing cultural values/beliefs, difficulty in understanding, or miscommunication between the OT practitioner and the child and his or her family/caregivers may lead to difficulty in not only compliance, but also achieving or establishing mutual and beneficial goals (Cook & Hussey, 2002) for the child.

The *physical* context includes the nonhuman and environmental conditions in which the assistive technology is being used, such as the furniture or devices within the classroom or building. The physical context also refers to the temperature (i.e., thermal heat, cold), noise (i.e., sounds, feedback cues), or light (i.e., the amount of light available). Assessing the physical context is vital to assistive technology implementation and can be crucial to a successful performance of an assistive device for a child. For example, if the room is too noisy, a child with decreased attention or auditory sensation may not be able to focus or hear the beeps of an electronic augmentative device, respectively. Or a child with low vision may require a room with greater illuminance in order to see the buttons on a modified keyboard of a computer.

The *personal* context includes the gender, age, educational status, and socioeconomic status of a child (AOTA, 2002). With the consideration that a child will continue to grow, the personal and temporal contexts are extremely important factors in the selection process of fitting the appropriate assistive device to the child. Should the OT practitioner purchase a new assistive device every few years as the child outgrows the previous device? If the family cannot afford to purchase numerous assistive devices, then should the OT select a device that can be modified as the child grows? An OT practitioner must consider the socioeconomic status of a child's family when choosing an assistive device. If cost is an issue, should the OT practitioner simply construct the assistive device? What state or federal funding options are available? Often times, finding appropriate funding will be a major obstacle in implementation of assistive technology. OT practitioners may have to be prepared to search for less expensive or low tech devices that will be as functional as an expensive high tech device.

The *temporal* context is closely related to the personal context in that it refers to the life stage of a child, and the duration and time with respect to days and years (AOTA, 2002). Certain assistive devices are designed for different age groups. For example, communication boards for infants are smaller and simple in design, compared to larger and more complex items/pictures on the communication board for an older child, and even more so for a teenager. Assistive devices may be used during certain times of the day (e.g., daytime, nighttime) or even certain times of the year (e.g., summertime, wintertime).

The *virtual* context is communication by means of computers, without physical contact. This context is becoming more relevant with the increase in computer technology and increase in accessibility, and popularity of e-mail and chatting online available to children. With the improvements in mainstream computer technology, more and more children with disabilities are now able to access online chatting and e-mail. Thus, specialized assistive devices for computers, especially high tech devices, are becoming increasingly available on the commercial market.

The *spiritual* context is often difficult to assess with a child, given that inspiration and motivation are constantly developing and being shaped as the child grows. Improved access to toys, communication, and self-care via high or low tech devices may become a positive source of inspiration or motivation for a child's functional performance outcomes.

The seven contextual factors described above collectively influence the functional performance of a child, and for successful implementation of assistive technology, the OT practitioner must consider all contextual areas for positive outcomes in occupational therapy intervention.

Role of the Occupational Therapy Assistant in Assistive Technology "Work"

The OT practitioner plays an important role in the planning, selection, implementation, treatment process, and family/caregiver training involved with assistive technology. Under the supervision of an OT, the occupational therapy assistant (OTA) may assist (depending on demonstrated level of competency and state and facility guidelines) with the evaluation and data collection, collaborate with the OT in providing occupational therapy services, and participate in management of the assistive technologies. Following the evaluation of the functional status of a child (i.e., physical evaluation, history intake, functional assessment) (AMA, 1996), goal development and treatment planning are initiated by introducing the appropriate assistive device to the child. The OT practitioner must observe the interaction between the child and device to determine its efficacy. The OTA must follow typical treatment protocols set forth by the supervising OT and treatment facility, and depending on the setting and the OTAs demonstrated level of competency, may make recommendations for any modifications and/or changes to the assistive device/aid until the desired functional outcome is achieved. With regards to goal-setting and assistive technology, OT practitioners may collaborate to prepare functional and measurable goals for a child to use assistive technology devices in a context specific manner, and within a given time frame. Goals can be numerous, however, are usually specific to functional areas, such as ADLs and play/leisure. Goals should be measurable, and be written with a specific assistive device in mind if the goal is to specifically address using a specific piece of equipment (goal #1), or broader if nonspecific assistive equipment is to be used in treatment (goal #2):

Goal 1: Child will use the adaptive fork with built-up handle to increase self-feeding for 30 minutes, 5 to 7 times a week with minimum assistance from the therapist.

Goal 2: Child will independently incorporate assistive equipment to increase participation in writing, art, and construction activities 50% of the time, 3 to 5 times a week.

As previously discussed, selecting the appropriate assistive device for treatment involves examining the purposefulness and meaningfulness of an assistive device to the child, examining issues and barriers to progress, and evaluating the environments in which the child participates on a daily basis. Additionally, the OT practitioner works within the guiding principles of specific frames of reference (please

refer to Chapter 3: A Brief Overview of Occupational Therapy Theories, Models, and Frames of Reference) and considers the child's strengths and challenges, existing short- and long-term goals, the relevant performance components in which the child will be using the device, as well as the problem list. Take Ingrid, who loves animals. She demonstrates decreased fine motor coordination and play participation. The OT practitioner wants to improve her fine motor skills in order to increase independence of play participation. Ingrid has many motorized toy animals, however is unable to operate the small on/off lever switch underneath the animal, which makes Ingrid frustrated and unhappy (Figure 23-2). What can the therapist do (Figures 23-3 and 23-4)?

As Ingrid is playing with the adapted toy dog, more generic questions that are pertinent to the selection of the switch are:

- Can the child approach, contact, and release the switch with adequate speed and control using his or her hand (Figure 23-5)?

- Can he or she do the above activity for a predetermined time period? OR: What is the baseline duration of time the child can play with the toy?

- Could the switch be modified, or could other switches be used? Could the switch be used with body parts other than the hand (Figure 23-6)?

- Does child have the potential ability to independently use this technology device?

- Is there a low tech alternative?

- Will the child use this assistive device at home and/or in the community?

- Will the child be able to transfer learning to use the switch in a play situation/context, to ultimately, an educational one?

There are numerous types of switches available today, each with distinct and common features that can be adapted in a variety of ways. Table 23-2 contains a description of ten common switches used by occupational therapy practitioners.

When choosing the most appropriate adaptive switch for a child, it is helpful to consider the following:

1. Choose a switch that will match a child's targeting ability, in terms of perception (i.e., for feedback), range of motion, strength, and muscle tone.

2. Choose a switch that will be most functional for the child, not just the device. Although certain switches may be designed for specific devices (i.e., a computer), switches can be used/adapted to improve a specific functional area of a child with a disability.

3. Choose a switch that will not cause any pain or fatigue for the child when using the switch, as well as any subsequent pain, fatigue, or other negative effects after using the switch.

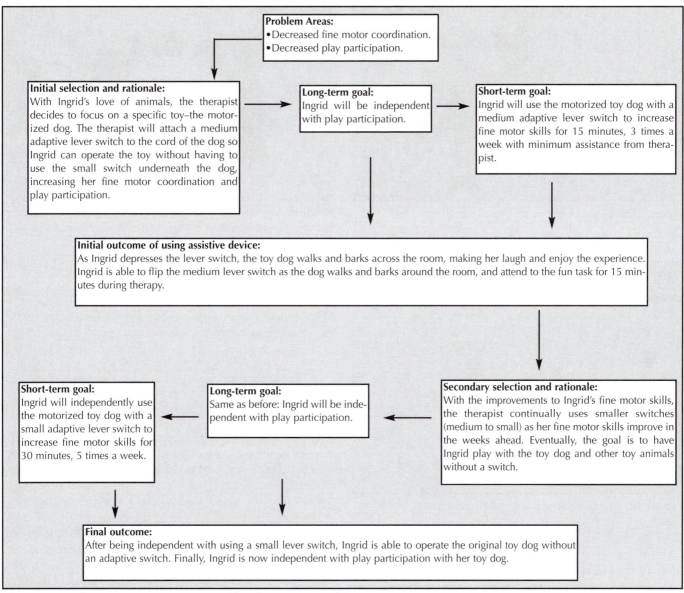

Problem Areas:
- Decreased fine motor coordination.
- Decreased play participation.

Initial selection and rationale:
With Ingrid's love of animals, the therapist decides to focus on a specific toy–the motorized dog. The therapist will attach a medium adaptive lever switch to the cord of the dog so Ingrid can operate the toy without having to use the small switch underneath the dog, increasing her fine motor coordination and play participation.

Long-term goal:
Ingrid will be independent with play participation.

Short-term goal:
Ingrid will use the motorized toy dog with a medium adaptive lever switch to increase fine motor skills for 15 minutes, 3 times a week with minimum assistance from therapist.

Initial outcome of using assistive device:
As Ingrid depresses the lever switch, the toy dog walks and barks across the room, making her laugh and enjoy the experience. Ingrid is able to flip the medium lever switch as the dog walks and barks around the room, and attend to the fun task for 15 minutes during therapy.

Short-term goal:
Ingrid will independently use the motorized toy dog with a small adaptive lever switch to increase fine motor skills for 30 minutes, 5 times a week.

Long-term goal:
Same as before: Ingrid will be independent with play participation.

Secondary selection and rationale:
With the improvements to Ingrid's fine motor skills, the therapist continually uses smaller switches (medium to small) as her fine motor skills improve in the weeks ahead. Eventually, the goal is to have Ingrid play with the toy dog and other toy animals without a switch.

Final outcome:
After being independent with using a small lever switch, Ingrid is able to operate the original toy dog without an adaptive switch. Finally, Ingrid is now independent with play participation with her toy dog.

Figure 23-2. Selecting assistive equipment within the occupational therapy process.

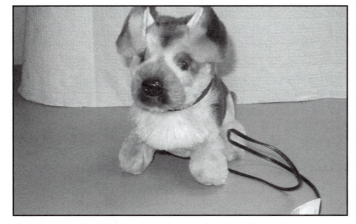

Figure 23-3. A switch-activated, adaptive dog. Front view.

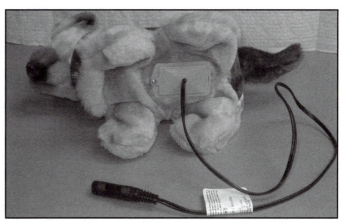

Figure 23-4. A switch-activated, adaptive dog. Bottom view.

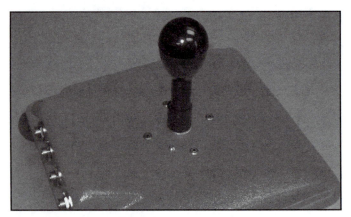

Figure 23-5. A joystick switch.

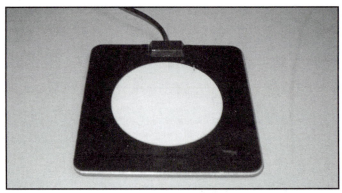

Figure 23-6. A plate switch. This thin, flat switch can activate any switch-adapted device by depressing the yellow circle (for visual contrast with black square) with a finger, hand, elbow, knee, foot, etc.

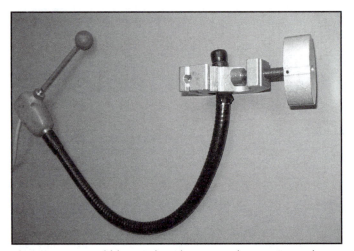

Figure 23-7. A wobble switch with gooseneck mounting and clamp.

4. Choose a switch that uses a child's body part (i.e., hand, feet, head) that will provide the best and most consistent control.

5. Choose a switch that can be conveniently placed/mounted within functional reaching distance for the child. Sometimes a switch will be mounted on the arm of a wheelchair, or even attached to a body part of the child (Figure 23-7).

Assistive technology should never be recommended or used without proper and appropriate caregiver and/or family training. Once implementation of assistive technology takes place, it is important to provide family/caregiver training to maximize the device/aid's functional purpose. Training involves instruction on proper use and maintenance of the assistive device, as well as any potential contraindications relative to the device. Family/caregiver train-

ing is provided to increase carryover for the child to use the assistive device across settings such as the treatment facility, home, and community.

Reflections for the OTA

Assistive technology should only be recommended or used with proper and appropriate caregiver and/or family training.

The OTA may, depending on demonstrated level of competency, assist with the construction/fabrication or ordering of assistive devices, and provide direct treatment and parent/caregiver training. A multitude of assistive technology devices may be purchased through healthcare suppliers, retail stores, or online. Budget and time restrictions, as well as the uniqueness of the child's functional limitations and problems may require individualized construction of the assistive technology device to ensure a better fit and enhanced solution to a specific problem (Ryan, 1993). To best suit each child, individualized construction of assistive devices necessitates that they be unique and diverse in their scope; from the simple fabrication of card holders for leisure pursuits to battery interrupters for use with motorized toys and portable listening devices.

A battery interrupter is one example of an individually constructed assistive technology device that the OTA, depending on demonstrated level of competency, can fabricate for a child. It is a mechanical device that is used to control a battery-powered product via an adaptive switch. Essentially, it is an interface that interrupts the circuit of a device, converting an ordinary product or toy into a potential assistive device. There are three basic parts to a battery interrupter: 1) the PC board, which is place between the batteries to stop the flow of electricity, 2) the switch, which

Table 23-2

Common Switches Used in Pediatric Assistive Technology

Type	*Description*	*Important Considerations*
Button Switch 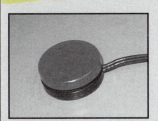	One of the most commonly used switches in assistive technology, this is a simple pressure switch that is usually round-shaped. It is a single switch that turns on/off a device from a push of a button.	Easy to operate with a large target area for children with decreased fine motor control. Durable and can be attached almost anywhere on the body, on walls, and/or on a tabletop. Comes in a variety of colors, sizes, shapes, and activation forces. Good for children with low vision in discriminating between switches, such as green for "proceed" and red for "stop". Has an audible click for activation feedback.
Lever Switch	This is also a simple pressure switch that flips in one direction to turn on/off a device. This single switch can be modified to keep the device on when the lever is depressed and turned off when the lever is released.	Comes in a variety of sizes and shapes. Good for children with decreased upper extremity range of motion. Has an audible click feedback.
Pillow Switch 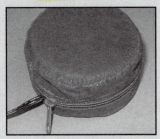	Similar to a button switch, this is a single, pressure switch that is covered by a cushy, soft-cloth casing (hence referred to as a pillow).	A child can squeeze, grasp, or push the switch to activate a device. Good for children with poor grasp control. Because of its soft covering, it is good for use with sensitive sites, such as the face or a postinjury site (may need to clean the covering to keep it hygienic). Comes in a variety of sizes. Has an activation click for auditory feedback (although sound usually reduced by cloth coverings). Although it can be unfavorable for children with tactile defensiveness, it can be used beneficially (i.e., desensitization).
Pneumatic Switch 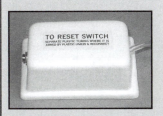	This is an air-pressure controlled switch. A child pushes a bulb-shaped switch, which forces the air into an apparatus box; that in turn automatically depresses a microswitch inside.	The bulb is usually rubber-lined so it has good tactile feedback. It comes in a variety of shapes (i.e., square, circular) and sizes (i.e., flat, round). A commonly used pneumatic switch is the Sip n Puff switch, which has two microswitches on either side of the apparatus box that performs two actions—one is with inhalation (the "sip") and the other is exhalation (the "puff"). This device is a pressure switch that can be used for dual switch actions (see rocker switch).
Sound/Voice-activated Switch	This non-pressure switch is operated through electrical sensors that respond to sound stimuli (i.e., hand clap, oral/verbal words). For example, a device is turned on when a child says, "on" and turns the device off when the child says, "off".	No physical movement needed. Need to assess environmental conditions as background noise may interfere. Also, this switch may not be appropriate in community locations such as the workplace, movie theater, or library.
Tilt Switch	This is a non-pressure, single switch that is usually attached to a body part. It is composed of a ball floating within liquid inside a tilting mechanism. When the mechanism is tilted to one side by moving a body part (i.e., a child tilts his/her head to the side), the ball connects the switch and the device turns on.	May be used with various parts of the body that are movable, including the fingers, arms, legs, or head. A certain amount of range of motion is needed (usually about 90 degrees). The weight of the switch itself can be a means for feedback, and can be used as a cuing mechanism.

Within the pneumatic switch image: TO RESET SWITCH / SEPARATE PLASTIC TUBING WHERE IT IS JOINED BY PLASTIC UNION & RECONNECT

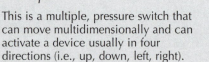

Common Switches Used in Pediatric Assistive Technology

Type	*Description*	*Important Considerations*
Joystick Switch 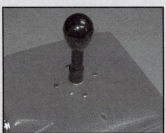	This is a multiple, pressure switch that can move multidimensionally and can activate a device usually in four directions (i.e., up, down, left, right). Depending on the type and complexity, this switch may also move diagonally.	Depending on the level of hand and upper extremity function, the joysticks can be modified with different size balls or even a "T"-post for hand/wrist placement on the horizontal bar of the "T". Recommended for children with a fair amount of upper extremity range of motion and control. A small ball or object is usually connected to the top of the switch for grip and control.
Rocker Switch 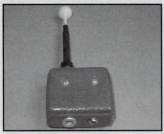	This is a pressure, dual switch. It is basically composed of two single switches, which pivots at the center of both switches.	Similar to the dual functionality of the sip and puff switch, the rocker switch is unique and beneficial for scanning selections, such as first moving through a list and secondly, selecting an item from the list. For example, a child can select the category "fruit", and then can move the switch down until it reaches "apple".
Wobble Switch	This is a pressure, single switch that can move and activate in any four directions (left, right, up, down). It is usually composed of a flexible wand with a ball attached on the end.	This switch can be used by multiple body parts, usually the head or elbow. May require children with moderate amount of range of motion to activate. Has an audible click for feedback. Usually will require mounting on a solid surface or support (i.e., gooseneck).
Proximity Switch	This is a non-pressure, single switch that responds by physical proximity of a body part, such as placing a hand near or over the switch box. The internal sensors are usually heat sensors that activate the device when a body part (i.e., hand, foot) nears the switch.	This switch is advantageous for children with little range of motion in the upper or lower extremities. Also, minimal strength is required to activate the switch. The sensor sensitivity can be adjusted for proximity distance and for length of proximity time. Proximity switches usually are more costly than other switches.
Photocell Switch 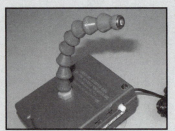	This is a non-pressure, single switch that operates by waving a hand or object part across a sensor. The sensor detects surrounding light levels, and is activated by movement by a body part (i.e., hand, foot) or non-human object (i.e., stick, reacher).	This switch requires children with limited range of motion or strength for activation of the switch. The sensor sensitivity is usually adjustable for the proximity and/or amount of movement required for the activation of the device. The physical environment must be assessed because different lighting levels may interfere with the operation of the switch. Like proximity switches, photocell switches are usually also more costly than other switches.

(Adapted from Burwell, 2001.)

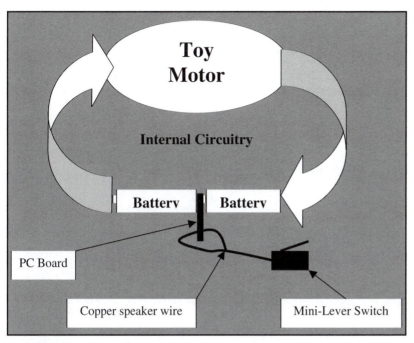

Figure 23-15. A conceptual design of a battery interrupter stopping the electricity flow of the battery-powered toy. The arrows represent the flow of electricity.

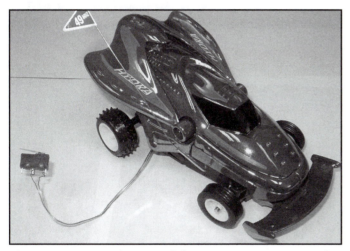

Figure 23-16. A mini-lever switch battery interrupter in use with a toy car. Side view.

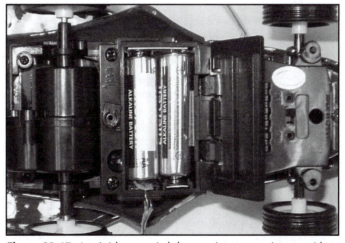

Figure 23-17. A mini-lever switch battery interrupter in use with a toy car. Bottom view.

controls the flow of electricity, and 3) the wiring to connect the PC board to the switch (Figure 23-15). When a child depresses the switch (or turns on the device), the current flows through the circuit and the battery current reaches the motor, making the device operational. When the child releases the switch (turning off the switch), the circuit is broken, making the device inoperative. Battery interrupters are appropriate for children with poor fine motor dexterity, low vision, and sensory integration deficits (i.e., tactile). For example, OT practitioners may use battery interrupters attached to a toy as a treatment option for children with tactile defensiveness. By attaching various tactile stimuli sheets (i.e., cotton cloths, sandpaper) to the switch, the child depresses the switches covered with the various stimuli. The child then experiences different tactile stimuli while playing with the toy (Figures 23-15 through 23-17).

Today, there are many high and low tech assistive technology devices available to diminish the impact of functional impairments, such as decreased functional mobility (i.e., grasp strength, coordination, muscle atrophy/weakness, joint limitations), cognition (i.e., decreased memory), and communication (i.e., decreased oral and auditory processes). As we continue further into the technological era, increasingly innovative assistive devices will be introduced

Environment:
-Work in a well-ventilated and well-light room, with a safe insulated electrical outlet.
-Recommend working on large flat tables.
-Remove any unnecessary clutter from the workstations.

Materials required:
1. Mini lever switch. Can be purchased at a local radio or electronic store.
2. Solder (rosin core)
3. 1 sheet of 1/32" thick dual-sided printed circuit (PC) board (copper-plastic/fiberglass-copper layers)
4. Copper speaker wire; 8-12" in length; 24 gauge; 2 conductor; non-stranded

Tools required:
1. Soldering iron
2. Tin Snips
3. Durable scissors
4. Wire cutter with wire stripper notch

Setting up the wiring:
1. With the wire cutter, splice both ends of the copper wire apart by cutting the wire lengthwise about one inch up the center of the wire. Both ends should be 'Y'-shaped.
2. Strip the plastic covering on all four ends of the wire by using the notch on the wire cutter. The copper wire on all four ends should be sticking out of the plastic covering.

| 1 |

Setting up the PC board:
1. With the tin snips, carefully cut out a rectangular piece of the PC board from the sheet, about ½ inch wide and 1 inch in length. The PC board may crack during the cutting so be careful with the sharp edges.
2. With the scissors, cut the edges cleanly so that no piece of copper/fiberglass is fraying out.

| 2 |

Solder the one end of the wire to the PC board:
1. With a dry towel or tissue, wipe the PC board surface clean.
2. Preheat the soldering iron.
3. Choose either end of the wire, and solder one side of the 'Y' to one side of the PC board by carefully feeding the solder into the tip of the soldering iron. The solder will melt into liquid metal and quickly dry to create a metal bond between the wire and PC board. Try to make this bond as flat as possible. Be careful not to inhale too much solder smoke.
4. Solder the other Y-side of the same end of the wire to the other side of the PC board. Make sure both wires are not in contact with each other.

| 3 |

Solder the other end of the wire to the lever switch:
1. With the copper tips of the wire, wrap one end of the wire through the hole of end of the metal connection.
2. Solder the connection to ensure a permanent bond.
3. Repeat the wrapping of the other end of the wire to the other end of the switch. Solder that connection. Make sure both wires are not in contact with each other.

| 4 |

Attaching the battery interrupter to the device:
1. With the device on, carefully stick the PC board of the battery interrupter between the batteries. If the device only runs on one battery, place the PC board at either end of the battery. This should turn the device off.
2. Now the toy/device is a potential assistive device. Turn on the device by depressing the lever. Simply turn off the device by releasing the lever.

| Complete |

Figure 23-18. Constructing a simple lever switch battery interrupter.

into today's society. Table 23-3 is beginning list of common high and low tech assistive devices used by OT practitioners.

Funding, Reimbursement, and Legislation

In order to provide cutting-edge services for children with disabilities, OT and assistive technology practitioners need to be familiar with current funding sources and eligibility requirements. Assistive technology services and adaptive devices can be costly and may be beyond the financial reach of some potential users. Fortunately, numerous funding options are available (Lazarro, 2001), including those for children and their families. With respect to assistive technology in pediatrics, there are three general types of funding sources available: public, private, and other (AMA, 1996; Cook & Hussey, 2002; Lazarro, 2001; MATP, 1998).

PUBLIC FUNDING

Federal Level: The Individuals with Disabilities Education Act (IDEA) entitles all children (aged 0 to 18), regardless of their disability, to a free and appropriate public education. Part B of IDEA (for children aged 3 to 18) requires local school districts/systems to provide access to assistive technology services and devices if documented in a child's Individualized Education Plan (IEP). Alternatively, parents/caregivers may elect to use their private insurance to obtain assistive technology services. Part C of IDEA mandates that infants and toddlers (aged 0 to 3 years) enrolled in Early Intervention (EI) programs be eligible for assistive technology services and devices if it is written in their Individualized Family Service Plan (IFSP).

State Level: Through funding at state departments of public health, uninsured children aged 0 to 18 are eligible for health coverage at very little or no cost to the family/caregiver, and are also eligible for medical diagnosis and evaluation (MATP, 1998). In addition, some states in the U.S. cover assistive technology services and devices through a program called the Children's Medical Services (CMS) (MATP, 1998).

Reflections for the OTA

In Massachusetts, under expanded Medicaid (called MassHealth in Massachusetts) eligibility guidelines, children aged 0-18 can enroll in a program with full or primary coverage for preventative care, depending on family/caregiver income. If a child is not eligible, he/she may enroll in a program called the Children's Medical Security Plan (CMSP). In addition to these health coverage options, Massachusetts offers the Early and Periodic Screening, Diagnosis, and Treatment (EPSDT) program, which provides a comprehensive

medical screen, including an assistive technology assessment, for any Medicaid-eligible child under the age of 18 (MATP, 1998). This program is designed to assess health problems/needs early in a child's life in order to prevent costly and more complex interventions/treatments in the future.

Infants and toddlers enrolled in EI programs funded through state departments of public health are also eligible for assistive technology services and devices (MATP, 1998). For instance, a Medicaid, program called the Early and Periodic Screening, Diagnosis, and Treatment (EPSDT) program provides expanded services to children with disabilities and has funding to purchase assistive technology devices for children aged 0-3. The OTA is encouraged to review individual state regulations regarding funding and provision of AT services and devices (Table 23-4).

PRIVATE FUNDING

Available federal and state funding for purchase of assistive technology devices is extremely beneficial to parents/caregivers. Assistive technology devices that the family/caregiver elects to purchase on a private basis calls upon the OT practitioner to be creative and innovative in finding the best fit. Finding and matching an assistive device that meets the family/caregiver's budget is important because evaluating and implementing the proper device, as well as the cost of follow-up and regular maintenance of such devices may be costly. For instance, high-tech devices, such as environmental control units and computers are costly to purchase and use for long periods of time. Having functional knowledge of the purpose, design, and cost of the assistive device empowers the family/caregivers to choose the most effective and least expensive option (Lazarro, 2001). In addition to self-pay, another private source of funding is through the family/caregiver's private health insurance. As every insurance policy is variable and different, it is up to the family/caregiver to review specific details on coverage for the assistive technology device.

OTHER SOURCES

Other sources for funding of assistive technology include local and community service clubs, private foundations (i.e., Easter Seals Society), and volunteer organizations. Independent living centers may also be resources for obtaining assistive equipment and the help and expertise of assistive technology specialists. Independent living centers may be located by contacting local or state rehabilitation agencies.

Due to a relatively small, but growing consumer market, implementing high tech assistive technology remains an expensive option when working with children. Searching for the appropriate funding must be comprehensive, and is often challenging when one considers the paperwork and phone calling involved in obtaining the most cost effective

Table 23-3

Assistive Technology Devices Commonly Used With the Pediatrics Population

Assistive Device/Aid Category

Activities of Daily Living
(Please refer to Chapter 15: Self-Care,
for pictures of ADL-related assistive
technology devices.)

Instrumental Activities of Daily Living
(Please refer to Chapter 15: Self-Care,
for pictures of IADL-related assistive
technology devices.)

Play and Leisure

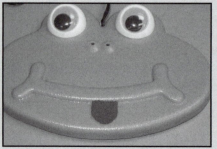

Common Examples of Items

Feeding
Plate guards
Scoop dish
Adapted silverware
• built-up handles
• bent forks
• weighted spoons
• rocker knife
• Velcro straps attached to
  silverware
Dycem™ and grips
Universal cuff
Electric mobile arm supports,
  feeding systems

Bathing
Grab bars
Long handled sponge with
  adaptive handle
Extended sink and tub faucet levers
Bath mat
Bath mitt
Shower stall chair, tub seat,
  extended tub bench
Shower hose
Electric Powered bath lift

Dressing
Dressing stick
Button hooks
Special clothing
Velcro™
Reachers

Toileting
Raised toilet seat
Commode
Grab bars, Arms

Functional Mobility
Bed rails
Manual wheelchairs
Walkers
Crutches
Power wheelchairs
Electric powered beds (adjustable beds)
Stair lift

Memory aids
Task reminders for daily schedule and medication routine

Reading
Mouthstick
Page turners
Book holders
Magnifying glass

Writing
Pen with wide and contoured grip
Pen holder
Raised line paper

Toys (Adapted toy switches, constructed toys)
Battery interrupters
Games
Computers, assorted software
Card Holder, adapted playing cards

Arts/Crafts
Modified gardening tools with built-up handles
(Please refer to Chapter 14: Childhood Occupations, for further information.)

Table 23-3 (continued)

Assistive Technology Devices Commonly Used With the Pediatrics Population

Assistive Device/Aid Category

Common Examples of Items

Social Communication

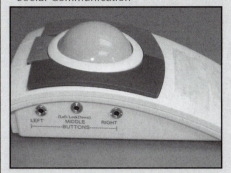

Augmentative/alternative communication (AAC) systems
Communication boards
> *Low-tech*: cardboard overlays, paper & pencil, typing aids
> *High-tech*: electronic keyboard overlays (i.e., Intellikeys™), laptops/computer tablets, electronics, human-computer interaction software
> AT devices: Mouthstick, head-pointer, universal cuff with typing aid

Sensory

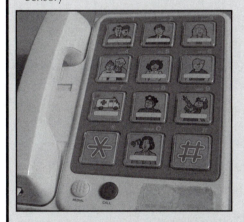

Auditory/Hearing
Assistive listening devices (i.e., hearing/amplification aids, cochlear implants)
Sound systems and noise reduction devices
Telecommunication devices (i.e., TTY, TDD).

Tactile
Adaptive switches (i.e., pillow switch). See Table 23-2: Common Switches.

Vision
Low-vision aids
Screen readers for visually-impaired
Screen magnification for computers
Magnifying glasses, large print
Braille
Lighting and alerting devices
Telephone alerting devices
(Please refer to Chapter 16: Visual Perceptual Dysfunction and Low Vision Rehabilitation for related information.)

Environmental Control

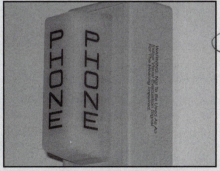

Environmental Control Units (ECUs)
X-10™ (http://www.x10.com)
Adaptive switches and buttons

Structural
Modifying pathways, installing lifts, automatic doors, and ramps for enhanced mobility
Increased lighting children with vision impairments
Visual alerts for children with hearing impairments

Seating, Positioning, Orthotics, and Prosthetics

Trunk, Upper and Lower Extremity Support Systems
Refer to Chapter 11: Positioning in Pediatrics
Refer to Chapter 24: Orthotics

Table 23-4

Legislation Relating to Assistive Technology

Year	Legislation	Description and Summary
1975	The Education for All Handicapped Children Act (P.L. 94-142)	This legislation mandates free and appropriate public education for all children with disabilities. It is the main federal source of funding for special education programs.
1988	The Technology-Related Assistance for Individuals with Disabilities Act (P.L. 100-407)	"The Tech Act" defines assistive technology services and devices, assists states in developing comprehensive, open-consumer programs on a state level, and provides appropriate technology resources to individuals with disabilities and their family/caregivers. Every state has federally funded Tech Act projects.
1990	The Americans with Disabilities Act (ADA) (P.L. 101-476)	The ADA guaranteed equal opportunity and full civil rights for individuals with disabilities in public accommodation, transportation, local and state government services, telecommunications, and employment.
1990	Individuals with Disabilities Education Act (IDEA) (P.L. 101-476)	The IDEA mandated assistive technology services be included in an IEP, and also included children and youth with traumatic brain injury and autism as eligible for special education.
1991	Individuals with Disabilities Education Act Amendments	The IDEA was amended to include assistive technology services to Part H for infants and preschoolers with disabilities.
1997	Individuals with Disabilities Education Act Amendments	The IDEA was amended to require that assistive technology be considered for every student who received special education services.

devices possible. However, the potential benefits of implementing assistive technology to enhance functional performance for the child with disabilities as well as to observe improvements in the well-being and self-esteem of the child who successfully uses, and feels good using assistive technology is well worth the effort.

Related Resources and Websites

In today's world of technology and information, there are a wealth of resources to access information about assistive technology on the World Wide Web (WWW), from community centers and educational institutions (i.e., universities), to private vendors. Additionally, every state in the US has a federally funded state assistive technology partnership (MATP, 1998). These partnerships serve as a valuable and beneficial resource for OT practitioners when searching for information on services and devices relating to assistive technology. When searching for information online, it is helpful to consider the following:

1. The last update of a website. Websites usually indicate the last update on bottom of the index page (first webpage). Non-updated websites may have outdated prices and information on assistive devices. You may need to hit F5 (on your keyboard) to refresh the website, or click on the 'refresh' button of the navigator button bar.

2. With regard to a specific assistive device, check to see if there is research to support the device, or if it has been tested for safety and usability. New models are constantly being introduced on the marketplace. Although price is important, safety should always be a priority.

3. Cross-check several websites and/or vendors. Always check several websites on assistive technology devices to compare prices and models. Prior to a purchase of an assistive device, you should be confident with the current competitive prices.

4. Source, quality, and reputation of the vendor. Websites that advertise and promote products may have different vendors. Feel free to inquire assistive technology specialists or attend conferences and expositions (see below) for the quality, service, and reputation of specific vendors and dealers.

Reflections for the OTA

Need help with assistive technology and don't know where to start? Every state has a federally funded assistive technology program, so start with your state assistive technology center!

The websites below provide useful information about pediatric-based assistive technology and occupational therapy:

Abledata: A national database of information on more than 17,000 products that are currently available for people with disabilities (http://www.abledata.com)

American Occupational Therapy Association (AOTA): The official website of the American Occupational Therapy Association. Provides literature and information on assistive technology-related issues, as well as a technology special interest section, which publishes a quarterly newsletter introducing or discussing current and upcoming technology in the field of occupational therapy (http://www.aota.org).

Assistive Technology Education Network (ATEN): the Florida Diagnostic and Learning Resources System (FDLRS) Specialized Center; the site offers tutorials that can be downloaded on a variety of assistive technology. (http://www.aten.scps.k12.fl.us)

Learning Disabilities Online: Provides an interactive guide regarding learning disabilities for children, parents, and teachers. (http://www.ldonline.org)

Massachusetts Assistive Technology Partnership (MATP): An organization in Boston, dedicated to increasing access and advocacy regarding assistive technology for people of all ages and all disabilities through a variety of consumer activities. (http://www.matp.org).

RESNA: Rehabilitation Engineering and Assistive Technology Society of North America - A professional organization that aims to promote advocacy, research, and education of people with disabilities through through the use of technology. Includes information on certification courses. (http://www.resna.org)

Spaulding Rehabilitation Hospital Assistive Technology Center (ATEC): An inpatient and outpatient assistive technology specialist center for assistive technology utilization, located in Boston, MA for persons of all ages (children, adults, geriatrics). (http://www.spauldingrehab.org)

Wisconsin Assistive Technology Initiative (WATI): A statewide project to help all school districts develop or improve their assistive technology services; provides good resources and links to other assistive technology-related sites. (http://www.wati.org)

Other useful sources for assistive technology products, education, and services include conferences and expositions, where vendors, dealers, and assistive technology specialists display their services and advertise their products. Below is a list of national conferences and expositions that include pediatric assistive technology.

Abilities Expo: National and regional expositions on independent and assisted living products and services. (http://abilitiesexpo.com)

American Occupational Therapy Association (AOTA): Annual national occupational therapy conference. See above. (http://www.aota.org)

Assistive Technology Industry Association (ATIA): Annual national conferences for the east coast. (http://www.atia.org)

California State University, Northridge: Center on Disabilities-International conference on technology and persons with disabilities. See below. (http://www.csun.edu/cod)

Closing the Gap: Annual conference on computer technology in special education and rehabilitation. (http://closingthegap.com)

Rehabilitation Engineering and Assistive Technology Society of North America (RESNA): Annual assistive technology convention and exposition. See above. (http://www.resna.org)

World Congress and Exposition on Disabilities: Annual international expositions and conferences. (http://wcdexpo.com)

Occupational therapy practitioners interested in becoming specialized in evaluating and providing assistive technology services and devices may receive further certification through distance learning programs, such as at the **California State University Center on Disabilities at Northridge, CA** (http://www.csun.edu/cod), or certification through various private organizations, such as the **Rehabilitation Engineering and Assistive Technology Society of North America (RESNA)** in Washington, D.C. (http://www.resna.org), which offers a certification program for assistive technology specialists.

Summary

This chapter provided an overview of the concepts and functional applications of assistive technology within the scope of occupational therapy, including the OT practitioner's role in the planning and implementation, treatment process, and family/caregiver training of assistive technology services. Use of assistive technology has gained increased awareness and support over the years. Today, OT practitioners integrate assistive technology into their treatment protocols in a variety of ways, depending on the short- and long-term goals of treatment and expected outcome of the child's functional performance. The goals of assistive technology implementation remains the same in all contexts, that is, OT practitioners use assistive technology as a tool or mechanism for enhancing functional performance and independence, while increasing the well-being and self-esteem of the child and the child's family/caregivers. Chapter 24 covers orthotics, which are functionally related to the subject of assistive technology, and will further the concept and applications of modern assistive technology.

ACKNOWLEDGMENT

I would like to thank the Spaulding Rehabilitation Hospital Assistive Technology Center (ATEC) for providing the adaptive switch photos.

Case Study

Edward is a 5-year-old boy of normal intelligence, diagnosed with mild cerebral palsy, resulting in speech and motor impairments. He has functional limitation with: 1) self-care skills, 2) communication, and 3) gross and fine motor development. He just entered kindergarten in a local district school nearby his home, which is located in a low-income housing project. Occupational therapy services were initiated on the first day of school.

1. What three assistive technology devices would be appropriate to use, purchase, or construct in order to meet each of his three functional needs in school? At home? In the community?

2. What are three short-term goals that include assistive technology, that would address each of the Edward's three functional limitations?

3. Which legislations are pertinent to Edward's situation, should he use assistive technology in the school?

4. How could you fund and document appropriate assistive technology for Edward?

5. Should the family/caregiver want to purchase private assistive technology for home use, what are two resources you could recommend with regards to finding the appropriate funding?

Application Activities

1. After purchasing the appropriate equipment (see Figures 23-15 and 23-18), build a battery interrupter in a laboratory session. Bring in a battery-operated toy or device (i.e., tape or CD player). At the end of the session, operate your device or toy with its newly built battery-interrupter.

2. Break into three groups. On a sheet of 9x12 paper, have each group design a communication board for a 10-year-old child who has a mild learning disability, decreased fine motor dexterity, and who needs to communicate with caregivers with all areas of ADLs. After 20 minutes, gather all groups together and discuss the positives and negatives of each of the three designs. To make this activity more fun and purposeful, vote for the best and most functional design, and give a prize to the winning group.

3. Purchase an environmental control unit (ECU). Connect three electric-powered items (i.e., light/lamp, fan, stereo) to the ECU and operate it for demonstration with the rest of the students in the class.

References

American Medical Association (AMA). (1996). *Guidelines for the use of assistive technology: Evaluation, referral, prescription* (2nd ed.). Chicago, IL.

American Occupational Therapy Association (1994). Uniform terminology for occupational therapy (3rd ed.). (1994). *American Journal of Occupational Therapy, 48*, 1047-1054.

American Occupational Therapy Association (1999). *Occupational therapy services for children and youth under the Individuals with Disabilities Education Act* (2nd ed.). Bethesda, MD: AOTA.

American Occupational Therapy Association (2002). Occupational therapy practice framework: Domain and process. *American Journal of Occupational Therapy, 56*, 609-639.

Burwell, C. M. (2001). The apprentice: A primer for assistive technology in the real world. http://www.geocities.com/at_apprentice/index.html.

Cook, A. M., & Hussey, S. M. (2002). *Assistive technologies: Principles and practice* (2nd ed.). St. Louis, MO: Mosby.

Hogan, D. P., Msall, M. E., Rogers, M. L., & Avery, R. C. (1997). Improved Disability Population Estimates of Functional Limitation Among American Children Aged 5-17. *Maternal and Child Health Journal, 1*(4), 203-216.

Jacobs, K. (1999). *Quick Reference Dictionary for Occupational Therapy* (2nd ed.). Thorofare, NJ: SLACK Incorporated.

Krantz, G. C., Christenson, M. A., & Linquist, A. (1998). *Assistive products: An illustrated guide to terminology*. Bethesda, MD: AOTA.

Kraus, L. E., Stoddard, S., & Gilmartin, D. (1996). Chartbook on disability in the United States. http://www.infouse.com/disabilitydata/p32.textgfx.html.

LaPlante, M. P., Hendershot, G. E., & Moss, A. J. (1992). *Assistive technology devices and home accessibility features: Prevalence, payment, needs, and trends* (no. 217). Hyattsville, MD: National Center for Health Statistics.

Lazarro, J. J. (2001). *Adaptive technologies for learning and work environments* (2nd ed.). Chicago, IL: American Library Association.

Massachusetts Assistive Technology Partnership (MATP). (1998). *Assistive technology: A basic training manual*. Boston, MA: MATP Center.

National Center for Health Statistics (NCHS) (2002). http://www.cdc.gov/nchs/fastats/disable.htm.

National Center for Education Statistics (NCES) (2001). http://nces.ed.gov/pubs2002/internet/6.asp.

Ryan, S. E. (1993). *The certified occupational therapy assistant: Principles, concepts and techniques*. Thorofare, NJ: SLACK Incorporated.

Trombly, C. (1995). Occupation: Purposefulness and meaningfulness as therapeutic mechanisms. *American Journal of Occupational Therapy, 49*, 960-972.

Trombly, C. (1995). *Occupational therapy for physical dysfunction*. Baltimore, MD: Williams and Wilkins.

U.S. Census Bureau (2002). http://quickfacts.census.gov/qfd/states/00000.html.

Wenger, B. L., Kaye, S., & LaPlante, M. P. (1996). *Disabilities among children*. Disability Statistics Abstract (15). Washington, DC: National Institute for Disability and Rehabilitation Research.

24

ORTHOTICS

Christy Halpin Wright, OTR/L, CHT
Nicole Jacobs, OTR/L, CHT

Chapter Objectives

- Explain the rationale behind occupational therapy practitioners providing splinting services.
- Identify the goals of pediatric splinting.
- Describe the role of the occupational therapy assistant in splint fabrication, pt. education, splint monitoring, and documentation.
- Describe what skills and knowledge base is necessary to begin splinting, including:
  a. Knowledge of anatomy
  b. Knowledge of pediatric development
  c. Knowledge of splinting tools and materials
- List techniques or splinting tips for splint fabrication specific to the pediatric population.

Introduction

When treating patients with upper extremity injuries and functional deficits, the ability to fabricate hand splints is important. As will be discussed, splint fabrication is a combination of science and art. There are many different types of splints and splinting classification systems used in occupational therapy. The most common classification system organizes splints into four categories: static, serial static, dynamic, and static progressive. Static splints are those supporting a joint or joints in one position (Colditz, 1995). Static progressive splints use inelastic components to apply torque to a joint in order to position it as close to end range

as possible. These inelastic components allow progressive changes in joint position without changes in the structure of the splint. Serial static splints provide a single position for a joint or joints, are changed frequently, and are always applied at the maximum range of the joint motion. Dynamic splints are splints that move a joint through application of the prolonged force of elastic traction. Splints are selected based on a combination of patient and occupational therapy (OT) practitioner factors. These factors include: skill level of the OT practitioner, cost, physical attributes of the splint, wearer compliance, and cognition.

An entry-level occupational therapy assistant (OTA) should possess fundamental skills in theory, design, and splint fabrication, as well as a basic understanding of upper extremity anatomy (Coppard, 1996; Schultz-Johnson, 2002). The level of splinting related skills and understanding of upper extremity anatomy will influence the degree to which an OTA may participate in the splinting process with children. At no time should an OTA fabricate or modify orthotics without the supervision of an occupational therapist (OT). This chapter will provide an overview of each of these fundamental skills as applied to the art and science of splint fabrication.

A Basic Review of Upper Extremity Anatomy

Splint fabrication and pattern design is based on an understanding of upper extremity anatomy. It is beyond the scope of this chapter to discuss the anatomy in detail. Instead, it is the intent of this chapter to review the basic

Figure 24-1.
Anatomical position.

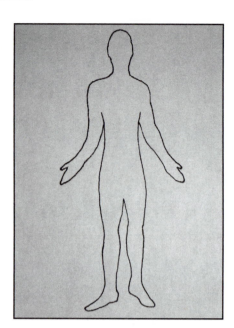

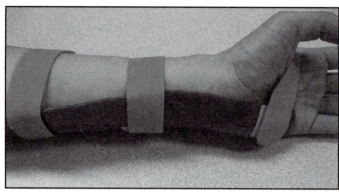

Figure 24-2. Ulnar gutter splint.

Figure 24-4.
Grasping arch.

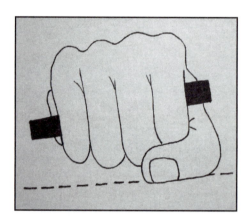

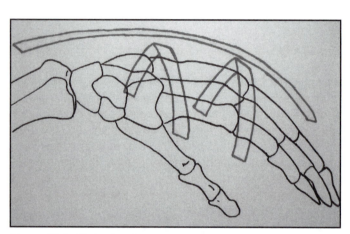

Figure 24-3. Skeletal arches.

information needed to begin splinting children's upper extremities. In order to understand written physician's orders, an OTA must possess knowledge of the terminology used to describe anatomy.

To begin, anatomical position refers to when the body is standing erect with the palms facing forward and with the thumbs out to the sides (Figure 24-1). The body is divided into three planes. The frontal plane divides the body into front and back. The transverse plane divides the body into top and bottom, and the sagittal plane divides the body into right and left sides. Other terms used to describe anatomical landmarks are volar (also called palmar) which pertains to the front of the hand when it is held in anatomical position. Dorsal describes the back of the hand where the knuckles are located. Radial refers to the thumb side of the hand and forearm, and ulnar refers to the small finger side of the hand and forearm. If a prescription/medical order reads: forearm based ulnar gutter splint with digits free, the doctor wants a

splint on the small finger side of the hand and forearm with the fingers not included. Figure 24-2 is an example of this splint.

There are three skeletal arches of the hand (Figure 24-3). The proximal transverse arch is formed by the distal row of carpal (wrist) bones and is relatively stable. The distal transverse arch is formed by the *metacarpal* (finger) heads and is more mobile. When the hand grasps, these arches deepen. The *longitudinal arch* is formed by the center carpals and the second and third metacarpal. This is a highly adaptable arch, because when the hand grasps an object, the thumb, ring finger, and small finger rotate and move around this arch to accommodate the object (Figure 24-4). The arch system may be altered by injury, abnormal muscle tone, or weakness of the intrinsic hand muscles. Certain injuries may cause flattening of the arches. The splint must be contoured to the arches in order to provide maximum functional potential and prevent *migration*.

The palmar creases of the hand serve as useful landmarks when fabricating a splint (Figure 24-5). These creases form in a direct relationship to the underlying structures. When fabricating splints, the OT practitioner must be aware of which joints underlie each crease. Splinting distal to a crease restricts motion of a specific joint, whereas splinting proximal to a crease allows motion of the joint (Hogan &

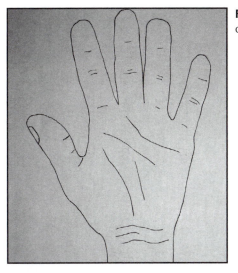

Figure 24-5. Palmar creases.

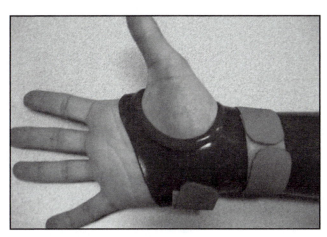

Figure 24-6. Volar cock-up.

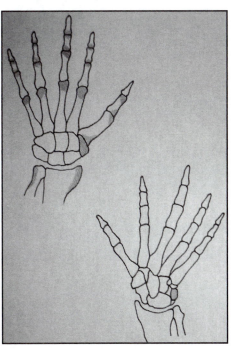

Figure 24-7. Boney prominences.

the prominences tends to be thin and easily irritated. Excess pressure in these areas may cause redness, pain, and eventual skin breakdown (Austin, 2003). The primary prominences at the elbow level are the olecranon process and the medial and lateral epicondyles. The forearm has two bony prominences. They are the ulnar styloid process and the styloid process of the radius. These are on the dorsal surface and may be easily irritated with dorsal or *circumferential splinting*. Other prominences prone to pressure sores include: the first CMC joint, dorsal thumb MP and IP joints, dorsal MP, PIP, and DIP joints of all digits, and the *pisiform* (Figure 24-7).

Using Orthotics in Pediatric Occupational Therapy Treatment

In order to determine when and why to use a pediatric splint, the purpose of the splint must first be identified. Pediatric splints are most commonly used for positioning, to increase function, to decrease hygiene problems, for protection of the extremity, or from self-injurious behavior (Charest, 2003; Hogan & Uditsky, 1998). Please refer to Table 24-1 for a problem-based splint selection chart.

SPLINTING FOR POSITION

Problems related to positioning may be the most obvious, yet the most difficult to splint. A positional splint may be used to correct contractures, provide stability or support, increase joint alignment, rest involved structures, and allow healing (Charest, 2003).

A contracture is tightening of soft tissues, which in turn leads to decreased range of motion (ROM) at a specific joint or joints. Splinting may help reduce contractures by either immobilizing or mobilizing the involved soft tissue. By immobilizing soft tissue at its maximum end range, shorten-

Uditsky, 1998). Beginning proximally and working distally, the creases are as follows: the proximal wrist crease, the distal wrist crease, the proximal palmar crease, the distal palmar crease, and the thenar crease. The thumb has two creases, the proximal and distal creases. There are three digital creases. The proximal, middle, and distal digital creases lay over the metacarpalphalangeal (MP), proximal interphalangeal (PIP), and distal interphalangeal (DIP) joints respectively. When a splint needs to immobilize only the wrist, the proximal and distal palmar crease must be cleared to allow full MP motion. The thenar crease must also be cleared to allow full thumb motion (Figure 24-6).

When fabricating and designing splints there are also bony prominences and associated features in the upper extremity that require attention. For instance, the skin over

Table 24-1

Problem-Based Splint Selection Chart

Problems	Splint Types	
Wrist Flexion	a.	Circumferential Wrist Positioning
	b.	Dorsal Wrist Cock-Up
	c.	Resting Hand
	d.	Volar Wrist Cock-Up with Radial Bare
	e.	Volar Wrist Cock-Up with Thumb Hole
Wrist Radial Deviation	a.	Dorsal Wrist Cock-Up
	b.	Long Thumb Spica
	c.	Radial Gutter
	d.	Volar Wrist Cock-Up with Radial Bar
Wrist Ulnar Deviation	a.	Dorsal Wrist Cock-Up
	b.	Neoprene Thumb-Abduction with Ulnar Gutter Insert
	c.	Ulnar Gutter
	d.	Volar Wrist Cock-up with Thumb Hole
Fisted Hand	a.	Circumferential Wrist Positioning
	b.	Dorsal Anti-Spasticity
	c.	Palmar Hygiene
	d.	Palm-Protector Cone Splint
	e.	Resting-Hand
	f.	Volar Anti-Spasticity
Thumb in Palm	a.	Hand-Based Serpentine
	b.	Long Thumb Spica
	c.	Modified Palmar Hygiene
	d.	Saddle Splint/Web Spacer
	e.	Standard Neoprene Thumb-Abduction Splint
	f.	Sof-Splint Thumb-Abduction Splint
	g.	Thumb Spica
	h.	Volar Wrist Cock-Up with Neoprene Thumb Abduction Loop
Nonweight-Bearing Through an Open Hand	a.	Clamshell
	b.	Inhibitive Weight-Bearing Mitt (IWM)
	c.	Mitt Weight-Bearing
	d.	Palmar Arch Orthosis

Modified from Hogan, L., & Uditsky, T. (1998). *Pediatric splinting: selection, fabrication and clinical application of upper extremity splints.* San Antonio, TX: Therapy Skill Builders.

ing may be prevented. Additionally, by mobilizing soft tissue over an extended period of time, lengthening of the soft tissue may occur. An unstable or hypermobile joint or joints decreases stability, which in turn will affect function (Charest, 2003; Hogan & Uditsky, 1998). A splint may provide the support needed to increase the overall function of the hand. Poor alignment of joints or repetitive use of joints may also lead to deformity. Abnormally positioned joints may not appear to be a problem at a young age, however; later in life when larger muscles and increased function place more demands on the joints, there is a risk for developing deformity. A splint may assist in deformity prevention by properly aligning these overused joints (Hogan &

Uditsky, 1998). When a joint or joints are painful and swollen, rest is needed. When pain and swelling occurs, active movement decreases and muscles become weak. For instance, a child may hold his/her hand in a position that feels less painful, but it may be one that could lead to a deformity. A splint may be fabricated to hold the hand in proper alignment until inflammation, edema, and/or pain have diminished. For example, a child with Juvenile Rheumatoid Arthritis may present with swollen, painful joints in the hand. A resting hand splint may position and rest the joints in a functional position, while providing relief to the painful joint (Figure 24-8).

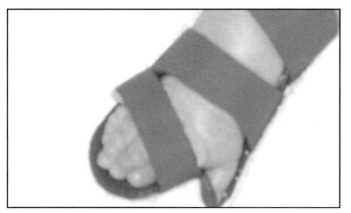

Figure 24-8. Resting hand splint.

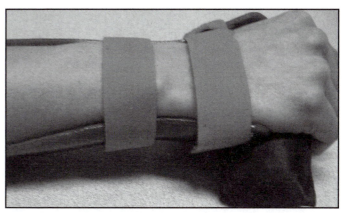

Figure 24-9. Gripping object with volar cock-up.

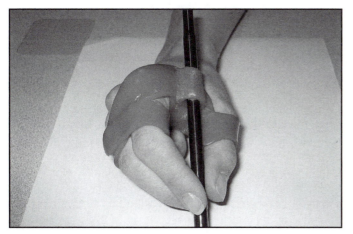

Figure 24-10. Pen/pencil holding splint.

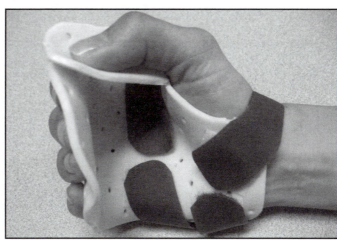

Figure 24-11. Hygiene-palm opening splint.

SPLINTING FOR FUNCTION

A functional splint may be fabricated to aid with or enhance existing function by providing support when there is weak or absent musculature. Prior to fabricating a splint for a child, it is important that the OT perform a full upper extremity functional evaluation to ensure that no independent function will be taken away by wearing a splint. The evaluation includes determining if, despite any problems, the upper extremities function, or if corrective splinting of certain joints will increase overall function. For example, if, due to muscle weakness, the wrist is positioned in extreme flexion, the child will have a weak grasp. If a splint is made to position the wrist in extension, the child's grip strength will improve (Figure 24-9).

If a child has difficulty with a particular task, the OT practitioner may fabricate a splint with a singular purpose in mind. For example, when a child has a hyper-mobile thumb, a splint may be fabricated to aide in holding objects, such as a pen or pencil (Figure 24-10).

SPLINTING FOR HYGIENE

Splints may be used to improve or prevent hygiene problems. The OT first determines the nature and extent of potential hygiene problems. Most frequently, and due to a tightly fisted posture, problems exist in the palm of the hand. A child may display red, irritated skin in the palm. If the skin breakdown is more severe, the OT practitioner may see peeling or flaking skin, and scabs or cuts from the fingernails digging into the palm. An unpleasant odor caused by sweat or inability to properly clean the hand may also be detected. In these cases, splinting may be used to open up and protect the palm (Figure 24-11).

SPLINTING FOR PROTECTION

Following injury or surgery, splinting may be used for protection. After surgery or injury, and once the pain and discomfort have subsided, a child may not understand that he/she is still injured and healing. For example, if a child has a healing wrist fracture, splinting may protect the injury during play activities. Further, and unlike a cast, the family/caregivers can remove the splint to address hygiene issues and perform range of motion (ROM) exercises during the healing process.

Sometimes it is necessary to splint children with developmental disabilities who are demonstrating self-abusive behaviors. These children may unknowingly risk their personal safety by doing things such as biting their skin or poking at their eyes. In these situations, children may benefit from splinting. For example, a child who seeks tactile input by continuously biting his/her hand may instead seek tactile input from other objects such as a soft toy, once provided with a splint that blocks elbow flexion (Figure 24-12). The OT practitioner must follow facility guidelines when fabricating a splint that might be considered a restraint. The wear, care, precautions, and purpose of a protective splint must be well documented and reviewed with the primary caregiver.

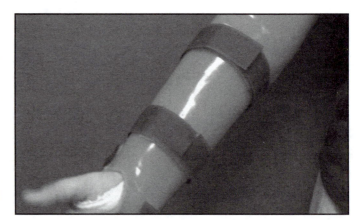

Figure 24-12. Elbow extension splint.

Planning and Implementing Orthotic Fabrication

It is easy to make the mistake of thinking that a pediatric splint is just a small adult splint. When splinting a child there are multiple needs to consider, including, anatomical structure, status of healing, tone, presence of edema, and personal compliance levels. Prioritizing these needs is essential when choosing the correct splint. The OT must first perform a thorough, personalized evaluation that assesses the general status of the hand or arm. The OT should focus on correcting one or two more significant problems through splinting, rather than trying to address all the problems at one time. The OTA may, depending on demonstrated level of competency, facility and state guidelines, and under the supervision of an OT, fabricate the actual splint. The level of supervision provided by the OT will depend on the OTA's level of experience and comfort not only with splinting, but also with children.

ANATOMIC STRUCTURES

Before an OT practitioner begins to fabricate a splint for a child, a strong understanding of anatomy and overall development, especially that of hand (function) is critical (please refer to Chapter 8: An Overview of Early Development and Chapter 18: The Development of Hand Skills). The OT must first assess the child to determine if all anatomic structures are present. If there are absent digits or structures, the *purchase* and fit of the splint will be more difficult to achieve. For example, a child with radial club hand may not have a thumb. The goal of the splint may be to stretch out the radial deformity at the wrist. Adequate purchase may be difficult because of the lack of digits and presence of baby fat. Sometimes, the immobilization of an additional joint may be required to ensure proper fit and purchase.

HEALING TIMEFRAMES

Children tend to heal more quickly than adults. This allows for shorter immobilization times following injury (Putnam & Fischer, 1996). However, adults, as compared children, are better able to follow precautions, thus may, for hygiene purposes, and to initiate therapy, be allowed to remove immobilization devices before soft tissues are completely healed. These protocols, directed towards adult splinting procedures will decrease the potential of developing contractures and stiffness. On the other hand, a child's soft tissue is more elastic than an adult's and may be immobilized without negative effect for as long as six to eight weeks (Charest, 2003). Because children cannot be counted on to follow through on maintaining specific precautions, and will not suffer adverse effects from prolonged immobilization, they can be casted or splinted until full healing occurs.

ABNORMAL TONE

Prior to fabricating a splint, the OT must also perform a full assessment of the child's tone. If the OT determines that spasticity is present, the splint must be made to be rigid and may require additional splinting material to prevent cracking and provide reinforcement (Charest, 2003) (Figure 24-13). There are also postures that the OT practitioner may place the joint in that will decrease tone and make splinting less difficult for all parties involved in the process,. These postures are usually similar to that of the desired position of the upper extremity in the splint. The OT practitioner must try to attain these postures prior to making the splint, to both aide in fabrication and to achieve the best position in the splint. It may be helpful for one OT practitioner to hold the arm in the desired position, while another fabricates the splint. For example, placing the arm in external rotation with the thumb adducted helps to decrease a flexor synergy pattern. This is the desired position in the splint and also helps decrease tone while splinting.

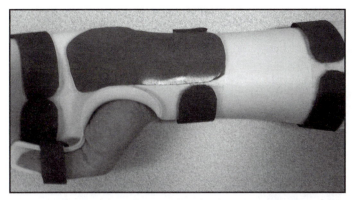

Figure 24-13. Reinforced resting hand splint.

SWELLING

Edema must not only be managed, but also accommodated for with splinting. As edema levels fluctuate, splints must be monitored closely to ensure proper fit.

COMPLIANCE

Compliance is dependent on a number of factors. First, the child must be willing to wear the splint; otherwise he or she will find ways not to. A significant factor to consider when fabricating a splint is the child's cognitive/developmental status. However, no matter what developmental age/level the child is functioning at, the family/ caregivers, and school personnel must encourage compliance with splinting wear, care, and precautions. This responsibility may fall solely on the family/caregivers if the child is very young or not involved in outside programming.

Permanent straps may be used to aide in keeping a splint on a baby or small child who cannot otherwise remove the splint (this is discussed in detail later in this chapter). If the child functions at a developmental level older than eight years, he or she can participate in splint donning, doffing, and overall care. This active participation may improve compliance by increasing the child's perceived level of independence and autonomy. Further, the more a child likes the splint, the more likely it is that he/she will wear it. Trying to make the splint as low profile and cosmetically pleasing as possible also increases the likelihood of wearing compliance. To increase compliance, the OT practitioner may choose to involve the child in the actual fabrication by allowing him/her to choose the color of thermoplastic and straps to be used. See Table 24-2 for more helpful hints.

Getting Started

Up to this point the process of selecting the type of splint to be fabricated, as well as an overview of goals and precautions associated with different types of splints have been discussed. To get started with the actual fabrication, the OT practitioner must first choose a material. It is important to understand the various types of materials that are currently available.

MATERIALS

Low temperature thermoplastics are most commonly used to fabricate splints. These thermoplastics are available through many rehabilitation vendors (see Table 24-6 following the Application Activity for a list of vendors). The materials are called low temperature because they soften in water heated between 135° and 180° F (Coppard, 1996). Once the material is pliable, it can be molded into a splint. Over 30 different types of low-temperature splinting materials are available, yet there is no one splinting material that is appropriate for all types of splint. When selecting a material, the OT practitioner must consider what the purpose of the material is to accomplish. To be a successful splinter, the OT practitioner must have knowledge of the types, as well as the characteristics, and working properties of the materials.

Thermoplastics are most commonly broken down into four main types: 1) elastic, 2) plastic, 3) rubber, and 4) plastic-rubber. Specific characteristics of thermoplastics are discussed below. It is better to have an understanding of the characteristics of each type of material rather than trying to memorize over 30 brand names. For example, if the OT practitioner has an understanding of elastic materials, he or she will be familiar with the working properties of each brand name that falls into the elastic category. Table 24-3 provides a summary of the properties of various thermoplastic materials.

Thermoplastics are broken down into two sub-categories. The first, handling characteristics refer to the thermoplastic when it is soft and workable. The second, performance characteristics, refer to the thermoplastic after it has hardened.

HANDLING CHARACTERISTICS OF THERMOPLASTICS

Drapability/Conformability

Drapability/conformability refers to the ability of thermoplastic material to intimately conform to the area or body part being splinted. When a material drapes or conforms easily it is said to have a high degree of drapability/conformability. These materials tend to pick up fingerprints and crease marks easily, so care must be taken in handling them when they are heated (Figure 24-14). An OT practitioner selects a highly conforming material for use with burn management, small bony areas, arches, and precise positioning (Hogan & Uditsky, 1998). Splints that are conformed exactly to the patient are more comfortable and reduce the likelihood of splint migration.

Table 24-2

Pediatric Splinting Tips

Compliance to Wear

- Permanent Strapping
- If developmentally able; child should assist with choosing colors and decorations for fabrication and be instructed in donning, doffing, and overall care of splint.
- Splint should be cosmetically pleasing.
- Splinting a favorite doll or stuffed animal so the child and his or her toy will have matching splints. The child can practice donning and doffing on the doll (see below).

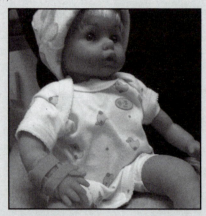

- Use colorful scraps of thermoplastic to make designs such as; flowers, smiling faces, rainbows and attach them to the splint.
- Decorate the splint with markers or stickers (see below).

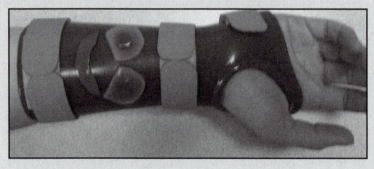

Fabrication

- Trace the pattern on a paper towel.
- Use an adult size pattern and shrink it down on a photocopier, or if possible, place child's hand directly onto copier to create an image.
- Use the uninvolved hand or the hand of a similar sized sibling if tracing the pattern on the involved extremity is too difficult.
- Use gravity for assistance.
- Keep hands moving along the splint material at all times, avoid being heavy handed and leaving fingerprints that may cause pressure spots.
- Use fingertips for small edges and finishing touches.
- Use a co-worker (as needed) to help maintain proper positioning while splinting.
- Choose a material that will best meet the needs of the splint as well as the clinician fabricating the splint.
- Prior to splinting, provide the child with a small piece of heated material. Encourage the child to play with the material, stretching and pulling it, and feeling the heat of it. This may help to reduce fears of the heated material during splint fabrication.
- Enlist a coworker, the caregiver, or yourself to try and distract the child. Have small toys or bubbles available to serve as distracters.

Table 24-3

Materials Reference Chart

Material Name	Conformability/ Drape	Resistance to to Stretch	Memory	Resistance to Fingerprints	Rigidity
ELASTIC MATERIALS					
Aquaplast Original	Maximum	Moderate	Maximum	Maximum	Moderate
Aquaplast Original Resilient	Moderate	Moderate	Maximum	Maximum	Moderate
Aquaplast ProDrape-T	Maximum	Minimal	Maximum	Maximum	Moderate
Aquaplast Resilient-T	Moderate	Moderate	Maximum	Maximum	Moderate
Aquaplast-T and Watercolors	Moderate	Moderate	Maximum	Maximum	Moderate
Encore	Maximum	Maximum	Maximum	Maximum	Moderate
Multiform Clear Elastic	Moderate	Moderate	Maximum	Maximum	Moderate
Orfit, soft	Maximum	Moderate	Maximum	Minimal	Minimal
Orfit, stiff	Minimal	Moderate	Maximum	Moderate	Minimal
Prism	Maximum	Moderate	Maximum	Maximum	Minimal
PLASTIC MATERIALS					
Clinic/Clinic D	Maximum	Moderate	Minimal	Minimal	Maximum
Kay Splint Basic I	Maximum	Minimal	Minimal	Moderate	Maximum
Kay Splint Basic II	Maximum	Moderate	Moderate	Moderate	Maximum
Multiform Plastic	Maximum	Minimal	Minimal	Minimal	Maximum
Orthoplast II	Maximum	Moderate	Minimal	Moderate	Maximum
Polyform	Maximum	Minimal	Minimal	Minimal	Maximum
RUBBER MATERIALS					
Ezeform	Moderate	Maximum	Moderate	Maximum	Maximum
Kay-Prene	Minimal	Maximum	Moderate	Maximum	Maximum
Kay-Splint IV	Moderate	Maximum	Maximum	Maximum	Moderate
Omega Plus	Minimal	Maximum	Moderate	Maximum	Maximum
Orthoplast	Minimal	Maximum	Moderate	Maximum	Moderate
San Splint	Minimal	Maximum	Moderate	Maximum	Maximum
Spectrum	Minimal	Moderate	Moderate	Maximum	Moderate
Synergy	Minimal	Maximum	Moderate	Maximum	Maximum
PLASTIC-RUBBER MATERIALS					
Kay Splint Basic III	Moderate	Moderate	Moderate	Moderate	Maximum
Polyflex II	Moderate	Moderate	Moderate	Moderate	Moderate
Preferred	Moderate	Moderate	Moderate	Moderate	Moderate

Modified from Hogan, L., & Uditsky, T. (1998). Pediatric splinting: selection, fabrication and clinical application of upper extremity splints. San Antonio, TX: Therapy Skill Builders. Also modified from North Coast Medical's thermoplastics chart.

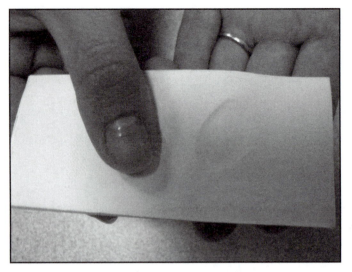

Figure 24-14. Fingerprinting material.

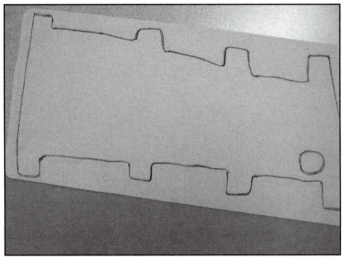

Figure 24-15. Pattern of anterior elbow splint with tabs.

Stretch

Stretch refers to the amount of resistance to being stretched the material offers, and its tendency to return to its original shape after stretch. When a material stretches easily it has a high degree of stretch. Materials that can be easily stretched have less control than materials with a high resistance to stretch. The OT practitioner selects materials with a high degree of stretch for small intricate splints, and avoids them when fabricating larger splints on patients who are uncooperative or who present with severe spasticity.

Memory

Memory refers to the ability of the heated material to return to its original shape after it has been stretched or previously molded. When a material can be reheated and remolded several times without excessive stretching, it is considered to have a high degree of memory. The OT practitioner selects a material with good memory if frequent remolding is anticipated.

Bonding

Bonding refers to the degree to which a material will stick to itself when properly heated. Self-bonding materials are considered to have a high degree of bond. Some materials have a coating that must be removed in order to create a permanent bond. If the coating on these materials is left in place, the material can be pried apart after cooling. This feature is helpful when molding a larger splint on a child who may move around a lot. For example, if a child needs an anterior elbow splint, the OT practitioner may cut the pattern out with tabs along both sides (Figure 24-15). The heated material is placed on the anterior surface of the elbow and the tabs are then pulled posterior and bonded to one another by pinching. This pulls the material tight, thus

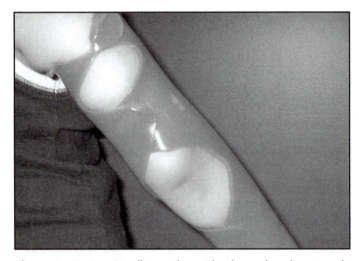

Figure 24-16. Anterior elbow splint with tabs ready to be popped and cut.

increasing precise molding. The OT practitioner then simply holds the arm in the desired position as the material sets. Once the material is hardened, the tabs are popped apart and cut off (Figure 24-16).

All thermoplastic materials form a stronger bond if the surfaces are prepared with solvent. *Bonding solvent* is a chemical agent that can be brushed onto both pieces of the plastic surface to be bonded.

Self-Finishing Edges

If the material is cut when warm, a *self-finishing edge* allows any cut edge to have a smooth texture. Some OT practitioners feel that use of self-finishing edges saves time because they do not have to manually roll or smooth the edges of the splint.

PERFORMANCE CHARACTERISTICS OF THERMOPLASTICS

Flexibility

Flexibility refers to a material's ability to withstand repeated stresses. A material that withstands repeated stresses is considered to have a high degree of flexibility. The OT practitioner selects a material with a high degree of flexibility for fabrication of circumferential splints because these splints must be pulled open for application and removal.

Rigidity

Rigidity refers to the strength of the splinting material. A material has a high degree of rigidity if it is strong and resists bending and cracking. The OT practitioner selects a material with a high degree of rigidity for large splints that need to support the weight of larger joints, or for children who present with spasticity.

Material Thickness

Thermoplastics come in several thicknesses, ranging from from 1/16" to 1/8". Although 1/8" thickness seems to be the standard for most splints, thinner thermoplastics are more commonly used for finger, arthritis, and pediatric splints. With pediatric splints, 1/16", 1/12", and 3/32" thick materials are most commonly used. These thinner materials minimize the weight of the splint and allow better conformability to smaller hands.

Solid Versus Perforated

Solid materials require less edge finishing than do perforated materials. This is because there are no holes to cut through during pattern making that would cause the edges to be rough. Some OT practitioners feel that the solid materials are more comfortable because the contact against the skin is more even. On the other hand, perforated materials allow for increased air circulation. Some OT practitioners feel that the presence of perspiration in a splint is a concern, and that perforations help to reduce it. Perforations also tend to make a splint less rigid, so it may be the best choice for a circumferential splint when the edges need to be pulled apart for donning and doffing.

Color

The color of the splint may affect a child's wearing compliance. Children often like to pick out a brightly colored splint. Unfortunately, not all thermoplastics come in colors; most continue to be white or beige. The elastic types of splinting materials tend to come in a wider selection of colors.

WORKING PROPERTIES OF THERMO-PLASTICS

Once the OT practitioner gains an understanding of the characteristics that define thermoplastics; flexibility, rigidity, material thickness, solid versus perforations, and color, he or she can better understand the working properties of each of the four types of thermoplastics. The working characteristics of thermoplastics are broken down into four types: 1) elastic, 2) plastic, 3) rubber, and 4) plastic-rubber.

Elastic

Elastic materials have excellent memory. They offer a high amount of conformability and a moderately high degree of stretch. Elastic materials resist most fingerprints. The finished product is moderately rigid. Because of the material's high degree of memory, it is a cost effective and time efficient splinting material for use when fabricating serial static splints.

Plastic

Plastic materials have a low degree of memory. They offer the maximum amount of conformability, drape, and stretch. Plastic materials retain fingerprints easily. The finished product is strong and rigid. Because of the high degree of conformability and stretch, this type of material is a good choice for intricate hand splints requiring a great deal of contouring and molding. These same characteristics make plastic materials hard to control. They are not a good choice for OT practitioners with limited splinting experience, for splints that need to cover a large surface area, or for splinting a child who is uncooperative, or a child presenting with spasticity.

Rubber

Rubber materials have a moderate degree of memory. They offer little drape and conformability. Rubber materials have a high degree of control and are resistant to stretch. Rubber is highly resistant to fingerprinting. The level of rigidity in the finished product varies with each individual brand of thermoplastic. Because of the high degree of control, and the ability to work aggressively with these materials without fingerprinting them, rubber materials are good choices for children presenting with spasticity or for large splints that do not require a close fit.

Plastic-Rubber

Plastic-rubber materials are recognized as the "middle of the road" splinting material. They offer a moderate degree of memory, control, conformability, and resistance to fingerprinting. Because of these characteristics, rubber-plastic materials are user friendly and a good choice for inexperi-

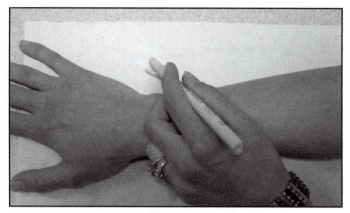

Figure 24-17. Hand flat on paper towel to trace pattern.

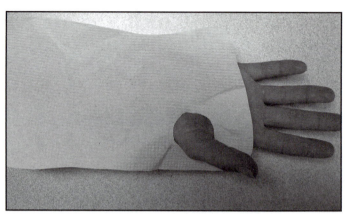

Figure 24-18. Paper towel pattern wrapped around hand to assess fit.

enced splinters, or for clinics that cannot afford to stock a wide variety of splinting materials.

Component Selection

When splinting the young pediatric population, it is important to keep in mind that most of these children have the tendency to mouth any object given to them. It is important to avoid fabricating a splint containing small pieces that may become detached and present a choking hazard. Outriggers and splints attachments are not recommended for young children because they contain small parts. Further, the construction features of an outrigger splint or splint attachment may cause injury to the eyes, ears, or elsewhere on the body if a child contacts these body parts with the splint. If a physician recommends a mobilization splint for an older child, outriggers made from thermoplastic tubing are a more appropriate choice than metal outriggers because the smooth tube encases the elastic components and contains no sharp edges.

SPLINT PATTERNS

When making splint patterns it is best to use industrial paper towels, because they are strong enough to not tear easily, but flexible enough to wrap around the hand to assess proper fit before tracing the pattern onto the thermoplastic. OT practitioners need to trace the outline of the child's hand on the paper towel, making certain that the hand is placed flat and in proper anatomical alignment (Figure 24-17). Of course, this may not always be possible, especially with the pediatric population, due to compliance issues or specific diagnosis. In these cases the OT practitioner may trace the contra-lateral extremity in order to prepare the pattern. Another option is to take a larger predrawn pattern and shrink it down on a photocopier, or if possible, place the child's hand directly onto the photocopier. After the pattern is traced onto the paper towel and cut out, it may

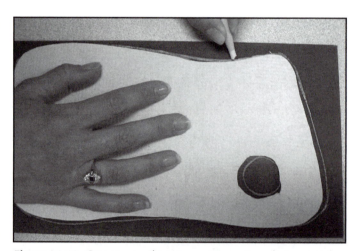

Figure 24-19. Grease pencil tracing pattern onto splint material.

be wrapped around the extremity to assess proper fit (Figure 24-18). The OT practitioner makes the appropriate adjustments prior to tracing it onto the thermoplastic material.

After making the pattern and assessing proper fit, the OT practitioner traces it onto the selected sheet of thermoplastic. A colored grease pencil works well for this process, as a pencil tends to break, and ink tends to leave permanent marks (Figure 24-19). The grease pencil glides well and makes a clear pattern. Grease pencil marks may be partially removed by rubbing them with a soft dry cloth or using rubbing alcohol. Both of these removal techniques work best before the material has been heated. These authors recommend trying to cut on the inside of the pattern, as this way the finished product will be free of all markings.

SPLINT MOLDING

OT practitioners are taught to avoid heavy handling and grabbing, and to cradle heated material to prevent fingerprinting. To ensure proper fit, OT practitioners are also taught to always mold the splint directly onto the patient. These rules cannot always be followed, especially when

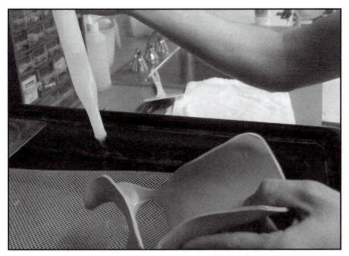

Figure 24-20. Spot heating splint material with baster.

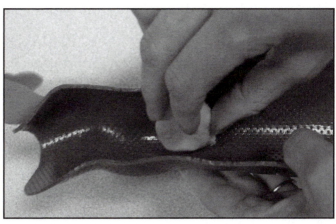

Figure 24-21. Putty being removed from splint after molding.

working with the pediatric population. For starters, it is very difficult to get a young child to sit perfectly still for at least four minutes while the splint hardens into a mold. It is also difficult to place the hot splinting material onto the child just after it comes out of the splint pan. Most children are frightened of the heat, so the OT practitioner is forced to let the material cool down for a few moments, thereby reducing working time. Another problem is the size of our adult hands. Children's splints are small and intricate; our hands are just too big for some of the conforming that is necessary to customize a splint. To minimize some of these challenges, it is important to know that there is nothing wrong with partially fabricating some of the splint on your hand or fingers, on the patient's contra-lateral limb, or even on the hand of a sibling. If molding the splint in this way, and, while the material still has some working time left, it is important to place the partially firm splint onto the patient's hand for the final molding. Please also refer to Table 24-2 for tips to help with pediatric splinting.

Once the splint is completed, minor adjustment may still be necessary. Because a pediatric splint is usually so small, using a heat gun or partial submersion into hot water may cause a complete splint meltdown. A good way to work around this problem is to use a kitchen baster to draw up hot water from the splint pan. For modification purposes, the OT practitioner may then slowly squeeze the baster to run the hot water on the exact spot that needs to be reheated for modification purposes (Figure 24-20).

PADDING

Various padding options are available, and most include an adhesive backing for easy application. Padding has either closed or open cells. These authors recommend using closed cell padding with the pediatric population because it resists absorption of odors, perspiration, and bacteria, and can easily be wiped clean. Open cell padding allows for absorption, thus making it more difficult to keep clean from bacteria, perspiration, and saliva. Sufficient space must be available for the padding; otherwise pressure between the splint and the skin may develop and lead to skin breakdown. If padding is to be used for comfort or to relieve any bony prominences, it should be applied prior to splint fabrication. The splint should be molded over the padding. Once the splint has cooled and set, the padding may be permanently attached to the splint material by using the self-adhesive backing.

Another padding option is to use therapy putty to pre-pad the bony prominence prior to splinting. Medium to firm resistance putty should be used because the heat from the splint will cause softening. By pre-padding an area in this way, a bubble is created in the splint to protect the potentially painful spot. Once the splint is completely cooled and formed, the putty is removed (Figure 24-21).

EDGE FINISHING

To prevent any pressure areas, the edges of a splint should be smoothed, rolled, or flared. The heated water from the splint pan or a heat gun is used to smooth, roll, or flare the edges of the splint. By heating the edge of the splint, the material softens. Once softened the palm of the hand is used to smooth and flare the edges from inside to outside (Figure 24-22). Smaller areas may necessitate that only the fingertips are used. By moistening the fingertips with water or lotion, finger imprints can be avoided. It is especially important not only to smooth, but also to flare the proximal edge of a forearm-based splint away from the skin. If the splint edge is not flared away, the constant rubbing caused by elbow movement will lead to skin breakdown. If fabricating an elbow splint, both proximal and distal borders should be flared to avoid skin breakdown.

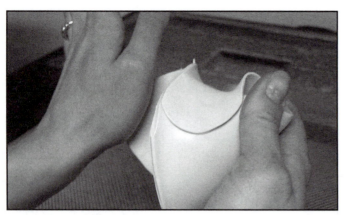

Figure 24-22. Flaring edges of splint.

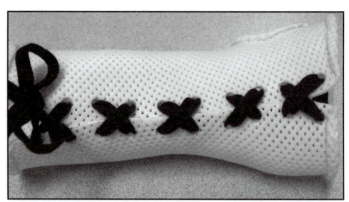

Figure 24-23. Circumferential wrist support using a shoelace for secure strapping.

STRAPPING

Many different strapping options are available. Choosing the proper texture, thickness, width, and color of Velcro® (Velcro USA, Manchester, NH) loop are important factors to consider when fabricating a splint. Velcro® loop comes in a variety of textures. Cushion strap most commonly comes in ¼" thickness. Soft Velcro® stretch loop, which provides a snug fit and secure closure, may be needed to secure circumferential splints. Standard loop is also readily available. Velcro® loop comes in a number of widths, ranging from ½" to 2". The width can be cut accordingly to fit a particular splint. The wider the strapping material, the more evenly the force is distributed. By dispersing the pressure over a larger surface area, the risk of pressure sores from the straps is reduced. Placing the straps circumferentially on the splint also helps to evenly distribute the force. When skin break down is a concern, soft, nonstretchable, ¼" thick strapping material is an excellent choice for pediatric splints. Most strapping material is available in a wide array of colors. Colored strapping helps with wearing compliance by both offering the child a choice, and adding to the visual appeal of the splint.

It seems as though many children have the unique gift of being escape artists. It does not matter how perfectly fabricated the splint is if the family/caregivers cannot keep it on the child. Simply adding more and more straps does not always ensure a lasting fit. Some techniques that these authors use to help keep a splint in place include:

- Place a sock over the child's hand and splint. This technique is supported by the "out of sight, out of mind theory". Alternatively, a sock puppet may be used if the splint is worn during the day and is not meant to be functional. This will not only help with wearing compliance, but also makes wearing the splint fun.

- Use shoelaces with or without a shoelace keeper. These authors recommend using this method with circumferential splints. By using this technique with circumferential splinting, the laces do not dig into the skin, as might happen with one-sided splints. To use this method, poke holes in either side of the splint, lace it up like a shoe, and secure it with a shoelace keeper or tie the shoelace string (Figure 24-23).

- Shoelace keepers are available in different colors and styles from drug stores and children's shoe stores.

- Dual-lock and Poly-lock fastening systems lock securely to themselves for high strength application. Dual-lock and Poly-lock fastening systems also mate with standard loop for high-retention attachment. This bond is extremely strong and can wear out the loop side of the Velcro® quickly, so extra straps must be supplied. Unfortunately, this bond is not only difficult for children to remove, but it can also be difficult for caregivers to remove.

- Some other ideas to keep splints in place include using a diaper clip, hook and eye fasteners, and even small luggage locks (Hogan & Uditsky, 1998). That said, it is important to be careful when using small parts or metal on a splint because children may hit themselves with it, or even mouth the small parts.

Once the straps are properly positioned, it is important to keep them in the proper position. For instance, a child may have several different caregivers donning and doffing the splint, which in turn, increases the chance of incorrect placement. One way to ensure proper strap placement is to permanently adhere one side of the strap to the splint. The most common way to permanently attach a strap is with rivets. Rivets are made of either metal or plastic, and come in various sizes. A hole is punched through the thermoplastic material and the strapping and the rivet is placed through the holes. To avoid potential skin breakdown or injury, it is important that the rivet be flush with the splint, both on the inside and outside surfaces. Moleskin may also be used to line the inside of the splint over the rivet (Figure 24-24). The OT practitioner may also fabricate rivets out of thermoplastic. After poking holes in both the strap and the splint, a small piece of thermoplastic is placed through both holes

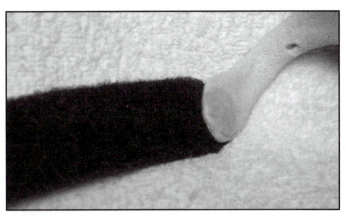

Figure 24-24. Permanently attaching strap with metal rivet lined with moleskin.

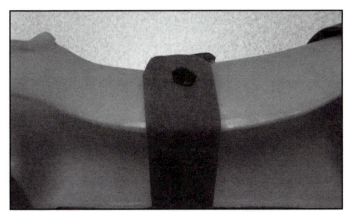

Figure 24-25. Permanently attaching strap with thermoplastic rivet.

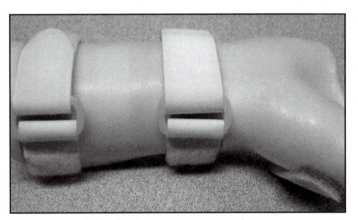

Figure 24-26. Self-adhesive D-ring strap on a long opponens splint.

and the material is pinched together. To avoid potential skin breakdown or injury, it is important that the rivet be flush with the splint both on the inside and outside surfaces (Figure 24-25).

Using self-adhesive D-ring straps is another option to adhere one side of the strap to the splint. These straps are readily available through most rehabilitation vendors. They offer the feature of being an all in one hook and loop strap (Figure 24-26). Another option to adhere a strap to a splint is to use a heat gun to heat the desired point of attachment on the splint. Once the thermoplastic becomes soft and tacky, the loop is pressed into the material to create a permanent bond. Because of its high degree of bond, this technique works best with material that has elastic or plastic properties.

The Role of the OTA in Fabricating Orthotics

As discussed earlier in the chapter, it is the responsibility of the OT to perform an initial evaluation and to determine the long and short-term goals of splinting. The OT should also provide documentation of precautions, special problems, contraindications and plans for re-evaluation. Prior to fabricating an orthotic device, and based on state and facility guidelines, the OTA must be checked off on all competencies for both splinting and pediatric care by the supervising OT. Once it has been determined that the OTA is proficient in splinting and the evaluation is complete, only then may the OTA design, fabricate, and apply the appropriate splint. The OTA, depending on demonstrated competency, may also provide caregiver education. The OT must provide adequate supervision and reassess the patient every 2 weeks. If deemed competent, the OTA may be responsible for continued care and splint modifications as needed.

ROLE OF THE OTA IN ORTHOTIC RELATED CHILD AND FAMILY/CAREGIVER EDUCATION

Once competency is demonstrated regarding splint fabrication and caregiver education, the OTA must discuss and provide all responsible family members/caregivers with written instruction in the wear, care, and precautions of splinting (Table 24-4). The OTA must provide a demonstration of splint application, and the family members/caregiver must be given the opportunity to practice applying the splint, as the correct wearing procedure may not be obvious (Gabriel, 1996). Providing the family/caregivers a photograph or written instruction showing the proper splint application may also be helpful. Another aide for ensuring correct application is to clearly mark the splint with cues. For example, a strap end could be marked 1 and the corresponding splint area could also be marked 1. This method indicates the exact point of attachment for caregivers to follow when applying the splint (Figure 24-27, Table 24-4).

The splint wearing schedule is prepared on a case by case basis, and depends on the purpose of the splint. All pediatric splints should be worn in the clinic for a 20-30 minute trial

Table 24-4

Hand Therapy Splint Instruction Sheet

Patient Name: Date:

Physician: Diagnosis:

Type of Splint:

Purpose:

Splint Wearing Schedule:

Remove Splint:

Splint Care: Please keep your splint area clean and dry. Wash splint daily with lukewarm water, mild soap, and a washcloth. An abrasive cleanser may also be used. Dry with a towel. Straps are hand washable, allow to air dry. Sleeves worn beneath splint should be washed daily by hand and air dried.

Splint Precautions: Tell or call therapist/ take off splint/ adjust straps immediately if any of the following happens:
1. New feelings of burning, or pins and needles
2. Redness/blisters/skin irritation (for example, edges of material/ straps/ or over boney regions)
3. Restriction of blood flow (noted by change in skin color or cold fingers)
4. Increased pain
5. Increased swelling (generalized or between straps)

Warning:
Your splint is temperature sensitive. Do not leave splint in the sun (window sill, car dashboard, radiator, oven or in hot water) as it will melt or lose its shape. An open flame from a stove or cigarette will cause the splint to melt. Be careful while cooking, smoking or near an open flame.

Please call _____ should you have any further questions.

Telephone #: _____

period prior to sending it home with the child and his family/caregivers. After this period of time, skin integrity must be assessed and modifications made as deemed appropriate by the OT practitioner. Once the splint has been fabricated, applied for a 20-30 minute trial period, and the appropriate wearing schedule determined, the child or parent/caregiver should slowly increase the splint wearing time until optimal wearing schedule is reached. For example, if the splint is to be worn for 23 hours per day, the parent/caregiver may start out with a two hour on and one hour off schedule. As the child's overall tolerance to splinting increases, the splint wearing time may increase until the 23 hour mark is met. The OT practitioner must also teach the parent/caregiver or child to monitor for any adverse skin reactions. If there is a red mark or irritation that remains for longer than 15 to 20 minutes after splint removal, then there is excessive pressure and the splint needs modification. The child or parent/caregiver must also monitor for any circulatory compromise or nerve compression potentially caused by the splint (please refer to Table 24-4).

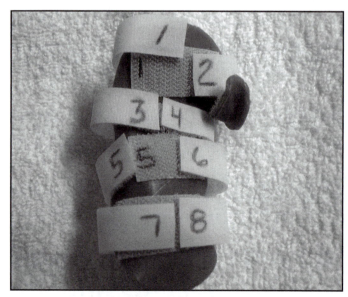

Figure 24-27. Marking straps with corresponding area on splint.

If splinting for hygiene, the splint should be worn up to 23 hours a day to maintain skin integrity (Hogan & Uditsky, 1998). If splinting for function, the splint should be worn while the child is at play or performing specific activities. If the splint is fabricated for protection or behavioral issues, it should be worn during waking hours when a specific behavior is more likely to occur. If splinting for positioning, the more serious the condition or injury, the more the child should wear the splint over a 24 hour period. For positioning splints that require an extended wearing schedule, night time wearing works well. This allows for prolonged stretch while sleeping, and removal during the day for passive range of motion or functional use of the hand.

The OTA must provide written and verbal instruction in the care of the splint, as proper care is necessary to ensure hygiene. Most splints made out of soft fabric, such as neoprene, can be washed by hand with a mild cleanser, or soap and water. Splints should be washed as needed; and with children's splints, this is more often than not. It is also important to remind family members/caregivers to be sure to allow for drying time, as soft splints need to air dry.

Thermoplastic material is temperature sensitive and will soften and lose shape when exposed to extreme heat sources. Heat sources include things such as the dashboard of a car in direct sunlight, a radiator, or even a dishwasher. The splint should be cleaned on a daily basis with soap and water, alcohol, or a gentle cleanser. The liners and straps should be replaced as needed.

Goal Development, Documentation, and Treatment Strategies

As previously discussed, the OT performs an evaluation prior to implementing splinting procedures. This evaluation must be thoroughly documented in accordance with facility guidelines. Table 24-5 provides an example of a sample splint fabrication evaluation form. The evaluation should include all relevant information regarding child's history, age, hand dominance, if any, the child's functional limitations, and the overall goals of the splint. The OT should also note the following: range of motion limitations, muscle tone, skeletal alignment, skin quality, boney prominences, or any other areas of concern in the areas to be splinted. The anatomical location of the splint, purpose, and type of splint should also be well documented. As part of the collaborative process between the OT and OTA, the OTA must fully understand the goals of the splint, the child's limitations, as well as boney landmarks to be paid close attention to during splinting.

The evaluation should also include a statement that the child and his/her parents/caregivers were given written, ver-

bal, and hands-on instruction in the wear, care and precautions of the splint. It is important for all parents/caregivers to receive this information so they have a point of reference from which to implement splint wearing. Finally, the fit of the splint should be assessed and documented prior to the child leaving the clinic. All of this information is important for future visits, so as to monitor the child's progress with splinting or to determine the need for modifications.

Upon follow up, documentation should include the patient's tolerance to splinting, any need for modifications or alterations, and any adjustments to the wearing schedule. If changes are made, the reason why these changes were made should also be well documented. It is also important to address and document whether or not the goals of the splint are being met. For example, is there an increase in ROM, is the child more functional with writing at school, and/or has the parent/caregiver found that the palm stays cleaner when the splint is used?

Reimbursement Procedures for Orthotics

Reimbursement for splinting differs depending on insurance policies and each type of (splinting) facility. The actual price of a splint is usually determined by the facility and takes into consideration the cost of the materials, as well as the OT practitioner's time. Every insurance company has guidelines as to how much of that cost they will reimburse. Insurance companies also have guidelines as to what type of documentation they require for reimbursement. Some insurance companies require a copy of the physician's referral along with the OT's evaluation. Other companies only require a phone call to the patient's Primary Care Physician (PCP). With so many insurances and so many policies, the family/caregiver should be encouraged to take an active role in being familiar with the coverage that their specific plan provides. Some insurance companies will only reimburse a particular treatment, or will only reimburse treatment that does not include splinting or durable medical equipment (DME). Other insurance companies may consider any splinting to be covered under the therapy umbrella; however, that therapy umbrella may only include six treatments within one calendar year. This can be difficult when splinting a child who may need constant adjustments or modifications due to growth or improvement in function. In these cases where full reimbursement is not offered, the balance of the cost falls on the child's parents/caregivers. Before initiating treatment, fabricating splints, or issuing equipment, the OT and the responsible party should be aware of what will be reimbursed, how to go about getting that reimbursement, and what the parent/caregiver is willing to pay for out of pocket. These cost constraints have forced OT practitioners to not only be more creative with their supplies but also to

---

Table 24-5

Hand Therapy Splint Fabrication and Evaluation Form

Patient Name: Date:
Physician: D.O.B.:
Job Title: Work Status: Dominance: R / L

History of Present Condition:
D.O.I.:
D.O.S.:

Examination Results:
Functional Level:
Pain:
Edema:
Sensibility:
Soft tissue/wound status/dressing:
Range of Motion/Strength:

Splint Goals: **Splint Plan:**
_____ Protect healing structures   _____ Immobilization Splint
_____ Increase Range of Motion   _____ Mobilization Splint
_____ Restrict Mobility   _____ Restriction Splint
_____ Correct Joint Alignment   _____ Nonarticular Splint
_____ Increase Function

Treatment: Type of Splint Fabricated/Function:

Assessment:
_____ Patient demonstrates understanding of purpose and proper use of splint
_____ Independent in use and care of splint:
_____Yes   _____No, requires assistance in:

Recommendations:
Further contact needed: _____ No _____Yes

Patient's Signature ————————————— Therapist's Signature —————————————————

---

be more frugal. OT practitioners are encouraged to educate themselves in less expensive splinting options that do not compromise the overall care of the child or the finished splint.

The OTA should have a strong grasp of the skills needed to fabricate a splint, educate caregivers, and document treatment. The OTA must possess this clinical knowledge, as well as skills in orthotic fabrication, to take on the challenge of splinting a child.

Summary

This chapter examined the realm of splinting within the occupational therapy profession. It addressed the rationale behind fabricating splints for the pediatric population, as well as the specific role of the OTA in the splinting process.

Case Study

JD is a 7-year-old, right-handed male who at age 3 months had a thrombosis from an IV, which was placed for pneumonia. He developed ischemia of his left hand, and

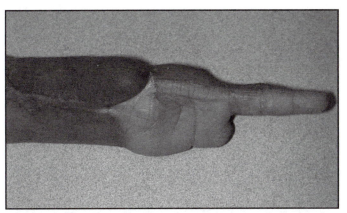

Figure 24-28. Hand after surgery prior to splinting.

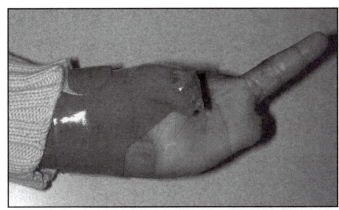

Figure 24-29. Thumb extension splint to improve pinching.

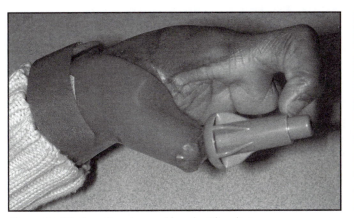

Figure 24-30. Functional use of hand with splint.

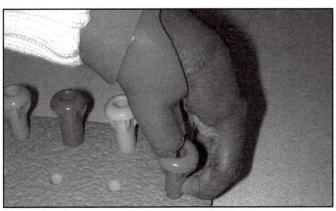

Figure 24-31. Functional use of hand with splint.

lost all digits, except his ring finger. Physical examination of the left upper extremity demonstrates a hypertrophic contracted scar along the radial aspect of the wrist. A well-developed ring finger is present. A stub of the proximal phalanx of the small finger is present. The hyperthenar muscles are well developed. JD has full active digital motion of the ring finger. He writes with his right hand. He is able to pick up a pen using the ring finger, by opposing this digit to his palm. The plan was to perform a debridement of the scar along the radial aspect of the wrist and a left groin pedicle flap in anticipation of a later toe to thumb transfer to provide JD with an opposable thumb. JD underwent the debridement and groin flap, which healed well. Unfortunately, upon having an arthrogram it was determined that JD was not a candidate for a toe to thumb transfer because of insufficient blood supply. The family was disappointed with this news but was willing to try a splint as a prosthesis. The splint was molded to extend JD's existing thumb and give him a functional pinch. Dycem® (Dycem Ltd., Bristol, England) was placed on the tip of the thumb splint. This provided a textured surface to assist in pinch.

DISCUSSION QUESTIONS

1. What are some other age appropriate functional activities that JD might be taught to do with his left hand?

2. Given JD's age, much involvement with splint care should he be expected to do?

3. How might you work with JD's family on accepting the prosthesis instead of a toe to thumb transfer? (Figures 24-28 through 24-31).

Application Activity

FABRICATING A WRIST SUPPORT

Purpose: This splint is used to immobilize the wrist.

Materials: 3/32, 1/12, or 1/16 inch splinting material. (Please refer to Table 24-3 for best type of material). Scissors, therapy putty or foam for boney prominences, hook and loop for straps, grease pencil, and paper towel to trace pattern.

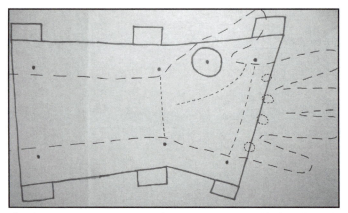

Figure 24-32. Wrist support splint pattern.

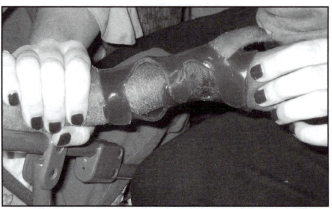

Figure 24-33. Splint fabricated before tabs are cut.

1. Begin by making the pattern. Using a paper towel make a mark along the ulnar and radial border of the distal palmar crease, just proximal to the index finger metacarpal.

2. Make a mark three quarters of the way up the forearm.

3. To make the thumbhole make a mark on either side of the thumb metacarpal.

4. Connect the marks (except for the thumbhole mark) to make the splint border. Then increase that border by one inch on both sides. Make a 1-inch circle around the thumb mark for the thumb hole.

5. To make the tabs that will aide in pulling the material circumferentially, add half an inch bumps in the pattern on both sides at the MP's, the wrist, and the most proximal portion of the splint.

6. Heat the material slightly, making it just soft enough to cut through it. Cut out the pattern.

7. Pre-pad the ulna styloid or any other bony prominences with therapy putty or foam.

8. Positioning is important to aide in molding and to decrease any tone. A gravity eliminated plane will make overall molding easier. Place the child's hand in supination with the wrist in extension. It is helpful to have a second OT practitioner to help maintain this position while molding the splint.

9. After the material is fully heated, place the material on the child positioning the thumb through the hole first to ensure proper fit and the best mold.

10. Next pull the tabs circumferentially and attach them together posteriorly. They will pull apart easily when the material is fully cooled. During molding it is important to form the material to the arches in the palm. This can be done by applying gentle pressure as you run your hand or thumb along the creases and over the contours of the hand. Keep in mind that both hands should be moving at all times, and heavy handling or grabbing of the material will result in fingerprinting and pressure spots.

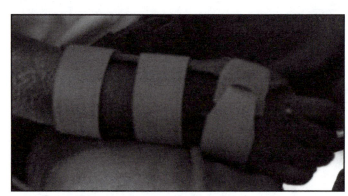

Figure 24-34. Wrist support on patient.

11. While the material is warm roll the distal edge for MP clearance and the proximal edge to prevent pressure along the forearm. Also roll the edges of the thumb hole to ensure comfort and prevent pressure spots with thumb use.

12. Once the material has fully cooled remove and trim as needed. It is also possible to roll the distal and proximal edge with the splint off the child. Remember when smoothing the edges use the palm of the hand and always use a gentle pressure from inside to outside.

13. Remove any theraputty or padding from the splint and check the overall fit of the splint. The MP creases of the fingers and the thumb should be cleared, and the ulna styloid or other boney prominences should now have a raised area from the thera-putty or padding. Make any necessary changes by spot heating and trimming.

14. Once the fit is satisfactory cut the tabs, smooth the edges, and apply the straps.

15. The straps are also applied circumferentially with one placed distal, one placed proximal, and one placed in the middle over the wrist crease area (Figures 24-32 through 24-36).

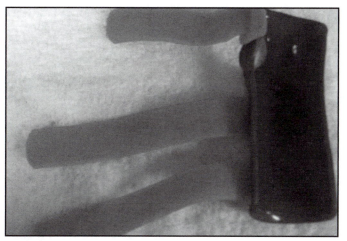

Figure 24-35. Wrist support.

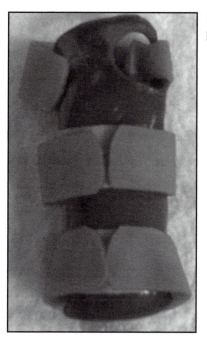

Figure 24-36. Wrist support.

Table 24-6
Splint Material Vendors

AliMed Inc.
297 High Street
Dedham, MA 02026-9135
(800) 225-2610

- Thermoplastics (limited selection)
- Prefabricated splints
- Strapping materials
- Various splinting supplies

North Coast Medical, Inc.
18305 Sutter Boulevard
Morgan Hill, CA 95037-2845
(800) 821-9319

- Thermoplastic materials
- Prefabricated splints
- Neoprene materials/supplies
- Strapping materials
- Padding materials
- Large selection of splinting supplies

Sammons Preston Rolyan
P.O. Box 5071
Bolingbrook, IL 60440
(800) 323-5547
Fax (800) 547-4333

- Thermoplastic materials
- Prefabricated splints
- Neoprene materials/supplies
- Strapping materials
- Padding materials
- Large selection of splinting supplies

Velcro USA
406 Brown Avenue
Manchester, NH 03108
(800) 225-0180
FAX (603) 669-8991

- Velcro products (including iron-on Velcro)

References

Austin, N.M. (2003). Anatomical principles. In M. A. Jacobs, N. Austin (Eds.), *Splinting the hand and upper extremity: principles and process* (pp. 19-47). Philadelphia: Lippincott Williams & Wilkins.

Charest, E. (2003). The pediatric patient. In M.A. Jacobs, N. Austin (Eds.), *Splinting the hand and upper extremity: principles and process* (pp. 434-445). Philadelphia: Lippincott Williams & Wilkins.

Colditz, J. (1995). Therapist's management of the stiff hand. In J.M. Hunter, E.J. Mackin, A.D. Callahan (Eds.), *Rehabilitation of the hand: Surgery and therapy* (pp. 1141-1159). St. Louis, MO: C.V. Mosby.

Coppard, B.M. (1996). Introduction to splinting. In B.M. Coppard, H. Lohman (Eds.), *Introduction to splinting: A critical thinking and problem solving approach* (pp. 1-20). St. Louis, MO: C.V. Mosby.

Gabriel, L. (1996). Splinting children who have developmental disabilities. In B.M. Coppard, H. Lohman (Eds.), *Introduction to splinting: A critical thinking and problem solving approach* (pp. 252-278). St. Louis, MO: C.V. Mosby.

Hogan, L. & Uditsky, T. (1998). *Pediatric splinting selection, fabrication, and clinical application of upper extremity splints*. San Antonio, TX: Therapy Skill Builders.

Putnam, M.D., Fischer, M. (1996). Forearm fractures. In C.A. Permer (Ed.), *Surgery of the hand and upper extremity* (pp. 599-635). New York: McGraw-Hill.

Schultz-Johnson, K. (2002). Static progressive splinting. *Journal of Hand Therapy, 15*(2), 163-178.

GLOSSARY OF TERMS

accommodations: changes that others make in interaction style, task demand or environmental conditions to facilitate another individual's ability to function in a specific environment or under certain conditions.

adaptive behavior: personal conduct that one is capable of modifying in age-appropriate ways to effectively address needs, demands and challenges.

adaptive response: an appropriate action in which the individual responds successfully to some environmental demand.

adolescence: period from 12 to 18 years.

Americans with Disabilities Act (ADA): a federal law mandating equal treatment and accommodation for those with limitations.

artful vigilance: when treating an individual, the therapist's ability to balance the need for adult direction and proximity for task facilitation and safety and the need for the individual to be free to explore, learn and challenge themselves independently.

asymmetrical tonic neck reflex (ATNR): present at birth and integrates between 4 and 6 months of age. Stimulus-turning head to right or left, which results in an extension pattern on the side to which the head is turned and a flexion pattern on the opposite side.

assistive device: any object or tool that improves or maximizes a person's functional independence in activities of daily living, work, play, and/or leisure.

assistive equipment: *see* assistive device.

assistive technology (AT): any item, piece of equipment, or product system, whether acquired commercially off the shelf, modified, or customized, that is used to increase, maintain, or improve functional capabilities of individuals with disabilities.

augmentative communication: a device or method that enhances a person's ability to communicate, such as an augmentative/alternative communication (AAC) board.

automatic writing: the stage of this learned motor skill in which the child can write with minimal attention. After mastering manuscript or cursive, the child becomes familiar enough with letter formation that they are able to remember how to form the letter from memory.

avoiding response: emerges around 1 month of age and is integrated at approximately 6 months of age. Stimulus is light, distally moving contact to the hand, which results in an extension and abduction of the fingers and withdrawal of the hand from the stimulus.

behavioral assessment: an approach to evaluation based on the analysis of samples of behavior, including the causes and consequences of the behavior.

best practice: occupational therapy services that are based on current research and sound clinical judgment.

bonding solvent: a solvent used for preparing thermoplastic material for a strong self-bond. This solvent is needed to bond coated thermoplastic, however, it can strengthen any type of thermoplastic bond.

Bundy's Model of Playfulness: graphic depiction of playfulness as determined by three elements, each in a continuum; intrinsic motivation, internal control, and freedom to suspend reality. A summation of each of the three elements determines the degree to which playfulness is present in a given transaction (Parham, L. D. & Fazio, L. S. (Eds.). (1997). *Play in occupational therapy for children*. St. Louis, MO: Mosby.).

carpals: wrist bones.

cephalocaudal development: motor development occurring in a head to toe direction.

circumferential splint: a splint that fits around the circumference of an extremity.

cognition: refers to the way that thought and information is processed.

collateral information: information gathered from sources that have contact with the client, such as teacher reports, prior evaluations or interview information from other family members.

comorbidity: refers to the presence of two or more concurrent diagnoses.

complex rotation: rotating an object 180 to 360 degrees, as demonstrated by turning a pencil around from eraser to lead end.

contexts: environments or milieu in which specific growth is presumed to develop and be nurtured.

copying: to reproduce a form or letter from a model such as copying from a book or the board.

crawling: the child moves with stomach on the surface, using the arms for most of the movement.

creeping: supporting weight on hands and knees while moving.

critical and sensitive periods: specific preprogrammed times at which people are most ready and available to learn and acquire new skills. Critical and sensitive periods are negatively influenced by deprivation of any sort.

cross-sectional study: a form of examination that involves sampling behavior from a broad range of subjects with similar characteristics at one point in time (e.g., surveying a large number of 11-year-olds across the state to examine cigarette smoking habits).

cultural context: refers to the customs and rituals practiced by different groups of people.

DAP note: a structured form of a narrative note. The acronym DAP stands for data, assessment and plan.

deprivation: denial of necessary supports in order to grow and mature.

directionality: the ability to interpret right and left directions in space.

disassociation: the separation between the radial and ulnar sides of the hand, the ulnar fingers are flexed into the palm while the radial side performs a precision task. Dissociation provides strength and stability to the radial side of the hand.

distal: body parts furthest from the center of body (i.e., fingers and toes).

dominance: development of a preferred hand for fine motor skills.

dynamical theory: based on the theory that brain structures work together and are interdependent in producing a specific movement pattern.

early childhood: period from 18 months until 5 to 6 years.

Early Intervention: refers to services provided to children, birth to 3 and their families.

enhanced sensory inputs: the provision of sensory stimuli at an intensity, frequency, or duration that is not readily obtained in the natural environment.

empathy: a capacity for taking another's point of view, the ability to feel what another is feeling.

environmental control unit (ECU): any device that allows those with limited or decreased physical or cognitive ability to operate other electronic devices by remote control.

extrinsic muscles: muscles located outside of the hand; they originate in the forearm and insert in the wrist or fingers.

Family-Centered Care Philosophy: consideration of, respect for, and active involvement of the child's family/caregivers in the planning, implementation, and decision-making processes of service provision.

fine motor skills: refers to the refined small motor skills executed with the hands and fingers.

finger to palm translation: moving an object from the finger pads to the palm of the hand. This activity occurs when a child picks up a piece of candy with the tips of the fingers and moves it to the palm.

flow: the state of joy and timelessness that accompanies total involvement with an activity that is a "just right challenge".

functional behavior: a response that is adaptive and allows a person to achieve a goal such as working or living independently.

gag reflex: a protective reflex present at birth. Stimulation to the back third of the tongue or pharyngeal area will evoke a gag.

gastroesophageal reflux (GER): the muscles at the lower end of the esophagus fail to contract enough to prevent reflux or backwash of the stomach contents into the esophagus, pharynx, and mouth.

gastrostomy tube: a feeding tube that goes into the stomach.

gavage feeding: feeding through a tube passed through the stomach.

grading: Systematically increasing or decreasing the demands of an activity to meet the needs or capabilities of an individual.

grasp: the act of obtaining and holding an object or stimulus.

grasp reflex: emerges at 1 month, continues to develop through the 4th month, and integrates between 6th and 10th months of age. Stimulus is a deep pressure to the palm that results in sudden flexion and adduction of all the joints of the fingers. As the grasp reflex becomes more fully developed (around 4 months of age), if only one finger is stimulated, flexion of only that finger is observed.

gravitational insecurity: an excessive, irrational fear of moving the head out of an upright position or having the feet leave the ground.

gross motor skills: refers to the large motor skills executed with the upper arms and legs.

growth and development: ordered changes in development that generally follows a set and predetermined timetable.

habituation: the nervous system process of becoming accustomed to a sensory stimuli to the point of no longer being actively aware of its presence.

high technology: devices or equipment with complex electrical components that require individualized adjustments and training for functional usage; usually not available or used by the common public.

homeostasis: a central nervous system state of balance where one is able to function optimally.

hypothesis: testable assumptions used to support or reject a theory.

IDEA: Individuals with Disabilities in Education Act.

ideation: the ability of an individual to conceive of a goal for an action and some general idea of how to achieve that goal.

IEP: Individual Education Plan.

IFSP: Individualized Family Service Plan.

infancy: Period from birth until 18 months.

imitation: 1) an attempt to match one's own behavior to another person's behavior; 2) to reproduce after watching someone draw a line, shape, form, letter, or word. This skill comes first in learning to draw.

inner drive: the innate, intrinsic desire of human organisms to seek out and achieve self-actualization through mastery over their environment.

integrated charting: type of charting that keeps all notes in chronological order, usually providing the most current information first.

intellectual functioning: a multifaceted capacity that generally includes ability to acquire and apply knowledge, to reason effectively and logically, to exhibit sound judgment, to be mentally alert, perceptive and intuitive, to be able to adapt to new situations and problems.

internal control: the extent to which an individual is in charge of his or her actions and, to some extent, the outcome of an activity; an essential element of play in Bundy's model of playfulness (Parham, L. D. & Fazio, L. S. (Eds.). (1997). *Play in occupational therapy for children*. St. Louis, MO: Mosby.).

intrinsic: in anatomy, denotes those muscles of the hand whose origin and insertion are both in the hand.

intrinsic motivation: a prompt to action that comes from within the individual and is not prompted by outside influences; drive to action that is rewarded by the doing of the activity itself rather than some external reward. Intrinsic motivation is widely accepted as an essential ingredient of play (Parham, L. D. & Fazio, L. S. (Eds.). (1997). *Play in occupational therapy for children*. St. Louis, MO: Mosby.).

instinctive grasp reaction: begins to emerge at 4 months and changes over the next 6 months so that by 10 months an automatic response no longer occurs. Stimulus is light contact to the radial or ulnar sides of the palm, resulting in pronation or supination toward the stimulus (4 to 6 months), then groping movements toward the stimulus (6 to 7 months) and finally, grasping the object 8 to 10 months).

IQ: an index of intelligence defined as a person's mental age divided by his chronological age and multiplied by 100.

jaw retraction: pulling back of the lower jaw.

jaw stabilization: active internal jaw control with minimal up/down jaw movements initially obtained by biting on the cup. Gradually develops using active jaw musculature by 24 months.

jaw thrust: strong downward movements of the lower jaw.

joint attention: the ability to focus on more than one task at a time (e.g., when a child plays a game and discusses events at school at the same time).

"just right" challenge: the optimum match between an individual's abilities and the task demands which makes the activity simultaneously accomplishable and yet challenging.

least restrictive environment: according to IDEA guidelines, children with disabilities are educated and must be allowed to participate to the fullest extent possible with children who are nondisabled.

lip retraction: pulling back of the lips and/or cheeks.

lip pursing: puckering the center of the lips; the lip corners may stay retracted.

long-term goals (LTGs): once achieved, often indicate a child is ready for discharge.

longitudinal arch: extends from the wrist to the end of the metacarpals. The palm makes a cup with finger flexion and flattens with finger extension.

loose associations: thinking (as reflected in speech) that moves haphazardly and rapidly from one fragmentary referent to another, so that ideas are touched on fleetingly rather than being logically developed.

low technology: devices or equipment with nonelectric or simple electronic systems that are commercially available to the public and require little training to use.

mashed foods: semi-solids with a slight texture that can be mashed with a fork.

mechanoreceptors: tactile receptors of the skin that respond to pressure or displacement of the skin or hair.

metacarpals: hand bones.

middle childhood: period from 6 to 12 years.

migration: passing from place to place. In splinting, refers to the splint moving from the anatomical place it was fitted to, to another place.

motor development: the acquisition of new and increasingly complex patterns of movement and movement related skills. Motor development is subdivided in gross and fine motor skill domains.

motor planning: the ability to plan and organize a motor action.

multisensory approach: involves using all the senses to help children learn: visual, auditory, kinesthesia, tactile, and olfactory.

munching: up and down jaw movements, the earliest form of chewing. Seen around 5 months, it is effective with foods that dissolve in saliva in the mouth.

nature vs. nurture: a proposed relationship between internal biology (nature) and environmental factors (nurture) and the influence they exert on development.

nasogastric feeding tube: a tube that goes through the mouth down to the stomach.

neurocognitive: thought processes highly related to the structure and functioning of the brain (e.g., attention, impulse control, and reasoning).

neurodevelopmental: behaviors that are dependent on the development of the brain and central nervous system (e.g., toilet training is dependent on neurodevelopment).

neuropsychological assessment: examination of the relationship between brain functioning and behavior that involves the use of specialized measurement devices, tests and procedures.

neurotransmitters: chemical "messengers" that travel throughout the brain and nervous system.

non-nutritive sucking: sucking period is shorter with a rest period. The respiration to suck ratio is 1:1.

norms: guidelines that professional and lay people track to follow specific phenomena such as physical growth.

occupation: "Activities…of everyday life, named, organized, and given value and meaning by individuals and a culture. Occupational is everything people do to occupy themselves, including looking after themselves…enjoying life…and contributing to the social and economic fabric of their communities…." (Law, M., Polatajko, H., Baptiste, W., & Townsend, E. (1997). Core concepts of occupational therapy. In E. Townsend (Ed.), *Enabling occupation: An occupational therapy perspective* (pp. 29-56). Ottawa, ON: Canadian Association of Occupational Therapists.)

occupational therapy practitioner: terminology that refers to occupational therapists and occupational therapy assistants.

oral gastric feeding tube: a tube that goes through the mouth down to the stomach.

opposition: rotation of the thumb toward the other fingers.

palm to finger translation: moving an object from the palm to the finger pads. Occurs when a small object is held in the palm and then moved from the palm to the distal surface of the radial fingers.

pencil grasp/hold: grip in which the pencil is held.

person first language: a respectful process that fosters positive attitudes towards individuals with disabilities and is reflected in documentation and spoken language emphasizing the person as an individual, not a disability (e.g., a child with hemiparesis).

physical context: refers to the physical space and potential (physical) barriers that people encounter in their lives.

pisiform: refers to the pea-shaped carpal (wrist) bone.

play: 1. An attitude or mode of experience that involves intrinsic motivation; emphasis on process rather than product and internal rather than external control; and an "as if" or pretend element; takes place in a safe, nonthreatening environment with social sanctions; 2. Any spontaneous or organized activity that provides enjoyment, entertainment, amusement, or diversion (Parham, L. D. & Fazio, L. S. (Eds.). (1997). *Play in occupational therapy for children*. St. Louis, MO: Mosby.).

playfulness: 1. The tendency to seek out opportunities for play or to respond to overtures of play with interest and pleasure; 2. A behavioral or personality trait characterized by flexibility, manifest joy, and spontaneity. *See also* Bundy's model of playfulness (Parham, L. D. & Fazio, L. S. (Eds.). (1997). *Play in occupational therapy for children*. St. Louis, MO: Mosby.).

praxis: the process of conceiving of, organizing, and carrying out intentional, goal-directed actions that are generally unfamiliar.

prenatal period: the approximately 38-42 week period between conception and birth.

problem-oriented charting: a type of charting that is organized by the problems that are being addressed by the therapy team. Practitioners from all disciplines document in the same section under the problem they are addressing.

proximal: refers to the regions closest to center of body (i.e., shoulders and hips).

psychoeducational assessment: psychological evaluation in a school or other setting, usually conducted to diagnose, remedy or measure academic or social progress or to otherwise enrich a student's education.

purchase: in splinting, refers to a secure grip applied to keep the splint from slipping.

pureed foods: foods that are blended to be smooth and thick.

radial side of the hand: refers to the thumb and index finger or the thumb, index and middle fingers.

reach: to extend the upper extremity in the direction of an object or stimulus.

release: the act of letting go of an object or stimulus.

retrospective study: a form of examination that relies on a person relating their understanding of events and behaviors in the past.

role fulfillment: the ability of the individual to perform purposeful activity (occupation) within a specific context or environment.

rooting reflex: head turning in response to tactile input to the side of the face, or lips. Present until around 4 months, may be longer in breast fed infants. The infant is seeking the source of food.

rotary chewing: up-and-down and side-to-side motions of the jaw in a circular motion; begins around 10 to 15 months of age.

Section 504: part of the Rehabilitation Act of 1973 that forbids discrimination against any person with a disability (physical or mental) in programs that receive federal funding.

self-finishing edge: a handling characteristic of thermoplastic that allows any cut edge to have a smooth surface.

sensory diet: an individualized program of regularly scheduled and as needed activities that facilitates an individual's ability to self-regulate arousal level and achieve a functional state of homeostasis.

sensory discrimination: a central nervous system function that assesses the salient qualities of incoming sensory inputs for skill use.

Sensory Integration: a central nervous system function, which organizes sensory information from the individual and the environment for regulation of behavior and performance of skill. This term also refers to a theory and an occupational therapy practice frame of reference.

sensory modulation: a central nervous system function that assesses incoming sensory inputs for relevance and value to regulate arousal level.

service competency: a method by which an OT can determine if an OTA is able to perform a certain evaluative, intervention, or documentation procedure. The OT evaluates the OTA's ability level and determines if it is sufficient to be performed without the direct supervision of the OT.

shift: using the finger pads to produce a slight linear adjustment of the object, i.e., adjusting the fingers on a pen so that the fingers are closer to the tip or moving a paper clip from the ulnar to radial digits.

simian crease or **transverse palmar crease**: a single crease extending across the palm of the hand from the ulnar to radial side; three creases are typically found in the palm. This crease is found in individuals with Down syndrome.

simple rotation: rotating an object by using the thumb in opposition to the fingers, the fingers usually act as a unit and the object is usually rotated less than 180 degrees (e.g., turning small knob on a lamp).

short-term goals (STGs): those small steps that take one closer to the long-term goals.

SOAP note: a structured form of a narrative note. The acronym SOAP stands for subjective, objective, assessment and plan.

social context: refers to the relationship milieu.

social or **emotional competency**: refers to the degree of success to which a child masters relational skills.

social and emotional development: learning to interpret, internalize and use information and cues generated from relational contexts.

somatic: relating to, or affecting the body.

source-oriented charting: type of charting that is organized by discipline in chronological order, with the most current information first. In this format, all occupational therapy notes are in one section and other disciplines each have their own section.

suck and swallow reflex: appears soon after birth; the mouth opens and sucking movements begin when light touch is applied to the corners or center of the lips. Present until around 6 months.

sucking: a rhythmic up-and-down movement of the tongue with less jaw movement, and tight lips.

suckling: an early form of sucking, forward-backward tongue movements, large up/down jaw excursions and loose lips.

suspension of reality: the degree to which an individual in play chooses to assume identities, act out events, or control materials in ways that diverge from the usual constraints of real life; an essential element of play in Bundy's Model of Playfulness (Parham, L. D. & Fazio, L. S. (Eds.). (1997). *Play in occupational therapy for children*. St. Louis, MO: Mosby.).

teratogens: outside forces such as disease or other negatives factors that impact development.

technology: *see* **low technology** and **high technology**.

theory: a set of related ideas that explain, describe or make predictions about specific phenomena.

3-jaw chuck finger position: the grip of the fingertips in which an object is held with the distal pads of the thumb, index, and middle fingers.

tongue lateralization: the movement of the tongue from side-to-side.

tongue retraction: strong pulling back of the tongue into the mouth.

tongue thrust: protrusion of the tongue from the mouth.

tonic bite: strong closure of the jaw in reaction to tactile input. Decreases around 8 to 10 months.

Total Parental Nutrition (TPN): intravenous feeding of specially prepared solutions.

traction response: present at birth; pulling the infant's arm into shoulder flexion leads to flexion of all the joints of the arm including the shoulder, elbow, wrist, and fingers. Within weeks, a pressing stimulus to the palm elicits this reflex.

transverse carpal arch: this arch is located where the bones of the carpals and metacarpals meet. This arch is fairly stable or fixed providing stability to wrist and metacarpal movements.

transverse metacarpal arch: this arch is at the level of the metacarpals (bones in the hands) and is mobile. The first, fourth and fifth metacarpals rotate around the second and third metacarpals forming a cupping of the palm to a flattened palm.

ulnar side of the hand: refers to the little and ring finger or the little, ring, and middle fingers.

vertical surfaces: inclined desk surfaces or easels placed on flat desks, or positions that place materials in a vertical orientation such as working at chalkboard, or lying on the floor. Vertical surfaces help to develop the hand and wrist positions needed for handwriting.

vertigo: a light-headedness or disorientation in response to movement or heights.

videofluoroscopic swallow study: often called a modified barium swallow. Child ingests a bolus of food saturated in barium and the swallow is video taped. Purpose is to determine if aspiration is occurring, and reason for aspiration.

INDEX

WAIT

...There's More!

SLACK Incorporated's Professional Book Division offers a wide selection of products in the field of Occupational Therapy. We are dedicated to providing important works that educate, inform and improve the knowledge of our customers. Don't miss out on our other informative titles that will enhance your collection.

Ryan's Occupational Therapy Assistant: Principles, Practice Issues, and Techniques, Fourth Edition
Sally Ryan, COTA, ROH and Karen Sladyk, PhD, OTR/L, FAOTA

624 pp., Soft Cover, 2005, ISBN 1-55642-740-9, Order #37409, **$57.95**

Ryan's Occupational Therapy Assistant: Principles, Practice Issues, and Techniques, Fourth Edition is a holistic book covering all aspects of OTA practice for both education and the NBCOT exam review. New features include evidence based treatment reviews and actual client records.

Quick Reference Dictionary for Occupational Therapy, Fourth Edition
Karen Jacobs, EdD, OTR/L, CPE, FAOTA and Laela Jacobs, OTR

600 pp., Soft Cover, 2004, ISBN 1-55642-656-9, Order #36569, **$26.95**

This definitive companion provides quick access to words, their definitions, and important resources used in everyday practice and the classroom. Used by thousands of your peers and colleagues, the *Quick Reference Dictionary for Occupational Therapy, Fourth Edition* is one of a kind and needed by all in the profession.

Foundations of Pediatric Practice for the Occupational Therapy Assistant
Amy Wagenfeld, PhD, OTR/L and Jennifer Kaldenberg, MSA, OTR/L

400 pp., Soft Cover, 2005, ISBN 1-55642-629-1, Order #36291, **$44.95**

OTA Exam Review Manual, Second Edition
Karen Sladyk, PhD, OTR/L, FAOTA

224 pp., Soft Cover, 2005, ISBN 1-55642-701-8, Order #37018, **$32.95**

Management Skills for the Occupational Therapy Assistant
Amy Solomon, OTR and Karen Jacobs, EdD, OTR/L, CPE, FAOTA

176 pp., Soft Cover, 2003, ISBN 1-55642-538-4, Order #35384, **$30.95**

The OTA's Guide to Writing SOAP Notes
Sherry Borcherding, MA, OTR/L and Carol Kappel, MT, OTA

224 pp., Soft Cover, 2002, ISBN 1-55642-551-1, Order #35511, **$27.95**

Best Practice Occupational Therapy: In Community Service with Children and Families
Winnie W. Dunn, PhD, OTR, FAOTA

400 pp., Soft Cover, 2000, ISBN 1-55642-456-6, Order #34566, **$47.95**

Children Adapt: A Theory of Sensorimotor-Sensory Development, Second Edition
Elnora M. Gilfoyle, D/Sc, OTR, FAOTA; Ann P. Grady, MA, OTR, FAOTA; and Josephine C. Moore, PhD, OTR, FAOTA, DSc(hon)

312 pp., Soft Cover, 1990, ISBN 1-55642-187-7, Order #30371, **$40.95**

Quick Reference Neuroscience for Rehabilitation Professionals: The Essential Neurologic Principles Underlying Rehabilitation Practice
Sharon A. Gutman, PhD, OTR

288 pp., Soft Cover, 2001, ISBN 1-55642-463-9, Order #34639, **$38.95**

Please visit
www.slackbooks.com
to order any of these titles!
24 Hours a Day...7 Days a Week!

Attention Industry Partners!
Whether you are interested in buying multiple copies of a book, chapter reprints, or looking for something new and different — we are able to accommodate your needs.

Multiple Copies
At attractive discounts starting for purchases as low as 25 copies for a single title, SLACK Incorporated will be able to meet all your of your needs.

Chapter Reprints
SLACK Incorporated is able to offer the chapters you want in a format that will lead to success. Bound with an attractive cover, use the chapters that are a fit specifically for your company. Available for quantities of 100 or more.

Customize
SLACK Incorporated is able to create a specialized custom version of any of our products specifically for your company.

Please contact the Marketing Manager of the Professional Book Division for further details on multiple copy purchases, chapter reprints or custom printing at 1-800-257-8290 or 1-856-848-1000.

*Please note all conditions are subject to change.

CODE: 328

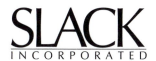

SLACK Incorporated • Professional Book Division
6900 Grove Road • Thorofare, NJ 08086
1-800-257-8290 or 1-856-848-1000
Fax: 1-856-853-5991 • E-mail: orders@slackinc.com • Visit www.slackbooks.com

Major Infant Reflexes

Reflex Name	Stimulation/ Response	Integration	Purpose	Consequences if not Integrated
Survival Reflexes				
Eye Blink*	In response to presentation of bright light or puff of air to the eyes, infant closes eyes or blinks.	Present throughout life.	Protects the eyes from bright light or from objects entering the eye.	May impede visual function.
Pupillary*	Pupils constrict when exposed to bright light and enlarge when exposed to dark or dim surroundings.	Present throughout life.	Protection against bright light as well as adaptation to varying visual environments.	May impede visual function.
Breathing	Inhale to obtain oxygen and exhale to expel carbon dioxide.	Present throughout life.	Protection; to ensure an even balance of oxygen intake and carbon dioxide output.	Necessary for survival.
Rooting	When cheek is stroked, infant turns head in direction of stimuli (touch) and opens its mouth.	Disappears by 3/4 months; replaced by a voluntary response to tactile stimuli.	To prepare baby to feed from bottle or breast.	May impede head, mouth, and tongue movements.
Suck	Touch or stimulation (i.e., placing something in mouth or taking something in mouth) initiates an automatic and rhythmic sucking pattern.	Permanent, although after 3-4 months, becomes a voluntary process.	Nutritional intake.	May impede ability to drink and feed.
Swallow	Liquids are taken in to mouth and then swallowed in a rhythmic pattern (such as, suck, suck, suck, swallow).	Permanent, although comes under voluntary control by 3-4 months.	Nutritional intake.	May impede ability to drink and feed.
Gag	Stimulation to the back third of tongue or pharyngeal region elicits a gag (choke).	Present throughout life, although most active until about 4-6 months.	Prevents babies from swallowing solid foods and serves a protective function throughout life.	May impede ability to drink and feed if over or under active.
Primitive Reflexes				
Babinski	Stroking to the bottom of the foot causes the infant to fan out and then curl up the toes.	Disappears at about 8-12 months.	Indicator that the infant's neurological system is developing normally.	If still present by age 2, may be an indicator that the nerve tracts connecting the spinal cord to the brain are damaged.
Gallant	Stroking on either side of spinal column from neck to mid/lower back (with infant in prone) causes infant to curve the back to the side being stroked.	Disappears at about 3-6 months.	Indicator that the infant's neurological system is developing normally.	May delay trunk and head stabilization.
Asymmetrical Tonic Neck (ATNR)	When placed supine, the infant's head is turned to either the right or left side. When head is turned to the right, the right leg and arm extend, while the left arm and leg flex (sometimes called the archer's position).	Disappears at about 4-6 months.	Indicator that the infant's neurological system is developing normally.	May be an indicator of delayed neurological development and may also impede voluntary upper extremity movement.
Symmetrical Tonic Neck (STNR)	When held in prone, baby's head flexes forward, causing muscle tone of the flexors in the upper extremities and of the lower extremities to increase. When held in supine, baby's head extends backwards, causing muscle tone of the extensors in the upper extremities and flexors of the lower extremities to increase.	Disappears at about 8-11 months.	Indicator that the infant's neurological system is developing normally.	May be an indicator of delayed neurological development and also impede voluntary movement.